Hypertension: Mechanism and Management

Hypertension: Mechanism and Management

Editor: Jayden Miller

FOSTER ACADEMICS
www.fosteracademics.com

www.fosteracademics.com

FOSTER ACADEMICS

Cataloging-in-Publication Data

Hypertension : mechanism and management / edited by Jayden Miller.
p. cm.
Includes bibliographical references and index.
ISBN 978-1-63242-597-3
1. Hypertension. 2. Hypertension--Treatment. 3. Blood circulation disorders. I. Miller, Jayden.
RC685.H8 H97 2019
616.132--dc23

Foster Academics,
118-35 Queens Blvd., Suite 400,
Forest Hills, NY 11375, USA

ISBN 978-1-63242-597-3 (Hardback)

Printed and bound in China.

Contents

Preface

The purpose of the book is to provide a glimpse into the dynamics and to present opinions and studies of some of the scientists engaged in the development of new ideas in the field from very different standpoints. This book will prove useful to students and researchers owing to its high content quality.

Hypertension is a persistent medical condition characterized by elevated blood pressure. It affects 16-37% of the world population. Excessive salt in the diet, alcohol consumption, smoking and excess body weight are factors that may lead to hypertension. Chronic kidney disease, endocrine disorder, narrowing of the kidney arteries or the disproportionate use of birth control pills may also trigger hypertension. One of the first treatment strategies for the management of hypertension is the integration of the right lifestyle changes with the correct medication course. Lifestyle changes may include weight loss, appropriate dietary modifications and regular exercise. A low sodium diet, DASH diet, green tea consumption and vegetarian diets are known to reduce blood pressure. Aerobic exercise, isometric resistance exercise, device-guided breathing and resistance exercise are considered effective physical exercise regimens. First-line medications, which are generally recommended for the management of hypertension, are calcium channel blockers, thiazide-diuretics, angiotensin receptor blockers, etc. This book explores all the important aspects of hypertension in the present day scenario. It provides significant information of this condition to help develop a good understanding of the treatment and management of hypertension. This book is appropriate for students seeking information in this area as well as for experts.

At the end, I would like to appreciate all the efforts made by the authors in completing their chapters professionally. I express my deepest gratitude to all of them for contributing to this book by sharing their valuable works. A special thanks to my family and friends for their constant support in this journey.

Editor

1

Factors Associated with Medication Nonadherence among Hypertensives in Ghana and Nigeria

Vincent Boima,[1,2] Adebowale Dele Ademola,[3,4] Aina Olufemi Odusola,[5] Francis Agyekum,[2] Chibuike Eze Nwafor,[6] Helen Cole,[7] Babatunde L. Salako,[8,9] Gbenga Ogedegbe,[7,10] and Bamidele O. Tayo[11]

[1] *School of Medicine and Dentistry, University of Ghana, P.O. Box 4236, Accra, Ghana*
[2] *Department of Medicine, Korle Bu Teaching Hospital, P.O. Box 77, Accra, Ghana*
[3] *Department of Paediatrics, Faculty of Clinical Sciences, College of Medicine, University of Ibadan, Ibadan PMB 5017, Oyo State, Nigeria*
[4] *Department of Paediatrics, University College Hospital, Ibadan PMB 5116, Oyo State, Nigeria*
[5] *Department of Medicine, General Hospital, Randle Avenue, Apapa PMB 1014, Lagos, Nigeria*
[6] *Cardiology Division, Department of Medicine, University of Port Harcourt Teaching Hospital, Port Harcourt PMB 6173, Rivers State, Nigeria*
[7] *Department of Population Health, NYU School of Medicine, 227 E. 30th Street, 6th Floor, New York, NY 10016, USA*
[8] *Department of Medicine, Faculty of Clinical Sciences, College of Medicine, University of Ibadan, Ibadan PMB 5017, Oyo State, Nigeria*
[9] *Department of Medicine, University College Hospital, Ibadan PMB 5116, Oyo State, Nigeria*
[10] *Global Institute of Public Health, New York University, New York, NY 10003, USA*
[11] *Department of Public Health Sciences, Stritch School of Medicine, Loyola University Chicago, 2160 South First Avenue, Maywood, IL 60153, USA*

Correspondence should be addressed to Adebowale Dele Ademola; dr_deboademola@yahoo.co.uk

Academic Editor: Francesco Cappuccio

Background. Blood pressure (BP) control is poor among hypertensives in many parts of sub-Saharan Africa. A potentially modifiable factor for control of BP is medication nonadherence (MNA); our study therefore aimed to determine factors associated with MNA among hypertensives in Ghana and Nigeria. *Methodology.* We conducted a multicenter cross-sectional study. Patients were recruited from Korle-Bu Hospital ($n = 120$), Ghana; and University of Port Harcourt Teaching Hospital, ($n = 73$) Apapa General Hospital Lagos ($n = 79$) and University College Hospital Ibadan ($n = 85$), Nigeria. *Results.* 357 hypertensive patients (42.6% males) participated. MNA was found in 66.7%. Adherence showed correlation with depression ($r = -0.208$, $P < 0.001$), concern about medications ($r = -0.0347$, $P = 0.002$), and knowledge of hypertension ($r = 0.14$, $P = 0.006$). MNA was associated with formal education ($P = 0.001$) and use of herbal preparation ($P = 0.014$). MNA was found in 61.7% of uninsured participants versus 73.1% of insured participants ($P = 0.032$). Poor BP control was observed in 69.7% and there was significant association between MNA and poor BP control ($P = 0.006$). *Conclusion.* MNA is high among hypertensives in Ghana and Nigeria and is associated with depression, concern about hypertensive medications, formal education, and use of herbal preparations. The negative association between health insurance and MNA suggests interplay of other factors and needs further investigation.

1. Introduction

Hypertension is a common but treatable public health problem globally. It is estimated to cause 7.5 million deaths annually, about 12.8% of all deaths worldwide [1]. Globally, the prevalence of hypertension in adults was approximately 40% in 2008 [2]. The number of people worldwide with hypertension rose from 600 million in 1980 to nearly 1 billion in 2008. The burden of hypertension is particularly high in sub-Saharan African countries. The reported prevalence of hypertension in Ghana ranges from 19% to 32.8% in rural areas and 25.5 to 48% in urban areas [3–5]. Similarly, recent studies in Nigeria showed that the prevalence of hypertension in rural areas ranges from 21 to 25% [6, 7] while in semiurban and urban areas the prevalence ranged from 27 to 46% [8–11]. Optimal blood pressure (BP) control with levels below 140/90 mmHg is associated with significant reduction in cardiovascular complications such as stroke and coronary heart disease [12, 13].

The increasing rates of hypertension in sub-Saharan Africa have been attributed to rapid epidemiologic transition from an agrarian lifestyle to a more westernized lifestyle, with increasing rates of obesity, unhealthy diet, and physical inactivity [3, 14]. Blood pressure control is generally poor among hypertensive patients in sub-Saharan Africa, and efforts to improve BP control are needed. Poor BP control among hypertensives in sub-Saharan Africa is related to the complex interplay of patient, provider, and socioeconomic factors in this region [3, 14]. For example, patients may lack knowledge about hypertension, or they may harbour beliefs that are discordant with those of the traditional medical model regarding the causes and treatment of hypertension. As a result, patients' beliefs may be discordant with practices associated with BP control potentially leading to poor medication adherence. Additionally, patients may exhibit poor medication adherence because they are unable to afford the cost of medications. Similarly, healthcare providers may have insufficient time and resources to provide the necessary education and treatment.

Of the patient factors that affect BP control, poor medication adherence is the most salient and little studied in sub-Saharan African countries including Nigeria and Ghana. Medication nonadherence (MNA) is a potentially modifiable risk factor for the improvement of BP control. Factors that may influence adherence include socioeconomic status, access to health insurance, depression, patient's knowledge of the disease, and beliefs about medications [15]. Past studies have reported a wide range of MNA in Ghana and Nigeria from 17.4 to 93%, making it difficult to compare the degree and factors associated with MNA in both countries [16–24].

In order to address these significant gaps in the adherence literature in sub-Saharan Africa, our study documents the levels and factors associated with MNA among hypertensive patients in the hospital setting in Ghana and Nigeria.

2. Methods

In this multicenter cross-sectional study, patients were recruited from four hospitals: Korle-Bu Hospital (n = 120), Ghana, and University of Port Harcourt Teaching Hospital, (n = 73) Apapa General Hospital Lagos (n = 79), and University College Hospital Ibadan (n = 85), Nigeria. Patients were eligible to be in this study if they were aged 18 years or older, were diagnosed hypertensive, and had been placed on medication for at least twelve months and provided informed consent. Hypertension was defined as systolic BP of ≥140 mmHg and/or diastolic BP of ≥90 mmHg [25] or patients already under treatment with antihypertensive medications. Patients were recruited from general outpatient or specialist medical clinics. The questionnaires were administered by the authors or trained research assistants. At each site, each consecutive patient who met the inclusion criteria was recruited. The same recruitment procedure was used in each center. Patient recruitment into the study took place between April and September 2013. Data collection was conducted by the authors and trained research assistants at each study site using a structured questionnaire. Blood pressure was measured with an Omron electronic BP machine, after at least 10 minutes rest, in the dominant arm of seated patients on three occasions at an interval of one minute. The average of the last 2 readings was recorded.

The dependent variables were medication adherence and BP control. Adherence to antihypertensive medications was measured using the 8-item Morisky medication adherence scale. Based on a pilot study in Korle Bu Ghana, the response options for the Morisky scale were modified from "never/rarely," "once in a while," "sometimes," "usually," and "all the time" to "Never/rarely" versus "sometimes/usually/all the time." Individual item scores were summed and those with a score of 8 were considered adherent to medication. Medium adherence corresponded to a score of 6–8, while a score of <6 was considered low adherence [26]. Medication nonadherence referred to a score of <8 (i.e., medium or low adherence). Blood pressure control was defined as systolic BP < 140 mmHg and diastolic BP < 90 mmHg [27].

Demographic and socioeconomic characteristics including age, gender, ethnicity, education, occupation, and income were recorded. Educational status was classified as none, primary, junior secondary, senior secondary, and tertiary. Monthly income was stratified as <$100, $101–300, $301–1000, $1001–3000, and >$3000. Clinical information regarding when the diagnosis of hypertension was made, for how long patients had been on antihypertensives, and presence of any associated comorbid conditions were obtained from patients' medical records. Beliefs about medication were measured using the modified beliefs about medication questionnaire (BMQ) [28]. The BMQ includes questions on beliefs about the necessity of taking medications (BMQ-necessity) and concerns about medications (BMQ-concern). The difference between the BMQ-necessity and BMQ-concern scores was also determined for each patient (BMQ necessity-concern score). Each question on the BMQ is based on a 5-point Likert scale with response options: "strongly agree," "agree," "disagree," "strongly disagree," and "uncertain." Pilot testing of the BMQ indicated that participants were more comfortable with 3 response options. We therefore modified the responses to "agree," "disagree," and "uncertain," The parameters were scored as disagree = 1, uncertain = 2, and agree = 3. The sum total of the BMQ-necessity score, BMQ-concern, and the difference between BMQ-necessity and concern scores was calculated [28]. The Patient Health Questionnaire 9 (PHQ-9) was used to assess depression in this study. For this scale, sores of 0, 1, 2, and 3 are assigned to response categories of "not at all," "several days," "more than half the days," and "nearly every day," respectively. The PHQ-9 total score ranges from 0 to 27. PHQ-9 scores of 0–4, 5–9, 10–14, 15–19, and 20–27 represent none to minimal, mild, moderate, moderately severe, and severe depression, respectively. Scores of >4 were classified as depression. A 17-item questionnaire based on the JNC 7 and adapted from previous studies was used to assess knowledge of hypertension [14, 29–31]. The questions were based on true or false responses to statements such as "high blood pressure cannot be cured but can be controlled," "high blood pressure can damage hearts," "a person who has high blood pressure should take more salt," and "management of high blood pressure must include medications, diet, and lifestyle modification." A score of 1 mark was given for each correct response and the final score was a sum total of the correct responses.

Data collected was entered into Statistical Package for Social Sciences (SPSS) software student version 17.0 and used for analysis. Descriptive statistics such as means, standard deviations, proportions, and percentages were used to summarize quantitative and qualitative variables, respectively. Inferential statistics including Chi-square analysis and Pearson's correlation were used to compute associations between variables. The student t-test was used to compare means. P values < 0.05 were considered significant and r-values of >0.15 were considered strong correlations. Ethical approval for the study was obtained from University of Ghana Ethical and Protocol Review Committee (EPRC), the University of Ibadan/University College Hospital Ibadan Ethical Review Committee, and the University of Port Harcourt Ethical Review Committee.

3. Results

As shown in Table 1, a total of 357 hypertensive patients were recruited for the study, of which 42.6% were men. Their mean age was 56.6 ± 13.2 years. The majority of the study participants (33.61%) were recruited from Korle Bu, while 20.4%, 22.1%, and 23.8% participants were recruited from Port Harcourt, Apapa, and Ibadan, respectively. There were significant differences in the age of participants, gender, and access to health insurance between sites. The cohort from Korle Bu had the highest proportion of females and participants who were more likely to have health insurance.

Nonadherence to medications was present in 66.7% of participants. Port Harcourt had the highest prevalence of MNA (95.9%), while Ibadan had the lowest (45.1%). Depression was present in 31.4% of the study participants, with 2.8% and 1.4% reporting moderately severe and severe depression, respectively. Depression was more prevalent in the cohort from Korle Bu (41.7%) and Port Harcourt (41.1%) compared to the other centres. Table 1 shows the distribution of patient characteristics by site.

3.1. Relationship among Depression, Beliefs about Medicines, and Medication Adherence. The mean age of patients who were nonadherent to medications was 54.5 ± 13.2 years while those who were adherent had a mean age of 60.9 ± 12.1 years ($P < 0.001$). Among the cohort from Korle Bu, those who were nonadherent were also significantly younger than subjects who were adherent, 55.3±13.4 years versus 61.3±13.7 years ($P = 0.037$). There was significant correlation between PHQ-9 score for depression and Morisky score in Korle Bu ($r = -0.230$, $P = 0.012$) and in the pooled data ($r = -0.203$, $P < 0.001$). The mean BMQ-concern score among participants who were nonadherent was 9.0 ± 2.7 compared to 7.5 ± 2.5 among those who were adherent. There was a significant negative correlation between BMQ-concern score and Morisky score in Ibadan ($r = -0.338$, $P = 0.002$) and in the pooled data ($r = -0.355$, $P = 0.000$). The BMQ-necessity-concern score was associated with MNA in the pooled data ($r = 0.336$, $P < 0.001$). Knowledge of hypertension was significantly but weakly correlated with Morisky score ($P = 0.006$, $r = 0.14$). Table 2 shows correlations among Morisky score and depression, beliefs about medication, knowledge of hypertension, and income by site.

3.2. Relationship among Socioeconomic Status, Income, Health Insurance, and Medication Adherence. Level of income did not show correlation with Morisky score ($r = 0.021$, $P = 0.744$). The majority of participants (56.3%) did not have any health insurance. MNA occurred in 47.7% of those who did not receive formal education compared with 70.9% of those who had some form of formal education ($P = 0.001$). MNA was noted in 61.7% of those who did not have health insurance and in 73.1% of those who had health insurance ($P = 0.032$). MNA was significantly more common among patients who used herbal preparation for the treatment of systemic hypertension ($P = 0.014$). There were no differences in medication adherence between patients who were married compared with those who were not. See Table 3 for a summary of characteristics by adherence.

3.3. Correlations of Blood Pressure Control. Blood pressure was controlled in 35.9% of study participants. There was variation in the proportion of patients with BP control across the study sites ranging from 9.6%, in Port Harcourt, to 54.1% in Ibadan. There was significant association between medication nonadherence and poor BP control in the pooled data ($P = 0.006$). Table 1 includes rates of BP control and medication adherence across sites. The cohort of patients from Port Harcourt had the highest level of MNA (95.9%) and the lowest proportion with BP control (9.6%, $n = 4$).

4. Discussion

We report a high prevalence of MNA (66.7%) among hypertensives in hospitals in Ghana and Nigeria. Patients who were nonadherent were significantly younger than patients who were adherent. There was significant negative correlation between depression and concerns about medication and medication nonadherence. Knowledge of hypertension was positively correlated with adherence. Patients who were adherent were less likely to use herbal preparations or to have received formal education and were more likely to have children. Level of income was not associated with adherence. Not unexpectedly, poor BP control was significantly associated with MNA. Access to health insurance surprisingly showed significant association with MNA. The proportion of patients who had uncontrolled BP was higher among patients who had health insurance, compared to patients without health insurance, but the finding was not significant. Further studies on the operation of the health insurance system are

Table 1: Distribution of study population characteristics by site.

Parameter	Korle Bu	P. Harcourt	Lagos	Ibadan	Pooled
Total (%)	120 (33.6)	73 (20.4)	79 (22.1)	85 (23.8)	357 (100)
Age (years)[a]	57.0 ± 13.7	47.4 ± 12.5	57.8 ± 9.8	62.9 ± 11.5	56.6 ± 13.2
Females (%)[a]	70 (58.3)	37 (50.7)	56 (70.9)	42 (49.4)	205 (57.5)
Insurance N (%)[a]	114 (95)	20 (27.4)	5 (6.3)	17 (20)	156 (43.7)
HTN with comorbidities (%)[a]	57.4	20.5	34.2	62.4	45.8
Depression (%)					
No (%)	70 (58.3)	43 (58.9)	60 (75.9)	72 (84.7)	245 (68.6)
Mild (%)	32 (26.7)	18 (24.7)	18 (22.8)	10 (11.8)	78 (21.8)
Moderate (%)	10 (8.3)	5 (6.8)	1 (1.3)	3 (3.5)	19 (5.3)
Mord-severe (%)	4 (3.3)	6 (8.2)	—	—	10 (2.8)
Severe (%)	4 (3.3)	1 (1.4)	—	—	5 (1.4)
Total (%)	**120 (100)**	**73 (100)**	**79 (100)**	**85 (100)**	**357 (100)**
BMQ-necessity [median (IQR)]	14 (11–15)	11 (9–13)	15 (13–15)	10.5 (7–13)	
BMQ-concern [median (IQR)]	7.5 (5–11)	11 (9–12.5)	7 (8-9)	7 (5–9)	
Knowledge about HTN [median (IQR)]	15 (14–16)	13 (11–14)	13 (12–15)	14 (13–15)	14 (13–15)
Nonadherence (%)	72.5	95.9	53.2	45.9	66.7
Medium adherence (%)	41.7	12.3	38.0	32.9	32.8
Low adherence (%)	30.8	83.6	15.2	12.9	33.9
Blood pressure control (%)[a]	27.7	9.6	53.2	54.1	35.9
Educational status					
None (%)	6.7	1.4	53.2	16.5	18.2
Primary (%)	7.5	31.5	19.0	21.2	18.2
Junior secondary (%)	31.7	12.3	8.9	1.2	15.4
Senior Secondary (%)	15.0	28.8	13.9	18.8	18.5
Tertiary (%)	39.2	26.0	5.1	42.4	29.7
Occupation[a]					
Petty trader (%)	24.6	12.3	45.5	13.1	23.9
JCS (%)	23.7	19.2	6.5	3.6	14.2
SCS (%)	11.0	15.1	2.6	14.3	10.8
Businessman (%)	11.0	20.5	22.1	17.9	17.0
Unemployed (%)	4.2	5.5	15.6	1.2	6.3
Housewife (%)	0.8	9.6	0	1.2	2.6
Others (%)	1.7	9.6	2.6	0	3.1
Artisans (%)	5.9	0.0	1.3	7.1	4.0
Retired (%)	16.9	8.2	3.9	41.7	18.2
Use of herbal preparation (%)[a]	15.8	35.6	11.7	9.4	17.5

[a] $P < 0.005$.
BMQ: beliefs about medication questionnaire; IQR: interquartile range; HTN: hypertension; JCS: junior civil servant; P. Harcourt: Port Harcourt; SCS: senior civil servant.

warranted while measures to improve medication adherence are required.

We report a high prevalence of MNA in our study population (66.7%), but our finding is within the range of MNA that has been documented in previous studies from sub-Saharan Africa. Most studies in Nigeria and Ghana have documented MNA ranging from 32.7 to 49.3% [16, 17, 20, 23]. There was however a study from Ghana that documented MNA of 93% before the availability of National Health Insurance [19]. Elsewhere in sub-Saharan Africa, MNA ranged from 10.3 to 87.5% [32–38]. Variation may be partly due to the different definitions or methods used to assess MNA. Most of the studies though based on self-report, utilized different definitions for MNA. An advantage of our study was that the same tool was used to assess MNA in the various sites. Furthermore we also observed significant association between MNA and BP control in our study which will further validate the tool that was adopted to assess MNA in our study.

Our study found significant correlation between beliefs about medication and adherence to antihypertensives. Patients who had concerns about antihypertensive medications were less likely to be adherent to their medications. These findings are consistent with previous studies on the relationship between medication adherence and beliefs about

TABLE 2: Correlation of medication adherence (Morisky score) with depression, beliefs about medication, knowledge of hypertension, or income by site and in the pooled data.

Parameter	Korle Bu		Port Harcourt		Lagos		Ibadan		Pooled	
	r	*P*	*r*	*P*	*r*	*P*	*r*	*P*	*r*	*P*
Depression (PHQ-9)	−0.230	0.012	0.051	0.667	−0.043	0.705	−0.035	0.749	−0.203	0.000
BMQ-necessity	0.142	0.124	−0.079	0.507	0.091	0.433	0.002	0.984	−0.087	0.103
BMQ-concern	−0.148	0.111	−0.286	0.014	−0.014	0.905	−0.336	0.002	−0.355	0.000
BMQ-necessity-concern	0.215	0.020	0.174	0.141	0.079	0.505	0.210	0.060	0.337	0.000
Hypertension knowledge scale	0.024	0.797	0.212	0.071	0.019	0.865	−0.030	0.783	0.144	0.006
Income	0.139	0.143	−0.057	0.634	−0.200	0.081	0.099	0.419	−0.067	0.226

BMQ-concern: beliefs about medication concern score; BMQ-necessity: beliefs about medication necessity score; BMQ-necessity-concern: beliefs about medication necessity-concern score; P = P value; r = Pearson's correlation coefficient.

medications [39]. Specifically, patients in our study had concerns about potential adverse effects of long term use of antihypertensives or felt that daily use of antihypertensive medications was a significant disruption of their lifestyles. Patients were also concerned that they may be becoming too dependent on their medications. Other studies have identified side-effects of antihypertensive medications as a reason for MNA in patients [19, 23, 35, 38]. Studies have also documented that forgetting to take medications is an important barrier to adherence [17, 23, 38]. In addition, adherence is usually better with medications that require less frequent administration [16, 36–38]. Health education specifically about antihypertensive medications including potential side-effects, and inquiry about side-effects the patient may be experiencing and use of medications that are associated with fewer side effects may lead to improvement in adherence. In addition, use of medications that do not cause more disruption of the patients' daily activities than necessary may also improve adherence.

Our study also found that depression was significantly associated with MNA, particularly among patients at Korle Bu, but also in the pooled data. To the best of our knowledge this study is the first to assess depression and MNA among hypertensives in sub-Saharan Africa. Depression has been associated with poor BP control and medication nonadherence in studies outside sub-Saharan Africa [40, 41]. In a study from the USA, antidepressants were associated with significantly longer initial persistence of antihypertensive therapy among patients with depression who developed hypertension [42]. Evaluation for depression and appropriate management of the depression may improve medication adherence among hypertensives in sub-Saharan Africa.

Patients who were not adherent were significantly younger than patients who were adherent. This pattern has been observed in adherence studies carried outside sub-Saharan Africa and has also been documented in Sub-Saharan Africa [26, 43, 44]. The reason for worse medication non adherence in younger patients is not clear. A potential reason may be that younger patients are not as concerned about their health compared with the older patients. Health education directed towards younger age group may improve outcomes among the younger patients.

Our study found positive and significant correlation between knowledge of hypertension and adherence to medications. Previous studies from Africa have associated lack of knowledge regarding the curability of hypertension and lifelong need for antihypertensives with MNA [18, 20, 23, 38]. Our data thus support the need for adequate health education on hypertension to improve MNA in the subregion. Furthermore, patients who reported using herbal preparations for the treatment of hypertension were more likely to show MNA. This is consistent with most studies on hypertension from sub-Saharan Africa that have associated the use of alternative medical therapy with MNA [17, 18, 20, 36, 38].

Studies from Nigeria have noted increasing adherence with increasing educational status but these associations were not significant [16, 23]. Literacy has also been associated with a higher BP control in Nigeria but this was also not significant [45]. Our study, however, found that patients who had received any form of formal education were more likely to show MNA than those who did not. It may be that educated participants in our study were more skeptical towards the use of antihypertensives. A similar observation was noted in a Ghanaian study which also found significant negative association between educational status and medication adherence [17]. Another study from the United States found higher adherence among men with lower levels of education than among more highly educated men [46]. Our data is consistent with a previous suggestion that health education on hypertension and its treatment should be provided for all hypertensive patients in our subregion irrespective of the patients' educational status [47].

In most studies from sub-Saharan Africa participants have identified inability to afford the cost of medications as an important barrier to medication adherence [17–19, 33, 36, 38]. A positive relationship between cost and MNA has also been found in studies outside of Africa [39] Studies have however not consistently demonstrated association of medication adherence with level of income. Our study did not find an association between MNA and income [23, 39, 43].

Table 3: Distribution of study population characteristics by adherence (N = 357).

Population Characteristics	Nonadherent N (%)	Adherent N (%)	P value
Gender			0.623
Male	104 (68.4)	48 (31.6)	
Female	134 (65.4)	71 (34.6)	
Study Site			<0.001
Korle-Bu	87 (72.5)	33 (27.5)	
Port Harcourt	70 (95.9)	3 (4.1)	
Lagos	42 (53.2)	37 (46.8)	
Ibadan	39 (45.9)	46 (54.1)	
Age	54.4 ± 13.2 years	60.9 ± 12.1 years	0.000
Educational status			0.006
None	31 (47.7)	34 (52.3)	
Primary	48 (73.8)	17 (26.2)	
Junior	42 (76.4)	13 (23.6)	
Secondary	47 (71.2)	19 (28.8)	
Tertiary	70 (60.6)	36 (34.0)	
Formal education			0.001
Yes	207 (70.9)	85 (29.1)	
No	31 (47.7)	34 (52.3)	
Marital status			0.967
Married	172 (66.9)	85 (33.1)	
Not married	66 (66)	34 (34)	
Children			0.04
Yes	217 (65.2)	116 (34.8)	
No	21 (87.5)	3 (12.5)	
Occupation			0.317
Employed	176 (68.5)	81 (38.5)	
Unemployed	59 (62.1)	36 (37.9)	
Cost of drug ($)			0.1
<10	58 (73.4)	21 (26.6)	
11–30	87 (65.9)	45 (34.1)	
31–50	36 (67.9)	17 (32.1)	
51–100	27 (69.2)	12 (30.8)	
>100	14 (45.2)	17 (50.8)	
Insurance			0.032
Yes	114 (73.1)	42 (26.9)	
No	124 (61.7)	77 (38.3)	
Use of herbal medication			0.014
Herbal med.	50 (80.6)	12 (19.4)	
No herbal med.	186 (63.5)	107 (36.5)	
Hypertension			0.006
Control	72 (56.7)	55 (43.3)	
Uncontrolled	163 (71.8)	64 (21.2)	
Comorbidities			0.874
No comorbidity	132 (69.8)	57 (30.2)	
DM or renal comorbidities	62 (62.6)	37 (37.4)	
Other comorbidities	38 (69.8)	23 (30.2)	

DM: diabetes mellitus.

One explanation may be that in many African studies, as in ours, only a negligible number belong to the high socioeconomic class, making it difficult to access MNA in the high socioeconomic class [23, 45]. On the other hand the lack of association between income and MNA may reflect an interplay of other factors that contribute to medication adherence. A study carried out in Nigeria in a setting in which antihypertensives were offered for free, noted that BP control was low though higher than in settings where medications were not given for free suggesting that MNA may not be entirely due to cost [48].

We found that access to National Health Insurance was significantly associated with MNA. In addition, BP tended to be higher in patients with access to health insurance than those who did not. Most of the patients who had access to National health Insurance were from Ghana. The Ghanaian patients also had the highest proportion of patients with depression and the depression may have contributed to the high proportion of patients with MNA in the Ghanaian patients in spite of the access to health Insurance. In addition, the way the health insurance system operates may also be contributory. In Ghana for instance, a three-month prescription from clinicians is usually dispensed in three tranches where patients are given a one month supply and asked to come back for refill of their medications for the other two months. Some patients do not return for refill of their medication because of lack of travel funds or lack of a system to remind them to go for the refill. This argues in favour of a critical review of the current national health insurance system in Ghana. Esunge and colleagues in Cameroon had suggested that factors that improved MNA among hypertensives in low resource settings were free medications, free hospital visits, free transportation, open discussion with medical staff, use of common dialects, and politeness of medical staff [49].

Another method that may contribute to improvement in medication adherence in low resource settings is the use of phone technology. Use of text messages has been associated with improvement in adherence to medications [50]. Use of phone technology reminders even in low resource settings may be useful in improving medication adherence in a large number of patients.

Strengths of our study include the multicenter nature of the study, and the use of uniform tools to assess medication non-adherence, depression, knowledge of hypertension, and beliefs about medication across the sites. Limitations of our study are that the study is hospital-based and most patients were from tertiary health centers. As such, the patients in our study are likely to have more comorbidities and to be more highly motivated than patients in the community. Therefore, proportion of patients who are non-adherent in the community may be higher than the observation in our study. Furthermore, MNA was assessed by verbal report and this may also potentially underestimate adherence because of recall bias or social desirability bias, and this may also apply to the other self-report measures. A more objective measure such as urine antihypertensive drug assay, may have demonstrated a higher degree of MNA. However, the study provides valuable information on the burden of MNA among hypertensives and the potential influence of factors such as beliefs about medications, depression, and health insurance on MNA.

5. Conclusion

We studied MNA among hypertensives in hospitals in Ghana and Nigeria. MNA was found in 66.7% of participants. MNA occurred in younger patients and in patients who had varying degrees of depression or were concerned about their medications. Knowledge of hypertension was positively and significantly correlated with adherence. MNA was associated with use of herbal preparations, and formal education. Expectedly adherence was significantly associated with BP control. We also found that MNA was associated with health insurance, and this may be related to either underlying depression or the mode of operation of the health insurance. The finding of significant association between health insurance and MNA underscores the need for studies to identify the underlying causes of this association. Treatment of depression in patients with hypertension and depression may improve outcomes. Patients irrespective of educational status need education concerning treatment of hypertension and side-effects of medication in addition to education on hypertension to improve MNA. Other methods to improve medication adherence such as use of phone technology should also be studied.

Acknowledgments

Vincent Boima, Adebowale Ademola, Francis Agyekum, Aina Olufemi Odusola, and Eze Nwafor are grateful to the Cardiovascular Research Training Institute (Fogarty International Center Grant no. 5D43TW009140) for training and funding support. The authors are also grateful to Professor Daniel T Lackland, Profssors Kennedy Cruickshank, Dr. Berthelsen Nathan, and Dr Pauline E. Osamor, for support in conceptualizing the study, and to Prof W. Chaplin for assistance with the statistics. The authors appreciate Miss Polina Krass for her assistance with data management.

References

[1] World Health Organization, *Global Health Risks: Mortality and Burden of Disease Attributable to Selected Major Risks*, 2009.

[2] G. Danaei, M. M. Finucane, J. K. Lin et al., "National, regional, and global trends in systolic blood pressure since 1980: systematic analysis of health examination surveys and epidemiological studies with 786 country-years and 5.4 million participants," *The Lancet*, vol. 377, no. 9765, pp. 568–577, 2011.

[3] W. K. Bosu, "Epidemic of hypertension in Ghana: a systematic review," *BMC Public Health*, vol. 10, article 418, 2010.

[4] C. Agyemang, M. A. Bruijnzeels, and E. Owusu-Dabo, "Factors associated with hypertension awareness, treatment, and control in Ghana, West Africa," *Journal of Human Hypertension*, vol. 20, no. 1, pp. 67–71, 2006.

[5] A. G. B. Amoah, "Hypertension in Ghana: a cross-sectional community prevalence study in Greater Accra," *Ethnicity & Disease*, vol. 13, no. 3, pp. 310–315, 2003.

[6] I. I. Ulasi, C. K. Ijoma, and O. D. Onodugo, "A community-based study of hypertension and cardio-metabolic syndrome in semi-urban and rural communities in Nigeria," *BMC Health Services Research*, vol. 10, article 71, 2010.

[7] M. E. Hendriks, F. W. N. M. Wit, M. T. L. Roos et al., "Hypertension in Sub-Saharan Africa: cross-sectional surveys in four rural and urban communities," *PLoS ONE*, vol. 7, no. 3, Article ID e32638, 2012.

[8] R. A. Adedoyin, C. E. Mbada, M. O. Balogun et al., "Prevalence and pattern of hypertension in a semiurban community in Nigeria," *European Journal of Cardiovascular Prevention and Rehabilitation*, vol. 15, no. 6, pp. 683–687, 2008.

[9] J. O. Awobusuyi, O. O. Kukoyi, M. A. Ibrahim, and M. Atiba, "Indices of kidney damage and cardiovascular disease risk factors in a semiurban community of Iloye, South-west Nigeria," *International Journal of Nephrology*, vol. 2011, Article ID 564050, 6 pages, 2011.

[10] E. K. Oghagbon, A. B. Okesina, and S. A. Biliaminu, "Prevalence of hypertension and associated variables in paid workers in Ilorin, Nigeria," *Nigerian Journal of Clinical Practice*, vol. 11, no. 4, pp. 342–346, 2008.

[11] I. I. Ulasi, C. K. Ijoma, B. J. C. Onwubere, E. Arodiwe, O. Onodugo, and C. Okafor, "High prevalence and low awareness of hypertension in a market population in Enugu, Nigeria," *International Journal of Hypertension*, vol. 2011, Article ID 869675, 5 pages, 2011.

[12] I. J. Brown, I. Tzoulaki, V. Candeias, and P. Elliott, "Salt intakes around the world: implications for public health," *International Journal of Epidemiology*, vol. 38, no. 3, pp. 791–813, 2009.

[13] World Health Organization, *Global Status Report on Noncommunicable Diseases 2010: Description of the Global Burden of NCDs, Their Risk Factors and Determinants*, 2011.

[14] J. Spencer, E. Phillips, and G. Ogedegbe, "Knowledge attitudes, beliefs, and blood pressure control in a community-based sample in Ghana," *Ethnicity & Disease*, vol. 15, no. 4, pp. 748–752, 2005.

[15] L. M. Lewis, A. M. Schoenthaler, and G. Ogedegbe, "Patient factors, but not provider and health care system factors, predict medication adherence in hypertensive black men," *The Journal of Clinical Hypertension*, vol. 14, no. 4, pp. 250–255, 2012.

[16] M. R. Akpa, D. I. Agomuoh, and O. J. Odia, "Drug compliance among hypertensive patients in Port Harcourt, Nigeria," *Nigerian Journal of Medicine*, vol. 14, no. 1, pp. 55–57, 2005.

[17] T. H. Harries, V. Twumasi-Abosi, J. Plange-Rhule, and F. P. Cappuccio, "Hypertension management in Kumasi: barriers and prejudice?" *Journal of Human Hypertension*, vol. 19, no. 12, pp. 975–977, 2005.

[18] M. Kabir, Z. Iliyasu, L. Abubakar, and M. Jibril, "Compliance to medication among hypertensive patients in Murtala Mohammed Specialist Hospital, Kano, Nigeria," *Journal of Community Medicine and Primary Health Care*, vol. 16, no. 1, 2005.

[19] K. O. Buabeng, L. Matowe, and J. Plange-Rhule, "Unaffordable drug prices: the major cause of non-compliance with hypertension medication in Ghana," *Journal of Pharmacy and Pharmaceutical Sciences*, vol. 7, no. 3, pp. 350–352, 2004.

[20] P. E. Osamor and B. E. Owumi, "Factors associated with treatment compliance in hypertension in southwest Nigeria," *Journal of Health, Population and Nutrition*, vol. 29, no. 6, pp. 619–628, 2011.

[21] K. B. Yusuff and O. Balogun, "Physicians' prescribing of anti-hypertensive combinations in a tertiary care setting in

southwestern Nigeria," *Journal of Pharmacy & Pharmaceutical Sciences*, vol. 8, no. 2, pp. 235–242, 2005.

[22] A. Oyati, A. Orogade, S. Danbauchi, and P. Azuh, "Awareness, Treatment and Control of Hypertension among Hypertensives in Zaria," *Journal of Medicine in the Tropics*, vol. 13, no. 2, 2011.

[23] C. O. Amira and N. U. Okubadejo, "Factors influencing non-compliance with anti-hypertensive drug therapy in Nigerians," *The Nigerian Postgraduate Medical Journal*, vol. 14, no. 4, pp. 325–329, 2007.

[24] J. O. B. Olubodun, A. O. Falase, and T. O. Cole, "Drug compliance in hypertensive Nigerians with and without heart failure," *International Journal of Cardiology*, vol. 27, no. 2, pp. 229–234, 1990.

[25] A. V. Chobanian, G. L. Bakris, H. R. Black et al., "Seventh report of the Joint National Committee on Prevention, Detection, Evaluation, and Treatment of High Blood Pressure," *Hypertension*, vol. 42, no. 6, pp. 1206–1252, 2003.

[26] D. E. Morisky, L. W. Green, and D. M. Levine, "Concurrent and predictive validity of a self-reported measure of medication adherence," *Medical Care*, vol. 24, no. 1, pp. 67–74, 1986.

[27] P. A. James, S. Oparil, B. L. Carter et al., "2014 evidence-based guideline for the management of high blood pressure in adults: report from the panel members appointed to the Eighth Joint National Committee (JNC8)," *Journal of the American Medical Association*, vol. 311, no. 5, pp. 507–520, 2014.

[28] R. Horne, J. Weinman, and M. Hankins, "The beliefs about medicines questionnaire: the development and evaluation of a new method for assessing the cognitive representation of medication," *Psychology and Health*, vol. 14, no. 1, pp. 1–24, 1999.

[29] S. Sanne, P. Muntner, L. Kawasaki, A. Hyre, and K. B. Desalvo, "Hypertension knowledge among patients from an urban clinic," *Ethnicity and Disease*, vol. 18, no. 1, pp. 42–47, 2008.

[30] O. C. Alebiosu, O. B. Familoni, O. O. Ogunsemi et al., "Original research: knowledge of diabetes and hypertension care among health care workers in southwest Nigeria," *Postgraduate Medicine*, vol. 121, no. 1, pp. 173–177, 2009.

[31] National High Blood Pressure Education Program, *The Seventh Report of the Joint National Committee on Prevention, Detection, Evaluation, and Treatment of High Blood Pressure*, National Heart, Lung, and Blood Institute, Bethesda, Md, USA, 2004, http://www.ncbi.nlm.nih.gov/books/NBK9630/?report=reader.

[32] N. G. Nkosi and S. C. Wright, "Knowledge related to nutrition and hypertension management practices of adults in Ga-Rankuwa day clinics," *Curationis*, vol. 33, no. 2, pp. 33–40, 2010.

[33] A. G. Elzubier, A. A. Husain, I. A. Suleiman, and Z. A. Hamid, "Drug compliance among hypertensive patients in Kassala, Eastern Sudan," *Eastern Mediterranean Health Journal*, vol. 6, no. 1, pp. 100–105, 2000.

[34] D. W. R. Lunt, P. R. Edwards, K. Steyn, C. J. Lombard, and G. S. Fehrsen, "Hypertension care at a Cape Town community health centre," *South African Medical Journal*, vol. 88, no. 5, pp. 544–548, 1998.

[35] M. D. Mweene, J. Banda, B. Andrews, M. M. Mweene, and S. Lakhi, "Factors associated with poor medication adherence in hypertensive patients in Lusaka, Zambia," *Medical Journal of Zambia*, vol. 37, no. 3, pp. 252–261, 2010.

[36] C. Konin, M. Adoh, I. Coulibaly et al., "Black Africans' compliance to antihypertensive treatment," *Archives des Maladies du Coeur et des Vaisseaux*, vol. 100, no. 8, pp. 630–634, 2007.

[37] E. E. Maro and J. Lwakatare, "Medication compliance among Tanzanian hypertensives," *East African Medical Journal*, vol. 74, no. 9, pp. 539–542, 1997.

[38] K. Peltzer, "Health beliefs and prescription medication compliance among diagnosed hypertension clinic attenders in a rural South African Hospital," *Curationis*, vol. 27, no. 3, pp. 15–23, 2004.

[39] T. Mathes, T. Jaschinski, and D. Pieper, "Adherence influencing factors—a systematic review of systematic reviews," *Archives of Public Health*, vol. 72, no. 1, p. 37, 2014.

[40] M. Lemstra and M. W. Alsabbagh, "Proportion and risk indicators of nonadherence to antihypertensive therapy: a meta-analysis," *Patient Preference and Adherence*, vol. 8, pp. 211–218, 2014.

[41] A. F. Rubio-Guerra, L. Rodriguez-Lopez, G. Vargas-Ayala, S. Huerta-Ramirez, D. C. Serna, and J. J. Lozano-Nuevo, "Depression increases the risk for uncontrolled hypertension," *Experimental and Clinical Cardiology*, vol. 18, no. 1, pp. 10–12, 2013.

[42] J. A. Schmittdiel, W. Dyer, C. Uratsu et al., "Initial persistence with antihypertensive therapies is associated with depression treatment persistence, but not depression," *Journal of Clinical Hypertension*, vol. 16, no. 6, pp. 412–417, 2014.

[43] P. Bovet, J.-P. Gervasoni, M. Mkamba, M. Balampama, C. Lengeler, and F. Paccaud, "Low utilization of health care services following screening for hypertension in Dar es Salaam (Tanzania): a prospective population-based study," *BMC Public Health*, vol. 8, article 407, 2008.

[44] M. A. Marentette, W. C. Gerth, D. K. Billings, and K. B. Zarnke, "Antihypertensive persistence and drug class," *The Canadian Journal of Cardiology*, vol. 18, no. 6, pp. 649–656, 2002.

[45] S. A. Isezuo, A. A. Sabir, A. E. Ohwovorilole, and O. A. Fasanmade, "Prevalence, associated factors and relationship between prehypertension and hypertension: a study of two ethnic African populations in Northern Nigeria," *Journal of Human Hypertension*, vol. 25, no. 4, pp. 224–230, 2011.

[46] J. Braverman and J. Dedier, "Predictors of medication adherence for African American patients diagnosed with hypertension," *Ethnicity and Disease*, vol. 19, no. 4, pp. 396–400, 2009.

[47] D. A. Oke and E. O. Bandele, "Misconceptions of hypertension," *Journal of the National Medical Association*, vol. 96, no. 9, pp. 1221–1224, 2004.

[48] B. L. Salako, F. A. Ajose, and E. Lawani, "Blood pressure control in a population where antihypertensives are given free," *East African Medical Journal*, vol. 80, no. 10, pp. 529–531, 2003.

[49] P. M. Esunge, "Patient compliance and the evaluation of drug trials for hypertension in rural Africa," *Ethnicity & Disease*, vol. 1, no. 3, pp. 292–294, 1991.

[50] S. Krishna, S. A. Boren, and E. A. Balas, "Healthcare via cell phones: a systematic review," *Telemedicine and e-Health*, vol. 15, no. 3, pp. 231–240, 2009.

2

Burden of Hypertension in the Capital of Afghanistan: A Cross-Sectional Study in Kabul City, 2015

Khwaja Mir Islam Saeed

Grant and Service Contract Management Unit (GCMU), Ministry of Public Health, Kabul, Afghanistan

Correspondence should be addressed to Khwaja Mir Islam Saeed; kmislamsaeed@gmail.com

Academic Editor: Roberto Pontremoli

Background. This study had the objective to assess the prevalence and associated factors of hypertension in an urban setting, Kabul city, Afghanistan. *Materials and Methods.* The World Health Organization's STEP-wise approach was adopted and used in Kabul in November 2015. The study analyzed a sample of 1172 adults in the age group of 25–70 years. Demographic, socioeconomic, and behavior data were collected using a structured questionnaire. Fasting venous blood sample was collected to assess the lipid profile and fasting blood sugar. *Results.* The study showed that the prevalence of hypertension among adult Kabul citizens was 32.3%. From this figure, 599 (51.1%) were females and 573 (48.9%) males with a mean age of 38.6 ± 12.2 years. Illiteracy rate was 49.6% and 77.5% were married. Smoking in adults were 8.1% and mouth snuff users were 9.8%. More than half (57.6%) of the study respondents were overweight and obese and 9.1% were recorded having raised blood sugar. In the multivariate logistic regression analysis, age, general obesity, central obesity, smoking, moderate physical activity, and taking fruits 3 days or less weekly were statistically significant predictors of hypertension. *Conclusions.* Burden of hypertension is increasing in main urban settings in Afghanistan. Integrated intervention focusing in main modifiable risk factors is needed to detect and prevent hypertension.

1. Introduction

Noncommunicable diseases (NCDs) are a major cause of morbidity and mortality globally. In contrary to the common misconception, the burden of these diseases is the worst in low- and middle-income countries where 80% of all NCDs occur, and it is rising rapidly [1, 2]. Hypertension (HTN) is one of those NCDs which is an important public health problem in both economically developed and developing nations [3]. As per World Health Organization report, about 40% of people aged more than 25 years had hypertension in 2008 [4]. Worldwide, 7.6 million premature deaths were attributed to high blood pressure [5]. It has been a main health challenge due to high frequency and associated risks for cardiovascular and kidney diseases such as myocardial infarctions, strokes, and renal failures [6] and even at the top end of the normal range increases the risk and is called silent killer [7, 8]. Predictors of hypertension include family history, age, race, obesity, and physical inactivity, lack of exercise, cigarette smoking, excessive salt intake, and excessive alcohol intake [9, 10]. Some of these risk factors are measurable and largely modifiable, and thus continuing surveillance of the levels of risk factors is of fundamental importance in NCDs control [11].

In Afghanistan, due to years of conflict, it has been difficult to make any accurate estimates of NCDs prevalence including hypertension. According to recent studies conducted in Kabul for adults more than 40 years old and in Jalalabad for adults more than 25 years old, the prevalence of hypertension was 46.2% and 28.4%, respectively [12, 13]. Furthermore, Iran, being a neighbor of Afghanistan and a middle-income country, has estimated the prevalence of hypertension to be 22.1% [14]. Pakistan, another neighboring country, recorded the prevalence of high blood pressure as 25.3% [15]. There is no reason to believe that Afghans are less susceptible to NCDs than people in Pakistan and Iran. Hence, further research in this area will be very beneficial to health authorities. The purpose of this study is to estimate the prevalence of hypertension and assess the predictors in urban Afghan adults.

2. Methods and Materials

To provide estimates of hypertension and other factors of NCDs in Kabul city, a provincial cross-sectional study was conducted in November 2015 using the WHO STEP-wise approach revised instrument. This instrument prescribes three steps for assessing behavioral risk factors, physical measurements, and biological risk factors [16]. All permanent residents and household members aged more than 25 years, including men and women who gave consent to participate, were included in the study. Temporary residents (resident < 6 months), inhabitants of institutionalized settings, and insecure areas were excluded. Assuming the highest prevalence (50%), 95% confidence interval (CI), and margin of error of 5%, a sample size of 385 subjects was calculated to include in the study. However, considering the proportion of other risk factors and design effect (D_{eff} of 2) of cluster sampling, the final sample size was increased to $(2 \times 600) = 1200$ for the city.

2.1. Sampling Strategy. The latest population census in Afghanistan was conducted in 1979 and hence is not useable now. Furthermore, the full and exact list of areas (villages) located in Kabul is not available. Consequently, it is difficult to estimate the overall population of residents in Kabul. However, a tentative estimate of the proportion of the study sample ($n = 1202$) among the general population of adult citizens was selected. The study team preferred to use the existing list the 2015 Expanded Programme for Immunization (EPI) of clusters as the sampling frame. This frame contains the estimated name of areas and number of households which is used for immunization. The strategy for approaching the 1200 households was determined to be cluster sampling of districts, clusters, areas, and households. At the first stage, from the list of 22 districts located in urban section of the city, the study team conventionally selected five districts using random numbers in the excel sheet. In the second stage from each selected district, the study team randomly selected the 2 clusters. Later on, the overall sample of 1200 households was divided among these selected areas according to the proportion to the size of household numbers in each areas. Finally, the households in each area were approached and selected systematically. Basically, therefore, the primary sampling unit was clusters of EPI, the secondary sampling unit was areas, and ultimate sampling unit was households. Lastly, within households, one adult individual with eligible criteria was chosen by the interviewer for enrollment in the study.

2.2. Data Collection. WHO STEP-wise tool contained questionnaires on demographic, behavioral, and physical measurements. Interviewers approached households, the final unit of sampling frame, for face to face data collection. A household was defined as a group of people who share the same food pot (not the same roof). In households with more than one eligible person, the study team used a lottery system to select only one respondent. In cases of refusal, the interviewer approached the next available household. Anthropometric measurements including height and weight were used to calculate body mass index (BMI). A BMI $\geq 30\,\text{kg/m}^2$ was considered as obese, 25–30 kg/m^2 as overweight, and 18.5–25 kg/m^2 as normal weight [17]. A waist circumference of 94 cm for men and 80 cm for women was defined as central obesity [18]. Systolic blood pressure (SBP) 140 mmHg and diastolic pressure (DBP) 90 mmHg were considered as hypertensive. Furthermore, SBP of less than 120 mmHg and DBP of less than 80 mmHg were calculated as being hypotensive while the group between the two were considered as prehypertensive [19]. Blood samples were collected the next morning after the respondent had fasted for 10–12 hours and were transported in cold boxes (2–8°C) from field to Central Public Health Laboratory (CPHL) in Kabul. Using Cry-vials, the samples were coded with ID number of the questionnaire. On arrival in CPHL, all serum samples were stored at −80°C and later on were tested for triglyceride, cholesterol, and glucose. A fasting blood sugar of ≥126 mg/dL was considered as diabetes mellitus [20]. *Epi-info*, version 7, and *SPSS*, version 20, were used for data management and analysis. The Institutional Review Board (IRB) reviewed the study protocol for technical and ethical approval and consent was taken from each individual before the interview. The results of physical and biochemical measurements communicated to required participants and the confidentiality of the information was maintained.

3. Results

The original total number of study participants was 1202 of which 30 records were taken from the study due to unavailability of sufficient epidemiological data or no blood; hence, analysis was conducted on 1172 records. Of these, 599 (51.1%) were females and 573 (48.9%) males with a mean age of 38.6 ± 12.2 years. Majority of the study participants were married (77.5%), while 60% of women were housewives and closely half of the respondents (49.6%) were illiterates (Table 1). Study subjects were reluctant to provide information on their income; however, it seems that just 7.6% had income of less than 10000 Afghani per month (150$).

Table 2 shows the prevalence of various behavioral risk factors for NCDs; 8.1% were current smokers and 46% of smokers had duration of 10 years. The general prevalence of snuff use was 9.8%; however, this figure is diluted due to low prevalence of snuff use in females (2%). Sixty-six percent had fruits and 65%% had vegetables less than three days per week. On average, the subjects were taking fruits 3.08 days per week and vegetables 3.10 days per week. Thirty-three percent of respondents reported to be using liquid oil for cooking in their kitchen while using solid ghee (52.1%) was more prevalent. Almost ten percent (9.4%) of the respondents practiced vigorous physical activity and 20.3% of subjects reported doing moderate physical activity. Approximately half (48%) of the respondents reported walking or using bicycle for 10 minutes per day. Forty-six percent of respondents (46.8%) recorded a reclining of three hours or more per day. About 57.5% of study respondents were overweight and obese and (60%) were suffering from central obesity. Only about 11.6% and 56.1% of the respondents had low or normal

TABLE 1: Frequency distribution of demographic characteristics of the study participants, Kabul city ($N = 1172$).

Variables	Categories	Female		Male		Total	
		N	%	*N*	%	*N*	%
Age	25–34	301	50.3	291	50.8	592	50.5
	35–44	158	26.4	131	22.9	289	24.7
	45–54	89	14.9	76	13.3	165	14.1
	55+	51	8.5	75	13.1	126	10.8
Level of education	Illiterate	370	62.8	205	36	575	49.6
	Primary and unofficial	86	14.6	116	20.4	202	17.4
	Secondary school	72	12.2	154	27	226	19.5
	High school and over	43	7.3	75	13.2	118	10.2
Job categories	Official employees	53	8.9	120	21.1	173	14.8
	Students	7	1.2	10	1.8	17	1.5
	Private business	5	0.8	50	8.8	55	4.7
	Worker/farmer	1	0.2	76	13.3	77	6.6
	Jobless	9	1.5	52	9.1	61	5.2
	Housework	356	59.7	12	2.1	368	31.6
	Unable to work	165	27.7	250	43.9	415	35.6
Monthly income in AFN	Less than 10000	5	3.8	11	13.9	16	7.6
	More than 10000	127	96.2	68	86.1	195	92.4
Marital status	Single	54	9.1	82	14.5	136	11.7
	Married	460	77.7	437	77.2	897	77.5
	Widow/widower	43	7.3	11	1.9	54	4.7
	Divorced	4	0.7	2	0.4	6	0.5

TABLE 2: Frequency distribution of behavioral risk factors for noncommunicable diseases among the study participants, Kabul city ($N = 1172$).

Variables	Categories	Female		Male		Total	
		N	%	*N*	%	*N*	%
Cigarette smoking status	No	595	99.5	480	83.9	1075	91.9
	Yes	3	0.5	92	16.1	95	8.1
Duration of smoking in years	<10 years	7	100	56	50.5	63	53.4
	10–20 years	0	0	36	32.4	36	30.5
	≥20 years	0	0	19	17.1	19	16.1
Mouth snuff status	No	585	98	467	82.1	1052	90.2
	Yes	12	2	102	17.9	114	9.8
Fruit taking[1] (days per week)	<3	372	64.7	378	68.1	750	66.4
	≥3	203	35.3	177	31.9	380	33.6
Vegetables taking[2] (days per week)	<3	406	68.8	350	61.6	756	65.3
	≥3	184	31.2	218	38.4	402	34.7
Type of kitchen oil	Liquid	174	29.2	214	37.7	388	33.3
	Solid	326	54.7	281	49.5	607	52.1
	Both	95	12.3	70	12.3	165	14.2
Vigorous physical activity[3]	No	550	92.1	507	88.9	1057	90.6
	Yes	47	7.9	63	11.1	110	9.4
Moderate physical activity[4]	No	449	75.1	481	84.5	930	79.7
	Yes	149	24.9	88	15.5	237	20.3
Pedal or bicycle for 10 minutes per day	No	403	67.3	206	36	609	52
	Yes	196	32.7	366	64	562	48
Reclining/siting (hours per day)	<3	296	52.1	301	54.3	597	53.2
	≥3	272	47.9	253	45.7	525	46.8

[1,2]One serving is amount of fruits or vegetables taken once, [3]physical activity in ten minutes caused high heart beats or respiration, and [4]physical activity in ten minutes caused moderate heart beats or respiration.

Table 3: Bivariate analysis of biodemographic and socioeconomic factors and hypertension among study participants in Kabul, Afghanistan.

Variables	Categories	Normotensive	Hypertensive	Odds ratio	CI 95% LL	CI 95% UL
Age in years	25–34	495 (83.6)	97 (16.4)	1	Reference	
	35–44	170 (58.8)	119 (41.2)	3.572	2.595	4.918
	45–54	85 (51.5)	80 (48.5)	4.803	3.301	6.988
	55 and over	43 (34.1)	83 (65.9)	9.85	6.422	15.108
Gender	Female	379 (63.3)	220 (36.7)	1	Reference	
	Male	414 (72.3)	159 (27.7)	0.662	0.517	0.847
Level of education	Illiterate	368 (64)	207 (36)	1	Reference	
	Literate	394 (72.2)	152 (27.8)	0.686	0.533	0.883
Monthly income (Afghanis)	≤150 USD	11 (68.8)	5 (31.2)	1	Reference	
	≥150 USD	141 (72.3)	54 (27.7)	0.843	0.28	2.538
Smoking	No	712 (66.2)	363 (33.8)	1	Reference	
	Yes	79 (83.2)	16 (16.8)	0.397	0.229	0.69
Snuffing	No	722 (68.6)	330 (31.4)	1	Reference	
	Yes	67 (58.8)	47 (41.2)	1.535	1.034	2.278
Strong physical activity	No	717 (67.8)	340 (32.2)	1	Reference	
	Yes	73 (66.4)	37 (33.6)	1.069	0.705	1.62
Moderate physical activity	No	642 (69)	288 (31)	1	Reference	
	Yes	147 (62)	90 (38)	1.365	1.014	1.837
Sedentary lifestyle in hours daily	<3 hours	405 (67.8)	192 (32.2)	1	Reference	
	≥3 hours	352 (67)	173 (33)	1.037	0.807	1.331
Fruits serving days per week	<3 days	523 (69.7)	277 (30.3)	1	Reference	
	≥3 days	244 (64.2)	136 (35.8)	1.284	0.989	1.668
Vegetables serving days per week	<3 days	512 (67.7)	244 (32.3)	1	Reference	
	≥3 days	272 (67.7)	130 (32.3)	1.003	0.774	1.299
Taking red meat in days per week	<2 days	121 (89)	15 (11)	1	Reference	
	≥2 days	589 (65.7)	308 (34.3)	4.218	2.424	7.34

blood pressure, respectively, while 32.2% had high blood pressure. Out of this group of high blood pressure, 29.4% were unaware of their status of hypertension. Nine percent (9.1%) were recorded as raised blood sugar and of these the prevalence of diabetes was 9.3% for females and 8.9% for males. Approximately 30% had high level of cholesterol and 41% had high level of triglycerides. Furthermore, high level of low density lipoprotein (LDL) and high level of high density lipoprotein (HDL) were 42.2% and 48%, respectively, among study subjects.

Outside the descriptive analysis on this study, the bivariate analysis was computed for demographic and socioeconomic variables. As Table 3 shows on the bivariate analysis, age, sex, level of education, smoking, moderate physical activity, and taking red meat were found to be significantly associated with high blood pressure.

Furthermore, Table 4 shows that body mass index (BMI), central obesity, use of table salt, and high blood sugar (diabetes mellitus) were found to be significantly associated with hypertension at P value level of 0.05 or more.

In the multivariate logistic regression analysis, age, general obesity, central obesity, smoking, moderate physical activity, and taking fruits less than 3 days or more weekly were statistically significant predictors of hypertension. Table 5 shows the adjusted odds ratio and 95% confidence interval along with P values.

4. Discussion

The main findings of this study were high level of hypertension among the adult population in Kabul city which is 32.2% despite being a low-income country. This finding is in line, and even higher, with other similar studies conducted elsewhere [13, 21, 22]. Mostly, attention is given on communicable diseases in the country while less focus is given to NCDs which impacts adversely on Afghanistan [23, 24]. In addition, the burden of hypertension in Kabul [12] in age group of 40 years and more was 46% which could be compared with same age group in this study. It appears that the high age groups are on greater risk of high blood pressure. About 29.4% of hypertension patients are unaware of their hypertension status indicating that more than one out of three cases of hypertension do not know that they have it. This finding is in agreement with other similar studies [25, 26].

Although many risk factors were significantly associated with hypertension in this study, at initial level however, few

TABLE 4: Bivariate analysis of pathophysiologic factors and hypertension among study participants in Kabul city, Afghanistan.

Variables	Categories	Normotensive	Hypertensive	Odds ratio	CI 95% LL	CI 95% UL
Basic mass index	Underweight	26 (78.8)	7 (21.2)	1	Reference	
	Normal weight	360 (77.4)	105 (22.6)	1.083	0.457	2.566
	Overweight	285 (66)	147 (34)	1.916	0.812	4.518
	Obese	122 (50.4)	120 (49.6)	3.653	1.528	8.736
Central obesity (pregnant excluded)	No	367 (78.3)	102 (21.7)	1	Reference	
	Yes	426 (60.6)	277 (39.4)	2.34	1.792	3.054
Use of table salt	No	541 (65.8)	281 (34.2)	1	Reference	
	Yes	192 (72.7)	72 (27.3)	0.722	0.531	0.981
Diabetes mellitus	No diabetic	739 (69.4)	326 (30.6)	1	Reference	
	Diabetic	54 (50.5)	53 (49.5)	2.225	1.49	3.322
Total cholesterol	<190 mg/dL	559 (68.4)	258 (31.6)	1	Reference	
	≥190 mg/dL	234 (65.9)	121 (34.1)	1.12	0.86	1.459
Low density lipoprotein (LDL)	<100 mg/dL	458 (67.6)	220 (32.4)	0.953	0.746	1.218
	≥100 mg/dL	335 (67.8)	159 (32.2)	0.988	0.771	1.266
High density lipoprotein (HDL) borderline 40 mg/dL for male and 50 mg/dL for female	<40 and 50 mg/dL	409 (67.2)	200 (32.8)	1	Reference	
	≥40 and 50 mg/dL	384 (68.2)	179 (32.3)	0.953	0.746	1.218
Triglycerides	<150 mg/dL	476 (68.9)	215 (31.1)	1	Reference	
	≥150 mg/dL	317 (65.9)	164 (34.1)	1.145	0.894	1.468

TABLE 5: Multivariable analysis of risk factors and hypertension among study participants in Kabul city, Afghanistan.

Variables	Categories	Adjusted Odds ratio	CI 95% LL	CI 95% UL	*P* value
Age	Lower age	1		Reference	
	Higher age	1.081	1.067	1.096	<001
General obesity	No	1		Reference	
	Yes	0.474	0.328	0.685	<001
Central obesity	No	1		Reference	
	Yes	0.531	0.377	0.747	<001
Oil for kitchen	Liquid			Reference	
	Solid	1.698	1.234	2.338	<001
Smoking	No	1		Reference	
	Yes	2.232	1.152	4.326	<05
Moderate physical activity	No	1		Reference	
	Yes	0.671	0.461	0.977	<05
Fruits days per week	Less			Reference	
	High	1.098	1.014	1.188	<05

predictors were independently associated with hypertension. Age was independently associated with hypertension and the burden got high proportions as age increases. This is in line with other studies where the risks of hypertension increase with age [27, 28]. Furthermore, general and central obesity were statistically associated with hypertension and odds were high among respondents who were overweight and obese. This finding is in accordance and supported by other studies in similar settings [12, 26]. Smoking was also independently associated with hypertension. This finding is in agreement with other similar studies where substance use was a significant predictor of hypertension [29, 30]. Moreover, moderate physical activity and diet in terms of taking fruits were associated with hypertension as protective factors [31, 32].

This study identifies high prevalence of hypertension and some of the major factors associated with hypertension for people living in the urban areas of Kabul city. Most of these factors are modifiable as well as protective and these could be targeted to improve the health of the citizens. For instance, projects in relation to smoking, encouragement of physical activity, taking more fruits, and reducing obesity will be very useful in health improvement. Intervention inspiring education campaigns to raise awareness on physical activity and healthy diet as protective factors against all NCDs is recommended. Currently, due to urbanization, Kabul city is overcrowded with very limited jogging as well as aerobic sport centres. Establishment of such facilities, which are lacking in urban settings particularly for women, is encouraged.

Limitations to this study included financial constraints which prevented listing of the households ahead of study, overestimation of hypertension due to free checking of blood pressure and blood testing, and the poor security situation which forced the research team to exclude some areas.

5. Conclusion

As a whole, the findings of this study are very important to policy makers and planners in terms of prevalence and risk factors such as age, smoking, obesity, low physical activity, and dietary habits. Thus, effective community-based precautionary and control strategies will contribute to prevent hypertension.

Competing Interests

The authors declare that there are no financial or nonfinancial competing interests of authors in this paper.

References

[1] Symposium on Non-Communicable Diseases in Ethiopia; The Harvard School of Public Health Multidisciplinary International Research Training (HSPH MIRT) Program, Addis Continental Institute of Public Health (ACIPH) and International Clinical Laboratories (ICL), Addis Ababa, Ethiopia, November 2012.

[2] World Health Organization, *Global Status Report on Noncommunicable Diseases: 2010*, World Health Organization, Geneva, Switzerland, 2011.

[3] P. M. Kearney, M. Whelton, K. Reynolds, P. K. Whelton, and J. He, "Worldwide prevalence of hypertension: a systematic review," *Journal of Hypertension*, vol. 22, no. 1, pp. 11–19, 2004.

[4] World Health Organization, "Global brief on hypertension," 2013, http://apps.who.int/iris/bitstream/10665/79059/1/WHO DCO WHD 2013.2 eng.pdf?ua=1.

[5] C. M. Lawes, S. V. Hoorn, and A. Rodgers, "Global burden of blood-pressure-related disease, 2001," *The Lancet*, vol. 371, no. 9623, pp. 1513–1518, 2008.

[6] Hypertension [webpage on the Internet] San Francisco: Wikimedia, http://en.wikipedia.org/wiki/Hypertension.

[7] World Health Organization & Centre for Disease Control, The Atlas of Heart Disease and Stroke, http://www.who.int/cardiovascular_diseases/resources/atlas/en.

[8] P. A. Sytkowski, R. B. D'Agostino, A. J. Belanger, and W. B. Kannel, "Secular trends in long-term sustained hypertension, long-term treatment, and cardiovascular mortality: the Framingham Heart Study 1950 to 1990," *Circulation*, vol. 93, no. 4, pp. 697–703, 1996.

[9] S. Fauci, E. Braunwald, D. L. Kasper et al., "Harrison's principles of Internal Medicine," in *Factors that Contribute to High Blood Pressure: The American Heart Association*, The McGraw-Hill Companies, New York, NY, USA, 17th edition, 2008.

[10] World Health Organization, *2008–2013 Action Plan for the Global Strategy for the Prevention and Control of Non-Communicable Diseases*, World Health Organization Press, Geneva, Switzerland, 2008.

[11] A. Krishnan, B. Shah, V. Lal, D. K. Shukla, E. Paul, and S. K. Kapoor, "Prevalence of risk factors for Non-Communicable Disease in rural area of Faridabad District of Haryana," *Indian Journal of Public Health*, vol. 52, pp. 117–124, 2008.

[12] K. M. I. Saeed, M. H. Rasooly, and N. J. Brown, "Prevalence and predictors of adult hypertension in Kabul, Afghanistan," *BMC Public Health*, vol. 14, no. 1, article 386, 2014.

[13] K. M. I. Saeed, "Prevalence of hypertension and associated factors in Jalalabad City, Nangarhar Province, Afghanistan," *Central Asian Journal of Global Health*, vol. 4, no. 1, 2015.

[14] A.-A. Haghdoost, B. Sadeghirad, and M. Rezazadehkermani, "Epidemiology and heterogeneity of hypertension in Iran: a systematic review," *Archives of Iranian Medicine*, vol. 11, no. 4, pp. 444–452, 2008.

[15] L. Degenhardt, H. A. Whiteford, A. J. Ferrari et al., "Global burden of disease attributable to illicit drug use and dependence: findings from the Global Burden of Disease Study 2010," *The Lancet*, vol. 382, no. 9904, pp. 1564–1574, 2013.

[16] R. Bonita, M. deCourten, T. Dwyer, K. Jamrozik, and R. Winkelmann, *Surveillance of Risk Factors for Noncommunicable Diseases: The WHO STEP-Wise Approach (WHO/NMH/CCS/01.2002)*, World Health Organization, Geneva, Switzerland, 2002.

[17] World Health Organization, *Obesity: Preventing and Managing the Global Epidemic*, WHO Technical Report Series no. 894, World Health Organization, Geneva, Switzerland, 2000.

[18] *The IDF Consensus Worldwide Definitions of the Metabolic Syndrome*, International Diabetes Federation, Brussels, Belgium, 2006, http://www.idf.org/webdata/docs/IDF_Meta_def_final.pdf.

[19] J. A. Whitworth, World Health Organization, International Society of Hypertension Writing Group, and World Health Organization, "2003 World Health Organization (WHO)/International Society of Hypertension (ISH) statement on management of hypertension," *Journal of Hypertension*, vol. 21, no. 11, pp. 1983–1992, 2003.

[20] Diabetes. Fact sheet no. 312, Updated January 2015, Geneva, Switzerland, World Health Organization, 2015, http://www.who.int/mediacentre/factsheets/fs312/en/.

[21] A. Awoke, T. Awoke, S. Alemu, and B. Megabiaw, "Prevalence and associated factors of hypertension among adults in Gondar, Northwest Ethiopia: a community based cross-sectional study," *BMC Cardiovascular Disorders*, vol. 12, article 113, 2012.

[22] N. K. Ibrahim, N. A. Hijazi, and A. A. Al-Bar, "Prevalence and determinants of prehypertension and hypertension among preparatory and secondary school teachers in Jeddah," *The Journal of the Egyptian Public Health Association*, vol. 83, no. 3-4, pp. 183–203, 2008.

[23] Health Management Information System (HMIS), *Annual Report 1393*, Ministry of Public Health, Kabul, Afghanistan, 2015.

[24] Disease early warning system (DEWS) surveillance, In: Annual Report, Kabul, Afghanistan, Afghan National Public Health Institute, Ministry of Public Health, 2015.

[25] T. P. Helelo, Y. A. Gelaw, and A. A. Adane, "Prevalence and associated factors of hypertension among adults in durame town, Southern Ethiopia," *PLOS ONE*, vol. 9, no. 11, Article ID e112790, 2014.

[26] F. Bonsa, E. K. Gudina, and K. W. Hajito, "Prevalence of hypertension and associated factors in Bedele Town, Southwest Ethiopia," *Ethiopian journal of health sciences*, vol. 24, no. 1, pp. 21–26, 2014.

[27] S. P. Manimunda, A. P. Sugunan, V. Benegal, N. Balakrishna, M. V. Rao, and K. S. Pesala, "Association of hypertension with risk factors & hypertension related behaviour among the aboriginal Nicobarese tribe living in Car Nicobar Island, India," *Indian Journal of Medical Research*, vol. 133, no. 3, pp. 287–293, 2011.

[28] H. Y. Jaddou, A. M. Batieha, Y. S. Khader, A. H. Kanaan, M. S. El-Khateeb, and K. M. Ajlouni, "Hypertension prevalence, awareness, treatment and control, and associated factors: results from a national survey, Jordan," *International Journal of Hypertension*, vol. 2011, Article ID 828797, 8 pages, 2011.

[29] A. Virdis, C. Giannarelli, M. F. Neves, S. Taddei, and L. Ghiadoni, "Cigarette smoking and hypertension," *Current Pharmaceutical Design*, vol. 16, no. 23, pp. 2518–2525, 2010.

[30] A. Pandey, N. Patni, S. Sarangi et al., "Association of exclusive smokeless tobacco consumption with hypertension in an adult male rural population of India," *Tobacco Induced Diseases*, vol. 5, no. 1, article 15, 2009.

[31] R. R. Dhungana, S. Devkota, M. K. Khanal et al., "Prevalence of cardiovascular health risk behaviors in a remote rural community of Sindhuli district, Nepal," *BMC Cardiovascular Disorders*, vol. 14, article 92, 2014.

[32] A. Vaidya and A. Krettek, "Physical activity level and its sociodemographic correlates in a peri-urban Nepalese population: a cross-sectional study from the Jhaukhel-Duwakot health demographic surveillance site," *International Journal of Behavioral Nutrition and Physical Activity*, vol. 11, no. 1, article 39, 2014.

3

Knowledge, Treatment, Control, and Risk Factors for Hypertension among Adults in Southern Iran

Sayed Fazel Zinat Motlagh,[1] Reza Chaman,[2] Sayed Rashid Ghafari,[1] Zafar Parisay,[1] Mohamad Reza Golabi,[1] Ahmad Ali Eslami,[3] and Amin Babouei[1]

[1]*Social Determinants of Health Research Center, Yasuj University of Medical Sciences, Yasuj, Iran*
[2]*Department of Community Medicine, School of Medicine, Yasuj University of Medical Sciences, Yasuj, Iran*
[3]*Department of Health Education and Promotion, School of Health, Isfahan University of Medical Sciences, Isfahan, Iran*

Correspondence should be addressed to Ahmad Ali Eslami; eslamiaa@gmail.com

Academic Editor: Hualiang Lin

Hypertension is the first and the most common risk factor to diseases such as cardiovascular, stroke, and renal diseases. The aim of this study was to determine the factors relevant to hypertension knowledge, treatment, and control in southern Iran. In this cross-sectional study, conducted in Kohgiluye Boyer-Ahmad province, south of Iran, a total of 1836 hypertension patients were randomly selected to participate voluntarily in the study. Hypertension treatment and its control were defined during study. In addition, knowledge about hypertension was measured by hypertension knowledge level scale (HK-LS). Treatment rates were 75.5 and 37.7 percent for female and male, respectively. Habitat, education, income, family history with hypertension, smoking, and time of diagnosis to the disease were found to be related to the treatment of the disease. Control rates were 30.7 and 31.4 for males and females, respectively. Habitat, education, and time of diagnosis to the disease were related to control. Over 50 percent of patients had average knowledge on hypertension. Considering the low rate of control and knowledge on hypertension among patients, health care providers should reinforce their services to improve appropriate knowledge level among elders and, also, plan comprehensive programs to promote health in order to encourage patients change and reform their life style.

1. Introduction

Rapid rise of noncommunicable diseases has been considered as a major health challenge in the present century, which threatens social and economic development of communities and people health [1]. Such diseases impose half of the burden of diseases cost in the world [2–4]. Following the present trend, it is predicted that patients will be responsible for over 70 percent of diseases by 2020 [1, 4, 5]. In this regard, hypertension has been considered as the first and the most common risk factor to cardiovascular diseases, stroke, and renal diseases; it has been known as a main modulated disability cause around the world [6, 7] so that hypertension caused at least 45 percent of mortality due to cardiovascular problems and 51 percent of stroke mortality rate [8]. Among 17 million deaths due to cardiovascular problems in the world [8], 9.4 million occur as a consequence of complications of hypertension [9]. In this regard, in Eastern Mediterranean Region where Iran is located, 26 percent of mortality results from hypertension [10].

On the other hand, statistics showed an increase in the prevalence of hypertension. The number of patients with hypertension has increased from 600 million cases in 1980 to 1 billion in 2008; over 40 percent of adults were known to have hypertension [11]. Also, it was suggested that, by 2025, 1.54 billion adults will suffer from hypertension [12]. In this regard, it was reported to be 14 to 34 percent in Iran [13–18] and various studies in other countries reported high rates of hypertension from 18 to 72 percent among males and females [19–27].

It is essential to control hypertension to minimize the side effects of hypertension. Rates reported for hypertension control were disappointing [28], which were suggested to be 13 to 56 percent around the world [23, 26, 29, 30]. An important component to control hypertension is knowledge, which is relative to lower rates of ceasing interventions, following the interventions behavior and better control on disease by patients. As a result, careful evaluation of hypertension has been considered as an inseparable part of general care of the patients [31].

Studies suggested low levels of knowledge on hypertension among patients [23, 24, 32], and lack of correct information and improper understanding of hypertension did not appertain to rural sites; it has been widely reported in urban environments and industrial countries, too [33, 34]. In Iran, studies on knowledge, treatment, and control of hypertension suggested low levels of the mentioned factors [15, 16]. In Isfahan healthy heart program, the effects of comprehensive self-care programs on improving knowledge, attitude, and treatment among patients with hypertension were investigated. The results from the program showed that factors such as knowledge, treatment pursuit, and hypertension control were 49.9, 43.8, and 15.8 percent, respectively [16]. Another study reported treatment and hypertension control as 33.35 and 35.10 percent [15].

Considering factors related to knowledge and hypertension management is an essential starting point to preventing high rates of cardiovascular mortality due to hypertension [35]. However, there is little information available on knowledge, treatment, and control of hypertension in southern Iran. Noticing the importance of the topic, the aim of this study was to determine the factors relevant to hypertension knowledge, treatment, and control in southern Iran.

2. Methods

2.1. Participants. This cross-sectional study was conducted on a sample of men and women with hypertension in urban and rural health centres in Kohgiluyeh and Boyer-Ahmad Province in southern Iran, in 2014. Patients met the inclusion criteria (six months past the definitive diagnosis disease doctor, a record in health centres, over the age of 30). To participate in the study the patients were invited by phone or visiting their location. Participants who could not communicate effectively with the study personnel or provide informed consent were excluded. Finally, out of the 2,400 patients invited to study, 1836 (76.52%) signed the consent form and voluntarily agreed to participate in the study.

2.2. Measures. Questionnaire included three sections that comprised the following questions: sociodemographic characteristics, hypertension-related information, and hypertension knowledge.

2.2.1. Sociodemographic Characteristics Variables. Sociodemographic data included data on age, gender, educational level (illiterate, elementary school, middle school, high school, diploma, and university), monthly family income (>5 million rials, 5 million rials to 10 million rials, 10 million rials to 15 million rials, and <15 million rials), marital status (single, married, divorced, or widowed/widower), employment status which was coded in 5 categories (employed, unemployed, farmer, retired, and housekeeper), physical activity, and smoking. (For smoking and hookah, nonsmoker and smoker were distinguished.)

Body Mass Index. Height (height was evaluated with an error close to 0.1 cm, using a SECA portable stadiometer with the individual in the standing position) and weight (weight measurements were taken with participants wearing light clothing and no shoes; weight was measured with an error close to 0.5 Kg using a SECA digital scale) were recorded by a nurse. Body mass index (BMI; calculated as weight/height^2) was divided into 4 categories: below normal weight ($BMI < 18.5$), normal weight ($18.5 \leq BMI < 25.0$), overweight ($25.0 \leq BMI < 30.0$), and obese ($BMI \geq 30.0$) [36].

2.2.2. Hypertension-Related Information. Hypertension-related questions included duration of hypertension, family history of HTN, and treatment of HTN which was defined as self-reported current use of antihypertensive medication. Control of HTN was defined as hypertensive participants' SBP < 140 mm Hg and DBP < 90 mm Hg among hypertensive participants who treated their HTN with drugs; that is, control in treatment was also analyzed. Hypertension was defined as systolic blood pressure (SBP) C140 mm Hg or diastolic blood pressure (DBP) C90 mm Hg according to the WHO criteria or history of previously diagnosed disease [37]; BP was measured in a sitting position after a minimum of 5 minutes of rest by using a standardized digital BP measuring machine (Omron Digital).

2.2.3. Hypertension Knowledge. Hypertension knowledge was ascertained by using Hypertension Knowledge Level Scale (HK-LS). This tool was developed from the Hypertension Knowledge Level Scale (HK-LS), a 22-item scale prepared by Erkoc et al. [37]. Hypertension Knowledge Level Scale (HK-LS) assessed respondents' knowledge in defining hypertension, lifestyle, medical treatment, drug compliance, diet, and complication of hypertension. Each item was a full sentence that was either correct or incorrect. And each item was prepared as part of a standard answer (correct, incorrect, or do not know). To assess the content validity of the scale to identify whether items were or were not representative of the knowledge level of hypertension, the opinions of experts were requested via an assessment form. The expert opinions were evaluated, and 2 items were excluded from the scale. All items were evaluated in terms of clarity and expression by considering the expert opinions, and relevant changes (definition (1 item), medical treatment (4 items), drug compliance (4 items), lifestyle (4 items), diet (2 items), and complications (5 items)) were made.

2.3. Statistical Analysis. Statistical analyses were performed using SPSS windows version 21.0 software (SPSS Inc., Chicago, Illinois, USA). *P* value < 0.05 was considered significant.

3. Results

The mean age of respondents was 66.26 years [SD: 12.36], ranging from 30 to 93 years. Almost, 722 participants were male (39.3%) and 1114 were female (60.7%). More than half of the participants (51.5%) were older than 60. Furthermore, 822 participants (44.8%) were living in cities and 1014 (55.2%) were living in villages. Regarding education, 1149 (66.2%) were illiterate, 362 (19.7%) were at elementary levels, 114 (6.2%) were at guidance level, 46 (2.5%) were at high school level, 90 (4.9%) finished high school, and 75 (4.1%) had academic education. With respect to marital status, 1488 participants (81%) were married. 191 (17.6%) were widows and 25 (1.4%) were single. Over 90 percent of participants had low income. In addition, 45.5 percent reported family history of hypertension. Also, 27.5 percent of the respondents reported regular physical activity (Table 1).

3.1. Hypertension Treatment and Control. As shown in Table 1, 222 male (30.7%) and 350 (31.4%) participants reported self-control on their hypertension. There was no significant difference between male and female participants ($P = 0.796$), though it was higher among females. There was a statistically significant correlation between habitat ($P = 0.000$), education ($P = 0.000$), income ($P = 0.002$), family history on hypertension ($P = 0.003$), smoking ($P = 0.006$), and diagnosis time ($P = 0.045$). Participants living in cities, with higher education and income levels, showed better control on their hypertension.

Treatment rate was high among participants. The treatment rates were 75.5% and 37.7% for females and males, respectively, while there was no statistically significant correlation between male and female participants ($P = 0.383$). 36.1 percent of participants who were under treatment showed regular use of their medications. 24.4 percent of participants under treatment reported control on their hypertension. There was a statistically significant correlation between age ($P = 0.000$), habitat ($P = 0.019$), education ($P = 0.004$), and diagnosis time ($P = 0.045$).

3.2. Knowledge. Table 2 represents patient's knowledge about hypertension. In general, 25.2 percent of participants showed high knowledge on hypertension (definition of hypertension, treatment pursuit, lifestyle, nutrition, and hypertension side effects).

This parameter was higher among male in comparison to females, participants with higher income in comparison to those with low incomes, among employees in comparison to other occupations, and among those with regular physical activities which was statistically meaningful.

4. Discussion

Improving knowledge, treatment, and control on hypertension could decrease high rates of mortality by cardiovascular diseases [38]. Results from our study showed that over half of the participants in the study were over 60 years old. Several studies reported a direct significance in the prevalence of hypertension and age, which corresponded to the results from the present study [14, 39–42]. The results, also, suggested higher hypertension risk with elders. Therefore, it seems essential to plan preventive interventions to control hypertension among older people. Results from the present study reported that hypertension remains mostly undiagnosed during the early years of prevalence so that over 45 percent of patients over 60 were diagnosed for hypertension less than 5 years ago, which suggest the careful consideration of screening and increasing public knowledge on hypertension and its symptoms.

Our results indicated treatment and control rates on hypertension to be 74.8 and 31.2 percent, which were higher in comparison to the results by Esteghamati et al. [16] (2007) in Isfahan where treatment and control on hypertension were 43.8 and 15.8 percent, respectively. This increase could result from implementing Family Physician program and offering health care services to the patients in Iran.

Chow et al. (2013) reported that the rate of treatment and control of hypertension in high-, average-, and poor-income countries is low [43]; results from the studies in Asia suggested similar findings [26, 44, 45]. Low rates of control and treatment of hypertension have been considered as a major risk to increase cardiovascular diseases and stroke [46], which suggested the necessity of efficient implementation of proper training programs and offering essential services to health care services by doctors and health experts, while majority of patients with diagnosed hypertension showed poor control on their disease. This gap has also been reported in several other studies [41, 43, 47]. It seemed that the only way used to control hypertension by patients was taking prescribed medicines; they avoided self-care behaviors such as regular physical activities, good nutrition, and weight control.

Results from the present study reported higher treatment and control of hypertension in females in comparison to males, which was in accordance with the results from other studies [14, 43, 47, 48]. As the patients grew older, the treatment of hypertension improved. It seems that patients were more sensitive to their disease when they grew older and tried medicines to treat their disease. It corresponded to the results from other studies [41, 43, 47].

Another finding from the present study suggested a statistically significant correlation between hypertension control and patients education. The higher their education level, the higher the control rate among patients so that patients having university degrees showed higher control on their hypertension which was in accordance with results from other studies [14, 26, 47, 49], though it was different from study by CHP-SNE which reported lower control on hypertension among individuals with lower education [50]. More than half of the participants reported average knowledge on hypertension, treatment pursuit, lifestyle, nutrition, and complication of hypertension. Only 25.2 percent of participants showed high knowledge on the disease. In comparison with other studies, the present study reported lower rates on the issue [34, 51–53]. Parmar et al. showed good rates of knowledge on hypertension among participants [52]. The difference could result from high number of illiterate participants living in villages.

TABLE 1: Percentage (%) of treatment and control of hypertension among hypertensive adults ($N = 1836$).

Variables	N	Control			Treatment		
		n	%	P	n	%	P
Gender							
Total	1863	572	31.2	—	1373	74.8	—
Male	722	222	30.7	$P = 0.796$	532	73.7	$P = 0.383$
Female	1114	350	31.4		841	75.5	
Age groups							
39–30	95	33	34.7		56	58.9	
49–40	262	84	32.1	$P = 0.135$	180	68.7	$P = 0.000$
59–50	534	183	34.3		401	75.1	
≥60	945	272	28.8		736	77.9	
Region							
Urban	822	308	37.5	$P = 0.000$	593	72.1	$P = 0.019$
Rural	1014	264	26		780	76.9	
Marital status							
Single	25	10	40		16	64	
Married	1488	472	31.7	$P = 0.251$	1104	74.2	$P = 0.138$
Divorced and widowed/widower	323	90	27.9		253	78.3	
Education level							
Illiterate	1149	322	28		891	77.5	
Primary school	362	129	35.6		258	71.3	
Secondary school	114	34	29.8	$P = 0.000$	76	66.7	$P = 0.004$
High school	46	22	47.8		32	69.6	
Diploma	90	28	31.1		60	66.7	
University	75	37	49.3		56	74.6	
Job							
Farmer	205	58	28.9		143	71.1	
Employed	111	42	37.8		84	75.7	
Retired	184	64	34.8	$P = 0.351$	137	74.5	$P = 0.659$
Unemployed	269	79	29.4		197	73.2	
Housekeeper	1071	329	30.7		812	75.8	
Income							
Poor	1655	495	29.9		1235	74.6	
Medium	148	61	41.2	$P = 0.002$	112	75.7	$P = 0.833$
Good	33	16	48.5		26	78.8	
Family history of hypertension							
Yes	832	289	34.7	$P = 0.003$	624	75	$P = 0.845$
No	1004	283	28.2		749	74.6	
Physical activity							
Yes	512	174	34	$P = 0.104$	380	74.2	$P = 0.730$
No	1324	398	30.1		993	75	
Tobacco							
Yes	253	61	24.1	$P = 0.009$	188	73.3	$P = 0.852$
No	1583	511	32.3		1185	74.9	
Body mass index (BMI)							
≤18.5	15	5	33.3		11	73.3	
25–18.5	655	214	32.7	$P = 0.612$	493	75.3	$P = 0.980$
30–25	736	229	31.1		547	74.3	
≥30	430	124	28.8		322	74.9	
Duration of diagnosis							
≤5	955	297	31.1		669	70.1	
5–9	366	130	35.5		293	80.1	
10–14	298	79	26.5	$P = 0.045$	235	78.9	$P = 0.000$
15–19	129	33	25.6		97	75.2	
≥20	88	33	37.5		79	89.8	

Table 2: Percentage (%) of knowledge of hypertension among hypertensive adults (N = 1836).

Variables	Weak		Average		Good		P
	N	%	N	%	N	%	
Gender							
Male	141	19.5	385	53.3	196	27.1	$P = 0.261$
Female	218	19.6	630	56.6	266	23.9	
Age groups							
39–30	22	23.4	39	41.1	34	35.8	$P = 0.019$
49–40	41	15.6	144	55	77	29.4	
59–50	100	18.7	300	56.2	134	25.1	
≥60	196	20.7	532	56.3	217	23	
Region							
Urban	149	18.1	452	55	221	26.9	$P = 0.189$
Rural	210	20.7	563	55.5	241	23.8	
Marital status							
Single	5	20	6	24	14	56	$P = 0.004$
Married	296	19.9	820	55.1	372	25	
Divorced and widowed/widower	58	18	189	58.5	76	23.5	
Education level							
Illiterate	234	20.4	663	57.7	252	21.9	$P = 0.000$
Primary school	72	19.9	206	57.9	84	23.2	
Secondary school	24	21.4	61	53.5	29	25.4	
High school	4	8.7	22	47.8	20	43.5	
Diploma	18	20	42	47.7	30	33.3	
University	7	9.3	21	28	47	62.6	
Occupation							
Farmer	35	17.4	114	56.7	52	25.9	$P = 0.001$
Employed	13	11.7	55	49.5	43	38.7	
Retired	34	18.5	88	47.8	62	33.7	
Unemployed	63	23.4	151	56.1	55	20.4	
Housekeeper	214	20	607	56.7	250	13.3	
Income							
Weak	322	20.1	20	13.5	7	21.7	$P = 0.005$
Average	927	56	73	49.3	15	45.5	
Good	396	23.9	55	32.2	11	33.3	
Family history of hypertension							
Yes	154	19.1	460	55.3	213	25.6	$P = 0.874$
No	200	19.9	555	55.3	246	24.4	
Tobacco							
Yes	33	27.5	66	55	21	17.5	$P = 0.028$
No	326	19	949	55.3	441	25.7	
Physical activity							
Yes	68	13.3	295	57.6	149	29.1	$P = 0.000$
No	291	22	720	54.4	313	23.6	
Body mass index (BMI)							
≤18.5	4	26.7	7	46.7	4	26.7	$P = 0.157$
25–18.5	143	21.8	364	55.6	148	22.6	
30–25	136	18.5	417	56.7	183	24.9	
≥30	76	17.7	227	52.7	127	29.5	
Duration of diagnosis							
≤5	183	19.2	522	54.7	250	26.2	$P = 0.714$
5–9	77	21	204	55.7	85	23.2	
10–14	60	20.1	169	56.7	69	23.2	
15–19	22	17.1	77	59.7	30	23.3	
≥20	17	19.3	43	48.9	28	31.8	

Another finding from the present study considered statistically significant correlation between patient's age and knowledge on the disease. It reported that the older the participants the less their knowledge on the issue, which was in accordance with results from other studies [34, 52]. It was concluded that age group of 30 to 39 had the higher knowledge on hypertension in comparison to other age groups, which could result from their higher education levels relative to other groups. Results from the present study in this regard suggested a meaningful relationship between education and knowledge: as the education among the patients improves, their knowledge on hypertension increases. It was in agreement with other studies [34, 52]. Low knowledge levels on hypertension were in relation to old age, low levels of education, and low income. Lack of training materials, poor screening, and poor consistency of health team were reported in these groups. It seems necessary to create proper training materials by health experts to improve patients' knowledge and, also, increase treatment rates and control on patients.

The strength of the present study was investigating a large urban and rural population with high rates of responding. However, as over 80 percent of the participants were over 50 years old and there was not a normal coverage to all possible age groups, it was considered as a limitation to the study.

5. Conclusion

Considering the low rate of knowledge and control of patients on hypertension, health care providers should reinforce their activities to help to improve patients' knowledge level, especially among elders, through focusing on identifying risk factors to hypertension, regular drug intake, good nutrition, physical activity, and changing and informing lifestyles of patients with hypertension.

Disclosure

This paper is a part of the Ph.D. dissertation of health education and health promotion supported by Isfahan University of Medical Sciences and Yasuj University of Medical Sciences.

Acknowledgments

The authors would like to thank Deputy of Research of Isfahan University of Medical Sciences and Yasuj University of Medical Sciences for financial support.

References

[1] World Health Organization, *Proceedings of the 15th Annual Conference of the Indian Society of Hypertension and 4th International CME on Atherosclerosis*, Hypertension and Coronary Artery Disease, World Health Organization (WHO), New Delhi, India, 2005.

[2] World Health Organization, *Global Recommendations on Physical Activity for Health*, World Health Organization, Geneva, Switzerland, 1st edition, 2010.

[3] S. H. Habib and S. Saha, "Burden of non-communicable disease: global overview," *Diabetes & Metabolic Syndrome: Clinical Research and Reviews*, vol. 4, no. 1, pp. 41–47, 2010.

[4] World Health Organization, *The Global Burden of Disease: 2004 Update*, WHO, 1st edition, 2008.

[5] S. G. Sepanlou, F. Kamangar, H. Poustchi, and R. Malekzadeh, "Reducing the burden of chronic diseases: a neglected agenda in Iranian health care system, requiring a plan for action," *Archives of Iranian Medicine*, vol. 13, no. 4, pp. 340–350, 2010.

[6] World Health Organization, *Global Health Risks: Mortality and Burden of Disease Attributable to Selected Major Risks*, WHO, 2013.

[7] M. Ezzati, A. D. Lopez, A. Rodgers, S. Vander Hoorn, and C. J. L. Murray, "Selected major risk factors and global and regional burden of disease," *The Lancet*, vol. 360, no. 9343, pp. 1347–1360, 2002.

[8] World Health Organization, "Causes of Death 2008," 2008, http://www.who.int/healthinfo/global_burden_disease/cod_2008_sources_methods.pdf.

[9] S. S. Lim, T. Vos, A. D. Flaxman et al., "A comparative risk assessment of burden of disease and injury attributable to 67 risk factors and risk factor clusters in 21 regions, 1990–2010: a systematic analysis for the Global Burden of Disease Study 2010," *The Lancet*, vol. 380, no. 9859, pp. 2224–2260, 2013.

[10] World Health Organization, "Report on the Regional Consultation on Hypertension Prevention and Control (Abu Dhabi, United Arab Emirates 20–22 December)".

[11] World Health Organization, "Global status report on no communicable diseases 2010," 2011.

[12] P. M. Kearney, M. Whelton, K. Reynolds, P. Muntner, P. K. Whelton, and J. He, "Global burden of hypertension: analysis of worldwide data," *The Lancet*, vol. 365, no. 9455, pp. 217–223, 2005.

[13] F. Amirkhizi, F. Siassi, S. Minaie, M. Jalali, M. A. Dorosty, and M. Chamari, "Assessment of blood pressure status and its relationship with anthropometric indices among women in rural areas of Kerman province, Iran," *Yafteh*, vol. 10, no. 2, pp. 31–38, 2009.

[14] A. Azizi, M. Abasi, and G. Abdoli, "The prevalence of hypertension and its association with age, sex and BMI in a population being educated using community-based medicine in Kermanshah: 2003," *Iranian Journal of Endocrinology and Metabolism*, vol. 10, no. 4, pp. 323–329, 2008.

[15] M. Ebrahimi, M. A. Mansournia, A. A. Haghdoost et al., "Social disparities in prevalence, treatment and control of hypertension in Iran: second National Surveillance of Risk Factors of Noncommunicable Diseases, 2006," *Journal of Hypertension*, vol. 28, no. 8, pp. 1620–1629, 2010.

[16] A. Esteghamati, A. Meysamie, O. Khalilzadeh et al., "Third national surveillance of risk factors of non-communicable diseases (SuRFNCD-2007) in Iran: methods and results on prevalence of diabetes, hypertension, obesity, central obesity, and dyslipidemia," *BMC Public Health*, vol. 9, no. 1, article 167, 2009.

[17] H. Fakhrzadeh, M. Nouri, R. Pour-Ebrahim, S. Ghotbi, R. Heshmat, and M. Bastanhagh, "Prevalence of hypertension and correlated risk factors among 25–64 aged inhabitants of Tehran University of medical sciences population lab region," *Iranian Journal of Diabetes and Metabolism*, vol. 3, pp. 37–43, 2004.

[18] A.-A. Haghdoost, B. Sadeghirad, and M. Rezazadehkermani, "Epidemiology and heterogeneity of hypertension in Iran: a systematic review," *Archives of Iranian Medicine*, vol. 11, no. 4, pp. 444–452, 2008.

[19] B. Altun, M. Arici, G. Nergizoglu et al., "Prevalence, awareness, treatment and control of hypertension in Turkey (the PatenT study) in 2003," *Journal of Hypertension*, vol. 23, no. 10, pp. 1817–1823, 2005.

[20] M. Dorobantu, R. O. Darabont, E. Badila, and S. Ghiorghe, "Prevalence, awareness, treatment, and control of hypertension in romania: results of the SEPHAR Study," *International Journal of Hypertension*, vol. 2010, Article ID 970694, 6 pages, 2010.

[21] A. D. Efstratopoulos, S. M. Voyaki, A. A. Baltas et al., "Prevalence, awareness, treatment and control of hypertension in Hellas, Greece: the hypertension study in general practice in hellas (HYPERTENSHELL) national study," *American Journal of Hypertension*, vol. 19, no. 1, pp. 53–60, 2006.

[22] P. M. Kearney, M. Whelton, K. Reynolds, P. K. Whelton, and J. He, "Worldwide prevalence of hypertension: a systematic review," *Journal of Hypertension*, vol. 22, no. 1, pp. 11–19, 2004.

[23] H.-S. Lee, Y.-M. Park, H.-S. Kwon et al., "Prevalence, awareness, treatment, and control of hypertension among people over 40 years old in a rural area of South Korea: the Chungju Metabolic Disease Cohort (CMC) study," *Clinical and Experimental Hypertension*, vol. 32, no. 3, pp. 166–178, 2010.

[24] W. J. Ma, J. L. Tang, Y. H. Zhang et al., "Hypertension prevalence, awareness, treatment, control, and associated factors in adults in Southern China," *American Journal of Hypertension*, vol. 25, no. 5, pp. 590–596, 2012.

[25] K. Wolf-Maier, R. S. Cooper, J. R. Banegas et al., "Hypertension prevalence and blood pressure levels in 6 European countries, Canada, and the United States," *The Journal of the American Medical Association*, vol. 289, no. 18, pp. 2363–2369, 2003.

[26] T. Xu, Y. Wang, W. Li et al., "Survey of prevalence, awareness, treatment, and control of hypertension among Chinese governmental and institutional employees in Beijing," *Clinical Cardiology*, vol. 33, no. 6, pp. E66–E72, 2010.

[27] B. Y. Yuvaraj, M. R. Nagendra Gowda, and A. G. Umakantha, "Prevalence, awareness, treatment, and control of hypertension in rural areas of Davanagere," *Indian Journal of Community Medicine*, vol. 35, no. 1, pp. 138–141, 2010.

[28] T. G. Pickering, "Why are we doing so badly with the control of hypertension? Poor compliance is only part of the story," *The Journal of Clinical Hypertension*, vol. 3, no. 3, pp. 179–182, 2001.

[29] G. C. R. Roca, L. M. A. Ródenas, J. L. L. Caro et al., "Control of hypertension in elderly patients receiving primary care in Spain," *Revista Española de Cardiología*, vol. 58, no. 4, pp. 359–366, 2005.

[30] Y. Wu, R. Huxley, L. Li et al., "Prevalence, awareness, treatment, and control of hypertension in China data from the China National Nutrition and Health Survey 2002," *Circulation*, vol. 118, no. 25, pp. 2679–2686, 2008.

[31] H.-R. Han, K. Chan, H. Song, T. Nguyen, J.-E. Lee, and M. T. Kim, "Development and evaluation of a hypertension knowledge test for Korean hypertensive patients," *The Journal of Clinical Hypertension*, vol. 13, no. 10, pp. 750–757, 2011.

[32] Y. Ostchega, C. F. Dillon, J. P. Hughes, M. Carroll, and S. Yoon, "Trends in hypertension prevalence, awareness, treatment, and control in older U.S. adults: data from the National Health and Nutrition Examination Survey 1988 to 2004," *Journal of the American Geriatrics Society*, vol. 55, no. 7, pp. 1056–1065, 2007.

[33] X. Li, N. Ning, Y. Hao et al., "Health literacy in rural areas of China: hypertension knowledge survey," *International Journal of Environmental Research and Public Health*, vol. 10, no. 3, pp. 1125–1138, 2013.

[34] S. Sanne, P. Muntner, L. Kawasaki, A. Hyre, and K. B. Desalvo, "Hypertension knowledge among patients from an urban clinic," *Ethnicity and Disease*, vol. 18, no. 1, pp. 42–47, 2008.

[35] J. J. Beunza, M. Á. Martínez-González, S. Ebrahim et al., "Sedentary behaviors and the risk of incident hypertension. The SUN Cohort," *American Journal of Hypertension*, vol. 20, no. 11, pp. 1156–1162, 2007.

[36] World Health Organization, "Obesity: preventing and managing the global epidemic: report of a WHO consultation," WHO Technical Report Series 894, World Health Organization, Geneva, Switzerland, 1999.

[37] S. B. Erkoc, B. Isikli, S. Metintas, and C. Kalyoncu, "Hypertension knowledge-level scale (HK-LS): a study on development, validity and reliability," *International Journal of Environmental Research and Public Health*, vol. 9, no. 3, pp. 1018–1029, 2012.

[38] N. C. Barengo, M. Kastarinen, R. Antikainen, A. Nissinen, and J. Tuomilehto, "The effects of awareness, treatment and control of hypertension on cardiovascular and all-cause mortality in a community-based population," *Journal of Human Hypertension*, vol. 23, no. 12, pp. 808–816, 2009.

[39] J. B. Jonas, V. Nangia, A. Matin, P. P. Joshi, and S. N. Ughade, "Prevalence, awareness, control, and associations of arterial hypertension in a rural central India population: the central India eye and medical study," *American Journal of Hypertension*, vol. 23, no. 4, pp. 347–350, 2010.

[40] I. I. Ulasi, C. K. Ijoma, B. J. C. Onwubere, E. Arodiwe, O. Onodugo, and C. Okafor, "High prevalence and low awareness of hypertension in a market population in Enugu, Nigeria," *International Journal of Hypertension*, vol. 2011, Article ID 869675, 5 pages, 2011.

[41] H. Wang, X. Zhang, J. Zhang et al., "Factors associated with prevalence, awareness, treatment and control of hypertension among adults in Southern China: a community-based," *PLoS ONE*, vol. 8, no. 5, Article ID e62469, 2013.

[42] K.-K. Zaw, T.-S. Latt, P.-P. Aung, T.-G. Thwin, and T.-K. Myint, "Prevalence of hypertension and its associated factors in the adult population in Yangon Division, Myanmar," *Asia-Pacific Journal of Public Health*, vol. 23, no. 4, pp. 496–506, 2011.

[43] C. K. Chow, K. K. Teo, S. Rangarajan et al., "Prevalence, awareness, treatment, and control of hypertension in rural and urban communities in high-, middle-, and low-income countries," *Journal of the American Medical Association*, vol. 310, no. 9, pp. 959–968, 2013.

[44] D. A. Ha, R. J. Goldberg, J. J. Allison, T. H. Chu, and H. L. Nguyen, "Prevalence, awareness, treatment, and control of high blood pressure: a population-based survey in Thai Nguyen, Vietnam," *PLoS ONE*, vol. 8, no. 6, Article ID e66792, 2013.

[45] J. Wang, L. Zhang, F. Wang, L. Liu, and H. Wang, "Prevalence, awareness, treatment, and control of hypertension in China: results from a national survey," *American Journal of Hypertension*, vol. 27, no. 11, pp. 1355–1361, 2014.

[46] World Health Organization, *World Health Statistics 2012*, World Health Organization, 2012, http://www.who.int/gho/publications/world_health_statistics/2012/en/index.html.

[47] M. Joffres, E. Falaschetti, C. Gillespie et al., "Hypertension prevalence, awareness, treatment and control in national surveys from England, the USA and Canada, and correlation with

stroke and ischaemic heart disease mortality: a cross-sectional study," *BMJ Open*, vol. 3, no. 8, Article ID e003423, 2013.

[48] M. Pereira, N. Lunet, A. Azevedo, and H. Barros, "Differences in prevalence, awareness, treatment and control of hypertension between developing and developed countries," *Journal of Hypertension*, vol. 27, no. 5, pp. 963–975, 2009.

[49] Y. Wu, E. S. Tai, D. Heng, C. E. Tan, L. P. Low, and J. Lee, "Risk factors associated with hypertension awareness, treatment, and control in a multi-ethnic Asian population," *Journal of Hypertension*, vol. 27, no. 1, pp. 190–197, 2009.

[50] S. Tian, G.-H. Dong, D. Wang et al., "Factors associated with prevalence, awareness, treatment and control of hypertension in urban adults from 33 communities in China: the CHPSNE study," *Hypertension Research*, vol. 34, no. 10, pp. 1087–1092, 2011.

[51] A. R. Demaio, D. Otgontuya, M. de Courten et al., "Hypertension and hypertension-related disease in Mongolia; findings of a national knowledge, attitudes and practices study," *BMC Public Health*, vol. 13, no. 1, article 194, 2013.

[52] P. Parmar, G. B. Rathod, S. Rathod, R. Goyal, S. Aggarwal, and A. Parikh, "Study of knowledge, attitude and practice of general population of Gandhinagar towards hypertension," *International Journal of Current Microbiology and Applied Sciences*, vol. 3, no. 8, pp. 680–685, 2014.

[53] X. Zhang, M. Zhu, H. H. Dib et al., "Knowledge, awareness, behavior (KAB) and control of hypertension among urban elderly in Western China," *International Journal of Cardiology*, vol. 137, no. 1, pp. 9–15, 2009.

4

The Hypertension of Hemophilia Is Not Explained by the Usual Cardiovascular Risk Factors: Results of a Cohort Study

Richard F. W. Barnes,[1] Thomas J. Cramer,[1] Afrah S. Sait,[1,2] Rebecca Kruse-Jarres,[3,4] Doris V. K. Quon,[5] and Annette von Drygalski[1,6]

[1]*Department of Medicine, Division of Hematology/Oncology, University of California San Diego, San Diego, CA, USA*
[2]*Department of Medicine, University of British Columbia, Vancouver, BC, Canada*
[3]*School of Medicine, Section of Hematology/Oncology, Tulane University, New Orleans, LA, USA*
[4]*Washington Center for Bleeding Disorders at Bloodworks NW, Seattle, WA, USA*
[5]*Orthopaedic Hemophilia Treatment Center, Orthopaedic Institute for Children, Los Angeles, CA, USA*
[6]*Department of Molecular and Experimental Medicine, The Scripps Research Institute, La Jolla, CA, USA*

Correspondence should be addressed to Richard F. W. Barnes; rlbarnes@ucsd.edu

Academic Editor: Claudio Borghi

Background. The etiology of the high prevalence of hypertension among patients with hemophilia (PWH) remains unknown. *Methods.* We compared 469 PWH in the United States with males from the National Health and Nutrition Examination Survey (NHANES) to determine whether differences in cardiovascular risk factors can account for the hypertension in hemophilia. *Results.* Median systolic and diastolic BP were higher in PWH than NHANES ($P < 0.001$) for subjects not taking antihypertensives. Those taking antihypertensives showed similar differences. Differences in both systolic and diastolic BP were especially marked among adults <30 years old. Differences between PWH and NHANES persisted after adjusting for age and risk factors (body mass index, renal function, cholesterol, smoking, diabetes, Hepatitis C, and race). *Conclusions.* Systolic and diastolic BP are higher in PWH than in the general male population and especially among PWH < 30 years old. The usual cardiovascular risk factors do not account for the etiology of the higher prevalence of hypertension in hemophilia. New investigations into the missing link between hemophilia and hypertension should include age of onset of hypertension and hemophilia-specific morbidities such as the role of inflammatory joint disease.

1. Introduction

About 1 in 5,000 male births in the United States results in hemophilia which is an X-linked bleeding disorder. In the 19th century, hemophilia was a rare disease in adulthood, with a median life expectancy of 11 years. Life expectancy increased when clotting factors were developed in the 1960s, with many patients surviving into middle age and beyond [1, 2]. The emergence of HIV in the early 1980s dramatically increased mortality among patients because the virus was disseminated in blood products. Today, with the advent of virally safe clotting factor preparations in the early 1990s, life expectancy approaches that of males in the general population [2, 3]. This has unmasked new comorbidities, such as the hypertension in hemophilia, that are incompletely characterized and poorly understood [4–8].

Bleeding in hemophilia most frequently manifests as spontaneous joint and muscle bleeding, resulting in progressive joint degradation. The most serious complications are intracranial hemorrhages (ICH) which are 20 to 50 times more frequent in patients with hemophilia (PWH) compared to the general male population [9] with a mortality rate up to 20% [10–12]. Hypertension is a major risk factor for ICH because the risk of ICH increases steeply with the stage of hypertension [9–11, 13, 14]. This is of particular clinical concern since there is increasing evidence that hypertension is more common in PWH compared to the general population [4–8, 15]. The reasons for the higher prevalence of hypertension in PWH remain obscure.

Hypertension in the general population is associated with age, BMI, cholesterol, kidney function, diabetes, smoking, HCV, and race [16]. Age, BMI, and diabetes were correlated with hypertension in PWH in two studies [6, 7], and renal function was inversely associated in one [7]. If hypertension is more prevalent among PWH than the general population, then it is reasonable to assume that one or more risk factors must be higher in PWH than among the general population. Alternatively, higher blood pressure among PWH could be explained if it increases more rapidly with a particular risk factor—the slope of blood pressure on the risk factor is steeper—than for other males. Our objective was to analyze the association between blood pressure and each of the usual risk factors to determine whether one or more risk factors could account for the hypertension of hemophilia.

Hypertension is a categorical variable that is derived from measurements of blood pressure (BP). We chose to analyze systolic and diastolic BP measurements, which are continuous variables and therefore provide greater statistical power [17]. We examined BP trends in relation to the usual cardiovascular risk factors by comparing a cohort of PWH against a randomly selected sample of males from the population of the United States. While previous studies have compared systolic BP or prevalence of hypertension against the general population [6, 8] or compared BP against the general male population adjusted for age in the Netherlands [5], this study focuses on a comparison of BP values adjusted for age between PWH and the general male population of the United States. In addition, we analyzed subjects treated with antihypertensive medications separately from untreated subjects.

2. Methods

2.1. Patients with Hemophilia. A retrospective data collection was performed for all male patients with hemophilia (PWH) aged 18 years and older seen regularly at three hemophilia treatment centers in the United States: University of California San Diego (2004–2014), Tulane University (2008–2011), and the Los Angeles Orthopaedic Hospital (2005–2012). Patient confidentiality safeguards and data acquisition methods were approved by the Institutional Review Boards of all three institutions. Only patients with complete data on age and race (Hispanic, white, black, and other) were included ($n = 469$). Data extracted included demographic information on age, ethnicity, hemophilia type and severity, positive tests for hepatitis C (HCV) or HIV by serology or reported history thereof, medication history, and smoking status.

Laboratory values of nonfasting patients were obtained during regular clinic visits. Data pertaining to diabetes (HbA1c, random blood glucose) and serum creatinine were recorded. The diagnosis of diabetes was defined according to the 2010 American Diabetes Association Standards of Medical Care in Diabetes as medication use for glycemic control, HbA1c > 6.5, or presence of ≥ 2 random glucose levels above 200 mg/dL [18]. Age, BMI (kg/m^2), and creatinine were recorded at the patient's final clinic visit. Renal function was determined by estimated glomerular filtration rate (eGFR) calculated using the CKD-EPI equation [19].

Blood pressure in all clinics was measured in accordance with the current recommendations of the American Heart Association [20]. In brief, blood pressures were obtained by licensed staff using calibrated automated manometers with subjects in a chair at rest, arm supported at heart level. The 3 most recent blood pressure measurements were used for analysis (the mean number of measurements was 2.6, 2.4, and 2.9 for University of California San Diego, Tulane University, and Los Angeles Orthopaedic Hospital, resp.).

PWH were divided into two groups: treated (those taking antihypertensive medications, $n = 118$) and untreated (those not taking such medications, $n = 342$).

2.2. Control Population. We compared the PWH to males drawn from the adult population of the United States during National Health and Nutrition Examination Surveys (NHANES). This is a series of surveys to evaluate the health status of the nation [21]. The data are freely available to the public (http://www.cdc.gov/nchs/nhanes/index.htm). Three cycles of NHANES (2007-2008, 2009-2010, and 2011-2012) were combined to give a large sample.

The age distribution of patients suffering from severe hemophilia is underrepresented in the older ages, and blood pressure varies with age as well as by race [16]. Therefore, in order to ensure comparable age distributions, we randomly selected untreated NHANES subjects to match untreated PWH by race (Hispanic, white, black, and other) and age-class (18–29, 30–39, 40–49, 50–59, 60–69, and 70–79 years) in the ratio of 5 NHANES subjects to each PWH. Similarly, for treated PWH we selected a comparison group of treated NHANES subjects in the same manner. Because there were few NHANES subjects under 40 being treated for hypertension, the actual ratio for treated subjects was 4.6 NHANES to each PWH.

2.3. Statistical Methods. The values of SBP, DBP, and continuous covariates were shown as medians and interquartile ranges because most were not normally distributed. Their values were compared by Wilcoxon tests. Categorical variables were compared by χ^2 tests.

We used analysis of covariance to test the proposition that the difference between the BP of PWH and NHANES subjects was due to one of the risk factors [22]. The outcome variables were log SBP and DBP. We used log SBP because it gave normally distributed residuals while SBP resulted in skewed residuals.

A binary variable Z distinguished NHANES subjects [$Z = 0$] and PWH [$Z = 1$]. The covariates were BMI, creatinine, glomerular filtration rate (eGFR), total cholesterol, diabetes (yes/no), HCV (yes/no), HIV (yes/no), smoking (never/former/current), and race (Hispanic, white, black, and other). HIV was dropped because too few NHANES subjects were positive. BMI and total cholesterol were transformed to logs and creatinine to log (1 + creatinine).

The BP analyses were run separately for young adults (18–29 years) and older adults (30–79 years) because exploratory analyses had shown differences between them in the associations with some covariates.

For each covariate X the regression model was log SBP on X, Z, age, and the interaction $X * Z$. When DBP was the outcome we used the quadratic form of age [23] with centered age, *Cage*, to avoid multicollinearity [22]. Thus the regression model was DBP on X, Z, *Cage*, *Cage*^{2}, and $X * Z$. If $P < 0.10$ for $X * Z$ interaction then an analysis of covariance was not possible because the slopes for NHANES subjects and PWH were not parallel [22]. If $P > 0.10$ for that interaction then the slopes were assumed to be equal and an analysis of covariance tested the hypothesis that the mean of the outcome, after adjustment for X and age, did not differ between PWH and NHANES subjects. That is, if the regression coefficient for Z differed from zero then we can assume that this particular risk factor could not account for the difference in BP between PWH and NHANES subjects. On the other hand, if the regression coefficient did not differ from zero then the higher BP value for PWH may be due to that particular risk factor.

Finally, having tested each covariate individually, we ran a full model with all covariates to test the proposition that these risk factors in combination explain the difference between PWH and NHANES subjects. Again, all interactions between Z and each covariate were tested. If it appeared that a particular covariate X caused the difference between PWH and NHANES subjects to disappear, then we also ran the full model without X in order to observe the effect of all risk factors with and without X.

3. Results

3.1. Demographics. There were 469 PWH of whom four-fifths had hemophilia A and 56% suffered from the severe form (see Table 1). About half were white and a quarter Hispanic.

Table 1: Demographics for the patients with hemophilia ($n = 469$).

		Frequency	
		n	%
Race	White	249	53.1
	Black	53	11.3
	Hispanic	115	24.5
	Other	52	11.1
Hemophilia type	A	371	79.1
	B	97	20.7
	Unknown	1	0.2
Hemophilia severity	Severe	263	56.1
	Moderate	65	13.9
	Mild	139	29.6
	Unknown	2	0.4
Inhibitor	Positive	28	6.0
	Negative	402	85.7
	Not tested	39	8.3

3.2. Blood Pressures and Cardiovascular Risk Factors. Both SBP and DBP values were significantly higher among PWH compared to NHANES subjects, whether subjects were taking antihypertensives or not. In PWH not taking antihypertensives median SBP and DBP were 125 and 78 mmHg (118 and 72 mmHg in NHANES) (Table 2), and in PWH taking antihypertensives SBP and DBP were 134 and 84 (127 and 76 mmHg in NHANES), respectively (Table 3); all $P < 0.001$. While PWH and NHANES subjects showed similar trends in BP by age, PWH had higher median BP values and 10th percentiles (Figures 1 and 2). The difference in 10th percentiles was particularly marked for DBP among treated PWH.

Despite their higher BP levels, PWH had better risk profiles, with lower BMI and total cholesterol and better renal function as reflected by creatinine and eGFR levels (Tables 2 and 3). Fewer PWH had ever smoked, and there were fewer diabetics among the PWH. On the other hand, as a consequence of virally contaminated blood products in earlier years, the prevalence of HCV and HIV was much higher.

In the regression models with adjustment only for age, log SBP and DBP remained higher among PWH than NHANES subjects, whether they were treated or untreated (Tables 4–7). When adjusting for age, BMI, renal function, cholesterol, smoking, diabetes, HCV, or race, only HCV emerged as a potential explanation for the higher BP values among PWH and then only for untreated subjects over 30 (Tables 4 and 6). The difference in BP between PWH and NHANES subjects was especially marked among the younger adults (Tables 4 and 6).

3.2.1. SBP for Untreated Subjects. The comparison between SBP curves for PWH and NHANES subjects illustrated that the difference between curves is much greater for young adults (18–29 years) compared to older adults (≥30 years) (Figure 3).

For young adults, after adjusting for age and each covariate alone (BMI, renal function, cholesterol, smoking, diabetes, HCV, and race) and then for all covariates together, the difference in SBP between PWH and NHANES subjects remained (Table 4). Similarly, the difference in SBP between PWH and NHANES subjects remained for subjects ≥ 30 years after adjusting for each of age, BMI, creatinine, eGFR, cholesterol, smoking, or race (Figure 3 and Table 4). However, in contrast to the young adults, the difference disappeared when the model was adjusted for HCV. When all covariates together were in the full model there was no difference between PWH and NHANES. When HCV was removed from the full model the difference reappeared, indicating that among the tested risk factors it was only HCV that might explain the difference in systolic BP among older adults not taking antihypertensives.

3.2.2. SBP for Treated Subjects. There were too few subjects in the young age group taking antihypertensive medications ($n = 5$ PWH) to justify analysis. For older adults taking antihypertensives the difference in SBP between PWH and NHANES subjects persisted after adjusting for each covariate alone and with all covariates together (Figure 4 and Table 5).

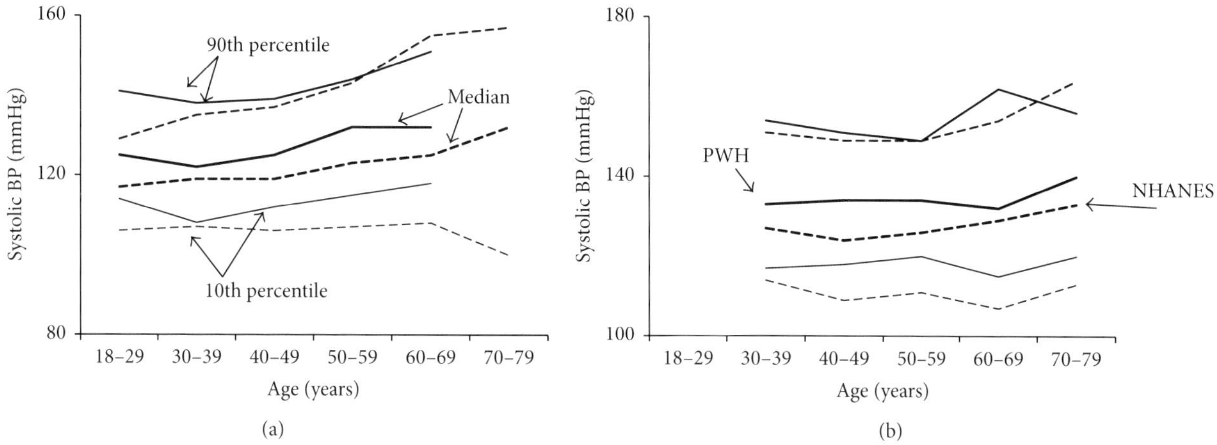

Figure 1: Systolic blood pressure as a function of age. Systolic blood pressure was higher among patients with hemophilia (PWH) compared to men of the general United States population (NHANES) at all ages, whether or not the subjects were taking antihypertensive medications. PWH are shown by solid lines and NHANES subjects by broken lines. Tenth percentiles, medians, and 90th percentiles are shown. The lower percentile lines show the 10th, while the upper percentile lines show the 90th. (a) Systolic blood pressure for untreated subjects. (b) Systolic blood pressure for treated subjects (taking antihypertensive medications).

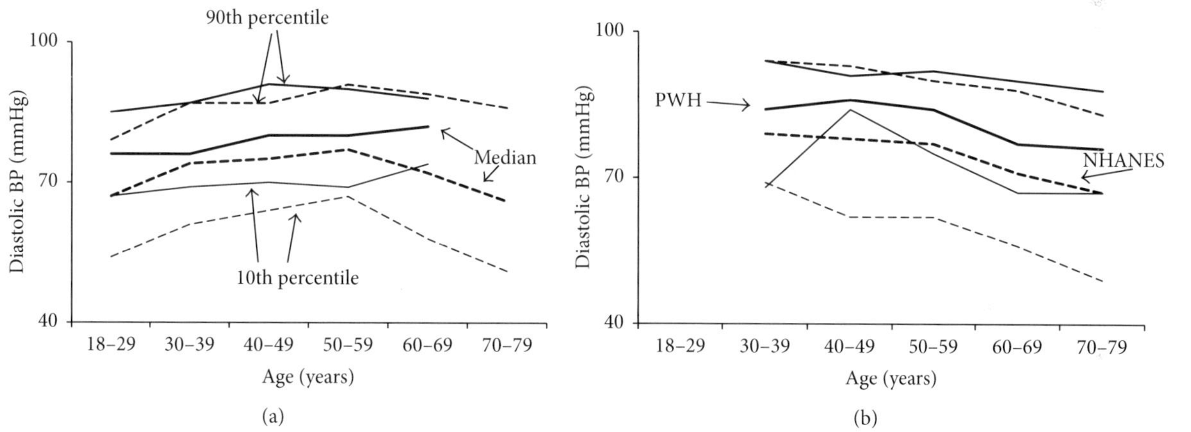

Figure 2: Diastolic blood pressure as a function of age. Diastolic blood pressure was higher among patients with hemophilia (PWH) compared to men of the general United States population (NHANES) at all ages, whether or not the subjects were taking antihypertensive medications. PWH are shown by solid lines and NHANES subjects by broken lines. Tenth percentiles, medians, and 90th percentiles are shown. The lower percentile lines show the 10th, while the upper percentile lines show the 90th. (a) Diastolic blood pressure for untreated subjects. (b) Diastolic blood pressure for treated subjects (taking antihypertensive medications).

3.2.3. DBP for Untreated Subjects. After adjusting for age and each covariate alone and then for all covariates together, the difference between PWH and NHANES remained for young adults (18–29 years) (Figure 5 and Table 6). Also, the difference between PWH and NHANES remained for subjects ≥ 30 years after adjusting for age, BMI, creatinine, eGFR, cholesterol, or smoking. However, as seen above with SBP, adjusting for HCV reduced the difference for subjects ≥ 30 years (Table 6). The interaction between Z (the binary variable that distinguished NHANES subjects from PWH) and race shows that the difference in DBP between PWH and NHANES subjects also depended upon race: the largest differences were among whites whereas black, Hispanic, and "other" did not show differences between PWH and NHANES (Table 8). When all covariates were included (the full model) the differences between PWH and NHANES for blacks, Hispanics, and "other" disappeared, but not for whites. The differences between PWH and NHANES reappeared when HCV was removed from that model (Table 9), indicating that among the tested risk factors it was only HCV that might explain the difference in diastolic BP among older adults not taking antihypertensives.

3.2.4. DBP for Treated Subjects. There were too few subjects in the young age group taking antihypertensive medications (n = 5 PWH) to justify analysis. For subjects ≥ 30 years, the difference between PWH and NHANES subjects persisted after adjusting for each covariate alone (Figure 6 and Table 7) and with all covariates together.

Table 2: Comparison of untreated (not taking antihypertensive medications) PWH and NHANES subjects.

(a)

Variable	NHANES Median (IQR)	n	PWH Median (IQR)	n	P
Systolic BP (mmHg)	118 (112–125)	1710	125 (118–134)	342	<0.001
Diastolic BP (mmHg)	72 (64–78)	1710	78 (73–83)	342	<0.001
BMI (kg/m^2)	26.9 (23.7–30.5)	1703	26.1 (22.9–29.3)	323	0.016
Creatinine (mg/dL)	0.92 (0.82–1.02)	1613	0.90 (0.75–1.00)	326	<0.001
eGFR (mL/min/1.73 m^2)	107 (94–119)	1613	112 (100–124)	326	<0.001
Cholesterol (total) (mg/dL)	188 (162–217)	1618	170 (146–196)	205	<0.001

(b)

Variable		NHANES n (%)	PWH n (%)	P
HIV	Positive	7 (0.5)	66 (20.5)	<0.001
	Negative	1464 (99.5)	256 (79.5)	
HCV	Positive	30 (1.9)	208 (63.8)	<0.001
	Negative	1590 (98.2)	118 (36.2)	
Diabetes	Positive	100 (5.9)	5 (1.5)	0.001
	Negative	1610 (94.2)	336 (98.5)	
Smoking	Current	473 (30.8)	42 (18.1)	<0.001
	Former	300 (19.5)	37 (16.0)	
	Never	765 (49.7)	153 (66.0)	

NHANES indicates subjects from the National Health and Nutrition Examination Survey of the general United States population; PWH, patients with hemophilia; IQR, interquartile range; BP, blood pressure; BMI, body mass index; eGFR, estimated glomerular filtration rate; and HCV, hepatitis C virus.

Table 3: Comparison of treated (taking antihypertensive medications) PWH and NHANES subjects.

(a)

Variable	NHANES Median (IQR)	n	PWH Median (IQR)	n	P
Systolic BP (mmHg)	127 (119–140)	539	134 (126–141)	118	<0.001
Diastolic BP (mmHg)	76 (67–83)	539	84 (76–89)	118	<0.001
BMI (kg/m^2)	30.6 (27.3–35.0)	534	27.7 (24.8–31.0)	115	<0.001
Creatinine (mg/dL)	0.99 (0.86–1.12)	508	0.90 (0.80–1.10)	116	0.007
eGFR (mL/min/1.73 m^2)	89 (73–101)	508	98 (74–108)	116	0.005
Cholesterol (total) (mg/dL)	186 (160–214)	509	164 (137–193)	85	<0.001

(b)

Variable		NHANES n (%)	PWH n (%)	P
HIV	Positive	2 (0.7)	33 (29.5)	<0.001
	Negative	281 (99.3)	79 (70.5)	
HCV	Positive	17 (13.4)	91 (81.3)	<0.001
	Negative	491 (96.7)	21 (18.8)	
Diabetes	Positive	178 (33.0)	31 (26.3)	0.188
	Negative	361 (67.0)	87 (73.7)	
Smoking	Current	109 (20.2)	16 (18.6)	0.166
	Former	192 (35.6)	23 (26.7)	
	Never	238 (44.2)	47 (54.7)	

NHANES indicates subjects from the National Health and Nutrition Examination Survey of the general United States population; PWH, patients with hemophilia; IQR, interquartile range; BP, blood pressure; BMI, body mass index; eGFR, estimated glomerular filtration rate; and HCV, hepatitis C virus.

4. Discussion

4.1. Blood Pressure Trends. Here we report the results of a large cohort study showing that the usual cardiovascular risk factors do not account for the higher blood pressure readings in hemophilia patients. We examined BP measurements while adjusting for age because the causes of hypertension are more likely to be revealed by examining its components—the two BP variables—than by examining hypertension itself. Furthermore, using continuous variables as outcomes is more likely to bring relationships with risk factors to light than if we were to use a binary outcome like hypertension [17].

This is the first study to examine systolic and diastolic measurements for PWH in separate treated (for antihypertensive medications) and untreated categories. PWH showed higher systolic and diastolic measurements than the general male population no matter which risk factor was included in the model.

Blood pressure measurements were higher for PWH even for subjects treated with antihypertensives. These observations imply that PWH are less responsive to such drugs, assuming comparable adherence to medications in both groups. However, since the treatment variable for PWH was based on charted use of medication, some patients may not have used the drugs as prescribed, while NHANES was self-reported drug use.

Although the 90th percentiles for PWH were similar to those for NHANES subjects, their 10th percentiles were higher. This indicates that the frequency distribution of BP covers a narrower range for PWH, with similar maxima but fewer low values. Among PWH the BP did not fall as much in diastole as among NHANES subjects, suggesting greater stiffness of the vascular walls. This phenomenon was particularly noticeable in treated subjects. These observations are new and are consistent with previous observations describing

TABLE 4: Analyses of covariance comparing log SBP values of untreated (not taking antihypertensive medications) PWH and NHANES subjects after adjusting for age and each covariate.

Covariate	Regression coefficient for Z (PWH versus NHANES)			r^2
	b	95% CI	P	
Young adults (18–29 years)				
No covariates (age + Z only)	0.069	0.050, 0.088	<0.001	0.085
log BMI	0.073	0.058, 0.088	<0.001	0.177
log (1 + Creatinine)	0.068	0.052, 0.084	<0.001	0.110
eGFR	0.068	0.052, 0.084	<0.001	0.110
log TotalCholesterol	0.079	0.060, 0.098	<0.001	0.094
Smoking status	0.071	0.052, 0.089	<0.001	0.087
HCV	0.066	0.048, 0.085	<0.001	0.104
Race	0.068	0.053, 0.083	<0.001	0.101
All covariates*	0.081	0.057, 0.105	<0.001	0.159
Older adults (30–79 years)				
No covariates (age + Z only)	0.031	0.013, 0.049	<0.001	0.041
log BMI	0.046	0.030, 0.061	<0.001	0.087
log (1 + Creatinine)	0.038	0.022, 0.054	<0.001	0.052
eGFR	0.037	0.020, 0.053	<0.001	0.052
log TotalCholesterol	0.036	0.017, 0.056	<0.001	0.060
Smoking status	0.035	0.017, 0.052	<0.001	0.043
HCV	0.012	−0.015, 0.039	0.384	0.051
Race	0.038	0.022, 0.053	<0.001	0.055
All covariates*	0.005	−0.027, 0.036	0.769	0.121
All covariates except HCV	0.049	0.029, 0.069	<0.001	0.111

Z indicates the binary variable that distinguishes PWH from NHANES ($Z = 1$ for PWH, $Z = 0$ for NHANES); PWH, patients with hemophilia; NHANES, subjects from the National Health and Nutrition Examination Survey of the general United States population; b, regression coefficient for Z representing change in log SBP per unit increase of the selected covariate; CI, confidence interval; r^2, square of the multiple correlation coefficient; BMI, body mass index; eGFR, estimated glomerular filtration rate; HCV, hepatitis C virus.

*Age, log BMI, eGFR, log TotalCholesterol, smoking status, HCV, and race.

TABLE 5: Analyses of covariance comparing log SBP values of treated (taking antihypertensive medications) PWH and NHANES subjects after adjusting for age and each covariate.

Covariate	Regression coefficient for Z (PWH versus NHANES)			r^2
	b	95% CI	P	
Older adults (30–79 years)				
No covariates (age + Z only)	0.047	0.017, 0.078	0.003	0.020
log BMI	0.038	0.011, 0.065	0.006	0.022
log (1 + Creatinine)	0.045	0.019, 0.072	<0.001	0.025
eGFR	0.044	0.018, 0.070	0.001	0.023
log TotalCholesterol	0.064	0.033, 0.095	<0.001	0.050
Diabetes	0.042	0.016, 0.068	0.001	0.024
Smoking status	0.042	0.012, 0.072	0.006	0.027
HCV	0.046	0.002, 0.090	0.039	0.023
Race	0.041	0.015, 0.066	0.002	0.041
All covariates*	0.053	0.001, 0.104	0.045	0.087

Z indicates the binary variable that distinguishes PWH from NHANES ($Z = 1$ for PWH, $Z = 0$ for NHANES); PWH, patients with hemophilia; NHANES, subjects from the National Health and Nutrition Examination Survey of the general United States population; b, regression coefficient for Z representing change in log SBP per unit increase of the selected covariate; CI, confidence interval; r^2, square of the multiple correlation coefficient; BMI, body mass index; eGFR, estimated glomerular filtration rate; HCV, hepatitis C virus.

*Age, log BMI, eGFR, log TotalCholesterol, diabetes, smoking status, HCV, and race.

TABLE 6: Analyses of covariance comparing DBP values of untreated (not taking antihypertensive medications) PWH and NHANES subjects after adjusting for age and each covariate.

Covariate	Regression coefficient for Z (PWH versus NHANES)			r^2
	b	95% CI	P	
Young adults (18–29 years)				
No covariates ($Cage + Cage^2 + Z$ only)	9.03	6.80, 11.25	<0.001	0.113
log BMI	8.59	6.80, 10.38	<0.001	0.167
log (1 + Creatinine)	8.91	7.06, 10.76	<0.001	0.159
eGFR	8.92	7.08, 10.77	<0.001	0.159
log TotalCholesterol	8.97	6.66, 11.28	<0.001	0.123
Smoking status	8.28	6.13, 10.43	<0.001	0.121
HCV	8.18	6.01, 10.35	<0.001	0.156
Race	8.52	6.77, 10.27	<0.001	0.162
All covariates*	10.38	7.43, 13.33	<0.001	0.163
Older adults (30–79 years)				
No covariates ($Cage + Cage^2 + Z$ only)	2.99	1.21, 4.77	0.001	0.035
log BMI	4.54	3.04, 6.03	<0.001	0.083
log (1 + Creatinine)	4.18	2.62, 5.73	<0.001	0.049
eGFR	4.10	2.54, 5.65	<0.001	0.047
log TotalCholesterol	4.03	2.14, 5.91	<0.001	0.050
Smoking status	3.15	1.43, 4.87	<0.001	0.039
HCV	2.45	−0.14, 5.04	0.064	0.045
Race	†			0.062
All covariates*	†			0.121
All covariates except HCV*	†			0.116

Z indicates the binary variable that distinguishes PWH from NHANES ($Z = 1$ for PWH, $Z = 0$ for NHANES); PWH, patients with hemophilia; NHANES, subjects from the National Health and Nutrition Examination Survey of the general United States population; b, regression coefficient for Z representing change in log SBP per unit increase of the selected covariate; CI, confidence interval; r^2, square of the multiple correlation coefficient; BMI, body mass index; eGFR, estimated glomerular filtration rate; HCV, hepatitis C virus.

*$Cage$, $Cage^2$, log BMI, eGFR, log TotalCholesterol, smoking status, HCV, and race.

†$Z*$race interaction was significant and therefore ANCOVA cannot be performed.

TABLE 7: Analyses of covariance comparing DBP values of treated (taking antihypertensive medications) PWH and NHANES subjects after adjusting for age and each covariate.

Covariate	Regression coefficient for Z (PWH versus NHANES)			r^2
	b	95% CI	P	
Older adults (30–79 years)				
No covariates ($Cage + Cage^2 + Z$ only)	6.40	3.75, 9.05	<0.001	0.165
log BMI	6.13	3.79, 8.47	<0.001	0.175
log (1 + Creatinine)	6.92	4.62, 9.21	<0.001	0.168
eGFR	6.73	4.45, 9.00	<0.001	0.172
log TotalCholesterol	8.53	5.97, 11.10	<0.001	0.224
Diabetes	6.60	4.34, 8.85	<0.001	0.179
Smoking status	6.57	3.95, 9.19	<0.001	0.164
HCV	6.97	3.13, 18.81	<0.001	0.170
Race	6.68	4.42, 8.95	<0.001	0.175
All covariates*	6.68	2.26, 11.10	0.003	0.239

Z indicates the binary variable that distinguishes PWH from NHANES ($Z = 1$ for PWH, $Z = 0$ for NHANES); PWH, patients with hemophilia; NHANES, subjects from the National Health and Nutrition Examination Survey of the general United States population; b, regression coefficient for Z representing change in log SBP per unit increase of the selected covariate; CI, confidence interval; r^2, square of the multiple correlation coefficient; BMI, body mass index; eGFR, estimated glomerular filtration rate; HCV, hepatitis C virus.

*$Cage$, $Cage^2$, log BMI, eGFR, log TotalCholesterol, diabetes, smoking status, HCV, and race.

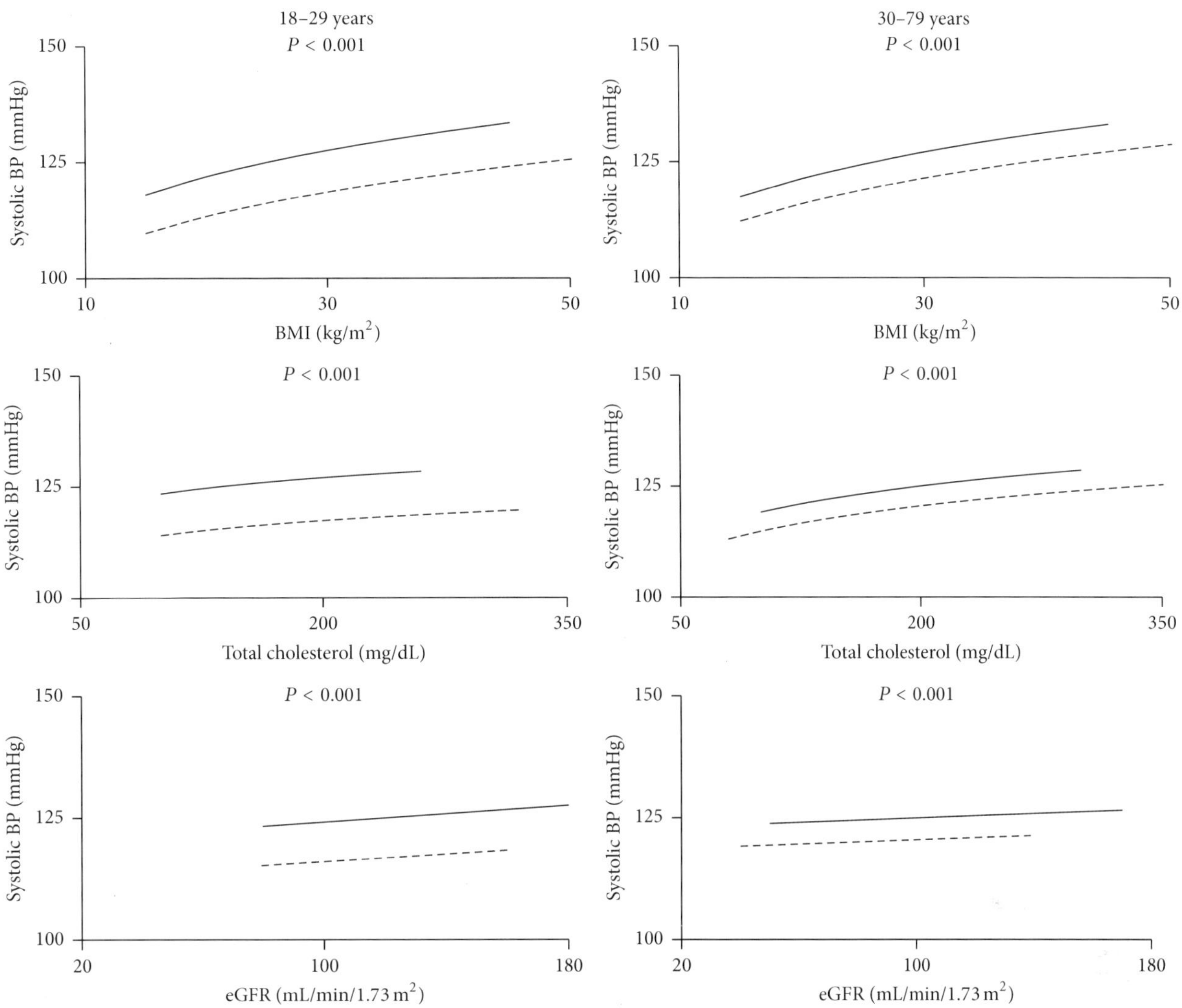

FIGURE 3: Systolic blood pressure for untreated subjects as a function of BMI, cholesterol, and estimated glomerular filtration rate (eGFR). The solid lines are the regression lines for PWH while the broken lines are for NHANES subjects. The P value for the difference between PWH and NHANES is shown.

impaired flow-mediated vessel dilation and decreased vascular endothelial function among PWH [24]. Thus PWH may suffer from systemic vascular changes that require further investigation. Towards that end, vascular remodeling in joints with evidence for systemic mediation was recently described as a unique feature of hemophilia [25], indicating vascular abnormalities of uncertain etiology that may be linked to the hypertension in PWH.

An unexpected finding was the marked elevated BP of the youngest age group, which is an alarming and worrisome finding, warranting future investigations in youth and children with hemophilia. With the exception of results from a small cohort study in the 1980s that found increased BP values in PWH [5], contemporary information regarding BP trends in PWH on a larger scale does not yet exist. Consequently, results from this study contribute important new information.

4.2. Risk Factors for Elevated Blood Pressures. Next, we examined whether one or more cardiovascular risk factors could explain the higher BP in PWH. First, one would expect to find at least one of the risk factors for high BP to be elevated in PWH. However, the converse was the case: PWH weighed less and had lower serum cholesterol, their serum creatinine levels and eGFR levels showed better kidney function, and they had lower rates of diabetes and smoking. Others have also found PWH to have better weight and cholesterol profiles [5, 26, 27], although one large study of PWH also noted that their diabetes and smoking rates were similar to the general population [26].

Second, BP levels were positively associated with cardiovascular risk factors such as age, BMI, and cholesterol, as would be expected. However the BP curves for PWH and NHANES subjects rose in parallel, and for all risk factors the BP curve for PWH was always above that for NHANES

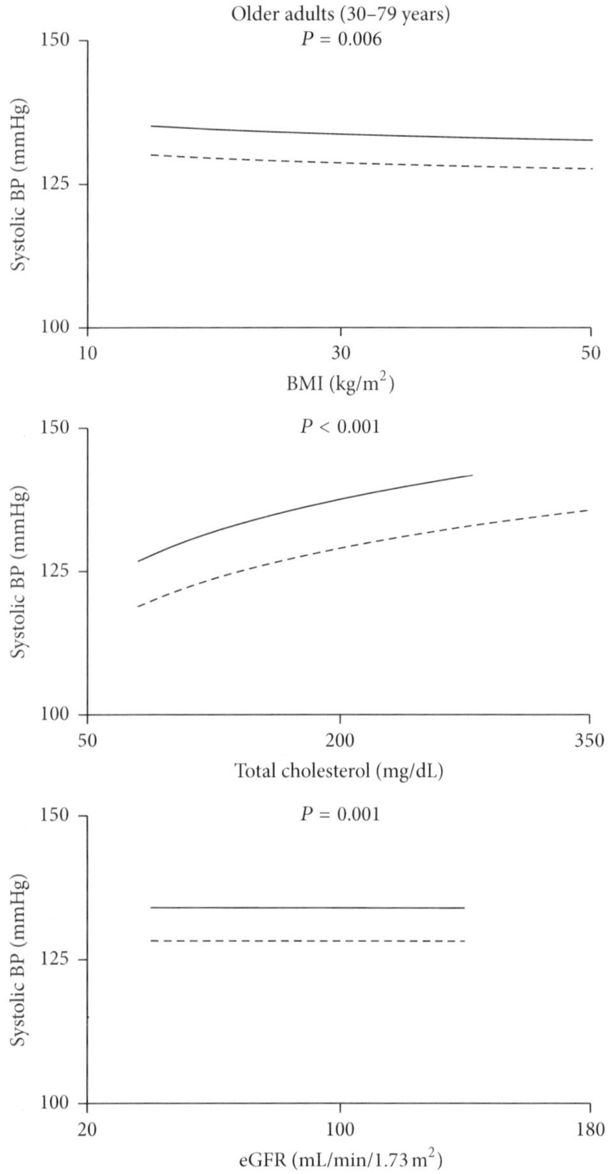

Figure 4: Systolic blood pressure for subjects treated with antihypertensive medications as a function of BMI, cholesterol, and estimated glomerular filtration rate (eGFR). The solid lines are the regression lines for PWH while the broken lines are for NHANES subjects. The P value for the difference between PWH and NHANES is shown.

Table 8: Estimated differences in diastolic BP between PWH and NHANES subjects by race for those models that had a significant interaction $Z*$race; older subjects (30–79 years) not taking antihypertensive medications.

Outcome	Variables in model	Race	Difference between PWH and NHANES (mmHg)	95% CI
DBP	Z, $Cage$, $Cage^2$, race, $Z*$race	White	5.88	3.39, 7.88
		Black	3.04	−2.95, 9.02
		Hispanic	1.76	−2.57, 6.08
		Other	0.80	−4.95, 6.54
DBP	Z, $Cage$, $Cage^2$, log BMI, eGFR, log TotalCholesterol, smoking status, HCV, race, $Z*$race	White	4.98	1.13, 8.84
		Black	0.17	−8.55, 8.88
		Hispanic	−0.31	−6.25, 5.63
		Other	0.58	−6.91, 8.07
DBP	Z, $Cage$, $Cage^2$, log BMI, eGFR, log TotalCholesterol, smoking status, race, $Z*$race	White	8.43	5.64, 11.22
		Black	3.34	−4.98, 11.66
		Hispanic	1.97	−3.32, 7.26
		Other	3.17	−3.82, 10.17

Z is the binary variable that distinguishes PWH from NHANES ($Z = 1$ for PWH, $Z = 0$ for NHANES); CI indicates confidence interval; $Cage$, centered age; BMI, body mass index; eGFR, estimated glomerular filtration rate; HCV, hepatitis C virus.

Table 9: Comparison of the effect of Z and HCV on blood pressure models after adjusting for all other covariates.

Outcome	Age-class	Treated?	P for Z	P for HCV
log SBP	18–29	No	<0.001	0.452
log SBP	30–79	No	0.769	<0.001
log SBP	30–79	Yes	0.045	0.668
DBP	18–29	No	<0.001	0.327
DBP	30–79	No	0.905	0.010
DBP	30–79	Yes	0.003	0.466

Z is the binary variable that distinguishes PWH from NHANES ($Z = 1$ for PWH, $Z = 0$ for NHANES); HCV, hepatitis C virus.

subjects. Higher BP among PWH cannot be explained by a steeper slope than for NHANES. Therefore, none of the usual cardiovascular risk factors could explain the higher BP in PWH.

Hypertension is well known to be one of the many consequences of HCV infection that include hyperglycemia, insulin resistance, diabetes mellitus, left ventricular mass index, disturbed lipid metabolism, endothelial dysfunction, inflammation, and vessel damage as well as greater vascular stiffness [28–33]. It is therefore not surprising that HCV appeared to contribute to some extent to higher BP. Interestingly, HCV only explained the higher BP in untreated PWH over 30 years. Subjects in this category infected with HCV had higher BP values than uninfected individuals after adjusting for other covariates. However, HCV did not explain higher BP among treated PWH where HCV prevalence was high (82.2% in PWH compared to 3.4% in NHANES subjects) or in young patients, where HCV prevalence was lower (36.4% in PWH compared to 0.5% in NHANES subjects). Thus, for PWH the

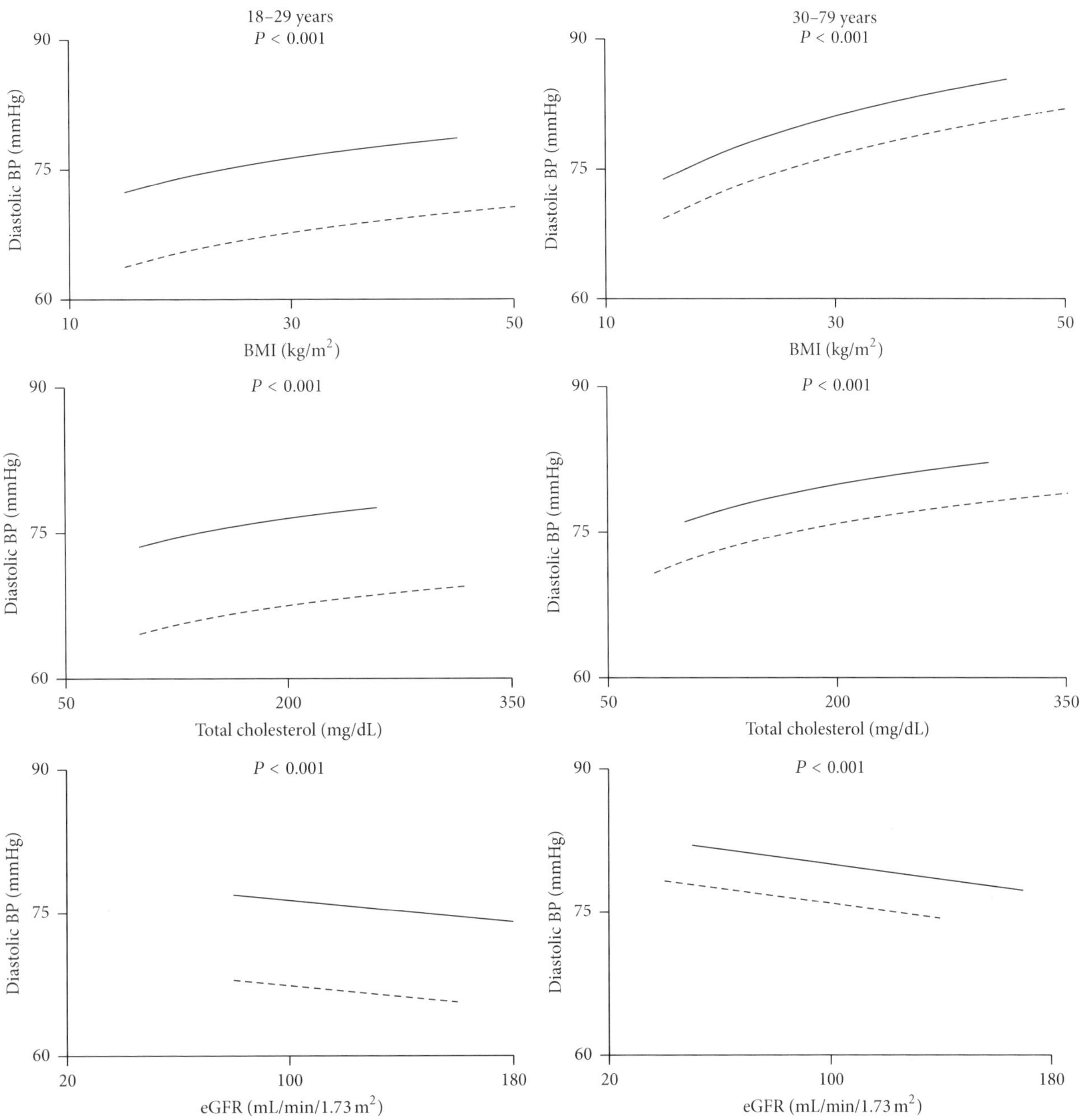

FIGURE 5: Diastolic blood pressure for untreated subjects as a function of BMI, cholesterol, and estimated glomerular filtration rate (eGFR). The solid lines are the regression lines for PWH while the broken lines are for NHANES subjects. The P value for the difference between PWH and NHANES is shown.

associations between BP and HCV varied with both age and treatment status and possibly with race. While HCV infection may contribute to higher BP in PWH, it does not fully explain the differences between PWH and NHANES.

The association between hypertension and insulin resistance (IR) remains obscure [34, 35]. Possibly a third factor may promote both IR and hypertension; for example, catecholamines are implicated in both carbohydrate metabolism and vascular resistance [35–37]. We could not examine the association between the homeostatic model assessment (HOMA) index, which is a measure of IR, and blood pressure because insulin concentrations were not measured in our cohort of PWH. However, the lower prevalence of diabetes among PWH suggests that IR may be less common compared to NHANES. Nevertheless, IR and its association with HCV should be examined in future studies of hypertension in PWH.

There is a long-standing debate whether PWH have poor renal function, possibly linked to renal bleeding [38–40]. We specifically examined this topic since hypertension is associated with poorer renal function in the general population [16]. As previously observed [7], PWH had superior

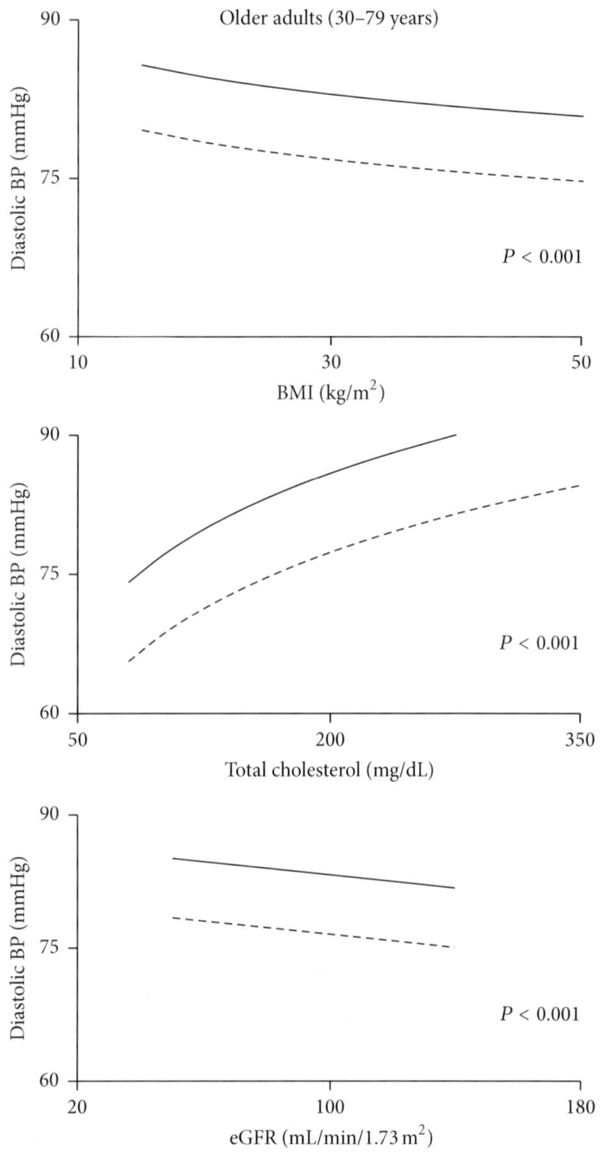

Figure 6: Diastolic blood pressure for subjects treated with antihypertensive medications as a function of BMI, cholesterol, and estimated glomerular filtration rate (eGFR). The solid lines are the regression lines for PWH while the broken lines are for NHANES subjects. The P value for the difference between PWH and NHANES is shown.

renal function despite having higher BP. This reinforces the argument that elevated BP levels in hemophilia are largely independent of the usual cardiovascular risk factors. However, since some studies have not found associations between hypertension and renal function in PWH [5, 6, 15], the questions concerning renal function, renal bleeding, and hypertension in hemophilia remain unresolved.

This study, like several others [4–6], was limited by the small number of patients because hemophilia is a rare disease. However, it contributes significantly to the accumulating evidence that the hypertension of hemophilia is an important comorbidity. Also, several other limitations have to be mentioned. First, BP measurements for NHANES subjects were taken on one day while PWH had frequent follow-up [26]. On the other hand, NHANES subjects with their single measurements outnumbered PWH by 5 : 1 and the large differences between PWH and NHANES subjects at all ages are strong evidence for higher values in hemophilia. Second, BP measurements were made by a large number of different people using a variety of equipment. It is unlikely that one group (PWH or NHANES) would have a systematic bias in one direction. But the variation in measurements is greater than if each group were measured by one provider using a single instrument, and that would reduce the power of statistical tests. Third, our regression models accounted for only a small proportion of the variance in SBP and DBP: much of the variation in BP for both PWH and NHANES subjects remains unexplained. Fourth, while HCV may explain some of the difference, we must be cautious since few NHANES subjects were infected.

5. Conclusion

We examined systolic and diastolic blood pressure in subjects that were divided into those taking or not taking antihypertensive medications. This study demonstrates that PWH suffer from higher BP levels than the general male population at all ages whether or not they are treated for hypertension. Further, their elevated BP levels cannot be easily explained by the usual cardiovascular risk factors. From a pragmatic clinical standpoint these findings are important since care paradigms for PWH need to develop a stronger focus on BP control to avoid the risk of mortality from ICH [9–12]. These findings are also important from a basic scientific standpoint: the etiology of the "Hypertension of Hemophilia" remains largely unresolved. Abnormal vascular stiffness and vascular remodeling in joints have been described in hemophilia [24, 25] and may be mediated systemically and are possibly related to the hypertension. Also, higher systolic and diastolic values seen among PWH in their twenties highlight questions about age of onset and, again, underlying etiology. New studies will be required to unravel the interrelations of vascular abnormalities, BP, and age of onset of hypertension among PWH.

Competing Interests

Doris V. K. Quon is a member of speakers' bureaux for Baxalta, Biogen, CSL, Grifols, and Novo Nordisk and also participates in advisory boards for Baxalta, Bayer, Biogen, and Novo Nordisk. Rebecca Kruse-Jarres is a paid consultant and participates in advisory boards for Baxalta, Bayer, Grifols, Novo Nordisk, Pfizer, and Roche and also receives research funding from Baxalta, Pfizer, and Roche. Annette von Drygalski has received honoraria for participating in scientific advisory board panels and for consulting and speaking engagements for Baxalta, Bayer, Biogen, CSL-Behring, Novo Nordisk, Grifols, and Pfizer and is also a cofounder and member of the Board of Directors of Hematherix LLC., a biotech company that is developing ^{super}FVa therapy for bleeding complications. The remaining authors declare no competing financial interests.

Acknowledgments

This work was supported by funding from Biogen ("Prevalence and Etiology of Subclinical Joint Bleeding and Joint Microbleeding in Adults with Hemophilic Arthopathy") and from Baxalta ("Cardiovascular Health in Hemophilia"), by a Career Development Award from the National Hemophilia Foundation/Novo Nordisk (Annette von Drygalski) and a scholarship from King Fahad Specialist Hospital Dammam, Saudi Arabia (Afrah S. Sait).

References

[1] S. A. Larsson, "Life expectancy of Swedish haemophiliacs, 1831–1980," *British Journal of Haematology*, vol. 59, no. 4, pp. 593–602, 1985.

[2] S. C. Darby, W. K. Sau, R. J. Spooner et al., "Mortality rates, life expectancy, and causes of death in people with hemophilia A or B in the United Kingdom who were not infected with HIV," *Blood*, vol. 110, no. 3, pp. 815–825, 2007.

[3] T. L. Chorba, R. C. Holman, M. J. Clarke, and B. L. Evatt, "Effects of HIV infection on age and cause of death for persons with hemophilia A in the United States," *American Journal of Hematology*, vol. 66, no. 4, pp. 229–240, 2001.

[4] S. Biere-Rafi, M. A. Baarslag, M. Peters et al., "Cardiovascular risk assessment in haemophilia patients," *Thrombosis and Haemostasis*, vol. 105, no. 2, pp. 274–278, 2011.

[5] F. R. Rosendaal, E. Briet, J. Stibbe et al., "Haemophilia protects against ischaemic heart disease: a study of risk factors," *British Journal of Haematology*, vol. 75, no. 4, pp. 525–530, 1990.

[6] D. E. Fransen van de Putte, K. Fischer, M. Makris et al., "Increased prevalence of hypertension in haemophilia patients," *Thrombosis and Haemostasis*, vol. 108, no. 4, pp. 750–755, 2012.

[7] A. von Drygalski, N. A. Kolaitis, R. Bettencourt et al., "Prevalence and risk factors for hypertension in hemophilia," *Hypertension*, vol. 62, no. 1, pp. 209–215, 2013.

[8] A. S. Sait, A. Kuo, R. Bettencourt, J. Bergstrom, M. Allison, and A. von Drygalski, "Risk assessment for coronary heart disease in patients with haemophilia: a single centre study in the United States," *Haemophilia*, vol. 20, no. 6, pp. 763–770, 2014.

[9] R. C. R. Ljung, "Intracranial haemorrhage in haemophilia A and B," *British Journal of Haematology*, vol. 140, no. 4, pp. 378–384, 2008.

[10] R. Nuss, J. M. Soucie, and B. Evatt, "Changes in the occurrence of and risk factors for hemophilia-associated intracranial hemorrhage," *American Journal of Hematology*, vol. 68, no. 1, pp. 37–42, 2001.

[11] N. Stieltjes, T. Calvez, V. Demiguel et al., "Intracranial haemorrhages in French haemophilia patients (1991–2001): clinical presentation, management and prognosis factors for death," *Haemophilia*, vol. 11, no. 5, pp. 452–458, 2005.

[12] C. Witmer, R. Presley, R. Kulkarni, J. M. Soucie, C. S. Manno, and L. Raffini, "Associations between intracranial haemorrhage and prescribed prophylaxis in a large cohort of haemophilia patients in the United States," *British Journal of Haematology*, vol. 152, no. 2, pp. 211–216, 2011.

[13] S. V. Antunes, P. Vicari, S. Cavalheiro, and J. O. Bordin, "Intracranial haemorrhage among a population of haemophilic patients in Brazil," *Haemophilia*, vol. 9, no. 5, pp. 573–577, 2003.

[14] H. C. Kim, C. M. Nam, S. H. Jee, and I. Suh, "Comparison of blood pressure-associated risk of intracerebral hemorrhage and subarachnoid hemorrhage: Korea Medical Insurance Corporation study," *Hypertension*, vol. 46, no. 2, pp. 393–397, 2005.

[15] H. L. Sun, M. Yang, A. S. Sait, A. von Drygalski, and S. Jackson, "Haematuria is not a risk factor of hypertension or renal impairment in patients with haemophilia," *Haemophilia*, vol. 22, no. 4, pp. 549–555, 2016.

[16] D. Lloyd-Jones and D. Levy, "Epidemiology of hypertension," in *Hypertension: A Companion to Braunwald's Heart Disease*, H. R. Black and W. Elliott, Eds., Elsevier/Saunders, Philadelphia, Pa, USA, 2013.

[17] L. Friedman, C. Furberg, and D. DeMets, *Fundamentals of Clinical Trials*, Springer, New York, NY, USA, 1998.

[18] American Diabetes Association, "Standards of medical care in diabetes—2010," *Diabetes Care*, vol. 33, supplement 1, pp. S11–S61, 2010.

[19] A. S. Levey, J. P. Bosch, J. B. Lewis, T. Greene, N. Rogers, and D. Roth, "A more accurate method to estimate glomerular filtration rate from serum creatinine: a new prediction equation. Modification of Diet in Renal Disease Study Group," *Annals of Internal Medicine*, vol. 130, no. 6, pp. 461–470, 1999.

[20] T. G. Pickering, J. E. Hall, L. J. Appel et al., "Recommendations for blood pressure measurement in humans and experimental animals: part 1: blood pressure measurement in humans: a statement for professionals from the Subcommittee of Professional and Public Education of the American Heart Association Council on High Blood Pressure Research," *Circulation*, vol. 111, no. 5, pp. 697–716, 2005.

[21] NCHS, *National Health and Nutrition Examination Survey, 2013-2014: Overview*, National Center for Health Statistics, Center for Disease Control and Prevention, Hyattsville, Md, USA, 2015.

[22] D. Kleinbaum, L. Kupper, A. Nizam, and K. Muller, *Applied Regression Analysis and Other Multivariable Methods*, Thomson Brooks/Cole, Belmont, Calif, USA, 2008.

[23] S. S. Franklin, W. Gustin, N. D. Wong et al., "Hemodynamic patterns of age-related changes in blood pressure: the Framingham Heart Study," *Circulation*, vol. 96, no. 1, pp. 308–315, 1997.

[24] M. T. Sartori, F. Bilora, E. Zanon et al., "Endothelial dysfunction in haemophilia patients," *Haemophilia*, vol. 14, no. 5, pp. 1055–1062, 2008.

[25] V. Bhat, M. Olmer, S. Joshi et al., "Vascular remodeling underlies rebleeding in hemophilic arthropathy," *American Journal of Hematology*, vol. 90, no. 11, pp. 1027–1035, 2015.

[26] D. E. Fransen van de Putte, K. Fischer, M. Makris et al., "Unfavourable cardiovascular disease risk profiles in a cohort of Dutch and British haemophilia patients," *Thrombosis and Haemostasis*, vol. 109, no. 1, pp. 16–23, 2013.

[27] A. A. Sharathkumar, J. M. Soucie, B. Trawinski, A. Greist, and A. D. Shapiro, "Prevalence and risk factors of cardiovascular disease (CVD) events among patients with haemophilia: experience of a single haemophilia treatment centre in the United States (US)," *Haemophilia*, vol. 17, no. 4, pp. 597–604, 2011.

[28] Z. M. Younossi, M. Stepanova, F. Nader, Z. Younossi, and E. Elsheikh, "Associations of chronic hepatitis C with metabolic and cardiac outcomes," *Alimentary Pharmacology and Therapeutics*, vol. 37, no. 6, pp. 647–652, 2013.

[29] C. P. M. S. Oliveira, C. R. Kappel, E. R. Siqueira et al., "Effects of Hepatitis C virus on cardiovascular risk in infected patients: A Comparative Study," *International Journal of Cardiology*, vol. 164, no. 2, pp. 221–226, 2013.

[30] M. Perticone, S. Miceli, R. Maio et al., "Chronic HCV infection increases cardiac left ventricular mass index in normotensive patients," *Journal of Hepatology*, vol. 61, no. 4, pp. 755–760, 2014.

[31] M. Perticone, R. Maio, E. J. Tassone et al., "Insulin-resistance HCV infection-related affects vascular stiffness in normotensives," *Atherosclerosis*, vol. 238, no. 1, pp. 108–112, 2015.

[32] F. Negro, D. Forton, A. Craxì, M. S. Sulkowski, J. J. Feld, and M. P. Manns, "Extrahepatic morbidity and mortality of chronic hepatitis C," *Gastroenterology*, vol. 149, no. 6, pp. 1345–1360, 2015.

[33] V. Katsi, I. Felekos, S. Skevofilax et al., "Cardiovascular disease and hepatitis C virus infection: an irrelevant statement or a hot relationship?" *Cardiology in Review*, vol. 23, no. 1, pp. 11–17, 2015.

[34] M. Modan, H. Halkin, S. Almog et al., "Hyperinsulinemia. A link between hypertension obesity and glucose intolerance," *The Journal of Clinical Investigation*, vol. 75, no. 3, pp. 809–817, 1985.

[35] S. Addison, S. Stas, M. R. Hayden, and J. R. Sowers, "Insulin resistance and blood pressure," *Current Hypertension Reports*, vol. 10, no. 4, pp. 319–325, 2008.

[36] E. Ferrannini, G. Buzzigoli, R. Bonadonna et al., "Insulin resistance in essential hypertension," *Munchener Medizinische Wochenschrift*, vol. 130, no. 1-2, pp. 3–10, 1988.

[37] E. Ferrannini, "Insulin resistance and blood pressure," in *Insulin Resistance: The Metabolic Syndrome X*, G. M. Reaven and A. Law, Eds., pp. 281–308, Humana Press, Totowa, NJ, USA, 1999.

[38] M. Small, P. E. Rose, N. McMillan et al., "Haemophilia and the kidney: assessment after 11-year follow-up," *British Medical Journal*, vol. 285, no. 6355, pp. 1609–1611, 1982.

[39] R. Kulkarni, J. M. Soucie, B. Evatt et al., "Renal disease among males with haemophilia," *Haemophilia*, vol. 9, no. 6, pp. 703–710, 2003.

[40] A. A. Hamed, M. H. Shalaby, N. S. El-Kinawy, A. A. Elamawy, and S. M. Abd El-Ghany, "Renal abnormalities among Egyptian children with hemophilia a using renal scintigraphy: relation to risk factors and disease severity," *Clinical and Applied Thrombosis/Hemostasis*, 2015.

5

A Proposed Middle-Range Theory of Nursing in Hypertension Care

Eva Drevenhorn

Department of Health Sciences, Faculty of Medicine, Lund University, Lund, Sweden

Correspondence should be addressed to Eva Drevenhorn; eva.drevenhorn@med.lu.se

Academic Editor: Siew H. Gan

Nursing in hypertension care comprises counselling about lifestyle changes, blood pressure measurement, and being a translator for the physician. For the patient, changing lifestyle means performing self-care. As not much in the form of research and guidelines for nurses is available, a middle-range theory of nursing in hypertension care was developed to guide nurses in their practice, in order to improve the nursing of patients and design studies for investigating nursing in hypertension care. Concepts are presented related to the patient (attitude and beliefs regarding health and sickness, autonomy, personality and traits, level of perceived vulnerability, hardiness, sense of coherence, locus of control, self-efficacy, and access to social support and network) and the nursing (applying theories and models for behavioural change in the consultation and using counselling skills, patient advocacy, empowerment, professional knowledge and health education, and supporting the patient). Then the concepts related to the consultation (communication, shared decision-making, concordance, coping, adherence, and self-care) are integrated with Orem's theory of nursing. Clinical and research implications of the theory are discussed.

1. Introduction

Nursing in hypertension care has been shown to comprise counselling about lifestyle changes, blood pressure measurement, and being a translator for the physician [1]. A more detailed description of the nursing interventions is presented by Hong [2]. When a nurse is a member of a team with other healthcare professionals in the care of the hypertensive patient, a reduction in blood pressure is seen [1]. This is a result of changed lifestyle, more correct intake of medication, and more frequent returns for follow-up visits. In this context for the patient, changing lifestyle and taking medicines mean performing self-care.

Patients with hypertension during pregnancy or other severe diseases are usually taken care of within specialised care, but adult patients with hypertension are mostly managed in primary care. Preferably the care is team-based so that the patients are met in a congruent way. The team can include, besides the nurse and physician, a physiotherapist or other professionals. The members of the team have to be aware that not many patients can identify any specific symptoms that are obviously connected with hypertension [3]; elevated blood pressure is most often detected when a patient is treated for some other ailment. The finding might surprise the patients, and then being faced with demands to perform self-care to adjust some figures on paper might be perceived as a real challenge. The nurse who sees the patient at visits to the clinic in primary care is presumed to have a health-promotional, holistic, and psychosocial approach in helping the patients to achieve blood pressure control.

Although nurses all around the world are involved in treating hypertensive patients, not many theoretical guidelines for nurses are available. There are theories of self-care and self-management of chronic illness in general, but not for hypertension specifically. A literature search found a theoretical framework for studying medication compliance in Chinese immigrants [4]. Otherwise the only papers found, with theoretical aspects, were a study that aimed to determine the effectiveness of a nurse's caring relationship according to Watson's Caring Model of blood pressure and quality of life [5], one that evaluated Orem's nursing self-care theory in hypertensive women (in Portuguese) [6], and another

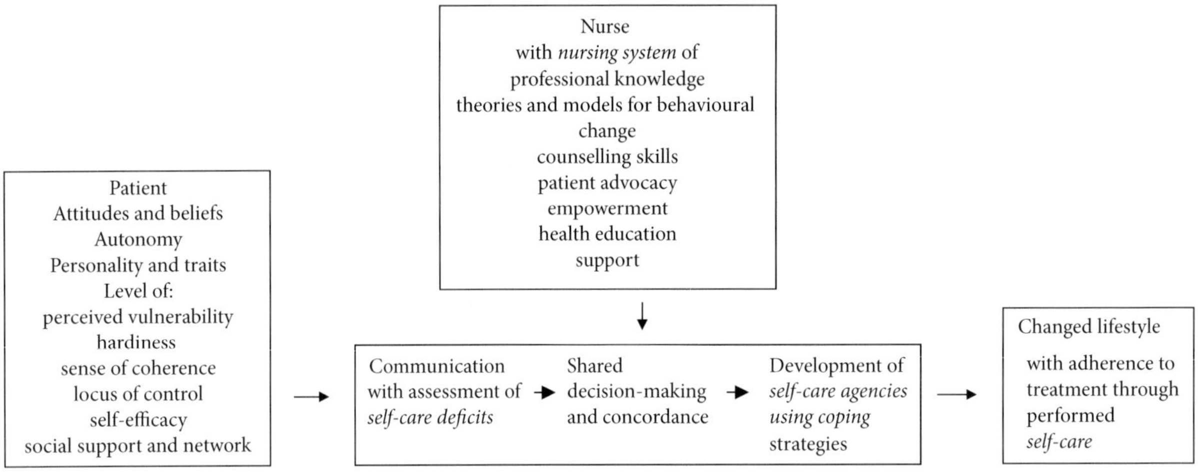

FIGURE 1: The constructed middle-range theory for nursing management of patients in hypertension care with the concepts involved in counselling about lifestyle changes and Orem's self-care deficit theory of nursing applied (shown in italics).

one that presented the middle-range theory of Attentively Embracing Story for practice implications with a client who had hypertension [7]. As these theoretical frameworks were not applied to embrace all aspects of nursing in hypertension care, a middle-range theory of nursing in hypertension care was judged to be needed to guide nurses in their practice, developing the nursing of patients and designing studies to investigate nursing in hypertension care. Former work in the development of the proposed theory has been presented [8, 9].

2. Methodology

A middle-range theory is to be developed inductively from research and practice [10] and can be combined with existing theories [11]. Theories deriving from other disciplines and practice research can also be integrated. With this background, a middle-range theory of nursing in hypertension care is proposed (Figure 1) with concepts related to the patient, nursing in hypertension care, the encounter between the patient and the nurse, the expected outcomes of this encounter, and the integration of an existing grand theory of nursing.

In the development process of the proposed theory, extensive literature search and review were conducted to find concepts that mirrored counselling on lifestyle change and taking medicines to help the patient to perform self-care. Measuring blood pressure was omitted as this is to be done in a standardised way, which is well defined in hypertension guidelines. As for nursing in general, pieces from other disciplines such as medicine, sociology, and psychology fit in well; the databases PubMed, Cinahl, PsycINFO, SocSci, and Eric were used in the literature search along with the Cochrane Library in 2001, 2005, and 2014 (Table 1). The great output from the initial searches in 2001 was diminished through a thorough review to grasp what might be relevant for nursing in hypertension care. To find any relevant paper which could give any new aspects to be taken into account when elucidating what might be of concern for the patient and nurse in hypertension care, a variety of keywords (both MeSH terms and free text keywords) were used: adaptation, attitude, communication, compliance, coping, counselling, educational models, emotions, empowerment, health behaviour, health education, health promotion, hypertension, lifestyle, motivation, nurse-patient relations, nursing, patient self-determination, self-care, self-efficacy, and social support. The words were used separately as well as combined in the same structured way in every database. The procedure was documented to make it possible to repeat or refine the literature search.

During the review reference lists were also used to find cited original literature. While reviewing the findings from papers, books, and dissertations, a drawing was made to get an overview of relationships between the concepts and the way or order they fit in. Gradually the proposed model was formed with the concepts relevant for the patient and nurse arranged to form the model (Figure 1). The background for choosing keywords consisted of studies on nursing in hypertension care for several years while obtaining bachelors', masters', and doctoral degrees. Moreover, personal experience as an advanced nurse in primary care running a nurse-led hypertension clinic was crucial. The theory was first presented as a part of the framework of the author's thesis and some years later it was decided to rewrite the framework into a paper to be diffused among colleagues for discussion and review. Some of the concepts included are well defined but others are less well developed and defined and also not used in research with patients with hypertension. The proposed theory is work in progress and further development is needed. The theory is presented on these assumptions.

3. Definitions of Concepts

In the paper research results from each concept are presented whenever any study with hypertensive patients involved has been found regardless of the study's age. First, concepts

Table 1: Searches made in the different data bases during the years. The searches in 2001 started from the year of the start of the respective database.

2001		2005		2014	
Database (covering years)	Number of relevant findings	Database (covering years)	Number of relevant new findings	Database (covering years)	Number of relevant new findings
PubMed (1966–2001)	520	PubMed (2002–2005)	15	PubMed (2006–2014)	4
Cinahl (1982–2001)	326	Cinahl (2002–2005)	11	Cinahl (2006–2014)	4
PsycINFO (1967–2001)	298	PsycINFO (2002–2005)	15	PsycINFO (2006–2014)	2
SocSci (1986–2001)	147	SocSci (2002–2005)	3	SocSci (2006–2014)	2
Eric (1966–2001)	0	Eric (2002–2005)	0	Eric (2006–2014)	0

related to the patient are presented followed by the concepts related to nursing in hypertension care, concepts related to the consultation where the patient and nurse meet, the integration with Orem's self-care deficit theory, and finally the expected outcome (Figure 1).

3.1. Concepts Related to the Patient. Concepts that are related to the patients' ability, disposition, and willingness to change lifestyle and take medicines are presented here. Factors comprising attitude and beliefs regarding health and sickness, autonomy, personality and traits and level of perceived vulnerability, hardiness, sense of coherence, locus of control, self-efficacy, and access to social support and network are of importance.

3.1.1. Attitude and Beliefs regarding Health and Sickness. An attitude is a psychological tendency that is expressed by evaluating a particular entity with some degree of favour or disfavour [12] and a value can be defined as a personal belief about the worth, desirability, goodness, truth, and beauty of a particular idea or object [13]. One's concept of health is tied into one's belief systems, which means that no patient will follow instructions that the person does not believe will work or will work towards a goal not valued. For that reason the patients' values can be considered the basis for decision-making on whether to perform lifestyle change or not. Patients hold ideas about whether hypertension is a disease or not, whether the drug is necessary evil or a help, and how the drug should be taken and its effects [14], and their perceptions of the cause of hypertension, experiences of symptoms, and beliefs about the treatment can influence their self-management [15]. Assessing these attitudes and beliefs is an important first step to develop a plan of care for the patient [16].

3.1.2. Autonomy. Autonomy is defined as self-government; that is, people are autonomous to the extent to which they are able to control their own lives [17]. The hypertensive patient is facing demands to make lifestyle changes that are to be lifelong and for that reason the decision has to be autonomously made [18]; otherwise the maintenance of the new behaviour is likely to decrease. It is therefore crucial that nurses can identify that the patient is sufficiently autonomous, which means that the patient can understand and retain the information relevant to the decision in question, believe the information, and weigh up the information to arrive at a decision.

3.1.3. Personality and Traits. A personality is a blend of two or more traits [19], which are factors that determine our conduct in many different situations and also when it comes to changing lifestyle. Traits are divided into the dimensions extraversion (active, assertive, enthusiastic), agreeableness (appreciative, forgiving, generous), conscientiousness (efficient, organised, responsible), neuroticism (anxious, tense, worrying), and openness (artistic, imaginative, insightful). States or moods are singular occurrences. Older adults, >65 years of age, who score high in conscientiousness are shown to perceive themselves as having health competence, which in turn was strongly related to health behaviours (exercise, dietary/health information, and relaxation/social support) [20]. Scoring high in conscientiousness might also promote self-control skills that can affect adherence to treatment [21]. Type A behaviour pattern, aggressively seeking to achieve more and more in less and less time, appears to increase blood pressure reactivity to external stressors in persons with mild hypertension [22].

3.1.4. Vulnerability. Vulnerability is defined in nursing literature as an externally evaluated risk (by a person outside the experience) or as an experiential state (as understood by the person herself) [23]. The individual's perceptions of self and challenges to self and of resources to withstand such challenges create the individual person's perceived vulnerability. The degree of vulnerability changes with the degree of environmental support and personal resources [24]. Psychological effects of vulnerability could give, among other things, a feeling of not belonging, helplessness, fear, anger, uncertainty, loss of control, isolation, anxiety/worry, and powerlessness. Likelihood to engage in positive action to change behaviour depends on whether the individual perceives himself as being well, chronically ill, or having an acute illness [25]. It is concluded that a hypertensive person can be placed between well and chronically ill, which means that motivation to learn about any aspect of healthcare is based upon the acceptance of self-responsibility for health. The person does not feel vulnerable or at any risk.

3.1.5. Hardiness. The concept of hardiness was first introduced as a personality characteristic with the dimensions of commitment (active involvement in one's life activities), control (belief in the ability to influence the course of one's life events), and challenge (change is normal and growth-producing) [26]. Hardy individuals have a higher sense of commitment to self and work, perceive life change as challenging rather than threatening, and maintain a sense of control in life rather than powerlessness. Hardy persons in hypertension and RA groups are reported to be more likely to participate in patient education programmes, and this was related to better physiological functioning [27].

3.1.6. Sense of Coherence. The theory of sense of coherence is a salutogenetic model (salute = health, genesis = origin) [28]. A person with generalised resistance-resources such as money, good self-strength, cultural stability, and social support can manage to make stressors understandable, that is, have a feeling of coherence. This also involves coping strategies, that is, a plan for behaviour, social support, and cultural factors. A person with a feeling of coherence has an attitude that expresses a long-lasting and deep faith in the world's predictability and thinks there is a high likelihood that things will turn out as well as you can reasonably expect. It does not imply that one is in control but that one is involved as a participant in the processes shaping one's destiny as well as one's daily experience. It is not important whether power is in our hands or elsewhere but that the location of power is where it is legitimately supposed to be.

3.1.7. Locus of Control. As psychosocial dynamics influence health behaviour, Rotter et al. [29] developed the idea that generalised expectancies and reinforcement make a person create a sense of locus of control over the events in his life. If the effect of reinforcement is perceived as not being entirely derived from a person's own actions but the result of luck, chance, or fate, as under the control of powerful others, it is labelled a belief in external control. If the person perceives that the event originated from his own behaviour or his own characteristics, it is termed a belief in internal control. It is reported that patients with hypertension who scored high on internal control adhered to their medication had a controlled blood pressure [30].

3.1.8. Self-Efficacy. Perceived self-efficacy refers to beliefs in one's capabilities to organise and execute the courses of actions required to produce certain practical attainments [31]. If people believe they have no power to produce results, they will not attempt to make things happen [32]. Perceived self-efficacy is a uniformly good predictor for diverse forms of behaviour. Efficacy beliefs affect performance both directly and by influencing intentions. Suggested areas for research include nonpharmacological treatment for hypertension, adherence to diet and medication regimens for lipid control, and interventions to improve exercise habits [33]. Effects of health literacy on self-efficacy and knowledge about health matters are also a factor to consider [34].

3.1.9. Social Support and Network. There is no universally accepted definition or conceptualisation of social support, but Lindsey [35] defines social support as provision of information that leads people to believe they are cared for, loved, esteemed, valued, and a member of a network of communication and mutual obligation. There are four types of social support: informational (provision of information that the person can use in coping with personal and environmental problems), appraisal (transmission of information relevant to self-evaluation), instrumental (access of the individual to behaviours that directly help in time of need), and emotional (provision of empathy and demonstration of love, trust, and caring). Social network that provides social support is defined as a group of people with whom the person has social connections, which may be formal or informal and can be described by size, density, and complexity. In studies high social network score is associated with lower systolic and diastolic blood pressure for both sexes [36]. In China it was found that social support, education, and duration of diagnosis of hypertension were significant predictors of treatment adherence [37].

3.2. Concepts Related to Nursing in Hypertension Care. Concepts of importance for the nurse when nursing patients in hypertension care are presented here. They involve applying theories and models for behavioural change in the consultation and using counselling skills, patient advocacy, empowerment, professional knowledge and health education, and supporting the patient.

3.2.1. Theories and Models for Behavioural Change. There are several theories and models developed to understand what determines behaviours. In healthcare the health belief model [38] is the most frequently used model in behaviour change. In this model goal-setting, decision-making, and social learning are integrated for making one's own decisions depending on positive or negative attitudes. Perceived susceptibility and barriers for behaviour change are included too. Other models that are useful for nurses in treating patients regarding lifestyle changes are, for example, the transtheoretical model (TTM) or stages of change model (SOC) [39] where the learner goes through a cycle from precontemplation to contemplation, preparation, and action to maintenance of new behaviour; the self-regulatory model (SRM) [40] where motivation for changing lifestyle is dependent on perceived threat; the protection motivation theory (PMT) [41] according to which judging the severity of health threats affects coping responses; or the health promotion model (HPM) [42] where perceived benefits, barriers to action, self-efficacy, interpersonal and situational influences affect behaviour change. In our own studies it was shown that nurses educated in the SOC model may have some help when using the model in counselling hypertensive patients [43].

3.2.2. Counselling Skills. The process of counselling can be defined as "the means by which one person helps another to clarify his life situation and to decide further lines of action" (p. 2) [44]. To act, the patient needs to be able to identify those things she has to do, stop doing, continue to do, and accept. Morrison and Burnard [45] suggest definitions of counselling as helping people to come to terms with a problem, enable a person to find solutions to problems, or help people to help themselves. Motivational interviewing (MI) [46] is a patient-centred goal-oriented counselling style for addressing the coercion of ambivalence about change. Using this counselling style is a way to preserve patient-centredness, empathy, and patient autonomy in the consultation. Own studies show that nurses after consultation training fulfilled more aspects of patient-centredness after the training [47] and were more focused and discussed lifestyle factors to a greater extent with their patients [48]. Furthermore effects on patients' weight parameters, physical activity, perceived stress, and the proportion of patients who achieved blood pressure control have been demonstrated [49].

3.2.3. Patient Advocacy. An advocate is "one who pleads the cause of another" (p. 439) [50]. The concept of advocacy is linked with concepts of morality, ethics, autonomy, and patient empowerment. Gadow [51] proposes that the concept of advocacy is the philosophical foundation and ideal of nursing. The nurse is uniquely suited for fundamental and existential advocacy distinct from just providing the patient with any correct and objective information and being paternalistic. Schwartz [52] states that the advocate should inform the patient and promote informed consent, empower the patient and protect autonomy, protect the rights and interests of the patient, ensure access to available resources, support the patients, and represent the views/desires of the patients and not just their needs.

3.2.4. Empowerment. The word empower means "to authorise, to license, to impart power, to enable, and to permit" and a definition of the concept of empowerment could be "in a helping partnership it is a process of enabling people to choose to take control over and make decisions about their lives" (p. 309) [53]. Rappaport [54] views empowerment as the vehicle by which problems in living may be handled, and it suggests a sense of control over one's life in personality, cognition, and motivation. The empowerment approach to health education seeks to increase patient autonomy and expand freedom of choice [55]. The nurse can contribute by doing assessments of patients' psychosocial health and appraisal of health and health risks. Personal empowerment is promoted by encouraging people to identify their values, needs, goals, and the resources they have to solve problems. Awareness, freedom, choice, and responsibility are the four pillars of empowerment. Nurses' counselling was found to contain both empowerment and nurse-centred features in a study in hypertension care, which alternated during the conversations but nurse-centred features were predominant [56].

3.2.5. Professional Knowledge. To be able to perform all the tasks that are included in nursing in hypertension care, the nurse has to be updated in the latest guidelines for hypertension treatment, both pharmacological and nonpharmacological. Being the leader of the team [1] around the patient, as often is the case, the nurse has to have knowledge about how to value the results of the patient's blood tests regarding, for example, blood lipids and also body measurements such as waist circumference and body mass index. The nurse also needs to be able to estimate the patient's individual risk profile.

3.2.6. Health Education. The importance of health teaching as a part of nursing has been recognised for a long time. A professional model for teaching in nursing practice consists of four components: social service ideal (characteristics of the profession), practice environment (environment that influences the practice), client state (nurse's view of the client), and nursing practice strategies (unique nursing interventions) [57]. This model is applicable in nursing in hypertension care as it encompasses a professional autonomy and spirit which the nurse must master as she is often managing the clinic on her own. She must also have understanding of man's physiological and psychosocial state to make an assessment of the patient to determine the nature of teaching needed. This encompasses a holistic view. The teaching can be performed individually or in group. Hypertensive patients were interviewed about their views on a working booklet used in consultations at nurse-led clinics where the nurses had received counselling training [58]. The booklet was reported to have been read several times by some patients, but a few patients did not remember receiving it. Individual health education in primary care is reported to give lower systolic and diastolic blood pressure and body mass index and improve self-efficacy regarding medication adherence [59].

3.2.7. Support. The patient often gets social support from, for example, their next of kin and friends, but the nurse also has to support the patient regarding the specific individual lifestyle problems the patient has. Support and MI skills can also be needed to help the patients to increase their self-efficacy to succeed in changing lifestyle [46]. This could also be expressed as interpersonal transactions that include the expression of positive affect of one person towards another, the affirmation of another's behaviours, perceptions, or expressed views, and the giving of symbolic or material aid to another person [35, 60].

3.3. Concepts Related to the Consultation and the Expected Outcome. In the consultation the patient and the nurse meet. Presented below are specific concepts related to this meeting and the expected outcome, where the nurse is communicating with the patient to reach a shared decision in concordance with the patient regarding the self-care the patient should perform. To be able to perform self-care the patient uses different coping strategies to adhere to the decided treatment.

3.3.1. Communication. Caring is an interpersonal process and builds the rapport between nurse and patient. A conceptual framework has been developed for classifying varieties of interpersonal intervention between nurse and patient

[45]. The authoritative interventions are prescriptive (to offer advice, make suggestions), informative (to offer information), and confronting (to challenge) and the facilitative ones are cathartic (to enable the release of emotion), catalytic (to "draw out"), and supportive (to encourage or validate). An interpersonally skilled person is one who can move appropriately and freely between the various categories as a means of guiding therapeutic action. All of these interventions can be found in MI [46] except the authoritative kind, which is seen as counterproductive for creating rapport with the patient. A client-centred approach means that the client himself is best able to decide how to find solutions to his problems in living [61]. All the skills of communication are also skills of counselling as listening, paraphrasing, challenging, and goal-setting [62]. Communication can be verbal or nonverbal. Interviewed hypertensive patients reported that the nurse listened and they had been guided and motivated to perform lifestyle changes after the nurses' counselling training [58]. There were more informed thoughts about how to manage lifestyle in this group compared to the control group.

3.3.2. Shared Decision-Making and Concordance. The Swedish Health and Medical Services Act [63] states that care should be given based on respect for patients' own decisions and their integrity. Toop from New Zealand states in a paper [64] that a patient-centred approach based on mutual participation has gained increasing support, and in the US the concept of sustained partnership between patient and clinician has been included in a definition of primary care. Mutual goal-setting is a process whereby nurse and patient collaboratively define a set of patient goals and agree on the goals to be attained. Goal-setting is an essential part of problem solving and the nursing process. Charles et al. [65] argue that the shared treatment decision-making model has four necessary characteristics: both the physician and patient are involved in the treatment decision-making process, they share information with each other, they take steps to participate in the decision-making process by expressing treatment preferences, and a treatment decision is made. Charles and contributors focus on physicians' interaction with patients but here the principles for decision-making are generally applicable.

Through the concordance website managed by the RPSGB concordance coordinating group the new concept will begin to grow [66]. The historical background was the problem of noncompliance with medication and growing knowledge about the beliefs that people hold about their medication and about medicines in general. These beliefs decide whether the individual will comply with a prescription or not. The concept can also be extended to other treatment modalities such as behaviour change. In the consultation concordance should be based on a negotiation between equals. Concordance implies the approach of bringing patients into a full therapeutic partnership, that a patient's decision-making preferences may change with time and circumstances, and that if the patient has relatively more authority or control in the consultation, the prescriber will have less. Moreover, the patient might choose a treatment other than that proposed by the prescriber and this is not a failure but a success of care, and if this happens, it is no basis for rejection of the patient. In MI the word concordance is not used, but the idea of the MI spirit means that the patients are viewed as valued partners whom the counsellor wants to help to make his or her own decisions regarding health matters [46]. Shared decision-making and concordance do not overlap but rather supplement each other.

3.3.3. Coping. Coping comprises the person's strategies to handle trying situations and demands that are appraised as taxing or exceeding the resources of the person [67], such as being diagnosed as having hypertension. A person can use strategies to handle the stress through acceptance, tolerance, medication, avoidance, and so forth or strategies to change the situation that caused the stress [68]. A vigilant coping strategy is directed to the problem in an effort to prevent or control it [67] and could mean information searching or systematic problem solving. Coping by avoidance could be jogging, relaxation, vacation, hobbies, wishful thinking, eating, drinking, smoking, using drugs or medications, or sleeping. Arora and McHorney [69] used questionnaires to study whether 2472 chronically ill (hypertension, diabetes, congestive heart failure, myocardial infarction, depression) persons preferred an active or passive role in medical decision-making. They found that patients using an active coping strategy preferred an active role in meetings with health professionals.

3.3.4. Adherence. There has been a shift through the years from using the term compliance to using adherence, though many authors still use the word compliance. Compliance has authoritative connotations, implying that the practitioner expects the patient to follow rules that are for the patient's own good [13] or that the patient is a passive responder to the clinician's authoritative demands [70]. Noncompliance means that the patient asserts the right of self-responsibility. Adherence can be defined as "the extent to which a person's behaviour (in terms of taking medications, following diets, or executing lifestyle changes) coincides with medical or health advice" according to Haynes in 1979 [71]. Expectancy of internal control over health and hypertension and knowledge of the treatment regimen are significant determinants of adherence. Poor adherence to treatment can also mean that the person actually has not changed his opinion, has not understood the message completely, is not convinced about having to change behaviour to avoid illness, or has not received any help to adopt other habits [72]. Sensitivity of symptoms is generally an indicator of disease and used as a motivator and guide for treatment. Hypertension is a good example of poor sensitivity and therefore a bad motivator for treatment adaptation [40]. Regarding adherence to medication Allen [73] states that the hypertensive patient feels well and there will be no increase in perceived well-being when medication is taken, which could contribute to noncompliance. The cost of the medication [74], especially among older people [75], is an important barrier to adherence.

3.3.5. Self-Care. Self-care can be defined as activities initiated or performed by an individual, family, or community to achieve, maintain, or promote maximum health [42]. Within the medical model, self-care has been defined as self-care in illness, compliance with therapeutic regimens, and active participation in rehabilitative activities. Self-care for health promotion requires that "clients have the knowledge and competencies that can be used to maintain and enhance health" (p. 98). A similar definition is used by Levin [76] meaning that self-care is a process where a lay person can function effectively in taking care of his or her own health promotion and prevention and disease detection and treatment. Within nursing the concept of self-management seems to encompass not only different coping strategies but also health-promotive actions, interaction with healthcare providers, adherence to treatment, monitoring health status, making care decisions, and management of the impact of the illness on health [77].

3.4. Integration with Existing Theory of Nursing. All the defined concepts related to nursing in hypertension care form the basis for nursing interventions, and the nurse makes an assessment of the patient's self-care demands in communicating with the patient to help the patient to change lifestyle, that is, to perform self-care. For that reason Orem's self-care deficit theory of nursing [78] is integrated as a natural ingredient in the proposed middle-range theory.

The self-care deficit theory of nursing consists of three parts: theory of self-care, theory of self-care deficit, and theory of nursing systems [78]. Presuppositions for the theory are that people develop and exercise intellectual and practical skills through learning and manage themselves to sustain motivation essential for continuing daily care of themselves. Self-care is an action of persons who have developed the capabilities to take care of themselves in their environmental situations. They have the agency or power to act to regulate internal and external factors that affect their own functioning and development, that is, in the interest of life, health, and well-being. The ability to perform self-care, the self-care agency as a specific power of individuals, differs depending on capabilities and circumstances related to the self-care demands and health disorders. Self-care deficit arises when capabilities for self-care, because of existing limitations, are not equal to meeting some or all of the components of their therapeutic self-care demands. In hypertension care the self-care deficit could mean that the patient has a lack of knowledge about or is not motivated to perform lifestyle changes or to start taking medicines. These deficiencies mean that the patient cannot develop appropriate self-care agency.

To meet the patient's self-care deficit, nurses produce systems of nursing actions, nursing agencies [78]. In hypertension care these agencies most often are supportive-educative to help the patient to regain his self-care. The supportive-educative system is the only system where a patient's requirements for help are confined to decision-making, behaviour control, and acquiring knowledge and skills. The nursing actions could be of long or short duration.

The concepts related to nursing (theories and models for behavioural change, counselling skills, patient advocacy, empowerment, professional knowledge, health education and support) form the nursing system in hypertension care which the nurse brings into the encounter with the patient. The patients in turn bring certain attitudes and beliefs, a view of health, need for autonomy, their own personality and traits, perceived vulnerability, hardiness, a sense of coherence, locus of control, self-efficacy, and social support and network into the encounter. All these factors affect behaviour and thus the patients' habits. In the interaction the nurse uses appropriate parts of the nursing system to assess the patient's self-care deficits. From the interaction in the patient-centred communication, shared decision-making should emerge, with goal-setting in concordance between the patient and the nurse. From the decisions made about performing self-care the patient has to develop self-care agencies to perform behaviour change through his own coping and with assistance from nursing agencies, that is, the nurse's interventions. The desired outcome is changed lifestyle with the goal of adherence to treatment and maintenance of new behaviour. This was demonstrated in our own research in measuring hypertensive patients' exercise of self-care agency [79] where counselling training gave an increase in the patients' self-care agency scores, which was significantly correlated with increased physical activity and improved satisfaction with information about medication [80], which mirrors adherence to treatment. From Turkey it is similarly reported that hypertensive patients' educational level and social insurance situation affect the measured self-care agency score [81].

4. Clinical and Research Implications

Nursing in hypertension care has been criticised for not being fully professionally performed and for not having any structure for the counselling in the consultations [82]. Nurses could have a prominent position in the treatment of hypertensive patients, but to achieve this, the standard of the nursing needs to be enhanced. For that reason, a theory can be necessary to give a basis for the nurses to be able to develop guidelines for their own practice.

In being patient-centred in their communication, nurses must see the individual patient with his or her needs. It is then necessary for the nurse to have knowledge about what factors may affect the patient, factors that might help or be less helpful for the patient to manage to perform necessary lifestyle changes or take medicines. A patient can have the idea that living a healthy life is not for him as he is predestined because of a heavy heredity for cardiovascular diseases. His attitude is to be careless and his beliefs are that it is not worthwhile to attend to his weight. He maintains his stance to preserve his autonomy. He gives the impression of being conscientious as he is efficient and organised. Regarding his hypertension, he feels powerless (vulnerable) and thus has a low level of hardiness. He has also a low sense of coherence as he has low self-strength and feels that he is lucky if he will reach the age of fifty (external locus of control). However, he would score high on self-efficacy because when he decides to do things, he has a strong belief in being successful. He has also social support from his family and a social network that would be of help if he could be motivated to change lifestyle. This is exemplified in Table 2. In meeting patients, the experienced nurse presumably gets an impression of the

Table 2: A schematic description of how the nurse could make use of the proposed theory in hypertension care. All counselling sessions with patients need not follow the same order, and one concept is not used just at one particular time; for example, communication and professional knowledge are used throughout the consultation. The treatment mentioned here is lifestyle change.

Process of the consultation	Concepts related to the meeting	Concepts related to the patient	Concepts related to the nurse
Creating rapport with the patient	Communication		
Who is this person?		Personality and traits	Counselling skills
Assessing the patient's individual risk profile and telling the patient the result	Assessment of the patient's self-care deficits		Professional knowledge
What has the patient to say?		Attitudes and beliefs regarding health and sickness Sense of coherence Perceived vulnerability Hardiness	
The patient has questions		Autonomy	Health education
Discussion of pros and cons of lifestyle change where the patient reaches a decision whether to make a change or not	Shared decision-making and concordance	Locus of control	Patient advocacy Theories and models for behavioural change
The patient is willing	Development of self-care agencies using coping strategies	Self-efficacy Social support and network	Empowerment Support
Follow-up	Adherence to changed lifestyle through performed self-care		

individual patient and can report most of the statements listed in the scenario above, but the nurse would probably not be able to give a theoretical background and relate to these concepts. To be able to study and put words on what nursing in hypertension care means, a theoretical foundation is necessary.

To integrate Orem's self-care theory is particularly relevant to patient teaching with development of self-care skills [13, 32] as this is the goal for hypertensive patients and there is acceptance of the theory with its application to a variety of client populations and clinical settings (Whetstone and Reid, 1991). For many patients with hypertension it is hard to understand how the figures describing their blood pressure level are going to affect their lives. Most patients do not have symptoms that are easy to relate to the diagnosis. This means that their challenge is more demanding than those of many other patients, and it is also a big challenge for the nurse to help the patient to understand the seriousness of the figures and to motivate the patient to perform the lifestyle changes that are needed. For that reason a more detailed and applied theory is needed for the nurse in hypertension care than using Orem's grand theory alone or even a middle-range explanatory theory of self-management behaviour [83].

Intervention studies on nursing in hypertension care have been performed and show that consultation training can give nurses a structure for the consultations [48] and that nurses can be more patient-centred in their counselling [47]. Using behavioural models as a theoretical framework has also been found to be of use [43]. Other research shows that integrating behavioural models with counselling technique as in MI [84] is helpful for healthcare providers of different professions. In doing this the provider gets a structure for the consultation and can be more effective in treating the patients. For nurses the application of a theory in hypertension care can give even deeper understanding of the patients' challenges and also of their own professional nursing actions.

Further research could be directed to different aspects of the application of the theory to clinical settings or to the theoretical relationships between the concepts. In clinical settings it would be of interest to study nurses' views on applying the theory in their practice and also hypertensive patients' views of how they perceive their treatment and their experiences of performing self-care. Intervention studies could be performed where the nursing care is based on the theory to see if this makes any difference on patient outcomes. The relationships between the concepts and a development of the different concepts need attention too. There are several questions to be answered such as what the differences between concordance and shared decision-making are, whether it is important to incorporate levels of hardiness, sense of coherence, and locus of control in the theory, and whether it makes a difference using the word patient-centredness in defining counselling skills instead of person-centredness. According to Higgins and Moore's definitions [85], this proposed theory is predictive, that is, anticipating a particular set of outcomes, and has the components of identified and defined concepts, assumptions that clarify the basic underlying truths, a context within which the theory is placed but lacks identified relationships between and among the concepts. For that reason, views from the world of nurses interested in the development of theorising nursing in hypertension care are most valuable.

References

[1] A. Bengtson and E. Drevenhorn, "The nurse's role and skills in hypertension care: a review," *Clinical Nurse Specialist*, vol. 17, no. 5, pp. 260–268, 2003.

[2] W.-H. S. Hong, "Evidence-based nursing practice for health promotion in adults with hypertension: a literature review," *Asian Nursing Research*, vol. 4, no. 4, pp. 227–245, 2010.

[3] M. Middeke, B. Lemmer, B. Schaaf, and L. Eckes, "Prevalence of hypertension-attributed symptoms in routine clinical practice: a general practitioners-based study," *Journal of Human Hypertension*, vol. 22, no. 4, pp. 252–258, 2008.

[4] W. Li, N. A. Stotts, and E. S. Froelicher, "Compliance with antihypertensive medication in chinese immigrants: cultural specific issues and theoretical application," *Research and Theory for Nursing Practice*, vol. 21, no. 4, pp. 236–254, 2007.

[5] B. Erci, A. Sayan, G. Tortumluoğlu, D. Kiliç, O. Şahin, and Z. Güngörmüş, "The effectiveness of Watson's caring model on the quality of life and blood pressure of patients with hypertension," *Journal of Advanced Nursing*, vol. 41, no. 2, pp. 130–139, 2003.

[6] N. V. Cade, "OREM's self-care deficit theory applied to hypertensive patients," *Revista Latino-Americana de Enfermagem*, vol. 9, no. 3, pp. 43–50, 2001.

[7] M. J. Smith and P. Liehr, "Attentively embracing story: a middle-range theory with practice and research implications," *Scholarly Inquiry for Nursing Practice*, vol. 13, no. 3, pp. 187–204, 1999.

[8] E. Drevenhorn, A. Bengtson, and K. Kjellgren, "Theoretical aspects of hypertensive patients' predispositions toward lifestyle change—a review," *European Journal of Cardiovascular Nursing*, vol. 2, no. 1, pp. 84-85, 2016.

[9] E. Drevenhorn, A. Bengtson, and K. I. Kjellgren, "Application of a nursing system in hypertension care," in *Proceedings of Poster Presentation at the International Council of Nurses*, Geneva, Switzerland, 2003.

[10] P. Liehr and M. J. Smith, "Middle range theory: spinning research and practice to create knowledge for the new millennium," *Advances in Nursing Science*, vol. 21, no. 4, pp. 81–91, 1999.

[11] L. Walker and K. Avant, *Strategies for theory construction in nursing*, Pearson, Essex, UK, 5th edition, 2014.

[12] A. H. Eagly and S. Chaiken, *The Psychology of Attitudes*, Harcourt Brace College Publishers, London, UK, 1993.

[13] C. J. Gleit, "Health values," in *Eaching in Nursing Practice—a Professional Model*, N. I. Whitman, Ed., pp. 103–114, Appleton&Lange, Norwalk, Conn, USA, 1992.

[14] L. Lisper, D. Isacson, P.-O. Sjödén, and K. Bingefors, "Medicated hypertensive patients' views and experience of information and communication concerning antihypertensive drugs," *Patient Education and Counseling*, vol. 32, no. 3, pp. 147–155, 1997.

[15] B. Bajorek, K. Lemay, P. Magin, C. Roberts, I. Krass, and C. Armour, "Patients' attitudes and approaches to the self-management of hypertension: perspectives from an australian qualitative study in community pharmacy," *High Blood Pressure & Cardiovascular Prevention*, vol. 24, no. 2, pp. 149–155, 2017.

[16] R. M. Peters and T. N. Templin, "Theory of planned behavior, self-care motivation, and blood pressure self-care.," *Research and Theory for Nursing Practice*, vol. 24, no. 3, pp. 172–186, 2010.

[17] H. Aveyard, "Is there a concept of autonomy that can usefully inform nursing practice?" *Journal of Advanced Nursing*, vol. 32, no. 2, pp. 352–358, 2000.

[18] P. Burnard, "Implications of client-centred counselling for nursing practice.," *Nursing Times*, vol. 91, no. 26, pp. 35–37, 1995.

[19] R. R. McCrae and O. P. John, "An introduction to the five-factor model and its applications," *Journal of Personality*, vol. 60, no. 2, pp. 175–215, 1992.

[20] G. R. Marks and S. K. Lutgendorf, "Perceived health competence and personality factors differentially predict health behaviors in older adults," *Journal of Aging and Health*, vol. 11, no. 2, pp. 221–239, 1999.

[21] J. S. Wiebe and A. J. Christensen, "Patient adherence in chronic illness: personality and coping in context," *Journal of Personality*, vol. 64, no. 4, pp. 814–835, 1996.

[22] D. G. Byrne, "Anxiety, neuroticism, depression, and hypertension," in *Personality, elevated blood pressure, and essential hypertension*, E. H. Johnson, W. D. Gentry, and S. Julius, Eds., pp. 67–85, Hemisphere Publishing Corporation, Washington, DC, USA, 1992.

[23] J. Spiers, "New perspectives on vulnerability using emic and etic approaches," *Journal of Advanced Nursing*, vol. 31, no. 3, pp. 715–721, 2000.

[24] A. C. Rogers, "Vulnerability, health and health care," *Journal of Advanced Nursing*, vol. 26, no. 1, pp. 65–72, 1997.

[25] N. I. Whitman, "Health status," in *Teaching in nursing practice - a professional model*, pp. 91–102, Appleton&Lange, Norwalk, Conn, USA, 1992.

[26] S. C. Kobasa, "Stressful life events, personality, and health: an inquiry into hardiness," *Journal of Personality and Social Psychology*, vol. 37, no. 1, pp. 1–11, 1979.

[27] S. E. Pollock, B. J. Christian, and D. Sands, "Responses to chronic illness: analysis of psychological and physiological adaptation," *Nursing Research*, vol. 39, no. 5, pp. 300–304, 1990.

[28] A. Antonovsky, *Health, Stress, and Coping*, Jossey-Bass Publishers, London, UK, 1979.

[29] J. B. Rotter, J. E. Chance, and E. J. Phares, *Applications of a Social Learning Theory of Personality*, Holt, Rinehart and Winston, Inc, New York, NY, USA, 1972.

[30] M. Taher, "Correlation between compliance regimens with health locus of control in patients with hypertension," *Medical Journal of the Islamic Republic of Iran*, vol. 29, p. 194, 2015.

[31] A. Bandura, "Self-efficacy: toward a unifying theory of behavioral change," *Psychological Review*, vol. 84, no. 2, pp. 191–215, 1977.

[32] C. J. Gleit, "Theories of learning," in *Teaching in nursing practice—a professional model*, N. I. Whitman, Ed., pp. 51–80, Appleton&Lange, Norwalk, Conn, USA, 1992.

[33] J. K. Allen, "Self-efficacy in health behavior research and practice," *Cardio-Vascular Nursing*, vol. 24, no. 6, pp. 37-38, 1988.

[34] C. Y. Osborn, "The mechanisms linking health literacy to behavior and health status," *American Journal of Health Behavior*, vol. 35, no. 1, pp. 28–118, 2011.

[35] A. M. Lindsey, "Social support: conceptualizations and measurement instruments," in *Instruments for clinical nursing*, M. Frank-Stromborg, Ed., pp. 107–120, Jones and Bartlett Publishers, London, UK, 1992.

[36] J. Siegrist, "Self, social structure, and health-promoting behavior in hypertensive patients," *Patient Education and Counseling*, vol. 26, no. 1-3, pp. 215–218, 1995.

[37] C. Ma, S. Chen, Y. Zhou, and C. Huang, "Treatment adherence of Chinese patients with hypertension: a longitudinal study," *Applied Nursing Research*, vol. 26, no. 4, pp. 225–231, 2013.

[38] N. K. Janz and M. H. Becker, "The health belief model: a decade later," *Health Education Journal*, vol. 11, no. 1, pp. 1–47, 1984.

[39] J. O. Prochaska and C. C. DiClemente, "Transtheoretical therapy: toward a more integrative model of change," *Psychotherapy*, vol. 19, no. 3, pp. 276–288, 1982.

[40] H. Leventhal, E. A. Leventhal, and R. J. Contrada, "Self-regulation, health, and behavior: a perceptual-cognitive approach," *Psychology & Health*, vol. 13, no. 4, pp. 717–733, 1998.

[41] R. W. Rogers and S. Prentice-Dunn, "Protection motivation theory," in *Handbook of health behavior research. Part I Personal and social*, D. Gochman, Ed., pp. 113–132, Plenum Press, New York, YN, USA, 1997.

[42] N. J. Pender, C. L. Murdaugh, and M. A. Parsons, *Health Promotion in Nursing Practice*, Appleton&Lange, Stamford, Conn, USA, 6th edition, 2011.

[43] E. Drevenhorn, A. Bengtson, J. K. Allen, R. Säljö, and K. I. Kjellgren, "Counselling on lifestyle factors in hypertension care after training on the stages of change model," *European Journal of Cardiovascular Nursing*, vol. 6, no. 1, pp. 46–53, 2007.

[44] P. Burnard, *Counselling Skills for Health Professionals*, Stanley Thornes Ltd, Cheltenham, UK, 3rd edition, 1999.

[45] P. Morrison and P. Burnard, *Caring and Communicating. The Interpersonal Relationship in Nursing*, Macmillan Press Ltd, London, UK, 2nd edition, 1997.

[46] W. R. Miller and S. Rollnick, *Motivational Interviewing: Helping People Change*, The Guilford Press, London, UK, 3rd edition, 2013.

[47] E. Drevenhorn, A. Bengtson, J. K. Allen, R. Säljö, and K. I. Kjellgren, "A content analysis of patient centredness in hypertension care after consultation training for nurses," *Internet Journal of Advanced Nursing Practice*, vol. 8, no. 2, 2006.

[48] E. Drevenhorn, A. Bengtson, and K. I. Kjellgren, "Evaluation of consultation training in hypertension care," *European Journal of Cardiovascular Nursing*, vol. 8, no. 5, pp. 349–354, 2009.

[49] E. Drevenhorn, A. Bengtson, P. M. Nilsson, P. Nyberg, and K. I. Kjellgren, "Consultation training of nurses for cardiovascular prevention a randomized study of 2 years duration," *Blood Pressure*, vol. 21, no. 5, pp. 293–299, 2012.

[50] J. Hewitt, "A critical review of the arguments debating the role of the nurse advocate," *Journal of Advanced Nursing*, vol. 37, no. 5, pp. 439–445, 2002.

[51] S. Gadow, "Existential advocacy: philosophical foundation of nursing," in *Nursing: Images and Ideals - Opening Dialogue with the Humanities*, S. F. Spicker and S. Gadow, Eds., pp. 79–101, Springer Publishing Company, New York, NY, USA, 1980.

[52] L. Schwartz, "Is there an advocate in the house? The role of health care professionals in patient advocacy," *Journal of Medical Ethics*, vol. 28, no. 1, pp. 37–40, 2002.

[53] C. M. Rodwell, "An analysis of the concept of empowerment," *Journal of Advanced Nursing*, vol. 23, no. 2, pp. 305–313, 1996.

[54] J. Rappaport, "The power of empowerment language," *Social Policy*, pp. 15–21, 1985.

[55] C. Feste and R. M. Anderson, "Empowerment: from philosophy to practice," *Patient Education and Counseling*, vol. 26, no. 1-3, pp. 139–144, 1995.

[56] M. Poskiparta, L. Liimatainen, T. Kettunen, and P. Karhila, "From nurse-centered health counseling to empowermental health counseling," *Patient Education and Counseling*, vol. 45, no. 1, pp. 69–79, 2001.

[57] M. D. Boyd et al., "A professional model for teaching in nursing practice," in *Teaching in Nursing Practice—a Professional Model*, N. I. Whitman, Ed., pp. 3–16, Appleton&Lange, Norwalk, Conn, USA, 1992.

[58] E. Drevenhorn, A. Bengtson, and K. I. Kjellgren, "To be motivated or only comply—patients' views of hypertension care after consultation training for nurses," *Health Education Journal*, vol. 74, no. 1, pp. 28–36, 2015.

[59] R. Hacihasanoğlu and S. Gözüm, "The effect of patient education and home monitoring on medication compliance, hypertension management, healthy lifestyle behaviours and BMI in a primary health care setting," *Journal of Clinical Nursing*, vol. 20, no. 5-6, pp. 692–705, 2011.

[60] C. A. Heany and B. A. Israel, "Social networks and social support," in *Health behavior and health education*, K. Glanz, F. M. Lewis, and B. K. Rimer, Eds., pp. 189–207, Jossey-Bass Publishers, San Francisco, Calif, USA, 2008.

[61] C. R. Rogers, *Client-Centered Therapy*, Constable, London, UK, 1999.

[62] R. Bayne and V. Tschudin, "Listening: some basic qualities and skills," in *Counselling and Communication Skills for Medical and Health Practitioners*, R. Bayne, P. Nicolson, and I. Horton, Eds., The British Psychological Society: Leiser, UK, 1998.

[63] HSL, "Hälso- och sjukvårdslagen (Health and medical service act, Socialstyrelsen)," The National Board of Health and Welfare 763, 1982.

[64] L. Toop, "Primary care: core values Patient centred primary care," *British Medical Journal*, vol. 316, no. 7148, pp. 1882-1883, 1998.

[65] C. Charles, A. Gafni, and T. Whelan, "Decision-making in the physician-patient encounter: revisiting the shared treatment decision-making model," *Social Science & Medicine*, vol. 49, no. 5, pp. 651–661, 1999.

[66] M. Marinker, "Concordance training framework and roleplays," http://www.medicines-partnership.org/professional-development/training-resources/framework–roleplays.

[67] R. S. Lazarus, *Emotion and Adaptation*, Oxford University Press, New York, NY, USA, 1991.

[68] R. S. Lazarus and S. Folkman, "The concept of coping," in *Stress and coping*, A. Monat and and R. S. Lazarus, Eds., pp. 189–206, Columbia University Press, New York, NY, USA, 1991.

[69] N. K. Arora and C. A. McHorney, "Patient preferences for medical decision making: who really wants to participate?" *Medical Care*, vol. 38, no. 3, pp. 335–341, 2000.

[70] S. D. Schaffer and S.-J. L. Yoon, "Evidence-based Methods to Enhance Medication Adherence," *The Nurse Practitioner*, vol. 26, no. 12, p. 44, 50, 52, 54, 2001.

[71] A. L. Stanton, "Determinants of adherence to medical regimens by hypertensive patients," *Journal of Behavioral Medicine*, vol. 10, no. 4, pp. 377–394, 1987.

[72] L. Nordenfelt, *Action, Ability and Health. Essays in the Philosophy of Action and Welfare*, Kluwer Academic Publishers, London, UK, 2000.

[73] H. Allen, "Promoting compliance with antihypertensive medication," *British Journal of Nursing (Mark Allen Publishing)*, vol. 7, no. 20, pp. 1252–1258, 1998.

[74] B. M. Egan, D. T. Lackland, and N. E. Cutler, "Awareness, knowledge, and attitudes of older americans about high blood pressure: implications for health care policy, education, and research," *JAMA Internal Medicine*, vol. 163, no. 6, pp. 681–687, 2003.

[75] E. Holt, C. Joyce, A. Dornelles et al., "Sex differences in barriers to antihypertensive medication adherence: findings from the cohort study of medication adherence among older adults," *Journal of the American Geriatrics Society*, vol. 61, no. 4, pp. 558–564, 2013.

[76] L. S. Levin, "Self-care: towards fundamental changes in national strategies.," *International journal of health education*, vol. 24, no. 4, pp. 219–228, 1981.

[77] H. B. Bosworth, B. J. Powers, and E. Z. Oddone, "Patient self-management support: novel strategies in hypertension and heart disease," *Cardiology Clinics*, vol. 28, no. 4, pp. 655–663, 2010.

[78] D. E. Orem, *Nursing. Concepts of Practice*, S. t. Louis, Ed., Mosby Year Book Inc, SLouis , Mo, USA, 5th edition, 1995.

[79] E. Drevenhorn, A. Bengtson, P. Nyberg, and K. I. Kjellgren, "Assessment of hypertensive patients' self-care agency after counseling training of nurses," *Journal of the American Association of Nurse Practitioners*, vol. 27, no. 11, pp. 624–630, 2015.

[80] E. Drevenhorn, A. Bengtson, P. Nyberg, and K. Kjellgren, "Effects on hypertensive patients' satisfaction with information about their medication after nurses' consultation training," *Pragmatic and Observational Research*, vol. 2014, no. 5, pp. 35–41, 2014.

[81] A. D. Akyol, Y. Çetinkaya, G. Bakan, S. Yarali, and S. Akkuş, "Self-care agency and factors related to this agency among patients with hypertension," *Journal of Clinical Nursing*, vol. 16, no. 4, pp. 679–687, 2007.

[82] U. B. Aminoff and K. I. Kjellgren, "The nurse—a resource in hypertension care," *Journal of Advanced Nursing*, vol. 35, no. 4, pp. 582–589, 2001.

[83] A. C. Blok, "A middle-range explanatory theory of self-management behavior for collaborative research and practice," *Nursing Forum*, vol. 52, no. 2, pp. 138–146, 2017.

[84] K. A. Vanbuskirk and J. L. Wetherell, "Motivational interviewing with primary care populations: a systematic review and meta-analysis," *Journal of Behavioral Medicine*, vol. 37, no. 4, pp. 768–780, 2014.

[85] P. A. Higgins and S. M. Moore, "Levels of theoretical thinking in nursing," *Nursing Outlook*, vol. 48, no. 4, pp. 179–183, 2000.

6

Associations of Short Sleep and Shift Work Status with Hypertension among Black and White Americans

Mirnova E. Ceïde,[1] Abhishek Pandey,[2] Joe Ravenell,[3] Margaret Donat,[2] Gbenga Ogedegbe,[3] and Girardin Jean-Louis[3]

[1] *Montefiore Medical Center, Department of Psychiatry and Behavioral Science, 111 East 210 Street, Bronx, NY 10467, USA*
[2] *Brooklyn Health Disparities Center, Department of Medicine, SUNY Downstate Medical Center, Brooklyn, NY 11203, USA*
[3] *Center for Healthful Behavior Change, Department of Population Health, NYU Langone Medical Center, New York, NY 10016, USA*

Correspondence should be addressed to Mirnova E. Ceïde; mirnova@gmail.com

Academic Editor: Charles Agyemang

Objective. The purpose of this study was to investigate whether short sleepers (<6 hrs) who worked the non-day-shift were at greater likelihood of reporting hypertension and if these associations varied by individuals' ethnicity. *Methods.* Analysis was based on the 2010 National Health Interview Survey (NHIS). A total of 59,199 American adults provided valid data for the present analyses (mean age = 46.2 ± 17.7 years; 51.5% were female). Respondents provided work schedule and estimated habitual sleep durations as well as self-report of chronic conditions. *Results.* Of the sample, 30.8% reported a diagnosis of hypertension, 79.1% reported daytime shift work, 11.0% reported rotating shift work, and 4.0% reported night shift work. Logistic regression analysis showed that shift work was significantly associated with hypertension among Blacks [OR = 1.35, CI: 1.06–1.72. $P < 0.05$], but not among Whites [OR = 1.01, CI: 0.85–1.20, NS]. Black shift workers sleeping less than 6 hours had significantly increased odds of reporting hypertension [OR = 1.81, CI: 1.29–2.54, $P < 0.01$], while their White counterparts did not [OR = 1.17, CI: 0.90–1.52, NS]. *Conclusions.* Findings suggest that Black Americans working the non-day-shift especially with short sleep duration have increased odds of reporting hypertension.

1. Introduction

Over the past thirty years, various hazards have been associated with working outside the conventional day shift, which is commonly referred to as shift work. Shift work has been linked to gastrointestinal disease [1], metabolic syndrome [2–4], cardiovascular disease [5–10], and cancer [11, 12]. Evidence shows that shift work has detrimental effects on mood, cognitive performance, and family life [13–15]. Additionally, recent studies suggest that circadian disruption caused by shift work may result in impaired glucose metabolism, type II diabetes, and hypertension [4, 16, 17].

Generally, shift workers are at greater risk for cardiovascular disease including obesity [18, 19], diabetes [4, 16, 20], hypertension [17, 21–25], and metabolic syndrome [2, 3, 26–29]. A 10-year follow-up study of Japanese factory workers found that those who were mainly shift workers had higher body mass index (BMI) and total cholesterol than their day shift counterparts [19]. In addition, individuals who switched from day to shift work had on average 1.03 kg/m^2 increased BMI [19]. A similar 14-year cohort study of Japanese male steel workers revealed that rotating shift work was an independent risk factor for increased systolic and diastolic blood pressure [25]. These results are consistent with a prospective cohort study of British workers who were studied over a period of 45 years [29]. Investigators demonstrated that males working the night/early morning shifts tended to have less favorable outcome for waist circumference, body mass index, triglycerides, HDL-C, and Hemoglobin A1C; however, systolic and diastolic blood pressure and total cholesterol were unaffected. By contrast, female workers mainly showed elevated triglyceride levels [29]. It is of interest to ascertain whether these associations are independent of the amount of habitual sleep duration, as shift work is known to result in shorter sleep duration (<6.5 hrs) [30], which is also linked to cardiovascular disease [31, 32].

Relatively little is known concerning ethnicity and its association with shift work and hypertension, an important cardiovascular disease. It is important to examine ethnic effects on such associations because of data suggesting that Black short sleepers may have an increased risk of hypertension [8]. Furthermore, data from the Nurses' Health Study II suggested that Black women on rotating shift schedules had a 46% increased risk of developing hypertension compared with their White counterparts [17]. The purpose of this study was to investigate whether short sleepers (<6 hrs) working the nonday shift were at greater risk of reporting hypertension. We also explored whether associations varied based on individuals' ethnicity.

2. Methods

2.1. Participants. A total of 59,199 Americans (age range: 18–85 years) who participated in the 2010 National Health Interview Survey (NHIS) provided sociodemographic and subjective data as well as data on self-reported chronic conditions for the present analysis. Analysis focused on associations among shift work, short sleep, and hypertension, while examining effects of ethnicity on these associations. Final weights provided by the CDC were applied to all analyses to adjust for the use of complex design in the NHIS. Of the sample, 82.8% were of White ethnicity and 17.2% were of Black ethnicity. Adults of both sexes were represented; 48.5% of the volunteers were men and 51.5% were women.

2.2. Procedures. NHIS is an ongoing, cross-sectional, in-person household interview survey conducted annually by the National Center for Health Statistics of the Centers for Disease Control and Prevention. The NHIS uses a multistage area probability design sampling noninstitutionalized representative of US civilian population. Probability samples of the adult population of all 50 states and the District of Columbia were obtained. The final sample was characterized by a response rate of 90%. Details on sample design can be found in Design and Estimation for the National Health Interview Survey [33].

During face-to-face interviews conducted by trained interviewers from the US Census Bureau, volunteers provided sociodemographic data and information about self-reported chronic conditions. The chronic conditions included hypertension and diabetes. Ethnicity was assessed by the standards recommended by Interagency Committee for the Review of the Racial and Ethnic Standards. Participants responded to the question "which one of these groups would you say BEST represents your race?"

Health risk data included smoking status and alcohol intake. Smoking status was defined as current, former, or never. Alcohol intake was assessed based on the responses to the following questions: "in your entire life, have you had at least 12 drinks of any type of alcoholic beverage?" Respondents who consumed <12 drinks in their entire life were classified as never-drinkers; those who consumed ≥12 drinks in any year or their entire life were classified as drinkers.

Self-reported diseases were defined based on affirmative responses to the following questions: "have you ever been told by a doctor or other health professional that you have [disease or condition]?" Thus, hypertension was defined by an affirmative response to the question: "have you ever been told by a doctor or other health professionals that you had hypertension?" Diabetes was defined by an affirmative response to the question: "other than during pregnancy, have you ever been told that you have diabetes?" Participants also estimated habitual sleep duration (using full hour units, i.e., 5 hours, 6 hours, and 7 hours); no information on specific sleep disorders was elicited during the interview. Habitual short sleep duration was coded as (<6 hours/night), which was referenced to 7-8 hours/night sleepers. Short sleep duration was defined as <6 hrs because this is consistent with a number of previous studies evaluating negative outcomes of short sleep [20, 31, 34–37]. Long sleep duration (>9 hrs) was not included in this study as it is less frequent than short sleep duration among shift workers [32, 35, 38]. Participants were also asked to rate their mood within the last 30 days prior to the interview. Using mood indices (e.g., feeling of sadness, hopelessness, worthlessness, and poor effort), a depression severity score was generated which was a composite score estimated using the K-6 scaling system [39]. Responses were used to generate a score ranging from 0 to 24. Scores ≥13 indicated a greater degree of emotional distress [40].

Surveys were conducted using computer-assisted personal interviewing (CAPI), which utilizes a computer program for data collection that guides the interviewer through the questionnaire. The interviewer enters survey responses directly into the computer. The program determines through a computer algorithm whether data entered by the user match against all possible responses to specific questions; the program also checks for consistency against other data collected during the interview and saves the responses into a survey data file [41].

2.3. Statistical Analysis. Since the NHIS dataset includes data from different samples using a multistage area probability sampling design, all analyses performed in this study were based on weighted statistics using the weights provided with the NHIS dataset. These final weights that accompany the dataset represent a product of weights for corresponding units computed in each of the sampling stages to account for variations in sampling strategies that might affect generalization of final results [41].

Frequency and measures of central tendency were used to describe the sample. In preliminary analyses, Pearson and Spearman correlations were used to explore relationships between variables of interest; only factors showing a P value <0.05 were considered in the final regression model [40]. ANOVA was used for group mean comparisons, and Chi square test was employed to assess differences in categorical variables.

Using multivariate-adjusted logistic regression analyses, we examined associations of shift work (evening, night, or rotating shift work schedules) and short sleep duration with hypertension stratified by ethnicity; stratified analysis was justified by preliminary analysis showing significant interaction between ethnicity and shift work status (Wald = 40.26; $P < 0.01$) and short sleep (Wald = 43.34; $P < 0.01$), even with adjustment for covariates. The first model assessed odds of

Table 1: Baseline data of participants in the 2010 National Health Interview Survey (NHIS).

	Sociodemographic, health risk, and medical characteristics of NHIS participants					
Variable	Whites (SE)	95% (CI) lower	95% (CI) upper	Blacks (SE)	95% (CI) lower	95% (CI) upper
Age (mean)	46.9 (0.2)	46.6	47.4	43.2 (0.4)	42.5	43.9
Female gender (%)	51.0 (0.4)	50.2	51.9	54.8 (0.9)	53.1	56.6
Completed high school (%)	87.7 (0.3)	87.0	88.3	85.0 (0.6)	83.7	86.2
Income > 35 K (%)	68.0 (0.5)	66.9	69.0	50 (1.1)	47.8	52.3
Ever smoked 100 cigs in life (%)	43.0 (0.5)	42.1	43.9	34.4 (0.9)	32.6	36.2
Current drinker (%)	81.8 (0.4)	81.0	82.6	70.4 (0.9)	68.5	72.1
Emotional distress (%)	2.7 (0.1)	2.5	3.0	3.2 (0.3)	2.7	3.9
Diabetes (%)	9.9 (0.2)	9.4	10.4	13.2 (0.5)	12.2	14.2
Hypertension (%)	29.7 (0.4)	29.1	30.5	37.9 (1)	36.1	39.8

SE: standard error, CI: confidence interval.

Table 2: Distribution of work schedules among white and black NHIS participants.

	Work schedules of white and black participants in the 2010 NHIS data					
Variable	Whites (SE)	95% (CI) lower	95% (CI) upper	Blacks (SE)	95% (CI) lower	95% (CI) upper
Regular daytime shift (%)	72.1 (0.5)	71.0	73.2	65.7 (1.2)	63.3	67.9
Regular evening shift (%)	4.9 (0.2)	4.5	5.5	8.0 (0.7)	6.7	9.6
Regular night shift (%)	3.2 (0.2)	2.9	3.6	5.9 (0.6)	4.8	7.1
Rotating shift (%)	9.5 (0.3)	8.8	10.2	13.2 (0.8)	11.7	14.8

SE: standard error, CI: confidence interval.

reporting hypertension among shift workers. The second model determined odds of reporting hypertension among shift workers who were also short sleepers. Covariates entered in the models were gender, age, income, education, tobacco use, alcohol use, emotional distress, and diabetes. BMI was not included as a covariate in the final models, as it was not statistically significant in preliminary univariate analyses. All analyses were performed using SPSS 20.0.

3. Results

Of the sample, 30.8% reported a diagnosis of hypertension, 79.1% reported daytime shift work, 5.9% reported evening shift, 11.0% reported rotating shift, and 4.0 % reported night shift work. Table 1 illustrates the demographic and comorbid characteristics of both White and Black participants. Blacks were more likely to report hypertension compared with their White counterparts (37.9% versus 29.7%). Table 2 illustrates the distribution of work schedules among White and Black participants. Of note, a higher percentage of Blacks worked the night shift (5.9% versus 3.2%) or rotating shift (13.2% versus 9.5%) schedules relative to their White counterparts.

In Table 3, logistic regression analysis shows that shift work was significantly associated with hypertension among Black shift workers, but not among White shift workers. Among White shift workers, age, tobacco use, and diabetes were significantly associated with increased odds of reporting hypertension. Among Black shift workers, male gender, age, alcohol use, and diabetes were associated with increased odds of reporting hypertension.

Table 4 shows results of logistic regression analysis of shift workers who were also classified as short sleepers (<6 hrs), referenced to those sleeping 7-8 hours. Analysis showed that Black shift workers classified as short sleepers had significantly increased odds of reporting hypertension. Analysis showed no significant increases in odds of reporting hypertension among White shift workers.

4. Discussion

The goal of this study was to evaluate whether shift workers who also experience short sleep duration are more likely to report hypertension among Black and White Americans. Our study showed that shift work was only significantly associated with increased odds of reporting hypertension among Black participants, but not among White shift workers. In addition, Black shift workers, reporting short sleep duration, had increased odds of reporting hypertension compared with Black shift workers with healthy sleep duration (7-8 hours). Of interest, these associations were not significant for White participants.

The lack of significant finding among White participants is inconsistent with previous findings especially in the context of European studies, which tend to show increased cardiovascular risk among White shift workers [3, 5, 6, 26, 29, 42–44]. We should note, however, that our findings are consistent with more recent studies regarding increased odds of hypertension among Black shift workers as opposed to White shift workers [17]. These discrepancies could not be explained by differences in sociodemographic and health risk characteristics on the basis of individuals' ethnicity. Logistic regression indicated that age, male gender, and diabetes were all

TABLE 3: Logistic regression analysis showing adjusted odds ratios (OR) and confidence intervals (CI) for hypertension among white (top pane) and black (bottom pane) shift workers.

Likelihood of reporting hypertension among white and black shift workers				
Variable	OR	95% CI lower	95% CI upper	*P*
White shift worker	1.01	0.85	1.20	0.88
Gender	0.83	0.75	0.93	<0.01
Age	1.06	1.06	1.07	<0.01
Income	0.97	0.84	1.12	0.65
Tobacco use	1.26	1.11	1.43	<0.01
Alcohol use	1.26	1.06	1.50	<0.01
Emotional distress	1.67	1.05	2.67	<0.05
Diabetes	3.74	3.10	4.52	<0.01
Variable	OR	95% CI Lower	95% CI Upper	*P*
Black shift worker	1.35	1.06	1.72	<0.05
Gender	1.23	0.97	1.56	0.09
Age	1.08	1.07	1.09	<0.01
Income	0.85	0.65	1.11	0.23
Tobacco use	1.24	0.96	1.60	0.10
Alcohol use	1.48	1.13	1.94	<0.01
Emotional distress	3.07	1.56	6.05	<0.01
Diabetes	6.28	3.99	9.88	<0.01

TABLE 4: Logistic regression analysis indicating adjusted odds ratios (OR) and confidence intervals (CI) for hypertension among white (top pane) and black (bottom pane) shift workers reporting short sleep duration.

Likelihood of reporting hypertension among white and black shift workers reporting short sleep				
Variable	OR	95% CI lower	95% CI upper	*P*
White shift worker with short sleep	1.17	0.90	1.52	0.23
Gender	0.79	0.69	0.91	<0.01
Age	1.06	1.06	1.07	<0.01
Income	0.93	0.77	1.11	0.41
Tobacco use	1.03	1.01	1.05	<0.01
Alcohol use	1.19	0.93	1.52	0.16
Emotional distress	1.52	0.87	2.67	0.14
Diabetes	3.58	2.74	4.67	<0.01
Variable	OR	95% CI lower	95% CI upper	*P*
Black shift worker with short sleep	1.81	1.29	2.54	<0.01
Gender	1.40	1.01	1.94	<0.05
Age	1.09	1.08	1.11	<0.01
Income	0.91	0.64	1.29	0.59
Tobacco use	1.26	0.91	1.75	0.17
Alcohol use	1.79	1.17	2.75	<0.01
Emotional distress	3.55	0.85	14.77	0.08
Diabetes	5.93	3.16	11.11	<0.01

significant contributors to increased odds of reporting hypertension among both White and Black participants. Tobacco use was a significant contributor to increased odds of hypertension in the White participants, and alcohol use was a significant contributor in Black participants. The fact that diabetes was the strongest predictor in our model accords with previous findings suggesting that nonconventional shift work increases the risk of hypertension and diabetes. Indeed, a recent laboratory study, which mimicked the conditions of shift work by combining sleep restriction and circadian rhythm disturbance, resulted in increased postprandial glucose and decreased resting metabolic rate [16]. These findings are consistent with a study of nurses which found a dose dependent relationship between years working on rotating shift and risk of diabetes [4].

Our findings and previous literature suggest a relationship between shift work and short sleep duration with the presence of hypertension. Still a mechanism linking short sleep duration and shift work to hypertension is lacking. One hypothesis postulates that short sleep duration leads to sympathetic activation, which in turn results in high blood pressure [45, 46]. Other theories propose a disturbance in the circadian rhythm as the catalyst for a variety of pathways that lead to hypertension [23, 47–49]. One such study noted that people who work rotating or night shift work tended to display impaired blood pressure dipping at night after just one night shift [50]. Others propose that disturbances in circadian rhythm may lead to impaired endothelial function perhaps via decreased nitric oxide [50] and/or myocyte hypertrophy and fibrosis in animal studies [51]. In healthy men, cortisol secretion is inhibited during the first 4 hours of sleep [52]. A study of textile factory workers found that hair cortisol levels and BMI were increased in shift workers [53]. Disturbances in the circadian rhythm related transcription factor CLOCK affect acetylation of glucocorticoid receptors resulting in increased translation of glucocorticoid receptors and subsequent effects on end organ systems [48]. It is likely that the combination of sympathetic activation, endothelial dysfunction, and increased cortisol activity all contribute to the development of cardiovascular disease in shift workers especially those with short sleep duration.

Our study has notable limitations. First, we relied on subjective report of hypertension, especially diagnosis of hypertension in the past, which could not be verified with objective data. Secondly, we did not have data on subjective sleep disturbance or report of insomnia. Based on the Penn State cohort, those with insomnia and short sleep duration have a higher incidence of hypertension. Poor sleepers without insomnia had a marginal increased hypertension after adjusting for obesity [54]. Also in the Penn State cohort nonobese people, with subjective sleep disturbance, had an increased incidence of obesity [55]. Thirdly, night shift workers and rotating shift workers were categorized as a singular non-day-shift group. Previous work has shown that permanent night shift workers may be exposed to more sleep deprivation and may have different health behaviors like tobacco use, which would affect the risk of hypertension [56, 57]. Fourth, important information was unavailable such as presence of antihypertensive medications and diagnosis of sleep apnea. Additionally, we utilized cross-sectional data; thus, we could not ascertain long-term effects of shift work on hypertension or whether incidence of hypertension would be greater among shift workers. A previous cohort study of Belgian workers found an increased incidence of metabolic syndrome as well as a dose-dependent relationship [27]. Likewise, we could not establish the mechanism by which short sleep duration and shift work influenced hypertension.

Notwithstanding the limitations described above, our study has several strengths. First, we used a population-based representative sample of US adults, which enhanced generalizability of our findings. Many studies in the past have been conducted in relatively homogenous populations in Scandinavia [3, 58, 59] or Asia [22, 23, 25, 60]. Second, we investigated the association between ethnicity and short sleep and hypertension among shift workers, which heretofore has not been undertaken. Future studies should explore those associations among Hispanic and Asian populations as well. Investigations should also include large prospective cohort studies in the US utilizing diverse populations to provide information on incidence of hypertension in shift workers with short sleep duration.

5. Conclusion

Minimizing health risks among shift workers is a daunting challenge, a fact that has captured the attention of national organizations like the Center for Disease Control and Prevention. Our study suggests the need to explore modifiable factors that may compound detrimental effects of shift work and short sleep including alcohol consumption and tobacco use, which are established risk factors for cardiovascular disease among shift workers [42, 61, 62]. One promising intervention in this area is the implementation of workplace smoking cessation programs, which may reduce cardiovascular risk among shift workers. Another target of intervention may involve increased opportunity for healthy sleep duration by maintaining individuals on rotating shifts rather than on permanent night shift, which could mitigate risk of hypertension in shift workers [63, 64]. Improving availability of health food options in the workplace and providing opportunities for physical activity may also prove beneficial, as shift workers tend to eat more energy-dense foods and have less opportunity for physical activity [65]. In sum, a particular focus on reducing identified risk factors among Black short sleepers is of utmost importance since they are more vulnerable to the cardiovascular hazards of shift work.

Acknowledgment

This research was supported by funding from the NIH (R25HL105444, K24HL111315, R01HL095799, and R01MD004113).

References

[1] J. LaDou, "Health effects of shift work," *The Western Journal of Medicine*, vol. 137, no. 6, pp. 525–530, 1982.

[2] B. Karlsson, A. Knutsson, and B. Lindahl, "Is there an association between shift work and having a metabolic syndrome? Results from a population based study of 27,485 people," *Occupational and Environmental Medicine*, vol. 58, no. 11, pp. 747–752, 2001.

[3] B. H. Karlsson, A. K. Knutsson, B. O. Lindahl, and L. S. Alfredsson, "Metabolic disturbances in male workers with rotating three-shift work. Result of the WOLF study," *International*

Archives of Occupational and Environmental Health, vol. 76, no. 6, pp. 424–430, 2003.

[4] A. Pan, E. S. Schernhammer, Q. Sun, and F. B. Hu, "Rotating night shift work and risk of type 2 diabetes: two prospective cohort studies in women," *PLoS Medicine*, vol. 8, no. 12, p. e1001141, 2011.

[5] T. Akerstedt and A. Knutsson, "Cardiovascular disease and shift work," *Scandinavian Journal of Work, Environment & Health*, vol. 23, no. 4, pp. 241–242, 1997.

[6] T. Akerstedt, A. Knutsson, L. Alfredsson, and T. Theorell, "Shift work and cardiovascular disease," *Scandinavian Journal of Work, Environment and Health*, vol. 10, no. 6, pp. 409–414, 1984.

[7] D. L. Brown, D. Feskanich, B. N. Sánchez, K. M. Rexrode, E. S. Schernhammer, and L. D. Lisabeth, "Rotating night shift work and the sisk of ischemic stroke," *American Journal of Epidemiology*, vol. 169, no. 11, pp. 1370–1377, 2009.

[8] K. L. Knutson, E. van Cauter, P. J. Rathouz et al., "Association between sleep and blood pressure in midlife: the CARDIA sleep study," *Archives of Internal Medicine*, vol. 169, no. 11, pp. 1055–1061, 2009.

[9] A. Knutsson, "Shift work and coronary heart disease," *Scandinavian Journal of Social Medicine, Supplement*, vol. 17, no. 44, pp. 1–36, 1989.

[10] A. Knutsson, "Increased risk of ischaemic heart disease in shift workers," *Occupational Medicine (Oxford, England)*, vol. 45, no. 1, p. 55, 1995.

[11] H. A. Kolstad, "Nightshift work and risk of breast cancer and other cancers—a critical review of the epidemiologic evidence," *Scandinavian Journal of Work, Environment and Health*, vol. 34, no. 1, pp. 5–22, 2008.

[12] A. N. Viswanathan, S. E. Hankinson, and E. S. Schernhammer, "Night shift work and the risk of endometrial cancer," *Cancer Research*, vol. 67, no. 21, pp. 10618–10622, 2007.

[13] M. Munakata, S. Ichii, T. Nunokawa et al., "Influence of night shift work on psychologic state and cardiovascular and neuroendocrine responses in healthy nurses," *Hypertension Research*, vol. 24, no. 1, pp. 25–31, 2001.

[14] L. G. P. M. van Amelsvoort, N. W. H. Jansen, G. M. H. Swaen, P. A. van den Brandt, and I. Kant, "Direction of shift rotation among three-shift workers in relation to psychological health and work-family conflict," *Scandinavian Journal of Work, Environment & Health*, vol. 30, no. 2, pp. 149–156, 2004.

[15] C. Vetter, M. Juda, and T. Roenneberg, "The influence of internal time, time awake, and sleep duration on cognitive performance in shiftworkers," *Chronobiology International*, vol. 29, no. 8, pp. 1127–1138, 2012.

[16] O. M. Buxton, S. W. Cain, S. P. O'Connor et al., "Adverse metabolic consequences in humans of prolonged sleep restriction combined with circadian disruption," *Science Translational Medicine*, vol. 4, no. 129, Article ID 129ra43, 2012.

[17] S. J. Lieu, G. C. Curhan, E. S. Schernhammer, and J. P. Forman, "Rotating night shift work and disparate hypertension risk in African-Americans," *Journal of Hypertension*, vol. 30, no. 1, pp. 61–66, 2012.

[18] K. R. Parkes, "Shift work and age as interactive predictors of body mass index among offshore workers," *Scandinavian Journal of Work, Environment and Health*, vol. 28, no. 1, pp. 64–71, 2002.

[19] Y. Morikawa, H. Nakagawa, K. Miura et al., "Effect of shift work on body mass index and metabolic parameters," *Scandinavian Journal of Work, Environment and Health*, vol. 33, no. 1, pp. 45–50, 2007.

[20] F. Zizi, A. Pandey, R. Murrray-Bachmann et al., "Race/ethnicity, sleep duration, and diabetes mellitus: analysis of the national health interview survey," *The American Journal of Medicine*, vol. 125, no. 2, pp. 162–167, 2012.

[21] F. Yamasaki, J. E. Schwartz, L. M. Gerber, K. Warren, and T. G. Pickering, "Impact of shift work and race/ethnicity on the diurnal rhythm of blood pressure and catecholamines," *Hypertension*, vol. 32, no. 3, pp. 417–423, 1998.

[22] Y. Morikawa, H. Nakagawa, K. Miura et al., "Relationship between shift work and onset of hypertension in a cohort of manual workers," *Scandinavian Journal of Work, Environment & Health*, vol. 25, no. 2, pp. 100–104, 1999.

[23] T. Kitamura, K. Onishi, K. Dohi et al., "Circadian rhythm of blood pressure is transformed from a dipper to a non-dipper pattern in shift workers with hypertension," *Journal of Human Hypertension*, vol. 16, no. 3, pp. 193–197, 2002.

[24] M. Tafil-Klawe, J. J. Klawe, P. Złomańczuk, B. Szczepańska, W. Sikorski, and M. Śmietanowski, "Daily changes in cardiac and vascular blood pressure components during breath holding episodes in obstructive sleep apnea patients after day-shift and night-shift work," *Journal of Physiology and Pharmacology*, vol. 58, supplement 5, part 2, pp. 685–690, 2007.

[25] Y. Suwazono, M. Dochi, K. Sakata et al., "Shift work is a risk factor for increased blood pressure in Japanese men: a 14-year historical cohort study," *Hypertension*, vol. 52, no. 3, pp. 581–586, 2008.

[26] M. Ha and J. Park, "Shiftwork and metabolic risk factors of cardiovascular disease," *Journal of Occupational Health*, vol. 47, no. 2, pp. 89–95, 2005.

[27] D. de Bacquer, M. van Risseghem, E. Clays, F. Kittel, G. de Backer, and L. Braeckman, "Rotating shift work and the metabolic syndrome: a prospective study," *International Journal of Epidemiology*, vol. 38, no. 3, pp. 848–854, 2009.

[28] A. Pietroiusti, A. Neri, G. Somma et al., "Incidence of metabolic syndrome among night-shift healthcare workers," *Occupational and Environmental Medicine*, vol. 67, no. 1, pp. 54–57, 2010.

[29] C. Thomas and C. Power, "Shift work and risk factors for cardiovascular disease: a study at age 45 years in the 1958 British birth cohort," *European Journal of Epidemiology*, vol. 25, no. 5, pp. 305–314, 2010.

[30] R. Ursin, V. Baste, and B. E. Moen, "Sleep duration and sleep-related problems in different occupations in the Hordaland Health Study," *Scandinavian Journal of Work, Environment and Health*, vol. 35, no. 3, pp. 193–202, 2009.

[31] J.-K. Choi, M.-Y. Kim, J.-K. Kim et al., "Association between short sleep duration and high incidence of metabolic syndrome in midlife women," *The Tohoku Journal of Experimental Medicine*, vol. 225, no. 3, pp. 187–193, 2011.

[32] M. M. Ohayon, M. H. Smolensky, and T. Roth, "Consequences of shiftworking on sleep duration, sleepiness, and sleep attacks," *Chronobiology International*, vol. 27, no. 3, pp. 575–589, 2010.

[33] S. L. Botman, T. F. Moore, C. L. Moriarity, and V. L. Parsons, "Design and estimation for the National Health Interview Survey, 1995–2004," in *Vital and Health Statistics. Series 2, Data Evaluation and Methods Research*, vol. 130, pp. 1–31, 1995.

[34] D. F. Kripke, L. Garfinkel, D. L. Wingard, M. R. Klauber, and M. R. Marler, "Mortality associated with sleep duration and insomnia," *Archives of General Psychiatry*, vol. 59, no. 2, pp. 131–136, 2002.

[35] G. Liang, E. Schernhammer, L. Qi, X. Gao, I. de Vivo, and J. Han, "Associations between rotating night shifts, sleep duration, and

telomere length in women," *PLoS ONE*, vol. 6, no. 8, Article ID e23462, 2011.

[36] L. Rafalson, R. P. Donahue, S. Stranges et al., "Short sleep duration is associated with the development of impaired fasting glucose: the Western New York health study," *Annals of Epidemiology*, vol. 20, no. 12, pp. 883–889, 2010.

[37] A. N. Vgontzas, D. Liao, S. Pejovic et al., "Insomnia with short sleep duration and mortality: the Penn State cohort," *Sleep*, vol. 33, no. 9, pp. 1159–1164, 2010.

[38] D. I. Tepas and A. B. Carvalhais, "Sleep patterns of shiftworkers," *Occupational Medicine*, vol. 5, no. 2, pp. 199–208, 1990.

[39] R. C. Kessler, P. R. Barker, L. J. Colpe et al., "Screening for serious mental illness in the general population," *Archives of General Psychiatry*, vol. 60, no. 2, pp. 184–189, 2003.

[40] R. C. Kessler, J. G. Green, M. J. Gruber et al., "Screening for serious mental illness in the general population with the K6 screening scale: results from the WHO World Mental Health (WMH) survey initiative," *International Journal of Methods in Psychiatric Research*, vol. 19, supplement 1, pp. 4–22, 2010.

[41] National Center for Health Statistics, "Data file documentation, National Health Interview Survey, 2009 (machine-readable data file and documentation)," National Center for Health Statistics, 2010, http://www.cdc.gov/nchs/nhis.htm.

[42] L. Tenkanen, T. Sjöblom, and M. Härmä, "Joint effect of shift work and adverse life-style factors on the risk of coronary heart disease," *Scandinavian Journal of Work, Environment & Health*, vol. 24, no. 5, pp. 351–357, 1998.

[43] H. Bøggild and A. Knutsson, "Shift work, risk factors and cardiovascular disease," *Scandinavian Journal of Work, Environment and Health*, vol. 25, no. 2, pp. 85–99, 1999.

[44] F. Tüchsen, H. Hannerz, and H. Burr, "A 12 year prospective study of circulatory disease among Danish shift workers," *Occupational and Environmental Medicine*, vol. 63, no. 7, pp. 451–455, 2006.

[45] T. G. Pickering, "Could hypertension be a consequence of the 24/7 society? The effects of sleep deprivation and shift work," *The Journal of Clinical Hypertension*, vol. 8, no. 11, pp. 819–822, 2006.

[46] S. Puttonen, M. Härmä, and C. Hublin, "Shift work and cardiovascular disease—pathways from circadian stress to morbidity," *Scandinavian Journal of Work, Environment and Health*, vol. 36, no. 2, pp. 96–108, 2010.

[47] T. Kino and G. P. Chrousos, "Circadian CLOCK-mediated regulation of target-tissue sensitivity to glucocorticoids: implications for cardiometabolic diseases," *Endocrine Development*, vol. 20, pp. 116–126, 2011.

[48] T. Kino and G. P. Chrousos, "Acetylation-mediated epigenetic regulation of glucocorticoid receptor activity: Circadian rhythm-associated alterations of glucocorticoid actions in target tissues," *Molecular and Cellular Endocrinology*, vol. 336, no. 1-2, pp. 23–30, 2011.

[49] R. Manfredini and F. Portaluppi, "Night shift and impaired endothelial function: circadian out-of-synch may play a role," *International Journal of Cardiology*, vol. 154, no. 1, pp. 94–95, 2012.

[50] W. Kim, H. H. Park, C. S. Park et al., "Impaired endothelial function in medical personnel working sequential night shifts," *International Journal of Cardiology*, vol. 151, no. 3, pp. 377–378, 2011.

[51] T. A. Martino, N. Tata, D. D. Belsham et al., "Disturbed diurnal rhythm alters gene expression and exacerbates cardiovascular disease with rescue by resynchronization," *Hypertension*, vol. 49, no. 5, pp. 1104–1113, 2007.

[52] E. D. Weitzman, J. C. Zimmerman, C. A. Czeisler, and J. Ronda, "Cortisol secretion is inhibited during sleep in normal man," *The Journal of Clinical Endocrinology and Metabolism*, vol. 56, no. 2, pp. 352–358, 1983.

[53] L. Manenschijn, R. G. P. M. van Kruysbergen, F. H. de Jong, J. W. Koper, and E. F. C. van Rossum, "Shift work at young age is associated with elevated long-term cortisol levels and body mass index," *The Journal of Clinical Endocrinology & Metabolism*, vol. 96, no. 11, pp. E1862–E1865, 2011.

[54] J. Fernandez-Mendoza, A. N. Vgontzas, D. Liao et al., "Insomnia with objective short sleep duration and incident hypertension: the Penn State Cohort," *Hypertension*, vol. 60, no. 4, pp. 929–935, 2012.

[55] A. N. Vgontzas, J. Fernandez-Mendoza, T. Miksiewicz et al., "Unveiling the longitudinal association between short sleep duration and the incidence of obesity: the Penn State Cohort," *International Journal of Obesity*, 2013.

[56] K. Nabe-Nielsen, A. H. Garde, F. Tüchsen, A. Hogh, and F. Diderichsen, "Cardiovascular risk factors and primary selection into shift work," *Scandinavian Journal of Work, Environment and Health*, vol. 34, no. 3, pp. 206–212, 2008.

[57] P. Knauth, "Speed and direction of shift rotation," *Journal of Sleep Research*, vol. 4, no. S2, pp. 41–46, 1995.

[58] H. Bøggild, P. Suadicani, H. O. Hein, and F. Gyntelberg, "Shift work, social class, and ischaemic heart disease in middle aged and elderly men; a 22 year follow up in the Copenhagen Male Study," *Occupational and Environmental Medicine*, vol. 56, no. 9, pp. 640–645, 1999.

[59] L. G. P. M. van Amelsvoort, E. G. Schouten, and F. J. Kok, "Impact of one year of shift work on cardiovascular disease risk factors," *Journal of Occupational & Environmental Medicine*, vol. 46, no. 7, pp. 699–706, 2004.

[60] Y. Fujino, H. Iso, A. Tamakoshi et al., "A prospective cohort study of shift work and risk of ischemic heart disease in Japanese male workers," *American Journal of Epidemiology*, vol. 164, no. 2, pp. 128–135, 2006.

[61] D. R. Smith, S. Devine, P. A. Leggat, and T. Ishitake, "Alcohol and tobacco consumption among police officers," *The Kurume Medical Journal*, vol. 52, no. 1-2, pp. 63–65, 2005.

[62] T. Kageyama, T. Kobayashi, N. Nishikido, J. Oga, and M. Kawashima, "Associations of sleep problems and recent life events with smoking behaviors among female staff nurses in Japanese hospitals," *Industrial Health*, vol. 43, no. 1, pp. 133–141, 2005.

[63] M.-H. Chung, T. B. Kuo, N. Hsu, K.-R. Chuo, H. Chu, and C. C. H. Yang, "Comparison of sleep-related cardiac autonomic function between rotating-shift and permanent night-shift workers," *Industrial Health*, vol. 49, no. 5, pp. 589–596, 2011.

[64] K. Viitasalo, E. Kuosma, J. Laitinen, and M. Härmä, "Effects of shift rotation and the flexibility of a shift system on daytime alertness and cardiovascular risk factors," *Scandinavian Journal of Work, Environment and Health*, vol. 34, no. 3, pp. 198–205, 2008.

[65] G. Atkinson, S. Fullick, C. Grindey, and D. Maclaren, "Exercise, energy balance and the shift worker," *Sports Medicine*, vol. 38, no. 8, pp. 671–685, 2008.

7

Prevalence of Primary Hypertension and Risk Factors in Grade XII Learners in KwaZulu-Natal, South Africa

Rajendra Bhimma ,[1] Elaene Naicker,[1] Verena Gounden,[2] Louansha Nandlal,[3] Cathy Connolly,[4] and Sudesh Hariparshad[5]

[1] *Department of Paediatrics and Child Health, Nelson R Mandela School of Medicine, School of Health Science, University of KwaZulu-Natal, Congella, Durban 4013, South Africa*
[2] *Department of Chemical Pathology, University of KwaZulu-Natal and National Health Laboratory Services, Inkosi Albert Luthuli Central Hospital, Durban, South Africa*
[3] *Department of Optics and Imaging, Nelson R Mandela School of Medicine, School of Health Science, University of KwaZulu-Natal, South Africa*
[4] *Department of Biostatistics, School of Public Health, University of KwaZulu-Natal, South Africa*
[5] *Department of Nephrology, Nelson R Mandela School of Medicine, School of Health Science, University of KwaZulu-Natal, Congella, Durban 4013, South Africa*

Correspondence should be addressed to Rajendra Bhimma; bhimma@ukzn.ac.za

Academic Editor: Franco Veglio

Hypertension in childhood leads to hypertension in adult life, the strongest risk factor being obesity. This study determined the prevalence of primary hypertension and its risk factors in Grade XII learners in KwaZulu-Natal, South Africa, from March 2016 to June 2017. Weight, height, body mass index (BMI), random finger prick cholesterol and glucose, and spot urine for an albumin : creatinine ratio were measured. An average of three separate blood pressure readings taken was at least 5 minutes apart. Five hundred and sixty-four learners had weight, height, and BMI; 536 had random blood glucose; and 545 had cholesterol and random spot urine albumin : creatinine ratios measured. Prehypertension was detected in 168 (29.7%) and hypertension in 77 (13.7%) of learners. Ninety (15.9%) were overweight and 75 (13,3%) were obese. Hypercholesterolaemia was present in 58 (10.8%) and a high spot random urine albumin : creatinine ratio in 5 (1.0%). None had a high blood glucose level. Both prehypertension and hypertension in all learners showed a significant increase with increasing BMI. Six (1.0%) learners had metabolic syndrome. Female learners in other racial groups (defined as Indian, mixed race, and White learners), overweight, and obese learners showed significantly higher rates of hypercholesterolaemia. We showed overweight and obesity as risk factors for prehypertension and hypertension. This presages the need for an appropriate diet and adequate exercise in a child's school career.

1. Introduction

Hypertension has over the recent decades become a global health problem [1]. The criteria for hypertension in children and adolescents are complex as it entails correcting for age-, gender-, and height-specific reference values and as such pose a challenge in clinical practice [2]. Thus, both hypertension and prehypertension, though prevalent in childhood and increasing in frequency, remain widely underdiagnosed [3]. The global prevalence of hypertension in children and adolescents has been reported as 1 - 5% [4].

It is well established that hypertension in childhood and adolescence leads to hypertension in adult life and it is an independent risk factor for cardiovascular disease with other risk factors such as hypercholesterolaemia, hypertriglyceridaemia, low high-density lipoprotein cholesterol, truncal (central) obesity, hyperinsulinaemia, and metabolic syndrome [5, 6]. The strongest risk factor for paediatric hypertension is obesity; other factors include a family history of hypertension and male sex [7]. This association between excess weight and hypertension in childhood has been reported in several studies [8]. The prevalence of obesity has been exponentially increasing across both developed and developing countries [9–11]. Sorof *et al.* reported a three times higher prevalence of hypertension in obese compared to nonobese adolescents in a school-based hypertension and obesity screening study [8]. Among all demographic and clinical factors analysed, increasing body mass index (BMI) was the most strongly associated with hypertension.

According to Sorof and colleagues [12] the development of effective strategies to manage primary hypertension in children and adolescents requires an understanding of the condition in site-specific, community, or regional settings as these may have a bearing on modifiable factors such as dietary intake and activity levels. Children who are overweight, born preterm, or small for gestational age and of Black race are at increased risk for developing hypertension [13]. In the developed world, salt intake is generally above the recommended intake among children and a similar trend is seen in the developing world. Although a positive sodium balance is needed for growth in the first year of life, persistence of high salt intake subsequently can have deleterious cardiovascular consequences [14]. This is relevant since blood pressure in childhood tracks into adulthood and high salt intake is often associated with increased consumption of sugar-sweetened beverages (predisposing children to weight gain) [13].

In a previous study undertaken by Bhimma et al. in the central Phoenix Region of KwaZulu-Natal, South Africa in 2012 [15], the prevalence of prehypertension and hypertension among school-going children aged ≥6 to <18 years was estimated to be 2.1% (0.8–3.5%) and 2.6% (1.1–4.1%), respectively, similar to the 3-5% indicated in other reports in the literature globally [12, 15–19]. The risk of high blood pressure was found to rise with an increase in age, weight, height, waist circumference, increased triglyceride levels and heart rate, and family history of high blood pressure and diabetes, as well as suspected substance abuse [15]. A lack of exercise and an increased consumption of soft drinks were further associated with an increased risk for hypertension, which may be related to the increase in BMI associated with these lifestyle factors.

The study by Bhimma et al. was done in a single region (Phoenix) in KwaZulu-Natal in a wide age range of learners (≥6 to <18 years) and risk factors such as biochemical measurements of blood glucose, triglycerides, and high-density lipoprotein cholesterol levels were not reported. Phoenix is predominantly an Indian area and not truly representative of the other regions of KwaZulu-Natal [15]. In the present study, the racial demographics are more representative of the Province and we recruited only Grade XII learners to determine the cumulative effect of the risk factors for hypertension over the schooling years.

The aim of this study was to determine the prevalence of primary hypertension and associated risk factors in Grade XII learners in KwaZulu-Natal, South Africa, using a study sample more representative of the demographics of this Province. It is hoped that this study will help formulate strategies that will provide guidelines to regional health care policy makers on how to curb the imminent epidemic of increasing overweight and obesity and associated hypertension in learners.

2. Materials and Method

This was an observational, cross-sectional study on the prevalence of primary hypertension in Grade XII learners in 15 randomly selected schools from 5 districts in KwaZulu-Natal, South Africa, conducted from March 2016 to June 2017. Age, sex, race, and place of residence were recorded for each learner.

Certified trained nursing staff accompanied by a medically qualified doctor undertook the following biometric measurements: weight (kg) and height (cm). Weight measurements were undertaken with the learner wearing his/her school uniform but without a coat and other items that may increase weight, using a calibrated scale (Salter Salter Ultra Slim Bathroom Scale, Model SS3R®) with measurements in kilograms to one decimal space. Height measurements were done with the learner standing upright on a flat surface against a straight wall without shoes, heels together and the learners heels, buttocks, shoulders, and head touching the vertical wall surface with their line of straight sight aligned horizontally using a soft portable tape and measured to the nearest one centimetre. The tape measure was fixed to a straight wall and calibrated using a one metre ruler to ensure that the height measured using the tape fixed to the wall and the ruler were the same. Internal validation was done by one of the investigators measuring their height at the hospital using a stadiometer and comparing it to the height taken at the site. A single certified trained nurse at each site was allocated to do the height and weight measurements to avoid observer bias, although this could not be totally eliminated between sites. BMI was calculated as weight/height^2 (kg/m^2) and categorized according to the Center for Disease Control and Prevention (CDC) age- and sex-specific growth charts [20]. Learners were classified as normal if the BMI was ≤85th percentile (BMI ≥ 18.5 kg/m^2 and <25 kg/m^2) for age and sex, overweight if the BMI was ≥85th percentile but <95th percentile (BMI ≥ 25 kg/m^2 and <30 kg/m^2), and obese if the BMI was ≥95th percentile (BMI ≥ 30 kg/m^2 and <35 kg/m^2).

All learners also had the following clinical and laboratory assessments done: blood pressure measurements (mmHg), urinary dipsticks analysis, random blood sugar (glucometer reading), random cholesterol, and a random urine albumin: creatinine ratio on a spot urine sample.

Blood pressure measurements were done using an appropriate size cuff with the child at rest and seated upright. The right arm was maintained in a relaxed position and supported with the cubital fossa at the level of the heart. An average of three separate readings taken at least 5 minutes apart was recorded and the definition of hypertension used in this study was based on the Fourth Report on the Diagnosis, Evaluation, and Treatment of High Blood Pressure in Children and Adolescents [21] which states that sustained systolic or diastolic blood pressure measurements should be in the 95th percentile for a respondent to be classified as hypertensive [22]. Systolic and diastolic blood pressures were measured using the oscillometric method, employing an automated blood pressure monitor Edan Model 3® done by the same individual to eliminate operator bias. Recommendations for cuff sizes published by the National High Blood Pressure Education

Working Group on Hypertension control in Children and Adolescents (1996) were followed. The width: length ratio of the inflatable bladder used was at least 1:2 with width covering a minimum of 40% of the arm at a point midway between the olecranon and acromion and length covering 80-100% of the circumference of the arm.

Hypertension is defined by the Forth Report on the Diagnosis, Evaluation, and Treatment of High Blood Pressure in Children and Adolescents which classifies BP as follows: normal if <90th percentile; prehypertension if ≥90th to <95th percentile or >120/80 mmHg in adolescents; Stage 1 HPT if between ≥95th to 99th percentile plus 5 mmHg; Stage 2 HPT if >99th percentile plus 5 mmHg [21].

Biochemical measurements of random blood glucose and random cholesterol levels were made by fingerpick testing using the Accutrend Plus Cobas® machine (Roche Diagnostics®, Germany). Hyperglycaemia was defined as a random glucometer reading >11.1 mmol/l of blood glucose and hypercholesterolaemia as a random cholesterol level ≥4.6 mmol/l [23].

A fresh spot random clean-catch midstream sample of urine collected in a sterile urine collector was used for measurement of albumin: creatinine ratio and urinary dipsticks analysis. Urinary dipsticks analysis was done using Combur 9 Test® dipsticks (Cobas, Roche Diagnostics®) according to the manufacture's specifications. Measurement for albumin: creatinine ratio was undertaken at the National Health Laboratory Services on the Advia 1800 Chemistry Analyser® (Siemens, Tarrytown, NY) at the Inkosi Albert Luthuli Central Hospital. For males a random spot urine albumin: creatinine ratio in the range 2.5-25 mg/mmol was defined as normal. Greater than this range was considered as frank proteinuria. For females, the normal range was 3.5-35 mg/mmol and greater than this range was defined as frank proteinuria. Metabolic syndrome was defined by three metabolic abnormalities including three of the following: obesity, hypertension, high random cholesterol, or hyperglycaemia [23].

The measurements were all done at the schools using a suitable venue that was allocated by the school Principal. The basic science students were involved in setting up and assisting the students with the completion of the questionnaires. All equipment and staff were transported to the sites. All measurements were made by a single observer at each site to eliminate interobserver error. At the time of data collection if a value for any of the parameters measured was abnormal, the staff alerted the doctor on site who gave the learner a referral letter to a health care centre stating the problem. This was done following a private discussion with the student and with their full consent. Learners diagnosed with hypertension, hypercholesterolaemia, or high blood sugar were referred to the nearest health care centre for further evaluation and appropriate treatment. Overweight and obese learners with normotension were referred to the dietetics department of their local hospitals or Inkosi Albert Luthuli Central Hospital. Inclusion criteria for the study were all available Grade XII learners from randomly selected schools in KwaZulu-Natal whose parents gave written informed consent and who assented to participate in the study. Exclusion criteria were failure to obtain consent and/or assent to participate in the study, learners with known chronic diseases such as chronic kidney disease, heart disease, and diabetes that were likely to be a known secondary cause of hypertension.

2.1. Data Collection. The study team is comprised of nurses and doctors from the Nephrology Units (adult and paediatric) at the Inkosi Albert Luthuli Central Hospital who volunteered to undertake the study as part of their commitment to the World Kidney Day (Theme: "Kidney Disease & Children. Act Early to Prevent It!") commemorated on the 10 March 2016. In addition, medically trained staff (nurses and doctors) working in peripheral hospitals, private hospital in the Durban Functional Region and basic science students undertaking their Masters in Science degree from the University of KwaZulu-Natal, School of Laboratory Medicine, volunteered their services. All data were collected on a data sheet and given a case number. No identifiers were used so that the data was totally anonymous. Information was captured on an Excel password protected spread sheet using Microsoft Office version 10® and transported into an SPSS® statistical package for further statistical analysis.

2.2. Statistical Analysis

2.2.1. Sample Size. The requisite sample size was determined using an estimation of population size in the area, with a minimum representative sample taken from each school. A sample size of 316 was required to estimate the level of hypertension in school children to within 5% with a probability of 95% and assuming an estimate of 10% hypertension in the population. Since schools were the sampling unit, a design factor of 1.5 was used to adjust for the correlation within schools which increased the sample size to 474. The sample size was also increased by 15% to account for incomplete data and consent refusal. Thus, the total sample size required for this study was 560 children.

Statistical analysis was performed using the IBM SPSS Statistics® software package. Histograms and box-whisker plots were used to visually assess data distributions and check for outliers. The Kolmogorov-Smirnov test was used to assess whether the distributions differ from normal distribution. Nonparametric statistics was used to describe and test associations for variables with significantly skewed data, whereas parametric and summary statistics were used for variables that conform to normal distribution. Comparisons were made between hypertensive and nonhypertensive groups using the 2 χ^2 test in case of categorical variables. Continuous variables were summarized as a mean ± standard deviation (SD), and comparisons among the groups were based on the Student t-test. Differences were considered statistically significant when $p < 0.05$. Statistical differences were also sought for blood pressure in subjects who were overweight or obese versus those that were normal.

2.2.2. Ethical Considerations. Permission to conduct this study was obtained from the Provincial Department of Health and Provincial Department of Basic Education. The school Principal was informed and permission obtained prior to

Table 1: Stratification of hypertension by gender, race, and body mass index.

	Normotensive	Prehypertensive				Hypertensive			
	n (%)	n (%)	OR	95% CI	p value	n (%)	OR	95% CI	p value
Total	319 (56.6)	168 (29.8)				77 (13.6)			
Gender									
Male	97 (47.6)	73 (35.8)	1,8	(1.2 - 2.6)	0,004	34 (16.7)	1,8	(1.1 - 3.0)	0,02
Female	222 (61.7)	95 (26.4)				43 (11.9)			
Race									
Black	275 (57.8)	144 (30.2)				57 (12.0)			
Other racial groups	44 (50.0)	24 (27.3)	1,0	(0.6 - 1.8)	0,9	20 (22.7)	2,2	(1.2 - 4.0)	0,01
BMI									
Normal	256 (64.2)	105 (26.3)				38 (9.5)			
Overweight	43 (47.8)	32 (35.6)	1,8	(1.1-3.0)	0,02	15 (16.7)	2,4	(1.2-4.6)	0,01
Obese	20 (26.7)	31 (41.3)	3,8	(2.1-6.9)	<0.001	24 (32.0)	8,0	(4.1-16.0)	<0.001

BMI: body mass index.
Other racial groups: comprised of South African, Indian, White, and mixed race.
OR: odds ratio.
CI: confidence interval.

study commencement to undertake the study on school premises. Ethical approval to conduct the study was obtained from the Biomedical Research Ethics Committee of the University of KwaZulu-Natal (BE032/16). Written informed consent was obtained from parents or legal guardians. This was achieved by learners at each site being briefed at least two weeks prior to data collection with a study information sheet and consent forms attached given to learners to hand over to their parents or legal guardian. In addition, all learners had to have a signed assent form before participation in the study.

3. Results

A total of 575 learners were willing to participate and present at school on the day of the study. All learners had a detailed history taken by the medical officer on site to exclude any chronic diseases that may result in the development of secondary hypertension. Eleven parents refused consent and these learners were excluded. Complete data for height, weight, BMI, and blood pressure was obtained in 564 learners that were included in the study (Figure 1). Random glucose and cholesterol were measured in 536 learners as 28 refused to have finger prick bloods done and spot urinary albumin: creatinine ratios were measured in 545 learners as the urine from 19 learners unfortunately leaked in transit to the laboratory. All learners were of South African nationality, White. Given the small numbers of learners in each of the racial groups other than Black Africans, Indian, mixed race, and White learners were grouped together as other race groups giving a total of 88 (15,6%) learners in this collective group (Figure 1). The mean age of learners was 17.8 ± 1.1 years with a range of 16.2 – 21.7 years.

The mean height of the learners was 1.72 ± 0.12 metres (range 1.62-1.83) for males and 1.61 ± 0.22 metres (range 1.52 – 1.74). One hundred and thirty-one (23.2%) learners were <5th percentile for age-for-height based on the Center for Disease Control and Prevention (CDC) age-and-sex specific growth charts [20].

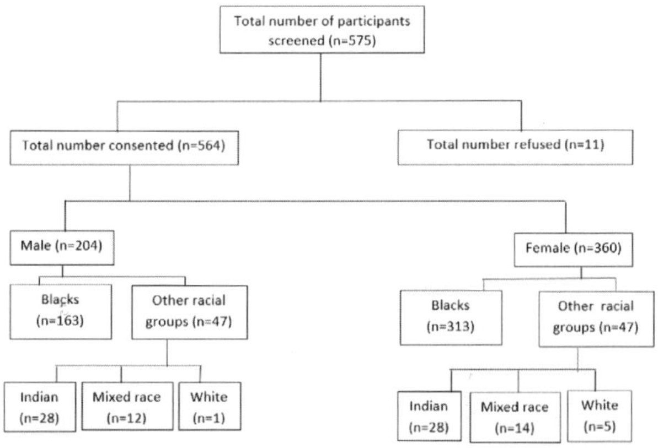

Figure 1: Study population of Grade XII learners from 15 schools in 5 different districts in KwaZulu-Natal.

Prehypertension was detected in 168 (29.7%) and hypertension in 77 (13.7%) of learners. The rates of elevated blood pressure (prehypertension and hypertension combined) in males and females were 52.5% and 38.3%, respectively. Males were more significantly likely to be prehypertensive compared to females (35.8% versus 26.4%, OR: 1.8, 95%CI: 1.2-2.6, $p < 0.004$), and also more likely to be hypertensive (16.7% versus 11.9%, OR: 1.8, 95% CI: 1.1-3.3, $p < 0.02$) (Table 1). On comparing Black African learners to other racial groups, there was no statistically significant difference with prehypertension in both groups. However, learners in the other racial groups were more likely to be hypertensive compared to Black African learners (22.7% versus 12.9%, OR: 2.2 95% CI: 1.2-4.0, $p < 0.01$). Thus, hypertension was significantly associated with race and sex (Table 1). None of the learners had a history of taking antihypertensive medication or had a previous diagnosis of hypertension.

The mean weight was 61.62 ± 14.64 kilograms (range 32.14-140.32). Fifty-four (9.6%) of learners were <5th percentile and 61 (10.8%) were >95 percentile for age-and

TABLE 2: Stratification of hypertension by body mass index, sex, and race.

		Normotensive	Prehypertensive				Hypertensive			
		n (%)	n (%)	OR	95% CI	p value	n (%)	OR	95% CI	p value
Black African[1]	BMI	275 (57.8)	144 (30.3)				57 (12.0)			
	Normal	224 (64.7)	90 (26.0)				32 (9.3)			
	Overweight	35 (52.2)	24 (35.8)	1.7	1.0-3.0	0.07	8 (11.9)	1.6	0.7-3.7	0.3
	Obese	16 (25.4)	30 (47.6)	4.7	2.4-9.0	<0.001	17 (27.0)	7.4	3.4-16.2	<0.001
Males	BMI	97 (47.6)	73 (35.8)				34 (16.7)			
	Normal	81 (51.9)	56 (35.9)				19 (12.2)			
	Overweight	10 (35.7)	11 (39.3)	1.6	0.6-4.0	0.3	7 (25.0)	3.0	1.0-8.9	0.049
	Obese	6 (30.0)	6 (60.0)	1.4	0.4-4.7	0.5	8 (40.0)	5.7	1.8-18.3	0.004
Females	BMI	222 (61.7)	95 (26.4)				43 (11.9)			
	Normal	175 (72.0)	49 (20.2)				19 (7.8)			
	Overweight	33 (53.2)	21 (33.9)	2.3	1.2-4.3	0	8 (12.9)	2.2	0.9-5.5	0.02
	Obese	14 (25.5)	25 (45.5)	6.4	3.1-13.2	<0.001	16 (29.1)	10.5	4.5-24.9	<0.001

OR: odds ratio.
CI: confidence interval.
[1]Other racial groups not included because of the small sample size.

sex-specific weight. Three-hundred and ninety-nine (70.7%) had a normal BMI, 90 (15.9%) were overweight, and 75 (13.3%) were classified as obese. None had a BMI >35 kg/m^2. Females were more likely to be overweight than males (OR: 1.4, 95%CI: 1.9-2.3, $p < 0.02$) and also more likely to be obese (OR: 1.8, 95% CI: 1.0-3.1, $p < 0.04$). On comparing Black African learners to those from other racial groups, the latter group was more likely to be overweight (OR: 2.2, 95% CI: 1.3-3.9, $p < 0.004$); however there were similar rates of obesity in both groups (OR: 1.2, CI 0.6-2.5, $p < 0.5$) (Table 1).

Both prehypertension and hypertension in all learners were associated with significantly higher BMI (Table 1). Prehypertension was 26.3% in learners with a normal BMI; 35.6% in those that were overweight; and 41.3% in obese learners (OR: 1.8, 95% CI 1.1-.30, $p < 0.02$ and OR: 3.7, 95% CI: 2.0-6.9, $p < 0.001$), respectively. Hypertension was 9.5% in learners with normal BMI; 16.7% in learners that were overweight; and 32.0% in obese learners (OR: 2.4, 95%CI: 1.2-4.6, $p < 0.01$ and OR: 8.1, 95% CI: 4.1-16.0, $p < 0.001$), respectively.

When stratified for race, there was no association of prehypertension or hypertension in Black African learners who were overweight when compared to those with normal BMI (OR: 1.6, 95% CI: 0.7-3.7, $p > 0.07$). However, both prehypertension and hypertension in Black African learners were significantly associated with obesity (OR: 4.7, 95% CI: 2.4-9.0, $p < 0.001$; OR: 7.4, 95% CI: 2.4-9.0, $p < 0.001$), respectively (Table 2). In learners in other racial groups, only hypertension was significantly associated with overweight (OR: 4.7, 95% CI 1.2-17.8, $p < 0.02$) and obesity (OR: 9.3, 95% CI: 2.1-42.1, $p < 0.004$). However, given the small numbers of learners in this group, the results must be treated with reserve. When hypertension and BMI were stratified by sex, both hypertension and hypertension were associated with overweight and obesity in females. However, in males only hypertension was associated with overweight and obesity (Table 2).

Hypercholesterolaemia was present in 58 (10.8%) of 536 learners. Thirty-four (6.3%) of learners with hypercholesterolaemia had normal blood pressure, 11 (2.1%) prehypertension, and 13 (2.4%) hypertension. Female learners in the other racial groups and overweight and obese learners showed an association with hypercholesterolaemia (Table 3). Only 6 (1.0%) of the 559 learners had all necessary criteria for the metabolic syndrome. There was no significant association when adjusted for race or sex.

Only 5 (1.0%) of 545 learners tested had a spot random urine albumin: creatinine ratio that was high. There was no significant association between learners with a high albumin: creatinine ratio and prehypertension or hypertension, sex, race, or BMI. Also, none of the learners had an abnormal blood glucose level.

Hypercholesterolaemia, random blood glucose, and spot urine albumin: creatinine ratios showed no signs of associated risk with hypertension.

4. Discussion

In our study, we found a high rate of prehypertension (29.7%) and hypertension (13.7%) in Grade XII learners in KwaZulu-Natal, South Africa. This is much higher than a report in a previous study undertaken by Bhimma et al. in the central Phoenix Region of KwaZulu-Natal, South Africa, in 2012; the prevalence of prehypertension and hypertension among school-going children aged ≥6 to <18 years was estimated to be 2.1% and 2.6%, respectively [15]. However in a study undertaken in grades 11 and 12 (i.e., pre- and matriculation years) in 10 schools (nine public schools and one private school) in nine provinces in South Africa over a ±9–10-year period, with more than 96% of learners being Black African, and mostly from penurious backgrounds, hypertension was reported in 12% of females and 16% of males [24], very similar to the findings in our study. Rates of hypertension in

Table 3: Stratification of cholesterol by hypertension, sex, race, and BMI.

	Cholesterol (n = 536) (missing = 28)					
	Normal (<4.5)		Abnormal (>=4.5)		Total	p value
	n	%	n	%	n	
Cholesterol	478	89%	58	11%	536	
Hypertension						
Both normal	269	89%	34	11%	303	0,06
Prehypertensive	146	93%	11	7%	157	
Hypertensive	63	83%	13	17%	76	
Sex						
Male	186	93%	13	7%	199	0,01
Female	292	87%	45	13%	337	
Race						
African	414	92%	34	8%	448	<0.001
Other racial groups	64	73%	24	27%	88	
BMI						
Normal	348	93%	28	7%	376	< 0.001
Overweight	73	83%	15	17%	88	
Obese	57	79%	15	21%	72	

Other racial groups: comprised of South African, Indian, White, and mixed race.

sub-Saharan Africa have been noted to be increasing among adults [25–27].

Detection of hypertension in children is important as it has been shown to have potentially severe consequences such as target organ damage including left ventricular hypertrophy, kidney damage and progression of chronic kidney disease, accelerated pathological vascular changes, and subtle neurological effects like reduced cognitive function [28, 29]. Whilst no long-term cohort studiers have directly linked hypertension in childhood to cardiovascular events in adults, it is well known that hypertension in childhood and adolescents tracks hypertension into adulthood [30].

Our study also found 15.9% of Grade XII learners to be overweight and 13.3% to be obese with females and learners from other racial groups being more likely to be overweight or obese. These findings are in line with other data from South Africa [31–33]. Previous studies have shown that the strongest risk factor for hypertension in childhood is obesity, male sex, and a family history of hypertension [7, 34]. These findings are supported by our study in which we showed overweight and obese learners to be more likely to be both prehypertensive and hypertensive compared to learners with normal weights as determined by BMI. Also, we showed that males were more likely to be both prehypertensive and hypertensive compared to female learners.

In adults, the rising rate of hypertension in sub-Saharan Africa has been associated with the rising rates of obesity, particularly in urban areas [10, 11]. These high rates of obesity-associated hypertension are probably due to the epidemiological transition to a more Westernised lifestyle with increased television viewing, Internet surfing and smart phones games, and other applications, leading to a more sedentary lifestyle, as well as dietary habits consisting of mainly processed foods. Indeed, a high consumption of energy-dense diets and a sedentary lifestyle account for the increasing burden of overweight and obesity in urban settings and now have also infiltrated into less developed areas [35]. There is substantial evidence that the risk of noncommunicable diseases such as coronary heart disease, ischaemic stroke, and type 2 diabetes mellitus increases steadily with increasing BMI [36].

The increasing prevalence of obesity is projected to increase worldwide to 50% and 60% by 2030 and 2050, respectively [37]. Although rates of hypertension are less clear, increasing BMI has been consistently associated with rising blood pressure throughout childhood [38–40]. This strong association of obesity-associated hypertension in less developed countries portends that these nations face similar difficulties to developed nations in overcoming lifestyle choices in combating obesity and hypertension.

In our study, there was no association of race on the rates of prehypertension in Grade XII learners. However, learners classified as belonging to other racial groups were more likely to be hypertensive compared to Black African learners (22.7% versus 12.0%, $p < 0.01$). This high risk for hypertension among minority groups (excluding Asians) has been demonstrated in several other studies [18, 41–43]. Our study had very few White learners and no Hispanic learners.

To help formulate strategies that will provide guidelines to regional health care policy makers submissions will also be made to the Department of Education and Department of Health to advise health care teams to do routine health screening in all learners, including blood pressure measurements. In addition, to sensitize health care workers to this looming epidemic, the data will be presented at local and international congresses, placed on hospital websites, as well as submitted to the lay press.

5. Study Limitations

This study has some limitations. Firstly, the criteria for the definition of hypertension in children are arbitrary and to a certain extent artificial. We used normative data from blood pressure in children and adolescents based on the Fourth Report on the Diagnosis, Evaluation, and Treatment of High Blood Pressure in Children and Adolescents [21]. Whether these normative data are applicable to children and adolescents in other parts of the world or to different ethnic backgrounds is unknown. Secondly, the numbers of Grade XII learners in the category other racial groups were relatively small (88 learners) and therefore comparisons may not have been sufficiently powered to show significant differences. Thirdly, in common with other studies [11, 44, 45], we used the average of three blood pressure measurements at a single visit taken at least five minutes apart with the leaner at rest. Ideally for the diagnosis of hypertension, blood pressure should be measured on at least three separate occasions with sustained systolic or diastolic blood pressure measurements above the 95th percentile for a respondent to be classified as hypertensive [21]. It is possible that the prevalence of hypertension would have been lower where these criteria were used to determine hypertension [46]. Fourthly we used BMI as the sole measure of obesity as in other reports [11, 12, 47, 48]. For more specific assessment of fat mass, other measurements estimating adiposity such as waist circumference, bioelectrical impedance, and MRI can be used. However for population-based studies, BMI correlates well with these other measures and remains widely used as a definition of obesity in hypertension research [11, 12, 47, 48]. Fifthly we were not able to accurately document levels of physical activity and substance abuse and consumption of processed food, all of which are variables indicative of hypertensive risk. Sixthly we could not accurately document the role of family history in our learners as many were unsure of the parents' blood pressure status and in many instances, parents failed to disclose their illnesses on the questionnaire form.

6. Conclusion

Our study showed a high prevalence of overweight and obesity as risk factors to prehypertension and hypertension in Grade XII learners in KwaZulu-Natal. To overcome this health care professionals, health authorities, and governments will need to educate learners on major lifestyle changes including *inter alia* improved dietary habits, doing more exercise with increased participation in sports, and encouraging to desist from smoking and others such unsavoury habits.

Acknowledgments

The authors thank Sanofi Genzyme for a donation of R20000 towards funding the study; the medical managers of the various hospitals for allowing medical and nursing staff time off to participate in data collection; Siemens Diagnostics for donating reagents for analysis of urine microalbumin and creatinine; and Roche and Astellas for sponsoring some of the equipment and meals for the participants. The authors would also like to thank the support staff of the Inkosi Albert Luthuli Hospital for their assistance in conducting the study.

References

[1] P. B. Balagopal, S. D. de Ferranti, S. Cook et al., "Nontraditional risk factors and biomarkers for cardiovascular disease: mechanistic, research, and clinical considerations for youth: a scientific statement from the american heart association," *Circulation*, vol. 123, no. 23, pp. 2749–2769, 2011.

[2] M. L. Hansen, P. W. Gunn, and D. C. Kaelber, "Underdiagnosis of hypertension in children and adolescents," *Journal of the American Medical Association*, vol. 298, no. 8, pp. 874–879, 2007.

[3] R. J. Cunningham 3rd., "Is pediatric hypertension underdiagnosed?" *Nature Clinical Practice. Cardiovascular Medicine*, vol. 5, no. 3, pp. 128-129, 2008.

[4] B. Falkner, "Hypertension in children and adolescents: epidemiology and natural history," *Pediatric Nephrology*, vol. 25, no. 7, pp. 1219–1224, 2010.

[5] S. Cook, M. Weitzman, P. Auinger, M. Nguyen, and W. H. Dietz, "Prevalence of a metabolic syndrome phenotype in adolescents: findings from the Third National Health and Nutrition Examination Survey, 1988–1994," *JAMA Pediatrics*, vol. 157, no. 8, pp. 821–827, 2003.

[6] C. L. Williams, L. L. Hayman, S. R. Daniels et al., "Cardiovascular health in childhood: a statement for health professionals from the Committee on Atherosclerosis, Hypertension, and Obesity in the Young (AHOY) of the Council on Cardiovascular Disease in the Young, American Heart Association," *Circulation*, vol. 106, no. 1, pp. 143–160, 2002.

[7] V. A. Moyer, "Screening for primary hypertension in children and adolescents: U.s. Preventive services task force recommendation statement," *Pediatrics*, vol. 132, no. 5, pp. 907–914, 2013.

[8] J. Sorof and S. Daniels, "Obesity hypertension in children: a problem of epidemic proportions," *Hypertension*, vol. 40, no. 4, pp. 441–447, 2002.

[9] A. M. Cali and S. Caprio, "Obesity in children and adolescents," *The Journal of Clinical ndocrinology & Metabolism*, vol. 93, no. 1, pp. 31–36, 2008.

[10] R. BeLue, T. A. Okoror, J. Iwelunmor et al., "An overview of cardiovascular risk factor burden in sub-Saharan African countries: a socio-cultural perspective," *Globalization and Health*, vol. 5, article 10, 2009.

[11] Z. Salman, G. D. Kirk, and M. D. Deboer, "High rate of obesity-associated hypertension among primary schoolchildren in Sudan," *International Journal of Hypertension*, vol. 2011, 2011.

[12] J. M. Sorof, D. Lai, J. Turner, T. Poffenbarger, and R. J. Portman, "Overweight, ethnicity, and the prevalence of hypertension in school-aged children," *Pediatrics*, vol. 113, no. 3, pp. 475–482, 2004.

[13] S. A. G. Lava, M. G. Bianchetti, and G. D. Simonetti, "Salt intake in children and its consequences on blood pressure," *Pediatric Nephrology*, vol. 30, no. 9, pp. 1389–1396, 2015.

[14] I. J. Brwon, I. Tzoulaki, V. Candeias, and P. Elliot, "Salt intakes around the world: implications for public health," *International Journal of Epidemiology*, vol. 38, pp. 791–813, 2009.

[15] R. Bhimma, M. Pillay, D. P. Naidoo et al., "Hypertension prevalence and risk factors in children and adolescents of school-going age in the Phoenix Area, Durban, South Africa," *Pediatric nephrology*, 2014.

[16] M. Antal, A. Regöly-Mérei, K. Nagy et al., "Representative study for the evaluation of age- and gender-specific anthropometric parameters and blood pressure in an adolescent Hungarian population," *Annals of Nutrition and Metabolism*, vol. 48, no. 5, pp. 307–313, 2004.

[17] E. Saleh, *Hypertension and its determinants among primary-school children in Kuwait: an epidemiological study*, 2000.

[18] R. Din-Dzietham, Y. Liu, M.-V. Bielo, and F. Shamsa, "High blood pressure trends in children and adolescents in national surveys, 1963 to 2002," *Circulation*, vol. 116, no. 13, pp. 1488–1496, 2007.

[19] P. Kardas, M. Kufelnicka, D. Herczyński, and K. Kawecka-Jaszcz, "Prevalence of arterial hypertension in children aged 9-14 years, residents of the city of Łódź," *Kardiologia Polska* 62, no. 3, pp. 211–217, 2005.

[20] C. L. Ogden, "Defining overweight in children using growth charts.," *Maryland medicine : MM : a publication of MEDCHI, the Maryland State Medical Society*, vol. 5, no. 3, pp. 19–21, 2004.

[21] B. Falkner, S. R. Daniels, J. T. Flynn et al., "The fourth report on the diagnosis, evaluation, and treatment of high blood pressure in children and adolescents," *Pediatrics*, vol. 114, no. 2, pp. 555–576, 2004.

[22] D. Batisky, "Blood pressure variability, prehypertension, and hypertension in adolescents," *Adolescent Health, Medicine, and Therapeutics*, p. 43.

[23] "National High Blood Pressure Education Program Working Group Report on Hypertension in the Elderly. National High Blood Pressure Education Program Working Group," *Hypertension*, vol. 23, no. 3, pp. 275–285, 1994.

[24] A. S. Carr and D. Elliot, "Otorhinolaryngology: Anesthesic Considerations," in *Pediatric Anesthesia Basic Principles-State of Art-Future*, B. Bissonnette, Ed., p. 1707, PMPH-USA, 1st edition, 2011.

[25] J. Addo, L. Smeeth, and D. A. Leon, "Hypertension in sub-Saharan Africa: a systematic review," *Journal of Hypertension* vol. 50, no. 6, pp. 1012–1018, 2007.

[26] Y. K. Seedat, "Recommendations for hypertension in sub-Saharan Africa," *Cardiovascular Journal of Africa*, vol. 15, no. 4, pp. 157-158, 2004.

[27] H. H. Vorster, "The emergence of cardiovascular disease during urbanisation of Africans," *Public Health Nutrition*, vol. 5, no. 1A, pp. 239–243, 2002.

[28] M. B. Lande, H. Adams, B. Falkner et al., "Parental Assessments of Internalizing and Externalizing Behavior and Executive Function in Children with Primary Hypertension," *Journal of Pediatrics*, vol. 154, no. 2, pp. 207–e1, 2009.

[29] C. M. Gallibois, N. A. Jawa, and D. G. Noone, "Hypertension in pediatric patients with chronic kidney disease: Management challenges," *International Journal of Nephrology and Renovascular Disease*, vol. 10, pp. 205–213, 2017.

[30] American Academy of Pediatrics, "National high blood pressure education program working group on high blood pressure in children and adolescents," *Pediatrics*, vol. 114, no. 2, 2004.

[31] M. E. G. Armstrong, M. I. Lambert, K. A. Sharwood, and E. V. Lambert, "Obesity and overweight in South African primary school children—the health of the nation study," *South African Medical Journal*, vol. 96, no. 5, pp. 439–444, 2006.

[32] S. P. Reddy, K. Resnicow, S. James, N. Kambaran, R. Omardien, and A. D. MBewu, "Underweight, overweight and obesity among South African adolescents: Results of the 2002 National Youth Risk Behaviour Survey," *Public Health Nutrition*, vol. 12, no. 2, pp. 203–207, 2009.

[33] J. Mukuddem-Petersen and H. Salome Kruger, "Association between stunting and overweight among 10-15-y-old children in the North West Province of South Africa: The THUSA BANA Study," *International Journal of Obesity*, vol. 28, no. 7, pp. 842–851, 2004.

[34] B. Aliarzadeh, C. Meaney, R. Moineddin et al., "Hypertension screening and follow-up in children and adolescents in a Canadian primary care population sample: a retrospective cohort study," *CMAJ Open*, vol. 4, no. 2, pp. E230–E235, 2016.

[35] Y. Tebekaw, C. Teller, and U. Colón-Ramos, "The burden of underweight and overweight among women in Addis Ababa, Ethiopia," *BMC Public Health*, vol. 14, no. 1, article no. 1126, 2014.

[36] "Global, W.H.O.O.S.a.t. and H.O.G. data. World Health Organization. Obesity. Situation and trends," http://www.who.int/gho/ncd/risk_factors/obesity_text/en/.

[37] "Africa, A.D.B.U.i. African Development Bank. Urbanization in Africa, 2012," https://www.afdb.org/en/blogs/afdbchampioning-inclusive-growth-across-africa/post/urbanization-in-africa-10143/.

[38] J. T. Flynn, "Pediatric hypertension: Recent trends and accomplishments, future challenges," *American Journal of Hypertension*, vol. 21, no. 6, pp. 605–612, 2008.

[39] R. Lauer, L. A. Barnes, R. Clark et al., "Highlights of the report of the expert panel on blood cholesterol levels in children and adolescents," *American Family Physician*, vol. 45, no. 5, pp. 2127–2136, 1992.

[40] R. V. Luepker, D. R. Jacobs, R. J. Prineas, and A. R. Sinaiko, "Secular trends of blood pressure and body size in a multi-ethnic adolescent population: 1986 to 1996," *Journal of Pediatrics*, vol. 134, no. 6, pp. 668–674, 1999.

[41] L. Chen, N. Simonsen, and L. Liu, "Racial differences of pediatric hypertension in relation to birth weight and body size in the United States," *PLoS ONE*, vol. 10, no. 7, Article ID e0132606, 2015.

[42] P. Muntner, A. Arshad, S. A. Morse et al., "End-stage renal disease in young black males in a black-white population: Longitudinal analysis of the Bogalusa Heart Study," *BMC Nephrology*, vol. 10, no. 1, article no. 40, 2009.

[43] A. W. Voors, T. A. Foster, R. R. Frerichs, L. S. Webber, and G. S. Berenson, "Studies of blood pressures in children, ages 5 to 14 years, in a total biracial community. The Bogalusa heart study," *Circulation*, vol. 54, no. 2, pp. 319–327, 1976.

[44] C. Agyemang, W. K. Redekop, E. Owusu-Dabo, and M. A. Bruijnzeels, "Blood pressure patterns in rural, semi-urban and urban children in the Ashanti region of Ghana, West Africa," *BMC Public Health*, vol. 5, article no. 114, 2005.

[45] W. E. Moore, J. E. Eichner, E. M. Cohn, D. M. Thompson, C. E. Kobza, and K. E. Abbott, "Blood pressure screening of school children in a multiracial school district: The healthy kids project," *American Journal of Hypertension*, vol. 22, no. 4, pp. 351–356, 2009.

[46] A. Chiolero, F. Cachat, M. Burnier, F. Paccaud, and P. Bovet, "Prevalence of hypertension in schoolchildren based on repeated measurements and association with overweight," *Journal of Hypertension*, vol. 25, no. 11, pp. 2209–2217, 2007.

8

Sociodemographic Characteristics, Dietary Practices, and Nutritional Status of Adults with Hypertension in a Semi-Rural Community in the Eastern Region of Ghana

Esi K. Colecraft,[1] **Matilda Asante**,[2] **Aaron K. Christian**,[3] **and Seth Adu-Afarwuah**[1]

[1]*Department of Nutrition and Food Science, University of Ghana, P.O. Box LG 134, Legon, Accra, Ghana*
[2]*Department of Dietetics, School of Biomedical and Allied Health Sciences, College of Health Sciences, University of Ghana, Accra, Ghana*
[3]*Regional Institute for Population Studies, University of Ghana, Legon, Ghana*

Correspondence should be addressed to Esi K. Colecraft; colecraft_s@hotmail.com

Academic Editor: Tomohiro Katsuya

Introduction. Hypertension is a major contributor to the global disease burden and mortality. Evidence suggests increasing hypertension prevalence in Ghana but there is limited public awareness and information on the characteristics of those with the disease. *Objective*. To describe the baseline characteristics of adults with hypertension who were randomized to receive either hypertension related nutrition education plus hospital-based standard of care or only the standard of care (control group) in Asesewa, a semi-rural community in the Eastern Region of Ghana. Only baseline data were used in the present analysis. *Methods*. A cross-sectional baseline survey was completed for 63 adults with confirmed hypertension diagnosis. Data on sociodemographic characteristics and diet were obtained through interviews and participants' body mass index (BMI) was computed. Pearson chi-square statistic was used to assess differences between those with both elevated diastolic blood pressure (DBP) and systolic blood pressure (SBP) and those with only elevated SBP. *Results*. Mean ± SD age of participants was 54.5±13.8 years. Approximately 71% of participants had both elevated SBP (>140 mmHg) and DBP (>90 mmHg) while the remaining 29% had only elevated SBP. The median number of times the food groups beneficial to hypertension management were consumed in the preceding week to the interview was 1 for green leafy vegetables, 1 for dairy products, 2 for fruits, and 4 for legumes. The median number of times for consuming harmful food groups was 3 for salted fish and 7 times for fats and oils. Signifcantly more participants in the age group above 50 than the younger participants had elevated SBP (83.3 vs. 16.7:P=0.027) and those with BMI equal to or greater than 25 were more likely to have both elevated SBP and DBP (P=0.047). *Conclusions*. Findings from this study have implications for the prevention and management of hypertension in this semi-rural population.

1. Introduction

The decision to render the phrase "*Control your blood pressure*" as the theme for 2013 World Health Day signified increasing recognition that elevated blood pressure (EBP) or hypertension is an important global public health concern [1]. Similarly, noncommunicable diseases were highlighted in the 2012 World Health Statistics report in which hypertension was estimated to contribute to more than one-half of the deaths from stroke and about 45% of deaths from heart disease [2]. The report also showed that while hypertension prevalence declined in most industrialized countries between 1980 and 2008, the opposite occurred in most African countries. With an estimated hypertension prevalence of nearly 37% in 2008, the African region had the highest prevalence of EBP. In Ghana, early reports suggested hypertension prevalence of less than 10% and less than 20% in rural and urban populations, respectively [3]. However, a 2010 systematic review revealed that, between 1970 and 2007, hypertension prevalence was between 19% and 48% [4]. While most studies generally reported lower hypertension prevalence for rural compared to urban localities, an assessment of hypertension prevalence in four rural communities in the Ga District of the Greater Accra Region reported rates of 25% and 37% among traders and farmers, respectively, leading to the authors' conclusion that hypertension is not only an urban concern in Ghana. Most Ghanaians with EBP in past studies were unaware that they had the condition [5].

Despite the increasing burden of hypertension in Ghana, there is limited context specific information on the sociodemographic and lifestyle risk factors of those affected. Identifying such risk factors is important for intervention planning, especially in a low resource context where lifestyle related preventive actions may be important in averting progression of mildly hypertensive or prehypertensive individuals to a more serious disease state requiring costly medical intervention.

Hypertension related deaths in low- and middle-income settings could potentially be reduced substantially by applying lessons learnt in high-income countries. One diet-based intervention that has been efficacious in reducing blood pressure among those with hypertension as well as preventing hypertension is the Dietary Approaches to Stop Hypertension (DASH) diet pattern developed in the United States and successfully adapted elsewhere including South Africa [6, 7]. The DASH diet promotes a dietary pattern that supplies nutrients shown to be "beneficial" (specifically, potassium, magnesium, and calcium) in the prevention and management of hypertension while minimizing "less beneficial" or "potentially harmful" nutrients (e.g., sodium and saturated fat and cholesterol) with respect to their effects on blood pressure [8]. The DASH dietary pattern emphasizes reducing sodium (salt) intake, increased consumption of fruits, vegetables, and low-fat dairy products and moderate consumption of whole grains, nuts, fish, and poultry. The DASH diet is based on evidence indicating that an increase in the consumption of fruits and vegetables has consistently been shown to be associated with lowering risk of hypertension [9]. Recommendations concerning reducing the consumption of meat and poultry are also consistent with the increasing number of studies indicating that their increased intake increases hypertension risk [10]. Epidemiological studies on the relationship between the consumption of whole grains and hypertension are far from being consistent. While some studies have found a lower risk of coronary heart disease others do not [11, 12]. Reduction in salt intake is strongly recommended as one of the top priority actions to tackle noncommunicable diseases and reduction of deaths from hypertension [13].

In 2015, a randomized controlled trial to test the impact of a nutrition education intervention based on the DASH diet principles on blood pressure was implemented among adults with blood pressure in Asesewa, a semi-rural township in the Eastern Region of Ghana. Baseline data collection on the study population (to facilitate pre- and postintervention comparisons of outcomes of interest) permitted the current analysis, which was aimed at describing the sociodemographic characteristics, dietary habits, and nutritional status of adults with hypertension enrolled in the nutrition education intervention study.

2. Methods

2.1. Study Area. The survey was carried out in Asesewa in the Upper Manya Krobo District in the Eastern Region of Ghana. Asesewa has a youthful population (50.9%) representing a broad-based pyramid with an elderly population of about 6%. Most people in the area (73.0%) are employed in the agricultural sector [14].

2.2. Study Design and Participants. This was a cross-sectional, baseline study of adults enrolled in the DASH-based nutrition education intervention study between February and July 2015. Potential participants were adults (>25 years old) who responded to announcements at places such as the main market, selected local churches, and the Asesewa Government Hospital at Asesewa for free blood pressure screening as well as adults attending outpatient services at the Asesewa Hospital, who had elevated BP.

Those screened with elevated blood pressure (systolic blood pressure (SBP) $\geq$ 140 mmHg and/or diastolic blood pressure (DBP) $\geq$ 90 mmHg) and those with EBP who were identified from the hospital OPD were asked to complete two consecutive follow-up measurements at the Asesewa Government Hospital to confirm the diagnosis. Persons with a confirmed diagnosis who agreed and signed the informed consent document after the study procedures had been explained to them were recruited into the study. Ethical approval for the study was granted by the Institutional Review Board of the University of Ghana Noguchi Memorial Institute for Medical Research. All participants signed or thumbprinted (if illiterate) a written informed document before being recruited.

2.3. Study Procedures. Blood pressure (BP) screening was done by trained project personnel using the digital Omron Blood Pressure Monitors (HEM-759-E, Omron Corporation, Kyoto, Japan), while the BP measurements to confirm hypertension diagnosis were completed by the nursing staff at the Asesewa Hospital. At enrolment, a pretested questionnaire was used to collect information on background sociodemographic characteristics, personal and family history of chronic diseases, and history of alcohol consumption and cigarette smoking. A 7-day food frequency questionnaire (FFQ) was used to obtain information about the number of times different food groups were consumed in the past 7 days. The FFQ was based on foods typically consumed in the locality and grouped in such a way to enable assessment of whether study participants' intake is in accordance with the DASH dietary pattern. Salted fish was added as a separate food group because it is a regular ingredient in Ghanaian cuisine which contributes significantly to salt intake with potential implications for hypertension. Additionally, participants' weights were taken to the nearest one kilogram with an Omron Body Composition Analyzer and Scale (Omron Healthcare, Inc., Vernon Hills, IL, USA). Participants' heights were taken with a Stadiometer to the nearest 0.1 centimetre. Anthropometric measurements were taken in duplicate and the averages computed.

2.4. Data Analysis. We performed statistical analysis by using Stata package 12 (STATA Corporation, Texas, USA). Body mass index (BMI) was computed from weight and height measurements and participants were categorized as underweight (BMI: < 18.5), normal weight (BMI: 18.5–24.9), overweight (BMI: 25.0–29.9), and obese (BMI: > 30.0). Descriptive statistics, mean ± SD for continuous variables and frequencies (%) for categorical variables, were used to summarize the data. The data on consumption of different food groups in the past week were skewed with some of the food groups having outliers; therefore median values were also computed. Bivariate analyses using Pearson Chi-Square Statistic were used to assess whether there were significant differences in sociodemographic characteristics, dietary intakes, and nutritional status between study participants with both elevated SBP and DBP and those with isolated only SBP.

3. Results

Sample. A total of 1165 adults were screened for hypertension and about 24% (n=282) had elevated systolic blood pressure. Only sixty-three adults with confirmed elevated systolic and diastolic blood pressure completed the baseline survey. Of these approximately 29% (16) had systolic hypertension only, while the remainder had both elevated systolic and diastolic blood pressure. Mean ± SD systolic and diastolic blood pressure of study participants were 151.9 ± 7.4 and 92.5 ± 7.7, respectively.

Sociodemographic Characteristics of Respondents. About 56% of the respondents were female, with a mean ± SD age of 54.5±13.8 years (Table 1). The majority were of Krobo ethnicity (76.2%) and Christian faith (90.5%). Approximately one-fifth of respondents did not have any formal education and only 17% had the tertiary level education. At the time of the survey, only a few (3.2%) of the participants were unemployed. The most common occupation was petty trading (38.1%) and about 22% of respondents had salaried occupations. Approximately 56% of the participants were married or lived with a partner (cohabiting). The mean household size was 5.1 (SD 2) persons.

Reported monthly household income was less than 200 Ghana Cedis (1 Ghana Cedi is approximately 0.23 US dollars) for the majority of participants and only 13% of households had incomes higher than 600 Ghana Cedis per month.

3.1. Nutritional Status of the Study Respondents and Family History of Chronic Conditions. The mean ± SD BMI of the respondents was 27.1 ± 5.3 with 38.1% and 25.4% of the respondents being overweight and obese, respectively. About one-fifth of study participants reported having at least one family member being overweight or obese. A family history of hypertension (55%) was the most common followed by stroke (23.8%). About 16% of the respondents reported a family history of diabetes and 8% had relatives that have suffered a heart attack.

3.2. Dietary Intakes of Respondents in the Preceding Week. Non-green leafy vegetables, roots and tubers, and cereals were the most frequently consumed foods by the respondents in the past week (Figure 1). The median frequencies of consumption of these foods were 16, 12, and 9, respectively.

Table 1: Selected background sociodemographic characteristics of study respondents.

Characteristic	n=63
Sex	
Female	55.6 (35)
Male	44.4 (28)
Age in years	54.5 ± 13.8
Ethnicity	
Krobo	76.2 (48)
Other	23.8 (15)
Religious affiliation	
Christianity	90.5 (57)
Islam and traditional religion	9.5 (6)
Marital status	
Married / Cohabiting	55.6 (35)
Single	44.4 (28)
Education	
No education	22.2 (14)
Primary	17.5 (11)
Junior High	38.1 (24)
Senior high/Technical and Vocational	4.8 (3)
Tertiary and above	17.4 (11)
Employment status	
Unemployed	3.2 (2)
Farming and fisher folks	17.5 (11)
Traders	38.1 (24)
Salaried workers	22.2 (14)
Artisans and labourers and others	19.0 (12)
Household size	5.1 ± 2.6
Households income	
≤ 200 GH	61.9 (39)
>200–600	25.4 (16)
>600	12.7 (8)

Values represent percentage (number) or mean ± standard deviation.

The median frequencies of consumption of legumes, green leafy vegetables, and fruits were 4, 1, and 2, respectively, in the past week.

Fish and seafood were the most consumed animal source of foods. Salted fish and fats/oils were consumed a median of 3 and 7 times, respectively, in the past week.

3.3. Comparison of Sociodemographic Characteristics, Family History of Chronic Disease, and Nutritional Status between Participants with Both High Systolic and Diastolic BP and Those with Only Isolated Systolic BP. Summary of comparisons of sociodemographic factors, family history of chronic diseases, and nutritional status between participants with both elevated SBD and DBP and those with only isolated elevated SBP using Pearson Chi-Square Statistic is shown in Table 2. A significantly greater proportion of respondents who were below 50 years had both elevated systolic and diastolic blood pressure (46.7% versus 16.7%; p=0.027) and a greater proportion of obese/overweight individuals had

TABLE 2: Comparison of sociodemographic, anthropometric, and family health characteristics between participants with both elevated SBP[1] and DBP[2] and those with only elevated SBP.

Characteristic	Hypertension Classification		P-Value[3]
	Both elevated SBP and DBP (n=45)	Isolated elevated SBP (n=18)	
Age in years			0.027
26–49	46.7 (21)	16.7 (3)	
50–95	53.3 (24)	83.3 (15)	
Education			0.502
No formal	20.0 (9)	27.8 (5)	
Some formal education	80.0 (13)	72.2 (13)	
Family history of at least one chronic disease			0.935
No	37.8 (17)	38.9 (7)	
Yes	62.2 (28)	61.1 (11)	
BMI			0.047
Normal (18.5–24.9)	28.9 (13)	55.6 (10)	
Overweight/obese (≥25)	71.1 (32)	44.4 (8)	

Values represent % (n). [1]Elevated systolic blood pressure (≥ 140 mmHg); [2]elevated diastolic blood pressure (≥ 90mmHg); [3]Pearson Chi-Square Statistic.

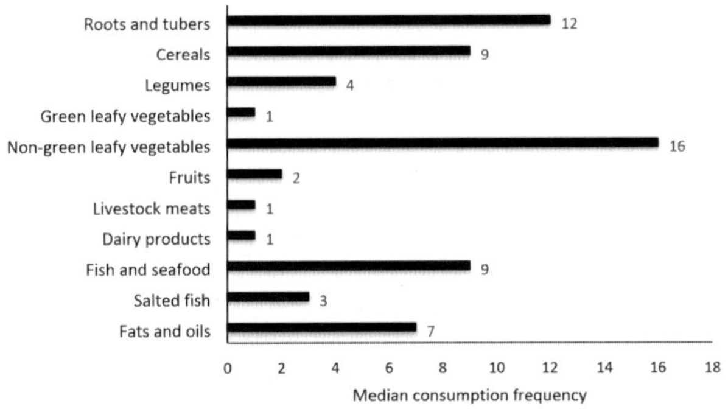

FIGURE 1: Respondents' median frequency of consuming foods from different food groups in the past seven days.

both elevated systolic and diastolic pressure compared to individuals within the normal body size (71.1% versus 44.4 %; p=0.047) (Table 2).

Other sociodemographic factors such as family history of hypertension, income, and dietary intakes showed no significant difference among the various categories.

4. Discussion

This study contributes to our current knowledge of the characteristics and potential predictors of hypertension among adults living in semi-rural communities in Ghana. It is important to note that less than 50% of those screened with elevated BP returned for the necessary confirmatory tests to determine their hypertension status. This apathy to follow-up on screening results may reflect lack of awareness about hypertension and its consequences which have been noted among socioeconomically disadvantaged individuals and communities [15]. Using data from the World Health Organizations' Study on Global Aging and Adult Health (SAGE), Lloyd-Sherlock et al. reported that compared to five (5) other low- and middle-income countries the Ghanaian sample had the lowest prevalence of hypertension awareness of just 23.3% compared to a range of about 38% for India and South Africa to 72.1% for Russian Federation [16]. The increasing hypertension prevalence [4] and the serious consequences of the diseases warrant that attention be given to public education efforts as a primary prevention measure to address this growing public health problem.

In this study, the age of the respondents was found to be significantly associated with either having both elevated systolic and diastolic blood pressure or having isolated elevated systolic blood pressure. Older adults (50 years and above) had elevated isolated systolic consistent with other findings; older respondents had elevated isolated systolic blood pressure. This was consistent with similar studies in rural and urban India [17]. Contrarily to our expectation a greater proportion of respondents below 50 years had both elevated systolic and diastolic high blood pressure compared to their older counterparts. There is, however, an increase in the incidence of young adults with hypertension in other populace [18].

These findings also buttress the need for the increased call for routine checks for high blood pressure among young adults as advocated for older adults. This is because, notably, young adults with elevated systolic and diastolic pressure are likely to have a slower rate of receiving an initial diagnosis than middle-aged and older adults in their study [19]. This can easily lead to a various health complication.

Also, more than half (55%) of the respondents in this study reported that they had a family history of hypertension. This is much higher than the 35.7 % reported in a study on the frequency of hypertension and prehypertension among adults in Hohoe, a municipality in the Volta region of Ghana [20]. A review of population-based studies on hypertension in Ghana indicated that hypertension was positively associated with a positive family history of hypertension

[21]. However, a study in Saudi Arabia, which examined the risk factors for diabetes and hypertension among expatriate workers, revealed that family history was not significantly associated with hypertension [22].

The predominant occupation of the respondents in this study was trading. This is likely to predispose them to hypertension due to the job-related stress and inappropriate food consumption and meal patterns. Concerning the level of income of the respondents, the majority of them were earning GHS200.00 or less. This low-income level may influence the dietary habits of the respondents and their ability to purchase foods beneficial for hypertension prevention and control [23, 24]. However, the systematic review by Addo and colleagues on hypertension in Ghana showed an inconclusive relationship between income level and hypertension [5].

Our study found significant differences in nutritional status (BMI) between participants with both elevated systolic and diastolic blood pressure and those with isolated SBP. The association between BMI and blood pressure is well established with several studies reporting higher likelihood of elevated BP among overweight and obese individuals [25–27]. A study assessing the determinants of isolated systolic hypertension in North India among both urban and rural areas showed that BMI was a significant independent predictor of isolated systolic hypertension [17]. In our study a significantly higher proportion of participants with both elevated SBP and DBP were overweight or obese compared to those with only isolated SBP. Similarly, a study conducted in South Korea found that having BMI ≥ 23 was associated with uncontrolled hypertension among elderly people [28]. Zhang and colleagues in their research among rural Chinese women also reported that although obese women had an increased risk of hypertension, "BMI was more related to isolated diastolic hypertension than to isolated systolic hypertension" [29].

The frequency of consuming food from various food groups was also found to be a contributory factor to having either an isolated elevated SBP or both elevated SBP and DBP. This research found out that respondents consumed fewer green leafy vegetables and fruits, which generally tend to be higher in potassium needed in the management of hypertension and had increased intake of fats and oils. A cross-sectional study on the prevalence and correlates of hypertension among rural populations in Sub-Saharan African revealed that frequent intake of fruit and vegetables was associated with lower blood pressure measures [30]. Additionally, a research in Chile showed that increased intakes of fruits and vegetables reduced the systolic blood pressure [31]. Some studies have identified lower income levels as a contributory factor to lower intake of fruits and vegetables and higher consumption of fatty foods [23, 32].

Generally, although the restriction of salted foods is considered an appropriate strategy for the control of high blood pressure adherence to this recommendation is often a challenge [33]. In the present study, the consumption of salted fish and fats and oils was higher than recommended for individuals with hypertension. It was observed that median salted fish consumption was about 3 times in the past week and while the present study did not show a significant relationship between salted fish consumption and having either both elevated SBP and DBP or isolated SBP, this link has been established in other studies. For example, among Japanese men, systolic blood pressure was significantly higher in the higher quintiles of salt intake while in India total dietary salt intake was a significant risk factor for hypertension even after controlling for potential confounders [34, 35]. Conversely, significant reduction in dietary sodium intake has been identified as an effective way of lowering SBP in Asian patients [36, 37]. Thus, measures to reduce salt intake may contribute to effective hypertension management in the study population.

Food groups such as legumes and green leafy vegetables that have potential benefits for hypertension management [38, 39] were minimally consumed by respondents in the week preceding the survey. Despite the benefits of legume consumption to hypertension management, results from this study corroborate others from even developed countries such as the United States reporting only about 8% adults consuming legumes on any given day [40].

The intake of dairy foods, which are good sources of calcium and potassium, was very low among the study participants. A systematic review and meta-analysis of elevated blood pressure and consumption of dairy foods showed that consumption of low-fat dairy foods was associated with a 13% reduction in risk of high blood pressure [41]. However, although the DASH diet recommends foods high in calcium, a study in rural African community did not find an association between the frequencies of consuming dairy products and the prevalence of hypertension [30].

The findings of this study provide useful information on dietary habits of people with hypertension in a low-income rural community which may inform hypertension management services. The study also points to the need for education and awareness among the general populace to foster better health-seeking behaviours for hypertension screening and management. Furthermore, lessons from this study will assist in developing programs for healthy ageing consistent with the World Health Organizations global strategy on ageing and health [2].

Acknowledgments

The study was partly funded by the University of Ghana Research Fund. The authors appreciate the contributions of Humphrey Thompson, Janet Carboo, and Claudia Ewa to the execution of this study and publication.

References

[1] WHO, *A global brief on hypertension: silent killer, global public health crisis*, World Health Organization, 2013.

[2] WHO, *World health statistics 2012 PArt III Global Health Indicators*, World Health Organization, 2012.

[3] J. O. M. Pobee, E. B. Larbi, D. W. Belcher, F. K. Wurapa, and S. R. A. Dodu, "Blood pressure distribution in a rural Ghanaian population," *Transactions of the Royal Society of Tropical Medicine and Hygiene*, vol. 71, no. 1, pp. 66–72, 1977.

[4] W. K. Bosu, "Epidemic of hypertension in Ghana: a systematic review," *BMC Public Health*, vol. 10, article 418, 2010.

[5] J. Addo, A. G. Amoah, and K. A. Koram, "The changing patterns of hypertension in Ghana: a study of four rural communities in the Ga District," *Ethnicity & Disease*, vol. 16, no. 4, pp. 894–899, 2006.

[6] F. M. Sacks, L. P. Svetkey, W. M. Vollmer et al., "Effects on blood pressure of reduced dietary sodium and the dietary approaches to stop hypertension (DASH) diet," *The New England Journal of Medicine*, vol. 344, no. 1, pp. 3–10, 2001.

[7] K. E. Charlton, K. Steyn, N. S. Levitt et al., "Diet and blood pressure in South Africa: Intake of foods containing sodium, potassium, calcium, and magnesium in three ethnic groups," *Nutrition Journal*, vol. 21, no. 1, pp. 39–50, 2005.

[8] L. J. Appel, T. J. Moore, and E. Obarzanek, "A clinical trial of the effects of dietary patterns on blood pressure," *The New England Journal of Medicine*, vol. 336, no. 16, pp. 1117–1124, 1997.

[9] F. J. He, C. A. Nowson, M. Lucas, and G. A. MacGregor, "Increased consumption of fruit and vegetables is related to a reduced risk of coronary heart disease: meta-analysis of cohort studies," *Journal of Human Hypertension*, vol. 21, no. 9, pp. 717–728, 2007.

[10] L. Borgi, G. C. Curhan, W. C. Willett, F. B. Hu, A. Satija, and J. P. Forman, "Long-term intake of animal flesh and risk of developing hypertension in three prospective cohort studies," *Journal of Hypertension*, vol. 33, no. 11, pp. 2231–2238, 2015.

[11] D. R. Jacobs, L. F. Andersen, and R. Blomhoff, "Whole-grain consumption is associated with a reduced risk of noncardiovascular, noncancer death attributed to inflammatory diseases in the Iowa Women's Health Study," *American Journal of Clinical Nutrition*, vol. 85, no. 6, pp. 1606–1614, 2007.

[12] M. K. Jensen, P. Koh-Banerjee, F. B. Hu et al., "Intakes of whole grains, bran, and germ and the risk of coronary heart disease in men," *American Journal of Clinical Nutrition*, vol. 80, no. 6, pp. 1492–1499, 2004.

[13] S. K. Ha, "Dietary salt intake and hypertension," *Electrolytes & Blood Pressure*, vol. 12, no. 1, pp. 7–18, 2014.

[14] GSS, *Final Report on Population and Housing Census*, Accra Ghana Statistical Service, Accra, Ghana, 2012.

[15] J. Hoebel, A. Starker, S. Jordan, M. Richter, and T. Lampert, "Determinants of health check attendance in adults: Findings from the cross-sectional German Health Update (GEDA) study," *BMC Public Health*, vol. 14, no. 1, article no. 913, 2014.

[16] P. Lloyd-Sherlock, J. Beard, N. Minicuci, S. Ebrahim, and S. Chatterji, "Hypertension among older adults in low and middle-income countries: prevalence, awareness and control," *International Journal of Epidemiology*, vol. 43, no. 1, pp. 116–128, 2014.

[17] T. Midha, M. Idris, R. Saran, A. Srivastava, and S. Singh, "Isolated systolic hypertension and its determinants-a cross-sectional study in the adult population of lucknow district in North India," *Indian journal of community medicine: official publication of Indian Association of Preventive & Social Medicine*, vol. 35, no. 89, 2010.

[18] T. De Venecia, M. Lu, and V. M. Figueredo, "Hypertension in young adults," *Postgraduate Medical Journal*, vol. 128, no. 2, pp. 201–207, 2016.

[19] H. M. Johnson, C. T. Thorpe, C. M. Bartels et al., "Undiagnosed hypertension among young adults with regular primary care use," *Journal of Hypertension*, vol. 32, no. 1, pp. 65–74, 2014.

[20] K. D. Nyavor, M. Kweku, I. Agbemafle et al., "Assessing the ownership, usage and knowledge of insecticide treated nets (ITNs) in malaria prevention in the hohoe municipality, Ghana," *Pan African Medical Journal*, vol. 28, no. 1, 2017.

[21] J. Addo, C. Agyemang, L. Smeeth, A. de-Graft Aikins, A. K. Edusei, and O. Ogedegbe, "A review of population-based studies on hypertension in Ghana," *Ghana Medical Journal*, vol. 46, supplement, no. 2, pp. 4–11, 2012.

[22] S. M. Ahmed, W. Sami, H. Alanazi, T. Aljarbaa, S. Alkhamis, and F. Almutiri, "A Study of Risk Factors for Diabetes & Hypertension among Expatriate Workers in Majmaah City, Saudi Arabia," *International Journal of Health and Rehabilitation Sciences (IJHRS)*, vol. 4, pp. 103–114, 2015.

[23] M. L. Loureiro and D. Rahmani, "Calorie labelling and fast food choices in surveys and actual markets: some new behavioural results," *AAEA & CAES Joint Annual Meeting*, pp. 4–6, 2013.

[24] S. P. M. Arruda, A. A. M. Da Silva, G. Kac, M. Z. Goldani, H. Bettiol, and M. A. Barbieri, "Socioeconomic and demographic factors are associated with dietary patterns in a cohort of young Brazilian adults," *BMC Public Health*, vol. 14, no. 1, article no. 654, 2014.

[25] C. Jackson, G.-C. Herber-Gast, and W. Brown, "Joint effects of physical activity and BMI on risk of hypertension in women: A longitudinal study," *Journal of Obesity*, vol. 2014, Article ID 271532, 2014.

[26] P. A. Cassano, M. R. Segal, P. S. Vokonas, and S. T. Weiss, "Body fat distribution, blood pressure, and hypertension. A prospective cohort study of men in the normative aging study," *Annals of Epidemiology*, vol. 1, no. 1, pp. 33–48, 1990.

[27] X. Lu, P. Shi, C.-Y. Luo et al., *Prevalence of hypertension in overweight and obese children from a large school-based population in Shanghai*, vol. 13, BMC Public Health, China, 2013.

[28] S.-H. Park, S.-J. Choi, K.-S. Lee, and H.-Y. Park, "Waist circumference and waist-to-height ratio as predictors of cardiovascular disease risk in Korean adults," *Circulation Journal*, vol. 73, no. 9, pp. 1643–1650, 2009.

[29] X. Zhang, S. Yao, G. Sun et al., "Total and abdominal obesity among rural Chinese women and the association with hypertension," *Nutrition Journal*, vol. 28, no. 1, pp. 46–52, 2012.

[30] S. De Ramirez, D. Enquobahrie, G. Nyadzi et al., "Prevalence and correlates of hypertension in rural Africa," *Journal of Human Hypertension*, vol. 24, pp. 786–795, 2010.

[31] L. Pienovi, M. Lara, P. Bustos, and H. Amigo, "Fruit and vegetable intake, and blood pressure. A population research," *Archivos Latinoamericanos de Nutrición*, vol. 65, no. 1, pp. 21–26, 2015.

[32] S. G. Ozcariz, C. De O Bernardo, F. Cembranel, M. A. Peres, and D. A. González-Chica, "Dietary practices among individuals with diabetes and hypertension are similar to those of healthy people: A population-based study Health behavior, health promotion and society," *BMC Public Health*, vol. 15, no. 1, article no. 479, 2015.

[33] U. A. Ajani, S. B. Dunbar, E. S. Ford, A. H. Mokdad, and G. A. Mensah, "Sodium intake among people with normal and high blood pressure," *American Journal of Preventive Medicine*, vol. 29, no. 5, pp. 63–67, 2005.

[34] K. Miura, N. Okuda, T. C. Turin et al., "Dietary salt intake and blood pressure in a representative Japanese population: Baseline analyses of NIPPON DATA80," *Journal of Epidemiology*, vol. 20, no. 3, pp. S524–S530, 2010.

[35] G. Radhika, R. M. Sathya, V. Sudha, A. Ganesan, and V. Mohan, "Dietary salt intake and hypertension in an urban South Indian population - [CURES - 53]," *Journal of the Association of Physicians of India*, vol. 55, no. JUNE, pp. 405–411, 2007.

[36] B. Zhou, H. Wang, W. Wang, X. Wu, L. Fu, and J. Shi, "Long-term effects of salt substitution on blood pressure in a rural north Chinese population," *Journal of human hypertension*, vol. 27, p. 427, 2013.

[37] F. J. He, M. Marciniak, E. Visagie et al., "Effect of modest salt reduction on blood pressure, urinary albumin, and pulse wave velocity in white, black, and asian mild hypertensives," *Hypertension*, vol. 54, no. 3, pp. 482–488, 2009.

[38] F. B. Hu, "Plant-based foods and prevention of cardiovascular disease: an overview," *American Journal of Clinical Nutrition*, vol. 78, no. 3, pp. 544S–551S, 2003.

[39] M. J. Orlich and G. E. Fraser, "Vegetarian diets in the Adventist Health Study 2: A review of initial published findings," *American Journal of Clinical Nutrition*, vol. 100, no. 1, 2014.

[40] D. C. Mitchell, F. R. Lawrence, T. J. Hartman, and J. M. Curran, "Consumption of Dry Beans, Peas, and Lentils Could Improve Diet Quality in the US Population," *Journal of the Academy of Nutrition and Dietetics*, vol. 109, no. 5, pp. 909–913, 2009.

[41] R. A. Ralston, J. H. Lee, H. Truby, C. E. Palermo, and K. Z. Walker, "A systematic review and meta-analysis of elevated blood pressure and consumption of dairy foods," *Journal of Human Hypertension*, vol. 26, no. 1, pp. 3–13, 2012.

9

A New Lebanese Medication Adherence Scale: Validation in Lebanese Hypertensive Adults

R. Bou Serhal,[1] **P. Salameh**,[2] **N. Wakim**,[1] **C. Issa**,[3] **B. Kassem**,[1] **L. Abou Jaoude**,[1] **and N. Saleh**[1]

[1]*Department of Epidemiology and biostatistics, Faculty of Public Health, Lebanese University, Fanar, Lebanon*
[2]*Faculty of Pharmacy, Lebanese University, Al Hadath, Lebanon*
[3]*Department of Nutrition and Dietetics, Faculty of Public Health, Lebanese University, Fanar, Lebanon*

Correspondence should be addressed to R. Bou Serhal; roulabouserhal@hotmail.com

Academic Editor: Tomohiro Katsuya

Background. A new Lebanese scale measuring medication adherence considered socioeconomic and cultural factors not taken into account by the eight-item Morisky Medication Adherence Scale (MMAS-8). *Objectives* were to validate the new adherence scale and its prediction of hypertension control, compared to MMAS-8, and to assess adherence rates and factors. *Methodology.* A cross-sectional study, including 405 patients, was performed in outpatient cardiology clinics of three hospitals in Beirut. Blood pressure was measured, a questionnaire filled, and sodium intake estimated by a urine test. Logistic regression defined predictors of hypertension control and adherence. *Results.* 54.9% had controlled hypertension. 82.4% were adherent by the new scale, which showed good internal consistency, adequate questions (KMO coefficient = 0.743), and four factors. It predicted hypertension control (OR = 1.217; p value = 0.003), unlike MMAS-8, but the scores were correlated (ICC average measure = 0.651; p value < 0.001). Stress and smoking predicted nonadherence. *Conclusion.* This study elaborated a validated, practical, and useful tool measuring adherence to medications in Lebanese hypertensive patients.

1. Introduction

Hypertension is an international public health burden that caused around 9,4 million deaths in 2010 [1]. In Lebanon, hypertension prevalence was 36,9% in adults aged 21 years and above [2]. Reducing sodium intake could significantly lower blood pressure in hypertensive and normotensive patients [3], as well as diminishing the risk of stroke and fatal coronary artery diseases in adults [4]. A wide variety of efficient medications to control hypertension is available [5]. Yet, low rates of controlled hypertension were observed. In USA, 47% of all hypertensive patients and 60% of treated hypertensive patients had controlled blood pressure [6], compared to, respectively, 27% [2] and 48.9% [7] in Lebanon. Patients with uncontrolled blood pressure had a higher risk of nonadherence to their medication [8], while adherent patients had lower systolic blood pressure and diastolic blood pressure [9].

Medication adherence was defined by the WHO as "the extent to which a person's behavior, taking medication, following a diet, and/or executing lifestyle changes, corresponds to agreed recommendations from a healthcare provider" [10]. In Lebanon, 22.4% of hypertensive patients were nonadherent to their medication [11]. Adherence amelioration was important to reduce hospitalization and mortality due to cardiovascular diseases [12], as well as resulting costs [13]. A precise evaluation of medication adherence and the factors that affect it is needed, with adequate tools to be used in routine clinical practice [14]. The eight-item Morisky Medication Adherence Scale (MMAS-8) is a subjective method, with a 93% sensitivity and a 53% specificity [15]. Even though it is frequently used in studies, as it is simple and not expensive, MMAS-8 does not take patients' cultural and socioeconomic factors into account, as well as their relationship with their healthcare providers, while these variables affect adherence. In this context, a new scale (Lebanese Medication Adherence

Scale: LMAS) was developed, taking into account factors related to the Lebanese culture. It evaluated psychological, occupational, economical, and annoyance factors.

The primary objective of this study was to validate the LMAS in Lebanese hypertensive adults, to assess its ability to predict hypertension control, and to compare it with MMAS-8. The secondary objective was to evaluate the adherence rate in Lebanese hypertensive adults, and to determine factors affecting antihypertensive adherence.

2. Methodology

2.1. Score Creation. The new score (LMAS) was inspired by the Morisky score, adding other variables affecting adherence, discussed by the investigators with physicians and community pharmacists in a focus group. The reasons why MMAS-8 was our source of inspiration were its simplicity and validity, as well as its common use among clinicians and researchers (in Lebanon and elsewhere) to asses antihypertensives adherence. MMAS-8 contains seven questions with dichotomic answer (yes/no) and one Likert scale question with five possibilities and measures forgetfulness, medication taking behavior, and secondary effects [16]. The Arabic version of MMAS-8 had already been validated in Lebanon [17].

LMAS assessed forgetfulness by a question evaluating its frequency, inspired by merging MMAS-8's questions regarding forgetfulness which investigate the past day, the past two weeks, and the general forgetting behavior. Moreover, a question regarding the frequency of reminders' (by caregivers, alarms, etc.) use to increase adherence was added, knowing that social interactions take a privileged place in the Lebanese culture and that reminders might affect adherence. Also inspired from MMAS-8, we included questions evaluating adherence change if the patients felt clinically better or worse, but behavior change if laboratory exams improved was added to LMAS. Furthermore, adherence when away from home was included in the new score, with an adaptation by adding suggestions of outdoor diner or lunch. A question regarding adherence during busy periods was also included in LMAS. In addition, economic factors, like adherence when health coverage does not pay for the medicine and delay in buying a new pills box when the old one becomes empty, were included in LMAS. Besides, adherence behaviors in case of boredom, if some food items were prohibited during treatment period, or if the patient or his neighbor (because these issues could be discussed often between Lebanese patients) experienced any secondary effects, were evaluated. Likewise, adherence behavior when the patients noticed that they took a lot of pills was tested. Consequently, LMAS contained 16 Likert scale questions with four options to answer each (coded from zero (less adherence) to three (higher adherence)) and was subject to validation.

2.2. Study Design, Procedure, Inclusion Criteria, and Sample Size. An observational cross-sectional study was conducted. Patients were recruited from the outpatient cardiology clinics of three hospitals in Beirut, visited at random dates in 2016, during patients' appointments. Patients matching the inclusion criteria were invited to participate in the study, after signing a written informed consent. Their blood pressure was measured twice, at a 10-minute interval, with their right hand placed at the level of the heart [18], with the validated digital sphygmomanometer "Omron M3 IT Intellisense" [19]. To reduce white coat effect, the surveyor measuring patients' blood pressure was not wearing any gown, and the measurement was done in the waiting area before the patient enters to the clinic. Controlled hypertension was defined by blood pressure lower than 130/80 mmHg for diabetic patients and lower than 140/90 mmHg for the others [20]. Patients also filled a questionnaire, and a fresh urine sample was collected, labelled by a code, preserved in a refrigerated box, and carried on the same day to the laboratory for analysis.

The INTERSALT equation was used to assess mean sodium intake of treated Lebanese hypertensive patients, as this equation had less bias [21]. To reduce cost, the INTERSALT equation was calculated in a group of patients for whom the measures of urinary sodium, potassium, and creatinine were taken. Only urinary sodium was measured for the rest of the patients, and the value of the INTERSALT equation was estimated by a statistical analysis using linear regression. Correlation between the two measures of INTERSALT (estimated and calculated) was determined by intraclass correlation coefficient. Mean daily sodium intake of hypertensive patients was then obtained based on the estimated values of INTERSALT equation.

Patients included were Lebanese, aged 18 years and above, with primary hypertension diagnosed at least six months ago, treated with antihypertensives for at least the past six weeks, and having signed the informed consent. Exclusion criteria were secondary hypertension, pregnant women, being hospitalized, dement, or mentally disabled, and patients with physical disability or any infection affecting blood pressure.

A ratio of 20 : 1 (number of subjects : number of items) was used to calculate sample size [22]. This corresponded to 320 patients for the 16 questions of the LMAS. 405 patients were included, to account for a maximum of 20% missing answers or incomplete questionnaires.

2.3. Variables Included in the Questionnaire. Sociodemographic characteristics of the patients were assessed. Lifestyle characteristics included BMI, physical activity (in minutes/week), stress level during the last three months, smoking status and amount (calculated in year-packs for cigarettes and shisha [23]), caffeine consumption (in g/day based on USDA database [24]), alcohol consumption (number of glasses consumed), diet type, and autoevaluation of salt consumption. Information concerning hypertension, as disease duration, baseline blood pressure, medication, comorbidities (including diabetes, high blood lipid levels, cardiovascular diseases, and psychiatric disorders), frequency of physician visits, secondary effects, and MMAS-8 and LMAS scores, was also collected.

2.4. Statistical Analysis. We used SPSS version 20 for data entry and analysis. To validate LMAS, an exploratory factor analysis with Varimax rotation was done, leading to the reduced dimension score (LMAS-14). Internal consistency of LMAS-14 was assessed using Cronbach alpha, which showed good internal consistency when it was >0.5. Sensitivity and specificity were shown by ROC curve, with hypertension control as a reference variable. Cut-off value was determined by Youden Index, defined as J = maximum (sensibility + specificity − 1). [25]. Logistic regression (backward LR method), with hypertension control as a dependent variable, was used to determine which score was a better predictor of hypertension control. Concordance between adherence measures of the two scores was evaluated by the intraclass correlation coefficient (considered good when it was >0.5).

To determine the factors affecting medication adherence, the dependent variable was adherence measured by LMAS-14. Each variable with p value ≤ 0.2 in bivariate analysis was included in the logistic regression (backward LR method). A cut-off of 6 was admitted to classify patients as adherent (MMAS-8 score between 6 and 8) and nonadherent (MMAS-8 score < 6). A cut-off value for classifying patients for the LMAS-14 was determined by ROC curve and Youden Index.

3. Results

3.1. Descriptive Statistics. Patients' mean age was 65 years; almost half (52.2%) were females and the majority resided in Beirut (47.2%). 12.9% had no health coverage. As for lifestyle, almost half of patients (42.2%) had a moderate stress level (Table 1).

Mean blood pressure measured was 132.94/80.75 (±15.36/12.02) mmHg. The majority of patients (54.9%) had controlled blood pressure. MMAS-8 showed that 86.1% of the patients were adherent to antihypertensive pills, while adherence rate using the LMAS-14 was 82.4% (Table 2).

3.2. LMAS Score Validation

3.2.1. Factor Analysis. Factor analysis was used to reduce the number of the score's questions and to study its principal components. After rotation, two questions were removed, as the correlation matrix showed they had correlation coefficients < 0.3 with other questions, and one of them had an anti-image correlation coefficient of 0.38 (<0.5). The new score, consisting of 14 questions, had a KMO coefficient of 0.743, showing adequate questions. The Bartlett test was significant (p value < 0.001), proving that the model was good. Anti-image correlation matrix showed positive values in the diagonals, proving that the questions were correlated; the majority of the values were above 0.8. In the principal component analysis, the used model explained 58.259% of the variance of the score's answers. Factor analysis showed a scale of four factors, with load > 0.4 (Table 3): the first (Cronbach alpha = 0.695.) included occupational factors that encouraged forgetting or stopping medication and consisted of five questions. The second, psychological factor (Cronbach alpha = 0.591), consisted of four questions. The third, annoyance factor (Cronbach alpha = 0.48), had three questions. Finally, the economical factor (Cronbach alpha = 0.48) consisted of two questions (Table 3).

3.2.2. Sensitivity, Specificity, and Cut-Off Value of LMAS-14. A cut-off value of 38 was determined for the LMAS-14, with a sensitivity of 82.9% and a specificity of 36.9%.

3.2.3. Prediction of Hypertension Control

(1) Daily Sodium Intake Estimation. Intraclass correlation coefficient between the variables was created by the estimation of INTERSALT (using urinary sodium measure) and the calculated INTERSALT was 0.807 for average measures (CI = [0.607–0.905]; p value < 0.001), proving a good correlation. We used the new variable in the following analysis. Mean daily sodium intake was 3.48 (±0.78) grams in hypertensive patients. No statistically significant difference in mean sodium intake (p value = 0.827 for Student's t-test) was found between patients declaring to follow a low salt diet (mean = 3.47 g/day) and those denying it (mean = 3.5 g/day).

(2) Predictors of Hypertension Control. Patients having a higher LMAS score had an OR of 1.217 (p value = 0.003) of achieving controlled blood pressure. Thus, having a longer disease duration (OR = 0.914; p value = 0.014) and a higher number of comorbidities (OR = 0.643; p value = 0.044) predicted lower hypertension control (Table 4).

3.2.4. Concordance between LMAS-14 and MMAS-8. Intraclass correlation coefficient showed good concordance between MMAS-8 and LMAS-14 scales (ICC average measure = 0.651; p value < 0.001).

3.3. Factors Affecting Adherence. A higher stress level (OR = 0.542; p value = 0.007) and being a past or actual smoker (OR = 0.506; p value = 0.013) decreased the probability of being adherent to antihypertensives by LMAS-14 (Table 5).

4. Discussion

Factor analysis allowed the selection of 14 questions divided in four factors for the LMAS-14. This is in accordance with the study that created the score by elaborating a scale divided in four factors [26]. Hypertension control rate was higher than other Lebanese studies in treated hypertensive patients [2, 7]. This could be due to recruiting study participants from outpatient clinics in Beirut hospitals, so these patients might have a better follow-up than the general population. Thus, results are lower than those (62.9%) found in a study at Beirut hospitals [11], probably due to the consideration of a lower cut-off for diabetic patients. Other countries had lower hypertension control rates [6, 22, 27–29].

Association between adherence to medication and hypertension control has already been demonstrated [7, 9]. LMAS-14 seems to be a better predictor of hypertension control in the Lebanese population; this could be due to taking into consideration the psychological and cultural factors. The good concordance between the two scores could be explained by the fact that LMAS-14 was inspired from MMAS-8 and both measure adherence. A higher number of comorbidities predicted lower hypertension control. This

Table 1: Sociodemographic and lifestyle characteristics.

Variable	Items	Mean/N	SD/%
Age		65.05	12.93
Sex	Male	197	48.8
	Female	207	51.2
Place of residence	Beirut	191	47.2
	Mount Lebanon	165	40.7
	North	4	1
	South	29	7.2
	Bekaa	16	4
Educational level	Illiterate	41	10.4
	Primary	101	25.7
	Complementary	81	20.6
	Secondary	68	17.3
	University	102	26
Frequency of physician's consultation	No routine consultation	131	32.9
	Once in six months	79	19.8
	Once in three months	151	37.9
	Once a month	32	8
	Once or more every two weeks	5	1.3
Health coverage	Self-payer	52	12.9
	Social security	132	32.7
	Cooperative of state employees	37	9.2
	Army	2	0.5
	General security	8	2
	Private insurance	121	30
	Nongovernmental organization	36	8.9
	Other	16	4
Socioeconomic status (crowding index)	Low socioeconomic status	9	3.6
	Moderate	111	44.8
	High	128	51.6
BMI	Underweight	2	0.5
	Normal	107	26.7
	Overweight	159	39.7
	Obese	133	33.2
Physical activity	No physical activity	285	71.1
	Lower than 150 min/week	24	6.0
	150 min/week or higher	92	22.9
Smoking	Never	199	49.1
	Stopped	78	19.3
	Still smoking	128	31.6
Stress level	Very low	10	4
	Low	49	19.7
	Moderate	105	42.2
	High	48	19.3
	Very high	37	14.9
Caffeine intake per day (mg)		67.67	53.17
Low sodium diet	No	143	36.6
	Yes	248	63.4

Table 2: Hypertension characteristics.

Variable	Items	Mean/*N*	SD/%
Mean systolic blood pressure		132.94	15.36
Mean diastolic blood pressure		80.75	12.02
Disease duration		9.45	7.05
Number of antihypertensive pills per day		1.97	1.06
Total number of pills per day		5.16	2.99
Comorbidities	No	127	31.7
	Yes	274	68.3
Secondary effects	None	240	60.5
	At least one	157	39.5
Hypertension control	Uncontrolled hypertension	141	45.1
	Controlled hypertension	263	54.9
MMAS-8	Nonadherent	56	13.9
	Adherent	348	86.1
LMAS-14	Nonadherent	71	17.6
	Adherent	333	82.4

Table 3: Questions, factors, and their internal consistency.

Factor	Cronbach alpha	Load	Question
Occupational	0.695	0.771	Do you forget to take your medication when you are busy (intensive work or travel)?
		0.722	Do you forget to take your medication if you are invited to lunch or dinner?
		0.712	Do you forget to take your medication?
		0.526	Do you get late when it comes to buying your medication packs when they become empty?
		0.438	Do you stop taking your medication if it forbids you from eating certain food that you love because of possible food-medication interaction?
Psychological	0.591	0.832	Will you stop taking your medication, without your doctor's consultation, if your neighbor/relative took a prescription like yours for a long term and it caused them side effects?
		0.709	Do you stop taking your medication without consulting your doctor if the laboratory tests show improvement during treatment period?
		0.685	Do you stop taking your medication without consulting your doctor if you do not feel better during treatment period?
		0.521	Do you stop taking your medication without consulting your doctor if you feel better during treatment period?
Annoyance	0.48	0.890	Do you decide to stop some of your medications without consulting your doctor if you noticed that you are taking too many medications every day?
		0.701	Do you stop your chronic treatment if you get bored of it?
		0.502	Do you stop taking your medication in case of side effects?
Economical	0.679	0.856	Do you stop taking your medication if your insurance does not cover it?
		0.833	Will you stop buying your medication packs if you considered them expensive?

Extraction method: principal component analysis. Rotation method: varimax with Kaiser normalization.

could be explained by the necessity, for patients with more comorbidities, to have a more complex treatment regimen with a wider variety of medication and thus to be less adherent to their medication and have lower blood pressure control. Having longer disease duration was a predictor of lower hypertension control, matching the findings of Sarfo et al. [30].

The mean sodium intake of our population was around 3.48 g/day, while a significant blood pressure decrease was observed with a mean sodium intake below 2 g/day [4]. The absence of statistically significant difference in mean daily sodium consumption, between patients declaring to follow a low sodium diet and those who do not, suggests either a social desirability bias or the inefficiency of those regimes.

This study showed higher adherence rates for LMAS-14 (82.4%) than another one in Beirut (77.6%) [11]. This could be due to a potential social desirability bias or due to the recruitment from hospitals clinics. Higher stress level predicted nonadherence to LMAS-14, concordant with a study in Beirut showing that anxiety reduced adherence [17].

Study strengths include sample size and control for sociodemographic, lifestyle, hypertension, comorbidities,

Table 4: Logistic regression for hypertension control.

Variables	Exp (*B*)	95% CI		*p* value
Physical activity duration	0.998	0.996	1.000	0.063
Disease duration	0.914	0.851	0.982	0.014
Number of comorbidities	0.643	0.418	0.989	0.044
LMAS-14	1.217	1.069	1.386	0.003

Omnibus test p value < 0.001; Hosmer-Lemeshow test p value = 0.491; Nagelkerke's R^2 = 0.215; overall predicted percentage = 69.6%. *Independent variables*: age, physical activity duration, disease duration, number of comorbidities, number of secondary effects symptoms, BMI, MMAS-8, LMAS_14, estimated INTERSALT, educational level, frequency of physician's consultation, and health coverage.

Table 5: Logistic regression for LMAS-14.

Variables	OR	95% CI		*p* value
Stress level	0.542	0.348	0.845	0.007
Smoking	0.506	0.297	0.864	0.013

Omnibus test p value < 0.001; Hosmer-Lemeshow test p value = 0.760; Nagelkerke's R^2 = 0.185; overall predicted percentage = 72.2%. *Independent variables*: age, number of antihypertensive pills, number of secondary effects, BMI, employment, adding salt to food at the table, food evaluation, frequency of physician's consultation, stress level, health coverage, crowding index, smoking, and estimated INTERSALT.

and adherence characteristics. To our knowledge, it is the first study in Lebanon that estimated daily sodium consumption and adjusted hypertension control predictors to it. We also obtained a validated scale measuring adherence, with good psychometric properties, concordant with Morisky score, and predicting hypertension control. Factors affecting adherence were also defined and were concordant with other studies.

However, some limitations are to be mentioned. A potential selection bias could be due to the recruitment done in cardiology outpatient clinics of three hospitals in Beirut. An overrepresentation of the Lebanese residing in Beirut and Mount Lebanon was also noted. A potential information bias could be due to the employment of subjective methods to measure adherence, but objective ones are expensive and are not available in Lebanon. Social desirability bias could have modified the classification of adherence in patients and its association with hypertension control. White coat effect was only prevented by the surveyors' dress code excluding hospital gowns and by the measurement technique, done outside the doctor's office in the waiting area, but baseline blood pressure before presentation to the clinic was not obtained, for the majority of the patients, due to the unavailability of sphygmomanometers at their house. Finally, financial constraints did not allow the measurement of all the necessary parameters for INTERSALT calculation to all patients; consequently, its estimation was done in the majority of patients who gave spot urine samples.

5. Conclusion

This study elaborated a validated, practical, and useful tool measuring adherence to medications in Lebanese hypertensive patients. Promotion of adherence to antihypertensives by physicians and public health actors is advantageous, as well as better stress management in Lebanese hypertensive patients. Further research is needed to estimate mean sodium intake in hypertensive patients and the consistence of their diets. A comparison between LMAS-14 and MMAS-8 using an objective measure of adherence might also be beneficial for future studies.

Abbreviations

MMAS-8: Eight-item Morisky Medication Adherence Scale
LMAS-14: Fourteen-item Lebanese Medication Adherence Scale.

Acknowledgments

The authors acknowledge the Lebanese University for paying the fees of laboratory tests and work field. They also acknowledge Jabre Ghorra Laboratory for laboratory tests. The authors also acknowledge all the physicians who were generous enough to let the surveyors include their patients in this study, as well as the hospitals that cooperated by permitting patients' enrollment at their outpatients clinics departments.

References

[1] S. Mendis, *WHO — Global status report on noncommunicable diseases 2014*, WHO, 2014, http://www.who.int/nmh/publications/ncd-status-report-2014/en/.

[2] D. Matar, A. H. Frangieh, S. Abouassi et al., "Prevalence, awareness, treatment, and control of hypertension in Lebanon," *The Journal of Clinical Hypertension*, vol. 17, no. 5, pp. 381–388, 2015.

[3] F. J. He, J. Li, and G. A. MacGregor, "Effect of longer term modest salt reduction on blood pressure: cochrane systematic review and meta-analysis of randomised trials," *British Medical Journal*, vol. 346, no. 7903, Article ID f1325, 2013.

[4] N. J. Aburto, A. Ziolkovska, L. Hooper, P. Elliott, F. P. Cappuccio, and J. J. Meerpohl, "Effect of lower sodium intake on health: Systematic review and meta-analyses," *BMJ*, vol. 346, no. 7903, Article ID f1326, 2013.

[5] P. A. James, S. Oparil, B. L. Carter et al., "2014 Evidence-based guideline for the management of high blood pressure in adults: report from the panel members appointed to the Eighth Joint National Committee (JNC 8)," *Journal of the American Medical Association*, vol. 311, no. 5, pp. 507–520, 2014.

[6] Q. Gu, V. L. Burt, C. F. Dillon, and S. Yoon, "Trends in antihypertensive medication use and blood pressure control among United States adults with hypertension: the national health and nutrition examination survey, 2001 to 2010," *Circulation*, vol. 126, no. 17, pp. 2105–2114, 2012.

[7] R. Farah, R. K. Zeidan, M. N. Chahine et al., "Predictors of Uncontrolled Blood Pressure in Treated Hypertensive Individuals: First Population-Based Study in Lebanon," *The Journal of Clinical Hypertension*, vol. 18, no. 9, pp. 871–877, 2016.

[8] A. M. Lulebo, P. B. Mutombo, M. A. Mapatano et al., "Predictors of non-adherence to antihypertensive medication in Kinshasa, Democratic Republic of Congo: a cross-sectional study," *BMC Research Notes*, vol. 8, no. 1, 2015.

[9] L. Villa, D. Sun, K. Denhaerynck et al., "Predicting blood pressure outcomes using single-item physician-administered measures: a retrospective pooled analysis of observational studies in Belgium," *British Journal of General Practice*, vol. 65, no. 630, pp. e9–e15, 2015.

[10] S. De Geest and E. Sabaté, "Adherence to Long-Term Therapies: Evidence for Action," *European Journal of Cardiovascular Nursing*, vol. 2, no. 4, pp. 323-323, 2016.

[11] M. Yassine, A. Al-Hajje, S. Awada et al., "Evaluation of medication adherence in Lebanese hypertensive patients," *Journal of Epidemiology and Global Health*, vol. 6, no. 3, pp. 157–167, 2016.

[12] S. Shin, H. Song, S.-K. Oh, K. E. Choi, H. Kim, and S. Jang, "Effect of antihypertensive medication adherence on hospitalization for cardiovascular disease and mortality in hypertensive patients," *Hypertension Research*, vol. 36, no. 11, pp. 1000–1005, 2013.

[13] A. Bitton, N. K. Choudhry, O. S. Matlin, K. Swanton, and W. H. Shrank, "The impact of medication adherence on coronary artery disease costs and outcomes: A systematic review," *American Journal of Medicine*, vol. 126, no. 4, pp. 357–e27, 2013.

[14] S. Garfield, S. Clifford, L. Eliasson, N. Barber, and A. Willson, "Suitability of measures of self-reported medication adherence for routine clinical use: A systematic review," *BMC Medical Research Methodology*, vol. 11, article no. 149, 2011.

[15] D. E. Morisky, A. Ang, M. Krousel-Wood, and H. J. Ward, "Predictive validity of a medication adherence measure in an outpatient setting," *The Journal of Clinical Hypertension*, vol. 10, no. 5, pp. 348–354, 2008.

[16] X. Tan, I. Patel, and J. Chang, "Review of the four item Morisky Medication Adherence Scale (MMAS-4) and eight item Morisky Medication Adherence Scale (MMAS-8)," *INNOVATIONS in Pharmacy*, vol. 5, no. 3, 2014.

[17] A. Al-Hajje, S. Awada, S. Rachidi et al., "Factors affecting medication adherence in lebanese patients with chronic diseases," *Pharmacy Practice*, vol. 13, no. 3, article no. 590, 2015.

[18] E. M. Frese, A. Fick, and H. S. Sadowsky, "Blood Pressure Measurement Guidelines for Physical Therapists , Cardiopulm," *Phys. Ther. J*, vol. 22, no. 2, p. 12, 2011.

[19] R. Asmar, J. Khabouth, J. Topouchian, R. El Feghali, and J. Mattar, "Validation of three automatic devices for self-measurement of blood pressure according to the International Protocol: The Omron M3 Intellisense (HEM-7051-E), the Omron M2 Compact (HEM 7102-E), and the Omron R3-I Plus (HEM 6022-E)," *Blood Pressure Monitoring*, vol. 15, no. 1, pp. 49–54, 2010.

[20] A. V. Chobanian, G. L. Bakris, H. R. Black et al., "The seventh report of the joint national committee on prevention, detection, evaluation, and treatment of high blood pressure: the JNC 7 report," *The Journal of the American Medical Association*, vol. 289, no. 19, pp. 2560–2572, 2003.

[21] M. E. Cogswell, C. Wang, T. Chen et al., "Validity of predictive equations for 24-h urinary sodium excretion in adults aged 18–39 y," *American Journal of Clinical Nutrition*, vol. 98, no. 6, pp. 1502–1513, 2013.

[22] V. Korb-Savoldelli, F. Gillaizeau, J. Pouchot et al., "Validation of a french version of the 8-item morisky medication adherence scale in hypertensive adults," *The Journal of Clinical Hypertension*, vol. 14, no. 7, pp. 429–434, 2012.

[23] N. Masters, C. Tutt, and N. Yaseen, "Waterpipe tobacco smoking and cigarette equivalence," *British Journal of General Practice*, vol. 62, no. 596, p. 127, 2012.

[24] "National Nutrient Database for Standard Reference Release 28," Tech. Rep., U.S.D. of A. Agricultural Research Service, 2016, https://ndb.nal.usda.gov/ndb/foods/show/4259?manu=&fgcd=Beverages.

[25] M. D. Ruopp, N. J. Perkins, B. W. Whitcomb, and E. F. Schisterman, "Youden index and optimal cut-point estimated from observations affected by a lower limit of detection," *Biometrical Journal*, vol. 50, no. 3, pp. 419–430, 2008.

[26] S. A. Assi, Y. Slaybi, P. Salameh, and N. Saleh, "Development of a scoring system to measure drug C," *Journal of Hypertension*, vol. 33, p. e281, 2015.

[27] H. Y. Jaddou, A. M. Batieha, Y. S. Khader, A. H. Kanaan, M. S. El-Khateeb, and K. M. Ajlouni, "Hypertension prevalence, awareness, treatment and control, and associated factors: results from a national survey, Jordan," *International Journal of Hypertension*, vol. 2011, Article ID 828797, 8 pages, 2011.

[28] A. A. Saeed, N. A. Al-Hamdan, A. A. Bahnassy, A. M. Abdalla, M. A. F. Abbas, and L. Z. Abuzaid, "Prevalence, awareness, treatment, and control of hypertension among Saudi adult population: a national survey," *International Journal of Hypertension*, vol. 2011, Article ID 174135, 8 pages, 2011.

[29] G. Tocci, A. Ferrucci, R. Pontremoli et al., "Blood pressure levels and control in Italy: Comprehensive analysis of clinical data from 2000-2005 and 2005-2011 hypertension surveys," *Journal of Human Hypertension*, vol. 29, no. 11, pp. 696–701, 2015.

[30] F. S. Sarfo, L. M. Mobula, G. Burnham et al., "Factors associated with uncontrolled blood pressure among Ghanaians: Evidence from a multicenter hospital-based study," *PLoS ONE*, vol. 13, no. 3, p. e0193494, 2018.

10

Epidemiology of Hypertension Stages in Two Countries in Sub-Sahara Africa: Factors Associated with Hypertension Stages

Kirubel Zemedkun Gebreselassie[1] and Mojgan Padyab[2]

[1]*Epidemiology and Global Health, Department of Public Health and Clinical Medicine, Umeå University, 901 85 Umeå, Sweden*
[2]*Centre for Population Studies, Ageing and Living Conditions Programme, Umeå University, Umeå, Sweden*

Correspondence should be addressed to Kirubel Zemedkun Gebreselassie; kirubelgebresilassie@yahoo.com

Academic Editor: Olugbenga Ogedegbe

Studies using the revised hypertension classification are needed to better understand epidemiology of hypertension across full distribution. The sociodemographic, biological, and health behavior characteristics associated with different stages of hypertension in Ghana and South Africa (SA) were studied using global ageing and adult health (SAGE), WAVE 1 dataset. Blood pressure was assessed for a total of 7545 respondents, 2980 from SA and 4565 from Ghana. Hypertension was defined using JNC7 blood pressure classification considering previous diagnosis and treatment. Multivariate multinomial logistic regression analysis using Stata version 12 statistical software was done to identify independent predictors. The weighted prevalence of prehypertension and hypertension in Ghana was 30.7% and 42.4%, respectively, and that of SA was 29.4% and 46%, respectively, showing high burden. After adjusting for the independent variables, only age (OR = 1.32, 95% CI: 1.14–1.53), income (OR = 1.9, 95% CI: 1.04–3.47), and BMI (OR = 1.16, 95% CI: 1.1–1.22) remained independent predictors for stage 1 hypertension in Ghana, while, for SA, age (OR = 2.27, 95% CI: 1.53–3.36), sex (OR = 0.28, 95% CI: 0.08–1), and BMI (OR = 1.15, 95% CI: 1.07–1.25) were found to be independent predictors of stage 1 hypertension. Healthy lifestyle changes and policy measures are needed to promptly address these predictors.

1. Introduction

Worldwide prevalence estimates for hypertension may be as much as 1 billion individuals, and approximately 7.1 million deaths per year may be attributable to hypertension. The World Health Organization reports that suboptimal systolic blood pressure (SBP) >115 mmHg is responsible for 62 percent of cerebrovascular disease and 49 percent of ischemic heart disease (IHD), with little variation by sex [1]. Hypertension has been identified as the leading risk factor for developing congestive heart failure [2], stroke [3], chronic kidney disease, and end stage renal disease [4] and is ranked third as a cause of disability-adjusted life-years [5].

The risk of developing these complications depends on the level of elevated blood pressure and has been seen in all age groups starting from blood pressure as low as SBP 115 and DBP of 75 [6]. Data from observational studies involving more than 1 million individuals have also indicated that death from both IHD and stroke increases progressively and linearly from levels as low as 115 mmHg SBP and 75 mmHg DBP upward especially in individuals ranging from 40 to 89 years of age, indicating need for new blood pressure classification [6]. The risk of coronary heart disease increased significantly in the high range prehypertension individuals (SBP 130–139 or DBP 85–89 mmHg) but not in the low range prehypertensive population (SBP from 120 to 129 or DBP 80 to 84 mmHg) [7].

Because of the new data on lifetime risk of hypertension and the highly increased risk of cardiovascular morbidity associated with levels of BP previously considered to be normal, the JNC 7 report has introduced a new classification that includes the term "prehypertension" for those with BPs ranging from 120 to 139 mmHg systolic and/or 80 to 89 mmHg diastolic. This new designation is intended to identify those individuals in whom early intervention by adoption of healthy lifestyles could reduce BP, decrease the rate of progression of BP to hypertensive levels with age, or prevent hypertension entirely [8]. Robust population-based data using these recent blood pressure categories are still needed to confirm prior estimates and inform policy decision makers in Sub-Saharan Africa.

Increasing urbanization has fueled social and economic changes in Sub-Saharan Africa, which have contributed to a surge in noncommunicable disease (NCD), including hypertension [9]. Epidemiological studies on hypertension in this region have been conducted over the years in an attempt to estimate the burden of hypertension, and these have reported variable rates within and between different population groups. In the first national Demographic and Health Survey, of 12,952 randomly selected South Africans aged 15 years, a high risk of hypertension was associated with less than tertiary education, older age groups, overweight and obese people, excess alcohol use, and a family history of stroke and hypertension [10]. Prehypertension was also more common in those aged 35 years compared with those aged <35 years and in overweight and obese people compared with people of normal weight [11]. Hypertension was defined in these studies as individuals with self-reported treated hypertension or with an average of 2 blood pressure measurements of at least 140/90 mmHg [9, 12, 13].

Prior studies on hypertension mainly focused on these dichotomous definitions of hypertension and did not examine the sociodemographic characteristics and risk factors for hypertension across full distribution of blood pressure. The current study follows the work of Basu and Millet on social epidemiology of hypertension in low- and middle-income countries from World Health Organization's Study on global AGEing and adult health (SAGE) [13]. Their work further showed additional variation in hypertension prevalence and social determinants of awareness when categorical definitions of hypertension were used compared to dichotomous definitions. Men had significantly lower probability of hypertension awareness than women at stage 1, but not at stage 2 [14]. This empirical study with an objective of studying social determinants and risk factors of different stages of hypertension tries to address this question. It determines the prevalence and independent predictors of different stages of hypertension in two countries in Sub-Saharan Africa, Ghana and South Africa.

2. Methods

2.1. Study Design and Population. We conducted a cross-sectional analysis of the Study on global AGEing and adult health (SAGE), WAVE 1 dataset which is a part of longitudinal survey program in WHO's multicountries study unit. The main SAGE surveys compile comparable longitudinal information on the health and well-being of adult populations and the ageing process from nationally representative samples in six middle- and low-income countries. We used the dataset of two Sub-Saharan countries, Ghana and South Africa. The SAGE study included nationally representative sample of persons aged 50 years and sample from younger adults aged 18–49 years as comparison which were also selected from both countries. Multistage cluster sampling was used [15]. The sampling design entailed two-stage probabilistic sample that yielded national and subnational estimates. In the first stage, a total sample of 600 enumeration areas (EA) in South Africa and 300 (EA) in Ghana were drawn from the master sample and used as the primary selection units (PSU). The second stage of the sample design was the selection of households from the EA's which formed the secondary sampling units. This stage of the process involved georeferenced aerial photograph maps of urbanized areas on which the locations of households were plotted. The total sample size of individuals was targeted to be 1000 people in the age group 18–49 years and 5000 people aged 50 years or older in each country.

2.2. Questionnaire. We recorded information about the household members from household and individual questionnaires; living place variable from the household questionnaire and sociodemographic characteristics, work history, blood pressure measurements, and risk factors including preventive health behaviors were taken from the individual questionnaire. Both the household and individual questionnaires were translated into six local South African and three local languages of Ghana. The respondents were interviewed face to face.

2.3. Blood Pressure Measurements and Classification. Blood pressure was measured three times while the respondent seated using automated OMRON R6 Wrist Blood Pressure Monitor, HEM-6000-E, Health Care Europe, B.V., Hoofddorp, The Netherlands. Such digital monitors have been shown to have high degree of agreement with mercury sphygmomanometers for systolic blood pressure [16, 17]. Average blood pressure was calculated arithmetically for the 3 measurements of each systolic and diastolic blood pressure. Missing values were excluded from being included in the study. Blood pressure classification was done using JNC 7 algorithm [1]. Prehypertension was defined as systolic blood pressure (SBP) measurement of 120–139 mmHg or diastolic blood pressure (DBP) of 80–89 mmHg. Stage 1 hypertension was defined as SBP of 140–159 mmHg or DBP of 90–99 mmHg and stage 2 as SBP of greater than or equal to 160 mmHg or DBP of greater than or equal to 100 mmHg. Accordingly normal pressure was defined as SBP of less than 120 mmHg and DBP of less than 80 mmHg.

All respondents were initially asked if they have ever been diagnosed with hypertension and if they did, whether or not they have been taking any kind of drugs or other treatment for the last 2 weeks and last 12 months. Normal blood pressure was defined as SBP <120 and DBP <80 mmHg and either no previous history of diagnosis or not taking antihypertensive medication. Those with SBP of 120 or more and DBP of 80 or more who did not have prior diagnosis nor treatment were designed as to have hypertension. They were subsequently stratified into three mutually exclusive different stages of hypertension. Those who reported as either having a diagnosis of hypertension previously or taking antihypertensive medication were excluded from analysis due to overlapping.

2.4. Sociodemographic Characteristics. All participants older than 18 years, of both sexes, were included in the study and classified as living in urban or rural area. Current marital status (married or single that included unmarried, widowed, or separated) was asked about using the individual questionnaire. Educational level was assessed by first asking whether respondents have been in any school, and those who answered yes were asked for the highest educational level completed according to the international standard classification of education [18]. Respondents were asked whether they had ever worked for pay, type of work, and employer. Occupation responses were written verbatim by the interviewer, then coded, and mapped to the International Standard Classifications of Occupations (ISCO) scheme [19]. Classification of income quintiles was based on permanent income estimates derived from household assets and characteristics of the dwelling upon which The 2001 WHO World Health Survey/SAGE WAVE 0 relied [15]. Recent alcohol intake was asked for by asking whether the respondents have consumed alcohol in the past 30 days. Response was documented as yes and no. Current smoking (yes or no), with provision for the collection of information on other forms of smoking apart from cigarettes, such as cigars, pipes, snuff, or chewing smokeless tobacco, was asked about. Question was formulated based on guidelines for controlling and monitoring the tobacco epidemic [20]. Work related and sport or leisure time physical activities were separately asked in a typical week. Vigorous or moderate physical activities required hard or moderate physical effort and caused an increase in breathing or heart rate for at least 10 minutes [21]. Fruit and vegetable servings in typical 24 hours were asked about. Inadequate intake was defined based on WHO recommendations and labeled as less than 5 servings (80 g per serving) on a typical day [22].

2.5. Anthropometric Measurements. Height was measured in centimeters after the respondents took off their shoes, put their feet and heels close together, stood straight, and stood forward with their back, head, and heels touching the wall. Next body weight was measured in kilograms. Body composition and fatness were assessed using WHO body mass index (BMI) derived from measured weight in kilograms and normalized by dividing by height in meters squared. It was categorized as underweight <18.5, normal weight 18.5–24.9, overweight 25 to 29.9, and obese greater than or equal to 30. Since abdominal obesity is highly correlated with atherosclerotic cardiovascular morbidity and mortality than BMI indices [23], waist circumference was also used to measure central obesity. The interviewer identified the top of the hip bone and after making sure the tape measure is parallel to the floor all the way around the body measured waist circumference (WC). The National Cholesterol and Education Program: Adult Treatment Panel III (NCEP: ATP III) guideline was used to designate central obesity: accordingly men with WC measurements greater than or equal to 102 cm and women with greater than or equal to 88 cm were considered to have one [24].

2.6. Statistical Analysis. Stata version 12 statistical software was used to analyze data after being cleaned. The individual and household data were merged together. Living place variable was taken from the household data while all the others were included from the individual dataset. To make sure the results of the individual country dataset represent the respective country population, weighting at the country level was done which was available in the SAGE dataset. Individual weights were poststratified according to the 2009 projected population estimates in Ghana and to the 2009 medium midyear population estimates in South Africa [25]. Weighted estimates of different stages of hypertension prevalence were reported as proportions of the actual sample size. Invalid blood pressure measurements such as values of diastolic blood pressure greater than systolic and those in the outliers were considered missing and excluded from analysis.

The associations between sociodemographic, biological, and health behavior variables and stages of hypertension (prehypertension, stage 1, and stage 2) were assessed in a two-step procedure where individuals with the different stages of hypertension were compared separately with those having normal blood pressure. In the first step, each variable was evaluated independently in a bivariate multinomial logistic regression analysis with different stages of hypertension as dependent variable to generate unadjusted OR with respondents' characteristics in each country separately. Those variables with P values less than 0.2 were retained and entered into multinomial logistic regression model in ascending stepwise manner to determine variables that were independently associated with the stages of hypertension. A probability level of $P < 0.05$ was considered significant. Age and BMI variables were entered in the multivariable multinomial models as continuous due to fewer numbers of people in the most upper and lower categories. All other variables were retained as categorical.

2.7. Ethical Approval. Informed consent was obtained from each respondent for interviews and measurements of anthropometrics. SAGE study received ethical clearance from WHO ethical review committee [26].

3. Results

The total sample size of the study was 8939, 3974 from South Africa and 4965 from Ghana. Participants who have been diagnosed previously with high blood pressure or who were already taking treatment were excluded from analysis due to overlap and difficulty to stratify them into mutually exclusive hypertension stages. Those with previous diagnosis of hypertension were 587 (12%) in Ghana and 1,111 (28%) in South Africa. Individuals taking antihypertensive medications were 396 (8%) in Ghana and 981 (25%) in South Africa. Completed interview response in South Africa was 2853 (96%) and 5057 (99%) in Ghana. Of these blood pressure was assessed for a total of 7545, 2980 (75%) respondents from South Africa and 4565 (92%) from Ghana which was included for analysis (Table 1). A higher number of study participants in Ghana were males (50.2%) compared to 48.5% in South Africa. More people lived in Urban areas in South Africa (69.7%) compared to only 44.4% in Ghana. In South Africa,

TABLE 1: Sociodemographic, health behavior, and biological characteristics (%) of study subjects, by country and hypertension stages.

$N = 7545$	Ghana ($n = 4565$)					South Africa ($n = 2980$)				
	Normal	Pre-HTN	Stage 1 HTN	Stage 2 HTN	Total (%)	Normal	Pre-HTN	Stage 1 HTN	Stage 2 HTN	Total (%)
Sociodemographic variables										
Age groups (years)	**					**				
18–49	28.1	32.6	20.5	18.8	762 (76.9)	28.2	31.7	16.2	23.9	334 (79.7)
50–59	20.1	23.2	28.3	28.4	1532 (9.4)	9.1	20.9	24.9	45.1	1242 (11.1)
60–69	18.5	24.7	23.1	33.7	1055 (6.3)	6.9	20.6	28.5	44.1	803 (5.7)
70–74	18.4	26.7	23.9	30.9	837 (5.1)	9.5	15	33.1	42.4	424 (2.5)
80+	19.0	27.6	24.5	29	374 (2.3)	5.8	20.4	29.6	44.2	171 (1.1)
Sex						*				
Male	26.2	29.3	20.7	23.8	2466 (50.2)	16.4	33.9	18.5	31.2	1361 (48.5)
Female	25.9	32.1	22.6	19.4	2099 (49.8)	31.3	25.1	18.4	25.3	1617 (51.5)
Living place						*				
Urban	23.6	30.3	24	22.2	1747 (44.4)	28.3	28.6	18.3	24.9	1890 (69.7)
Rural	28	31.1	19.8	21.1	2818 (55.6)	14.7	31.4	18.2	35.7	1084 (30.3)
Marital status										
Married	25.6	28.1	23.8	22.5	1758 (26.6)	28.9	29.1	19.5	22.6	1346 (46.5)
Single	26.3	31.8	20.8	21.1	2782 (73.4)	20	29.4	17.8	32.8	1578 (53.6)
Educational level	*					**				
No school	21.9	27.6	22.1	28.4	2337 (31.1)	7.7	20.8	22.4	49.1	647 (7.3)
<6 yrs	29.3	30.3	23.5	17	498 (12.8)	5.5	23.4	22.2	48.9	556 (13.9)
Primary	26.4	29.3	24.8	19.6	567 (20.1)	10.4	28.9	22	38.7	557 (13.9)
Secondary	21.8	41.3	21	15.8	244 (10.9)	35.2	26.2	17.4	21.3	391 (27.7)
High school	29.5	32.3	18.2	20.1	737 (20.7)	40.3	19.2	18.4	22.1	221 (29.1)
University	36.8	28.8	18.2	16.3	154 (4.4)	41.7	27.1	11.6	19.6	143 (8.1)
Occupation	*									
Public sector	23.6	34.1	21.8	20.6	380 (7.2)	26.9	30.1	10.7	32.4	395 (19.8)
Private	26.7	20.1	24.1	29.1	180 (5.2)	13.4	32.7	23	31	1421 (53.1
Self-employed	25	32.3	22	20.7	3564 (80.8)	44	31.8	10.5	13.8	106 (4)
Informal	25.2	24.0	15	35.8	332 (6.8)	33.9	16.9	18.9	30.3	592 (23.1)
Income	**									
Quintile 1 (poorest)	33.4	28.3	21.5	16.9	939 (15.6)	20	30	21.2	28.8	640 (19.6)
Quintile 2	33	29	16.9	21.1	932 (18)	28.3	23.6	22.8	25.3	631 (20)
Quintile 3	19.3	31	20.8	28.8	922 (19.4)	27.4	19.6	17.3	35.6	545 (20.2)
Quintile 4	18.8	34.8	24.6	21.8	921 (22.2)	21.1	35.6	13	30.4	551 (19.5)
Quintile 5 (richest)	28.2	29.6	23.2	19.1	845 (24.9)	23.7	37.7	17.7	20.9	595 (20.8)
Biological variables										
BMI (kg/m^2)	**					**				
Underweight	31	33	14.4	21.5	670 (9.3)	21.1	35.7	8.2	35	130 (3.5)
Normal	30.6	29.4	19.8	20.2	2543 (54.4)	35.9	35.6	12.2	16.4	777 (36.1)
Overweight	21.4	32.8	22.2	23.6	889 (24.2)	32.4	21.2	21.4	25	849 (30)
Obese	10.8	30.4	33.4	25.3	444 (12.1)	5.7	23.2	25.7	45.4	1148 (30.5)
Waist circumference	*									
Normal	27.9	29.9	20.2	22	3608 (76.7)	24.5	32	18.4	25.1	1574 (63.2)
Abnormal	20.2	32.8	26.2	20.9	930 (23.3)	20	25.2	20.8	34	1180 (36.9)
Health related behaviors										
Smoking	*									
No	25.9	31.4	22.2	20.5	3416 (84.1)	26.5	32.3	16.9	24.4	1819 (67.6)

TABLE 1: Continued.

N = 7545	Ghana (n = 4565)					South Africa (n = 2980)				
	Normal	Pre-HTN	Stage 1 HTN	Stage 2 HTN	Total (%)	Normal	Pre-HTN	Stage 1 HTN	Stage 2 HTN	Total (%)
Yes	26.2	27.6	18.8	27.5	1143 (15.9)	19.1	23.2	22.2	35.6	1077 (32.4)
Current alcohol use										
No	25.9	31.7	20.7	21.7	1181 (44.3)	25.4	21.2	31.2	22.2	347 (33.5)
Yes	28.2	27.2	22.7	22	1492 (55.7)	14.9	27.8	18.5	38.8	489 (66.5)
Work related physical activity	*					*				
High	25.5	33.5	19.9	21.2	1868 (44.7)	30.7	15.6	27	26.7	306 (12.4)
Moderate	29	28.7	22.5	19.7	1400 (27.5)	33.3	28.1	14.5	24.1	852 (36.3)
Low	23.5	28.5	23.7	24.3	1289 (27.8)	16	33.6	19.3	31.1	1734 (51.4)
Fruit intake/day	*					**				
0-1	25.7	27.9	23.9	22.5	1726 (32.3)	17.6	24.9	21.1	36.4	1476 (46.3)
2–4	28	31.9	19.8	20.3	2374 (57.8)	29.8	34.2	17.4	18.6	1305 (50.2)
>=5	13.7	32.7	24.7	29	402 (9.9)	37.8	9.2	7	46	79 (3.5)
Vegetable intake/day	*					**				
0-1	29.9	24.1	24.5	21.5	1112 (24.9)	14.9	24.8	24.4	35.9	1160 (35.7)
2–4	24.1	32.4	21.2	22.3	3269 (74.3)	30.8	32.7	15.3	21.2	1592 (60.6)
>=5	21.8	36.2	29.8	12.2	57 (0.9)	5.4	10.1	21.7	62.9	116 (3.7)
Blood pressure number	957	1205	1108	1295	4565	301	647	738	1294	2980
Weighted prevalence (%)	26.1	30.7	21.6	21.6		24.1	29.4	18.5	28.1	

$^{*}P < 0.2$, $^{**}P < 0.05$.
n = number of observations in the sample.
All percentages (%) are put as weighted estimates of the sample to represent population.

the proportion of obesity was 30.5% as compared to 12.1% in Ghana. Income quintile distribution was similar in both countries. Only 26.1% of the respondents in Ghana and 24.1% in South Africa fulfilled the definition of normal blood pressure. Prehypertension was more prevalent in Ghana (30.7%) than South Africa (29.4%). The weighted prevalence of hypertension (both stages 1 and 2) was 42.4% in Ghana and 46% in South Africa. The age group distribution across stages of hypertension was similar in both countries, the majority of prehypertensive individuals being in the age group of 18 to 49. Obese individuals constituted 45.4% of stage 2 hypertension in South Africa while they constituted only 25.3% of stage 2 hypertension in Ghana.

Prehypertension was significantly associated in Ghana with income distribution (OR = 1.9, 95% CI: 1.11–3.23) and BMI category (OR = 2.64, 95% CI: 1.11–6.3) in the bivariate multinomial analysis when compared with normal blood pressure measurement while in South Africa age (OR = 2.66, 95% CI: 1.34–5.28) and educational level (OR = 0.18, 95% CI: 0.05–0.63) only had a significant association (Table 2). Income and BMI remained to have a significant association with stage 1 hypertension. In addition age emerged as a new variable with significant correlation with stage 1 hypertension in Ghana in the bivariate analysis (OR = 1.71, 95% CI: 1.25–2.33). In South Africa stage 1 hypertension was significantly associated with age of the study participants (OR = 6.02, 95% CI: 2.61–13.88), educational level (OR = 0.09, 95% CI: 0.02–0.49), type of occupation (OR = 4.32, 95% CI: 1.06–17.55), BMI category (OR = 11.72, 95% CI: 2.35–58.43), and number of vegetable servings per day in the bivariate multinomial analysis (OR = 0.3, 95% CI: 0.11–0.82). Age, income, and BMI remained to be significantly associated with stage 2 hypertension in the bivariate multinomial analysis in Ghana. In addition educational level (OR = 0.07, 95% CI: 0.02–0.35) became a significant correlate with stage 2 hypertension. In South Africa factors significantly associated with stage 2 hypertension were age, living place, educational level, and fruit and vegetable intake.

4. Multinomial Logistic Regression Model with Pooled Multivariable Analysis

4.1. Ghana. For the multinomial logistic regression analysis, 10 independent variables which were associated with hypertension stages at level of P value < 0.2 in the bivariate analysis were retained in the model. These were age, educational level, type of occupation, income quintile, smoking status, BMI category, abdominal waist circumference, work related physical activity, and fruit and vegetable intake per day. Those with P values <0.05 in the multivariable model were considered statistically significant and were considered independent predictors of hypertension stages (Figure 1). At prehypertension level BMI (OR = 1.08, 95% CI: 1.03–1.14), income (OR = 2,24, 95% CI: 1.27–3.97), and number of vegetable intakes per day were found to be independent predictors after being adjusted for the other variables in the model. Income and BMI remained independent predictors

Table 2: Association between sociodemographic, health behavior, and biological variables with stages of hypertension (pre-HTN, stage 1, and stage 2) compared to normal blood pressure: bivariate multinomial analysis.

N = 7545	Ghana (n = 4565)			South Africa (n = 2980)		
	Pre-HTN OR (95% CI)	Stage 1 OR (95% CI)	Stage 2 OR (95% CI)	Pre-HTN OR (95% CI)	Stage 1 OR (95% CI)	Stage 2 OR (95% CI)
Age groups (years)						
18–49	1	1	1	1	1	1
50–59	1 (0.78–1.29)	1.93 (1.47–2.54)*	2.12 (1.59–2.83)	2.06 (1.04–4.09)	4.77 (2.13–10.67)	5.88 (3.01–11.48)
60–69	1.15 (0.86–1.54)	1.71 (1.25–2.33)*	2.72 (2.02–3.67)	2.66 (1.34–5.28)	7.19 (3.38–15.28)	7.57 (3.87–14.82)
70–74	1.25 (0.94–1.66)	1.78 (1.26–2.51)*	2.51 (1.8–3.51)	1.4 (0.57–3.44)	6.02 (2.61–13.88*)	5.25 (2.39–11.5)*
80+	1.25 (0.8–1.97)	1.77 (1.1–2.84)*	2.29 (1.47–3.57)*	3.17 (1.19–8.43)*	8.95 (3.5–22.89)	9.09 (3.77–21.93)
Sex						
Male	1	1	1	1	1	1
Female	1.11 (0.78–0.58)	1.1 (0.75–1.61)	0.82 (0.56–1.21)	0.39 (0.14–1.09)	0.52 (0.19–0.44)	0.43 (0.17–1.06)
Living place						
Urban	1	1	1	1	1	1
Rural	0.86 (0.6–1.24)	0.69 (0.47–1.03)	0.8 (0.51–1.25)	2.12 (0.82–5.49)	1.92 (0.75–4.88)	2.76 (1.14–6.68)*
Marital status						
Married	1	1	1	1	1	1
Single	1.1 (0.71–1.72)	0.85 (0.55–1.3)	0.91 (0.59–1.4)	1.46 (0.49–4.34)	1.32 (0.46–3.77)	2.1 (0.8–5.52)
Educational level						
No school	1	1	1	1	1	1
<6 yrs	0.82 (0.45–1.49)	0.8 (0.44–1.44)	0.45 (0.25–0.8)	1.58 (0.38–6.53)	1.39 (0.44–4.34)	1.4 (0.47–4.15)
Primary	0.88 (0.52–1.49)	0.93 (0.53–1.64)	0.57 (0.33–0.98)*	1.03 (0.28–3.84)	0.73 (0.2–2.66)	0.58 (0.17–1.95)
Secondary	1.5 (0.77–2.9)	0.95 (0.48–1.92)	0.56 (0.26–1.2)	0.27 (0.07–1.05)	0.17 (0.05–0.61)	0.09 (0.03–0.3)
High school	0.87 (0.52–1.45)	0.61 (0.35–1.07)	0.53 (0.3–0.92)	0.18 (0.05–0.63)*	0.16 (0.04–0.7)	0.09 (0.02–0.33)
University	0.62 (0.25–1.56)	0.49 (0.18–1.34)	0.34 (0.11–1.06)	0.24 (0.05–1.13)	0.09 (0.02–0.49)*	0.07 (0.02–0.35)*
Occupation						
Public sector	1	1	1	1	1	1
Private	0.52 (0.17–1.57)	0.97 (0.29–3.23)	1.25 (0.38–4.09)	2.18 (0.4–12.03)	4.32 (1.06–17.55)*	1.93 (0.49–7.64)
Self-employed	0.89 (0.47–1.72)	0.95 (0.49–1.85)	0.95 (0.46–1.97)	0.65 (0.06–7.18)	0.6 (0.07–5.23))	0.26 (0.03–2.33)
Informal	0.66 (0.27–1.62)	0.64 (0.27–1.55)	1.63 (0.6–4.39)	0.45 (0.07–2.99)	1.4 (0.22–8.72)	0.74 (0.16–3.51)
Income						
Quintile 1 (poorest)	1	1	1	1	1	1
Quintile 2	1.04 (0.6–1.79)	0.79 (0.44–1.41)	1.26 (0.74–2.14)	0.56 (0.14–2.26)	0.76 (0.17–3.43)	0.62 (0.18–2.14)
Quintile 3	1.9 (1.11–3.23)*	1.67 (0.94–2.96)	2.95 (1.76–4.95)	0.48 (0.1–2.37)	0.6 (0.11–3.15)	0.9 (0.2–4.12)
Quintile 4	2.19 (1.3–3.68)	2.03 (1.14–3.64)*	2.29 (1.32–3.97)*	1.13 (0.28–4.6)	0.58 (0.15–2.29)	1 (0.27–3.73)
Quintile 5 (richest)	1.24 (0.72–2.12)	1.27 (0.74–2.21)	1.33 (0.73–2.42)	1.06 (0.25–4.43)	0.7 (0.2–2.42)	0.61 (0.18–2.06)
Biological variables						
BMI (kg/m^2)						
Underweight	1	1	1	1	1	1
Normal	0.9 (0.51–1.6)	1.39 (0.76–2.55)	0.95 (0.53–1.71)	0.59 (0.12–2.87)	0.88 (0.16–4.68)	0.27 (0.05–1.38)
Overweight	1.44 (0.76–2.74)	2.23 (1.09–4.56)*	1.58 (0.77–3.26)	0.39 (0.07–2.06)	1.71 (0.28–10.53)	0.47 (0.08–2.77)
Obese	2.64 (1.11–6.3)*	6.62 (2.79–15.69)	3.37 (1.37–8.26)*	2.42 (0.53–11.03)	11.72 (2.35–58.43)*	4.81 (0.98–23.54)
Waist circumference						
Normal	1	1	1	1	1	1
Abnormal	1.52 (0.97–2.38)	1.79 (1.12–2.87)*	1.31 (0.8–2.13)	0.96 (0.25–3.75)	1.38 (0.38–5.04)	1.66 (0.49–5.56)
Health related behaviors						
Smoking						
No	1	1	1	1	1	1
Yes	0.87 (0.56–1.34)	0.83 (0.51–1.36)	1.33 (0.85–2.07)	1 (0.33–3.04)	1.83 (0.57–5.84)	2.02 (0.69–5.95)

TABLE 2: Continued.

N = 7545	Ghana (n = 4565)			South Africa (n = 2980)		
	Pre-HTN OR (95% CI)	Stage 1 OR (95% CI)	Stage 2 OR (95% CI)	Pre-HTN OR (95% CI)	Stage 1 OR (95% CI)	Stage 2 OR (95% CI)
Current alcohol use						
No	1	1	1	1	1	1
Yes	1.27 (0.77–2.1)	0.99 (0.6–1.65)	1.08 (0.66–1.76)	0.44 (0.1–1.93)	0.98 (0.15–6.56)	0.33 (0.08–1.42)
Work related physical activity						
High	1	1	1	1	1	1
Moderate	0.75 (0.49–1.15)	1 (0.63–1.58)	0.82 (0.5–1.33)	1.66 (0.35–7.95)	0.5 (0.08–2.93)	0.83 (0.19–3.62)
Low	0.92 (0.57–1.5)	1.29 (0.75–2.23)	1.24 (0.72–2.16)	4.14 (0.9–19.13)	1.38 (0.26–7.42)	2.24 (0.56–8.98)
Fruit intake/day						
0-1	1	1	1	1	1	1
2–4	1.05 (0.72–1.53)	0.76 (0.5–1.16)	0.83 (0.55–1.25)	0.81 (0.28–2.32)	0.49 (0.17–1.38)	0.3 (0.11–0.81)*
>=5	2.2 (1.06–4.56)	1.94 (0.91–4.14)	2.42 (1.29–4.54)	0.17 (0.02–1.34)	0.15 (0.02–1.03)	0.59 (0.07–4.65)
Vegetable intake/day						
0-1	1	1	1	1	1	1
2–4	1.67 (1.09–2.57)	1.07 (0.69–1.68)	1.28 (0.78–2.12)	0.64 (0.24–1.68)	0.3 (0.11–0.82)*	0.29 (0.11–0.72)*
>=5	2.07 (0.58–7.43)	1.67 (0.36–7.63)	0.78 (0.22–2.7)	1.13 (0.19–6.74)	2.46 (0.29–20.65)	4.86 (0.66–35.82)

*$P < 0.05$.

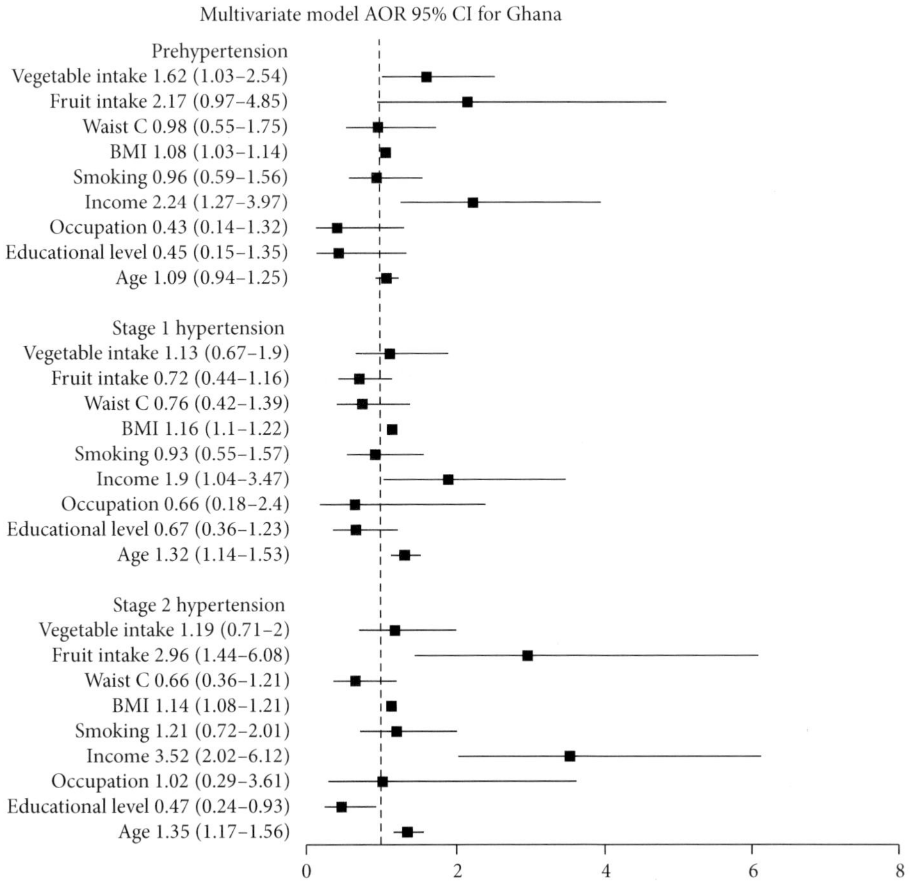

FIGURE 1: Adjusted odds ratios and 95% confidence intervals for stages of hypertension, Ghana.

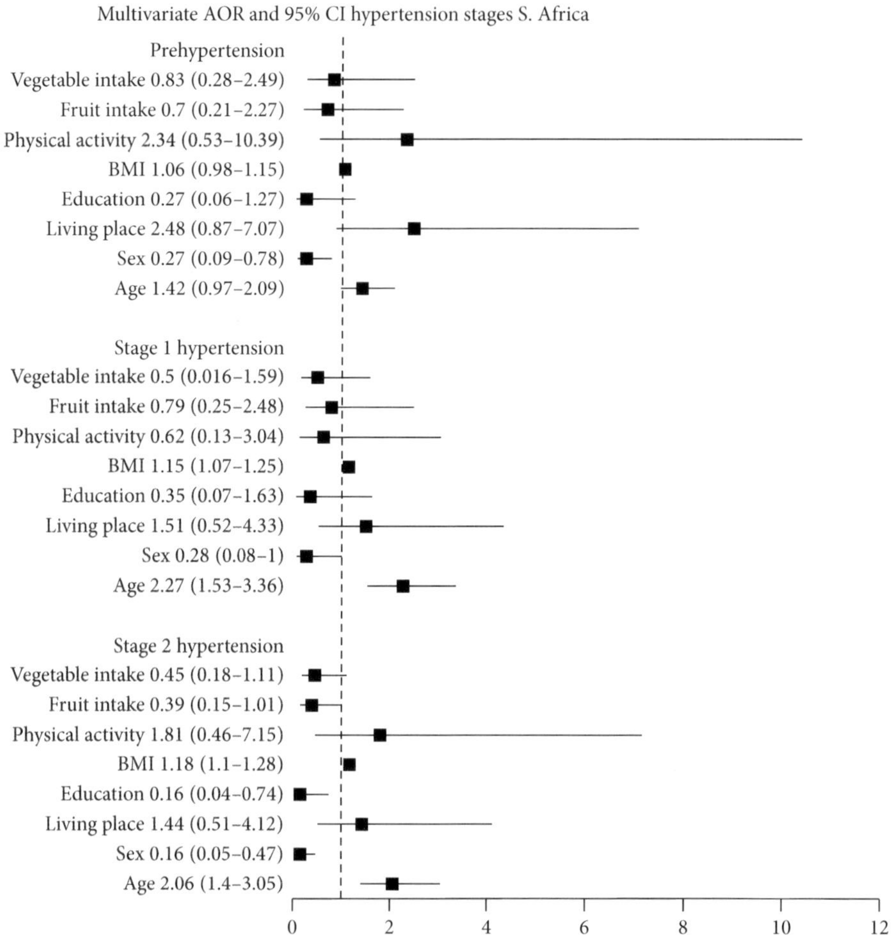

FIGURE 2: Adjusted odds ratios and 95% confidence intervals for stages of hypertension, South Africa.

for stage 1 hypertension as well. There was 32% increased risk of having stage 1 hypertension for every age increase by one year (OR = 1.32, 95% CI: 1.14–1.53). Age (OR = 1.35, 95% CI: 1.17–1.56), income (OR = 3.52, 95% CI: 2.02–6.12), and BMI (OR = 1.14, 95% CI: 1.08–1.21) remained as independent predictors for stage 2 hypertension as well. In addition higher educational level emerged as a protective variable against stage 2 hypertension in the model (OR = 0.47, 95% CI: 0.24–0.93).

4.2. South Africa. Eight variables which were associated with stages of hypertension in the bivariate analysis at probability level of $P < 0.2$ were retained in the multinomial logistic regression model. These were age, sex, living place, educational level, BMI category, work related physical activity, and fruit and vegetable servings per day (Figure 2). Only sex (OR = 0.27, 95% CI: 0.09–0.78) remained independent predictor of prehypertension in the multivariate logistic regression model after being adjusted for the other variables. Age and BMI emerged as independent predictors of stage 1 hypertension (OR = 2.27, 95% CI: 1.53–3.36 and OR = 1.15, 95% CI: 1.07–1.25). Sex remained as an independent predictor of stage 1 hypertension (OR = 0.28, 95% CI: 0.08–1). Being female resulted in 72% lower risk of having stage 1 hypertension than being male (OR = 0.28, 95% CI: 0.08–1). Age (OR = 2.06, 95% CI: 1.4–8.7), sex (OR = 0.16, 95% CI: 0.05–0.47), and BMI (OR = 1.18, 95% CI: 1.1–1.28) remained independent predictors of stage 2 hypertension in the final model. Educational level emerged as an independent predictor of stage 2 hypertension. Those with high school education tended to have 84% lower odds of stage 2 hypertension compared to those with no education (OR = 0.16, 95% CI: 0.04–0.74).

5. Discussion

The study has showed high burden of prehypertension and hypertension stages in the Sub-Saharan African countries, Ghana and South Africa. The weighted prevalence of hypertension (including both stages 1 and 2) was higher in South Africa (46%) compared to Ghana (42.4%). The high prevalence of hypertension in the current study is mostly due to higher age distribution of participants. More than 85% of respondents in Ghana and around 90% South Africans were in the age group more than 50, as part of the WHO SAGE study. The probability that a middle-aged or elderly individual will develop hypertension in his or her lifetime is 90% [27], explaining the higher prevalence in this study. Higher prevalence of hypertension (77.3%) than the current study was also reported in hypertension and associated factors in older adults study in South Africa [28]. Comparing the two countries South Africa had higher prevalence of hypertension that could be explained by higher proportion of people living in urban area (69.7% in South Africa and 44.4% in Ghana) and increased number of obese people (30.5% in South Africa and 12.1% Ghana). In addition lower rate of physical activity and fruit intake per day was reported in South Africa.

The weighted prevalence of prehypertension was higher in Ghana (30.7%) than South Africa (29.4%). Higher reports were made from the PURE hypertension trial done on 153,996 adults aged 35 to 70 years, from 628 communities in 3 high-income, 10 upper-middle and low-middle-income, and 4 low-income countries of 36.8% [12]. These are groups of people with increased cardiovascular risk but who do not need pharmacologic treatment unless there is another compelling medical indication such as diabetes or chronic kidney disease [29]. They have higher likelihood of progression to overt hypertension and need lifestyle changes as a treatment such as weight reduction, physical activity, and decreased salt intake [30]. Progression from prehypertension to stage 1 hypertension was positively related to male gender, higher waist circumference, and having parents with hypertension in population-based study Keelung, Taiwan [31]. Identifying these individuals has high public health importance as such measures taken could delay or prevent progression or development of hypertension.

The weighted prevalence of stage 1 hypertension in Ghana was higher (21.6%) than in South Africa (18.5%) and the weighted estimate of stage 2 hypertension was higher in South Africa (28.1%) and Ghana (21.6%). Prior studies on these two countries were mainly done on dichotomized blood pressure classification using SBP of 140 mmHg or DBP of 90 mmHg and more. According to hypertension in South African adults, results from the Demographic and Health Survey, 1998, the prevalence rate of hypertension was 11% in males and 14% in females when blood pressure cut-off point (160/95 mmHg) was used [32]. In the current study BMI was an independent predictor for prehypertension in both Ghana and South Africa which was a similar finding in the study done in the Ashanti region of Ghana which showed age (OR = 1.56, 95% CI: 1.12–2.18; $P < 0.01$), obesity (OR = 2.71; 95% CI: 1.40–5.24; $P < 0.001$), and sex (OR = 2.36, 95% CI: 1.77–3.15; $P < 0.001$) being independent predictors of prehypertension on multivariable logistic regression [11]. In addition income became one of the strongest predictors for prehypertension in Ghana in our study, with higher income quintiles associated with higher levels of prehypertension. This was similar with household characteristics for older adults and study background from SAGE Ghana WAVE 1, which showed people with the higher income quintiles generally reported more hypertension (income quintile 5, wealthiest = 26.7%, versus quintile 1, poorest = 5.5%) and received more current and chronic therapy [15]. Other studies in US and Canada have shown the opposite effect; inverse linear relationship between household income and hypertension prevalence in the United States, but no evidence of such a relationship in Canada, was seen due to similar burden of hypertension across different socioeconomic classes [33]. Middle-income was a high correlate in another study in urban India [34]. Getting income data reliably was difficult as income was generated from ho usehold assets and converted later to quintiles, hence requiring cautious interpretation of result. The proportion of both overweight and obese was higher in the 4th and 5th income quintiles than the lower ones (23% and 30%, resp.) which could explain the high prevalence of prehypertension in the group.

Being in the higher BMI category contributed significantly to having prehypertension and could be related to the low physical activity of the current study participants [35]. Those with the lowest work related physical activity had the highest rates of prehypertension. South Africa has one of the lowest rates of insufficient physical activity (49% in adult women and 43% in adult men) compared to global figure of 17% and Africa's coverage of about 10% [36]. Some of the explanations were high rate of urbanization, increased mechanized labour, and television watching [37]. The very low report of physical activity contributing to both obesity and prehypertension needs to be addressed in South Africa by clinicians, public health specialists, patients, and policy makers at the government level.

We have tried to see the social determinant and risk factors for different hypertension stages (1 and 2) separately and whether they differ in the two countries and across different hypertension stages in the same country. The study has showed only age, income, and BMI remaining as independent predictors of stage 1 hypertension in Ghana. We found educational level and number of fruit intakes per day having an inverse relationship to stage 1 hypertension in South Africa in the bivariate multinomial analysis. This is similar with the first demographic and health survey study: determinants and treatment of hypertension in South Africa which showed higher risk of having hypertension with less than tertiary education [10]. Adults with no education or less than primary school were more than 50%, and the highest report of stage 1 hypertension was seen in this group in the current study. Curriculum reforms and models to increase opportunity of education in the postapartheid education system are undergoing [38] and should be further strengthened.

Increasing fruit and vegetable intake was seen to have significant blood pressure lowering effect in stage 1 and stage 2 hypertension. This effect was not seen in the final model. The finding is consistent with other trials that demonstrated the greatest benefit of dietary changes at lower stages of hypertension [30]. The DASH (Dietary Approaches to Stop Hypertension) trials introduced the DASH diet which is comprised of four-five servings of fruit, four-five servings of vegetables, two-three servings of low-fat dairy per day, and <25 percent fat [39]. Drop in average systolic blood pressure by 11.4 mmHg and diastolic blood pressure by 5.5 mmHg in hypertensive individuals has been seen as early as two weeks, with the DASH diet. Increasing fruit intake is thus highly recommended in individuals especially with lower stages of hypertension to prevent progression of disease. Countries should be working on ways to make availability of fruits accessible and affordable. The weighted estimate of people taking the recommended fruit intake was very low (9.9%) in Ghana and (3.5%) South Africa. Vegetable intake was even much worse (0.9%) in Ghana and (3.5%) in South Africa. The wide confidence interval and attenuated beneficial effects of fruits and vegetables could be attributed to the very little proportion of people in these categories making the expected statistical association loose.

Though smoking cigarette was one of the most important risk factors for cardiovascular disorders and acute myocardial infarction in the INTERHEART Africa study [40], it was associated only in the bivariate analysis when studied individually. The effect was lost when multiple variables were retained in the regression model in both countries at every stage of hypertension. The incidence of hypertension increases in those who smoke 15 or more cigarettes per day [41] and could be the reason why strong association was not seen as only less than 2% individuals (Ghana) and around 7% (South Africa) smoked more than 15 cigarettes per day. Other studies have also documented "lower blood pressure measurements in those habitual smokers than nonsmokers due to weight loss and some vasodilatory effect of cotinine a metabolite of nicotine" [42, 43].

Only increasing age, income, BMI, and educational level were found to be independent risk factors for stage 2 hypertension in the final model in Ghana. There was no significant variation of stage 2 hypertension between sexes in Ghana, although it is known that men had higher systolic blood pressure measurements in early adulthood, while older women have steeper age-related rate of rise [27]. This could be in part due to the higher proportion of women who are overweight and obese in both countries.

This particular study has assessed the burden of hypertension in Sub-Saharan African countries. It focused mainly on risk factors and social determinants across different stages of hypertension among the two countries. This helps to identify newly emerging associated risk factors at different stages of hypertension and helps to be able to recommend measures accordingly. As it is always said "Prevention is better than Cure," we also recommend identifying individuals and treating accordingly at pre- and early hypertension stages, where the maximum benefit of lifestyle changes can be seen. These include having regular and intense physical exercise, reduction of body weight which can decrease average SBP by 5–20 mmHg for every 10 kg weight loss [1], increasing the opportunity to have basic education for all, and educating people with higher income in Ghana who are at high risk of prehypertension and subsequent overt hypertension due to probable acculturation to change their lifestyle. Government bodies at policy level and health specialists need to design methods to improve diagnosis and treatment of hypertension at earlier stages in respective countries.

6. Limitation

One of the major limitations of the current study was high number of missing and some invalid values in the original dataset. Missing and invalid blood pressure measurements accounted for 8% in Ghana and 25% in South Africa. They were excluded during the data cleaning period and not included in analysis. Alcohol consumption was an independent variable with the highest missing values (63%) in Ghana and (35%) in South Africa. This could be the reason for not seeing the expected protection from moderate dose of alcohol against hypertension and increased risk from excess dose [44]. The other components of therapeutic lifestyle changes that include intake of salt, saturated fat, and amount of calories [45] were not included in the SAGE questionnaire and their association with hypertension was not studied. The current study as any other cross-sectional studies determines only associations that are statistically significant without inferring causality. Further cohort studies that examine risk and causality are recommended. And finally using the JNC 7 blood pressure classification that was originally designed for US population and using its blood pressure cut-off points for Sub-Saharan population could impose risk of overgeneralization. Blood pressure cut-off points at which cardiovascular morbidity starts should be looked for in Sub-Saharan Africa context and guidelines should develop in the future.

Abbreviations

AOR: Adjusted odds ratio
BP: Blood pressure
BMI: Body mass index
CVD: Cardiovascular disorder
CI: Confidence interval
DASH: Dietary approaches to stop hypertension
DBP: Diastolic blood pressure
EA: Enumeration area
HTN: Hypertension
IHD: Ischemic heart disease
ISCO: International standard classification of occupation
JNC 7: Joint national committee 7 for hypertension
NCD: Noncommunicable disease
NCEP: ATP III: National Cholesterol Education Program: Adult Treatment Panel III
OR: Odds ratio
PSU: Primary selection unit
SA: South Africa
SAGE: Study on global AGEing and adult health
SBP: Systolic blood pressure
WC: Waist circumference
WHO: World Health Organization.

Acknowledgments

The authors wish to thank the WHO SAGE study group, Umeå International School of Public Health (UISPH), particularly Kjerstin Dahlblom, Nawi Ng, and Jennifer Stewart Williams, and Swedish Institute (SI) scholarships.

References

[1] A. V. Chobanian, G. L. Bakris, H. R. Black et al., "The seventh report of the joint national committee on prevention, detection, evaluation, and treatment of high blood pressure: the JNC 7 report," *Journal of the American Medical Association*, vol. 289, no. 19, pp. 2560–2572, 2003.

[2] F. Palano, F. Paneni, S. Sciarretta, G. Tocci, and M. Volpe, "The progression from hypertension to congestive heart failure," *Recenti Progressi in Medicina*, vol. 102, no. 12, pp. 461–467, 2011.

[3] J. A. Staessen, R. Fagard, L. Thijs et al., "Randomised double-blind comparison of placebo and active treatment for older patients with isolated systolic hypertension," *The Lancet* 350, no. 9080, pp. 757–764, 1997.

[4] J. Coresh, G. L. Wei, G. McQuillan et al., "Prevalence of high blood pressure and elevated serum creatinine level in the United States: findings from the third national health and nutrition examination survey (1988–1994)," *Archives of Internal Medicine* vol. 161, no. 9, pp. 1207–1216, 2001.

[5] M. E. Hendriks, F. W. N. M. Wit, M. T. L. Roos et al., "Hypertension in Sub-Saharan Africa: cross-sectional surveys in four rural and urban communities," *PLoS ONE*, vol. 7, no. 3, Article ID e32638, 2012.

[6] S. Lewington, R. Clarke, N. Qizilbash, R. Peto, and R. Collins, "Age-specific relevance of usual blood pressure to vascular mortality: a meta-analysis of individual data for one million adults in 61 prospective studies," *The Lancet*, vol. 360, no. 9349, pp. 1903–1913, 2002.

[7] L. Shen, H. Ma, M.-X. Xiang, and J.-A. Wang, "Meta-analysis of cohort studies of baseline prehypertension and risk of coronary heart disease," *American Journal of Cardiology*, vol. 112, no. 2, pp. 266–271, 2013.

[8] C. Lenfant, A. V. Chobanian, D. W. Jones, and E. J. Roccella, "Seventh report of the Joint National Committee on the prevention, detection, evaluation, and treatment of high blood pressure (JNC 7): resetting the hypertension sails," *Hypertension* vol. 41, no. 6, pp. 1178–1179, 2003.

[9] P. Kotwani, D. Kwarisiima, T. D. Clark et al., "Epidemiology and awareness of hypertension in a rural Ugandan community: a cross-sectional study," *BMC Public Health*, vol. 13, no. 1, article 1151, 2013.

[10] K. Steyn, D. Bradshaw, R. Norman, and R. Laubscher, "Determinants and treatment of hypertension in South Africans: the first demographic and health survey," *South African Medical Journal* vol. 98, no. 5, pp. 376–380, 2008.

[11] C. Agyemang and E. Owusu-Dabo, "Prehypertension in the Ashanti region of Ghana, West Africa: an opportunity for early prevention of clinical hypertension," *Public Health*, vol. 122, no. 1, pp. 19–24, 2008.

[12] C. K. Chow, K. K. Teo, S. Rangarajan et al., "Prevalence, awareness, treatment, and control of hypertension in rural and urban communities in high-, middle-, and low-income countries," *Journal of the American Medical Association*, vol. 310, no. 9, pp. 959–968, 2013.

[13] W. K. Bosu, "Epidemic of hypertension in Ghana: a systematic review," *BMC Public Health*, vol. 10, article 418, 2010.

[14] B. D. Capistrant and P. Kowal, "Social epidemiology of hypertension stages," *Hypertension*, vol. 62, no. 6, article e41, 2013.

[15] R. B. Biritwum, G. Mensah, N. Minicuci et al., "Household characteristics for older adults and study background from SAGE Ghana Wave 1," *Global Health Action*, vol. 6, no. 1, Article ID 20096, 2013.

[16] A. M. B. Menezes, S. C. Dumith, R. B. Noal et al., "Validity of a wrist digital monitor for blood pressure measurement in comparison to a mercury sphygmomanometer," *Arquivos Brasileiros de Cardiologia*, vol. 94, no. 3, pp. 345–370, 2010.

[17] H. Takahashi, M. Yoshika, and T. Yokoi, "Validation of Omron RS8, RS6, and RS3 home blood pressure monitoring devices, in accordance with the European Society of Hypertension International Protocol revision 2010," *Vascular Health and Risk Management*, vol. 9, pp. 265–272, 2013.

[18] S. L. Schneider and I. Kogan, "The International Standard Classification of Education 1997: challenges in the application to national data and the implementation in cross-national surveys," in *The International Standard Classification of Education (ISCED-97): An Evaluation of Content and Criterion Validity for 15 European Countries*, pp. 13–46, MZES, 2008.

[19] L. Wirth, Copyright International Labour Organization 2001 First published 2001 Second impression 2001 Publications of the International Labour Office enjoy copyright under Protocol 2 of the Universal Copyright Convention, Nevertheless, short excerpts from them may be reproduced without authorization, 2001.

[20] World Health Organization, *Guidelines for Controlling and Monitoring the Tobacco Epidemic*, World Health Organization, 1998.

[21] T. Armstrong and F. Bull, "Development of the World Health Organization Global Physical Activity Questionnaire (GPAQ)," *Journal of Public Health*, vol. 14, no. 2, pp. 66–70, 2006.

[22] World Health Organization, *Global Health Risks: Mortality and Burden of Disease Attributable to Selected Major Risks*, World Health Organization, 2009.

[23] J. I. Recio-Rodriguez, M. A. Gomez-Marcos, M. C. Patino-Alonso, C. Agudo-Conde, E. Rodriguez-Sanchez, and L. Garcia-Ortiz, "Abdominal obesity vs general obesity for identifying arterial stiffness, subclinical atherosclerosis and wave reflection in healthy, diabetics and hypertensive," *BMC Cardiovascular Disorders*, vol. 12, article 3, 2012.

[24] A. M. Gotto, "NCEP ATP III guidelines incorporate global risk assessment," *The American Journal of Managed Care*, supplement, pp. 1–3, 2003.

[25] W. He, M. N. Muenchrath, and P. R. Kowal, *Shades of Gray: A Cross-Country Study of Health and Well-Being of the Older Populations in SAGE Countries, 2007–2010*, Economics and Statistics Administration, US Census Bureau, 2012.

[26] N. Naidoo, S. Abdullah, A. Bawah et al., *Ageing and Adult Health Status in Eight Lower-Income Countries: the INDEPTH WHO-SAGE Collaboration*, Global Health Action, 2010.

[27] A. S. Fauci, *Harrison's Principles of Internal Medicine*, McGraw-Hill Medical, New York, NY, USA, 2008.

[28] K. Peltzer and N. Phaswana-Mafuya, "Hypertension and associated factors in older adults in South Africa," *Cardiovascular Journal of Africa*, vol. 24, no. 3, pp. 67–71, 2013.

[29] S. Chaturvedi, "The seventh report of the joint national committee on prevention, detection, evaluation, and treatment of high blood pressure (JNC 7): is it really practical?" *National Medical Journal of India*, vol. 17, no. 4, p. 227, 2004.

[30] L. J. Appel, M. W. Brands, S. R. Daniels, N. Karanja, P. J. Elmer, and F. M. Sacks, "Dietary approaches to prevent and treat hypertension: a scientific statement from the American Heart Association," *Hypertension*, vol. 47, no. 2, pp. 296–308, 2006.

[31] Y.-H. Chiu, S.-C. Wu, C.-D. Tseng, M.-F. Yen, and T. H.-H. Chen, "Progression of pre-hypertension, stage 1 and 2 hyper-

tension (JNC 7): a population-based study in Keelung, Taiwan (Keelung Community-based Integrated Screening No. 9)," *Journal of Hypertension*, vol. 24, no. 5, pp. 821–828, 2006.

[32] K. Steyn, T. A. Gaziano, D. Bradshaw, R. Laubscher, and J. Fourie, "Hypertension in South African adults: results from the demographic and health survey, 1998," *Journal of Hypertension*, vol. 19, no. 10, pp. 1717–1725, 2001.

[33] M. S. Kaplan, N. Huguet, D. H. Feeny, and B. H. McFarland, "Self-reported hypertension prevalence and income among older adults in Canada and the United States," *Social Science and Medicine*, vol. 70, no. 6, pp. 844–849, 2010.

[34] S. Yadav, R. Boddula, G. Genitta et al., "Prevalence & risk factors of pre-hypertension & hypertension in an affluent North Indian population," *Indian Journal of Medical Research*, vol. 128, no. 6, pp. 712–720, 2008.

[35] S. Mora, I.-M. Lee, J. E. Buring, and P. M. Ridker, "Association of physical activity and body mass index with novel and traditional cardiovascular biomarkers in women," *The Journal of the American Medical Association*, vol. 295, no. 12, pp. 1412–1419, 2006.

[36] J. Joubert, R. Norman, E. V. Lambert et al., "Estimating the burden of disease attributable to physical inactivity in South Africa in 2000," *South African Medical Journal*, vol. 97, no. 8, pp. 725–731, 2007.

[37] E. V. Lambert, M. I. Lambert, K. Hudson et al., "Role of physical activity for health in communities undergoing epidemiological transition," *World Review of Nutrition and Dietetics*, vol. 90, pp. 110–126, 2001.

[38] J. D. Jansen, "Curriculum Reform in South Africa: a critical analysis of outcomes-based education," *Cambridge Journal of Education*, vol. 28, no. 3, pp. 321–331, 1998.

[39] L. J. Appel, T. J. Moore, E. Obarzanek et al., "A clinical trial of the effects of dietary patterns on blood pressure," *Journal of Materials Science: Materials in Medicine*, vol. 8, no. 4, pp. 1117–1124, 1997.

[40] K. Steyn, K. Sliwa, S. Hawken et al., "Risk factors associated with myocardial infarction in Africa: the INTERHEART Africa Study," *Circulation*, vol. 112, no. 23, pp. 3554–3561, 2005.

[41] T. S. Bowman, J. M. Gaziano, J. E. Buring, and H. D. Sesso, "A prospective study of cigarette smoking and risk of incident hypertension in women," *Journal of the American College of Cardiology*, vol. 50, no. 21, pp. 2085–2092, 2007.

[42] K. A. Perkins, L. H. Epstein, B. L. Marks, R. L. Stiller, and R. G. Jacob, "The effect of nicotine on energy expenditure during light physical activity," *The New England Journal of Medicine*, vol. 320, no. 14, pp. 898–903, 1989.

[43] N. L. Benowitz and D. S. Sharp, "Inverse relation between serum cotinine concentration and blood pressure in cigarette smokers," *Circulation*, vol. 80, no. 5, pp. 1309–1312, 1989.

[44] H. C. Bucher, L. Bujanda, J. M. Marimon et al., "Mortality and light to moderate alcohol consumption after myocardial infarction," *Lancet*, vol. 353, no. 9160, pp. 1272–1273, 1999.

[45] J. A. Iestra, D. Kromhout, Y. T. van der Schouw, D. E. Grobbee, H. C. Boshuizen, and W. A. van Staveren, "Effect size estimates of lifestyle and dietary changes on all-cause mortality in coronary artery disease patients: a systematic review," *Circulation* vol. 112, no. 6, pp. 924–934, 2005.

11

Evaluation of 24-Hour Arterial Stiffness Indices and Central Hemodynamics in Healthy Normotensive Subjects versus Treated or Untreated Hypertensive Patients: A Feasibility Study

Stefano Omboni,[1] Igor N. Posokhov,[2] and Anatoly N. Rogoza[3]

[1] *Clinical Research Unit, Italian Institute of Telemedicine, 21048 Solbiate Arno, Italy*
[2] *Hemodynamic Laboratory, P.O. Box 69, Nizhny Novgorod 603009, Russia*
[3] *Department of New Methods of Diagnostics, Russian Cardiology Research and Production Complex, Moscow 121552, Russia*

Correspondence should be addressed to Stefano Omboni; stefano.omboni@iitelemed.org

Academic Editor: Junichiro Hashimoto

Objective. Central blood pressure (BP) and vascular indices estimated noninvasively over the 24 hours were compared between normotensive volunteers and hypertensive patients by a pulse wave analysis of ambulatory blood pressure recordings. *Methods.* Digitalized waveforms obtained during each brachial oscillometric BP measurement were stored in the device memory and analyzed by the validated Vasotens technology. Averages for the 24 hours and for the awake and asleep subperiods were computed. *Results.* 142 normotensives and 661 hypertensives were evaluated. 24-hour central BP, pulse wave velocity (PWV), and augmentation index (AI) were significantly higher in the hypertensive group than in the normotensive group (119.3 versus 105.6 mmHg for systolic BP, 75.6 versus 72.3 mmHg for diastolic BP, 10.3 versus 10.0 m/sec for aortic PWV, −9.7 versus −40.7% for peripheral AI, and 24.7 versus 11.0% for aortic AI), whereas reflected wave transit time (RWTT) was significantly lower in hypertensive patients (126.6 versus 139.0 ms). After adjusting for confounding factors a statistically significant between-group difference was still observed for central BP, RWTT, and peripheral AI. All estimates displayed a typical circadian rhythm. *Conclusions.* Noninvasive assessment of 24-hour arterial stiffness and central hemodynamics in daily life dynamic conditions may help in assessing the arterial function impairment in hypertensive patients.

1. Introduction

In recent years, great emphasis has been placed on the role of arterial stiffness and central blood pressure (BP) as independent predictors of the development of cardiovascular (CV) diseases [1–3]. Consequently, the assessment of arterial stiffness and central hemodynamics is recommended as additional tests for the clinical evaluation of hypertensive patients (based on history, physical examination, and findings from routine laboratory tests), particularly for those at risk of CV complications [4].

Regional and local arterial stiffness may be measured directly and noninvasively, at various sites along the arterial tree, by assessing pulse wave velocity (PWV) and augmentation index (AI) [1]. Central BP is derived from noninvasive techniques of measurement of radial or carotid pulses [5].

The most widely employed methods for evaluating pulse waveforms are those based on applanation tonometry and transfer functions, although recently oscillometric ambulatory blood pressure monitoring (ABPM) devices using specific algorithms for pulse wave analyses have been proposed for assessing arterial stiffness [6–9]. At present, oscillometry is an affordable technique and may allow a comfortable, accurate, repeated, and prolonged estimation of arterial stiffness and central hemodynamics over the 24 hours in daily life conditions [9]. The most recent studies seem to indicate reliability and feasibility of ambulatory arterial stiffness evaluation based on analysis of brachial oscillograms [10, 11].

In the present study we aimed at assessing the feasibility of determining central BP and various indices of arterial stiffness over the 24 hours by a noninvasive, clinically validated technology of pulse wave analysis based on oscillometric BP measurements, integrated in an ambulatory BP (ABP) monitor [10, 12]. Potential differences in arterial hemodynamics and stiffness were sought between healthy normotensive volunteers and hypertensive patients evaluated in a real-life context.

2. Materials and Methods

2.1. Study Population and Design. Treated or untreated hypertensive outpatients and untreated healthy volunteers, aged 18 years or more, were included in the study. Healthy individuals were eligible for inclusion into the study in absence of arterial hypertension (office systolic, SBP < 140 mmHg, and office diastolic, DBP < 90 mmHg plus 24-hour average SBP < 130 mmHg and DBP < 80 mmHg), blood test abnormalities (including impaired fasting glucose, impaired glucose tolerance, or dyslipidemia), obesity, and other major cardiovascular risk factors. Both healthy subjects and hypertensive patients were excluded in case of previous or current cardiovascular disease or any other concomitant significant systemic condition. All individuals were submitted to an ABPM, preceded by an office automatic BP measurement with the same device used for ambulatory monitoring. Office BP was measured in the sitting position after 5-minute rest: three measurements were obtained at 2 min intervals and the average of the three measurements was taken as the reference for office BP.

Hypertensive patients were recruited among consecutive patients with a known history of high BP presenting at the outpatient clinic of the Cardiology Research Complex, Moscow. Healthy volunteers were recruited among the staff and personnel at the Russian Railroad and at the Russian Navy. The study was conducted according to Good Clinical Practice guidelines and the Declaration of Helsinki, and the protocol was approved by the ethics committees of the centers involved. Written informed consent was obtained from all patients and controls prior to their inclusion into the study. All individuals were recruited and studied between September 2008 and December 2012.

2.2. ABP Measurement. ABPM was performed noninvasively over the 24 hours by the BPLab electronic, oscillometric, automated BP monitor (BPLab Gmbh, Germany). The device accuracy in measuring BP has been previously successfully tested in a validation study [13]. Additionally, the device has passed validation also for estimation of vascular indices against the most commonly noninvasive device, recommended as reference standard, the SphygmoCor [12, 14], in accordance with the ARTERY guidelines [15].

Current international guidelines were followed for proper ambulatory recording performance [16]. The optimal adult cuff was wrapped around the nondominant arm and the patient was asked to keep her/his arm still during the automatic BP measurements. The device was programmed to measure BP every 15–30 min during daytime (from 06:00 to 22:00) and every 30–60 min during nighttime (from 22:00 to 06:00). Each recording started in the morning and was preceded by verification of the accuracy of oscillometric BP measurements against auscultatory technique in every subject. After fitting the device, patients were sent home and asked to resume normal life and to come back 24 hours later for removal of the instrumentation.

2.3. Measurement of Ambulatory Arterial Stiffness and Central Hemodynamics. The BPLab BP monitor makes use of brachial oscillometric BP waves for a noninvasive estimation of central BP and arterial stiffness [10, 12–14]. The Vasotens principle of oscillometric pulse wave analysis is based on plethysmography and on recording the pulsatile pressure in the brachial artery. During BP measurement, the pressure waveforms in the cuff are digitalized and stored in the device memory while performing step-by-step deflation. Thereafter, signal processing is performed using a special mathematical algorithm, which is based on a specially developed transfer function that utilizes a modification in a certain frequency range within the acquired pulse signal to derive the aortic pressure wave. The modulus and phase characteristics of the Vasotens transfer function have been published previously [12]. The difference in time between the first wave and the second wave (i.e., the reflected wave) correlates to the distance, according to the manufacturer's instructions, and allows calculation of the pulse wave velocity (PWV). A detailed description of the Vasotens methodology may be found in previous publications [10, 12, 17].

The following indices were derived. The reflected wave transit time (RWTT) represents the transit time of pulse wave along a corresponding artery and is the reciprocal of PWV [10]. In case of a stiff artery, the magnitude of this index is reduced. The method used to estimate this parameter is based on the identification of the reflected wave on the pulse curve in sphygmogram records by original Vasotens algorithm. Since measures of arterial stiffness depend on BP and heart rate (HR) values [1], RWTT is usually normalized to a SBP of 100 mmHg and a HR of 60 bpm by a regression analysis of 24-hour RWTT to 24-hour SBP and 24-hour HR in each individual. PWV indicates the pulse wave speed in the arterial tree: if the artery is stiff, the speed is increased [1]. PWV was also normalized by BP and HR, applying the same methodology used for RWTT. The augmentation index (AI) is defined as the percentage ratio of the pressure increment caused by the reflected wave to the direct wave [1]. Normally, the reflected component in peripheral waves is always smaller than the direct component and AI is negative. In case of high arterial stiffness, the addition of the reflected component caused by different timing may exceed the direct component and the index becomes positive. AI is strongly dependent on HR, so the index is corrected for a HR of 75 bpm as described above. Additionally, AI was calculated from the central waveform reconstructed by transfer function analysis. Finally, we calculated the ambulatory arterial stiffness index (AASI), as one minus the slope of regression of DBP relative to SBP [18].

2.4. Statistical Analysis. The analysis of 24-hour BP recordings was preceded by removal of artifacts according to the previously described editing criteria [19]. Recordings were considered valid when at least 70% of expected measurements were available, as recommended by current guidelines [16, 19]. All the BP and arterial stiffness indices estimated in each

TABLE 1: Demographic and clinical data of healthy subjects and hypertensive patients.

	Healthy subjects ($n = 142$)	Hypertensive patients ($n = 661$)	P value
Age (years, means ± SD)	41.8 ± 8.8	58.1 ± 14.9	0.0001
Gender (n, %)			
Males	*97 (68.3)*	*292 (44.2)*	*0.0001*
Females	*45 (31.7)*	*369 (55.8)*	
Height (cm, means ± SD)	172.6 ± 9.2	170.8 ± 10.2	0.050
Weight (kg, means ± SD)	84.9 ± 16.5	78.6 ± 11.6	0.0001
BMI (kg/m^2, means ± SD)	28.4 ± 4.6	26.9 ± 2.9	0.0001
Antihypertensive treatment (n, %)	0 (0.0)	159 (24.1)	0.0001
Office SBP (mmHg, means ± SD)	122.5 ± 7.5	135.2 ± 11.9	0.0001
Office DBP (mmHg, means ± SD)	78.7 ± 8.0	78.5 ± 8.0	0.807
24-hour SBP (mmHg, means ± SD)	115.3 ± 6.7	129.3 ± 11.6	0.0001
24-hour DBP (mmHg, means ± SD)	71.3 ± 4.9	74.3 ± 6.6	0.0001
Daytime SBP (mmHg, means ± SD)	118.3 ± 6.8	132.1 ± 11.5	0.0001
Daytime DBP (mmHg, means ± SD)	74.0 ± 4.9	76.7 ± 6.8	0.0001
Nighttime SBP (mmHg, means ± SD)	103.1 ± 8.2	120.1 ± 15.7	0.0001
Nighttime DBP (mmHg, means ± SD)	60.9 ± 6.2	66.3 ± 8.6	0.0001

BMI: body mass index; SBP: systolic blood pressure; DBP: diastolic blood pressure.
Data are reported as means ± SD or as absolute (n) and relative (%) frequencies. The P values refer to the statistical significance of the difference between the two study groups.

single BP measurement were averaged for any given subject in order to obtain the 24-hour mean value. Additionally, the daytime and nighttime subperiods were defined according to sleeping times reported in the individual patient's diary cards: average measures for such awake and asleep periods were then computed.

Mean values obtained in each individual subject were averaged for the whole study population, separately for the healthy normotensive and hypertensive group. Differences in hemodynamic indices were assessed by analysis of variance, without adjustment (crude estimate) and after accounting for age, gender, body mass index (BMI), antihypertensive drug treatment, and mean ABP (adjusted estimate). Adjustment for mean ABP was not applied to normalized RWTT and normalized PWV, because these measures were already normalized to a SBP of 100 mmHg and to central BP. Comparison of categorical variables was made by a Chi-square test. To check the relation between the studied parameters, Pearson's correlation coefficient (r) was determined. The level of statistical significance was kept at 0.05 throughout the whole study. Data are shown as mean ± SD or as mean and 95% confidence interval for continuous variables and as absolute (n) and relative (%) frequencies for discrete variables.

3. Results

3.1. Demographic and Clinical Characteristics of the Study Population. Overall, 916 people were recruited and performed an ABP recording, of which 182 were healthy volunteers and 734 were hypertensive patients. In the control group, 40 subjects were not considered eligible for inclusion in the analysis because either of ABP recordings did not meet quality criteria ($n = 10$) or office or ABP were elevated. In the hypertension group valid ABP recordings could not be obtained in 73 patients. Thus, in summary, 803 subjects were included in the analysis, of which 142 were controls and 661 were patients with arterial hypertension. The average percentage of valid readings obtained over the 24 hours was 93.9% in the healthy control and 93.1% in the hypertensive group. The average number of valid readings available during the day was 32.9 ± 9.4 in the control group and 26.7 ± 5.6 in the hypertension group, while the corresponding figure for the nighttime period was 7.6 ± 2.6 and 8.2 ± 2.6.

Comparison of the baseline clinical characteristics of the two groups showed that hypertensive patients were older, were more often females, were thinner, had higher office SBP values, and had higher ABP than healthy controls (Table 1). A quarter (24.1%) of the hypertensive patients were regularly taking BP lowering medications.

3.2. Ambulatory Central BP and Arterial Stiffness Parameters. Both 24-hour central SBP and DBP were significantly higher in hypertensives than in healthy controls (Table 2). RWTT was significantly lower, whereas aortic PWV and peripheral and aortic AIs were significantly higher, in the hypertension group (Table 2). Also the AASI was significantly higher in hypertensive than in normotensive healthy subjects. After adjustment for confounding factors, a statistically significant between-group difference was still observed for central BP, RWTT, and AI, only.

When indices were assessed separately for the awake and asleep periods, before adjustment, all of them were

TABLE 2: Unadjusted (crude) and adjusted (by age, gender, body mass index, antihypertensive drug treatment, and 24-hour SBP and DBP) estimates for 24-hour BP and arterial stiffness parameters in healthy subjects and hypertensive patients.

	Crude estimate (mean, 95% confidence interval)	*P* value	Adjusted estimate (mean, 95% confidence interval)	*P* value
Aortic SBP (mmHg)				
Healthy subjects ($n = 142$)	105.6 (103.9, 107.2)	0.0001	108.3 (106.5, 110.0)	0.0001
Hypertensive patients ($n = 661$)	119.3 (118.6, 120.1)		118.7 (118.0, 119.5)	
Aortic DBP (mmHg)				
Healthy subjects ($n = 142$)	72.3 (71.2, 73.4)	0.0001	71.4 (70.2, 72.6)	0.0001
Hypertensive patients ($n = 661$)	75.6 (75.1, 76.1)		75.8 (75.3, 76.3)	
RWTT (ms)				
Healthy subjects ($n = 142$)	139.0 (137.2, 140.8)	0.0001	134.5 (132.5, 136.5)	0.0001
Hypertensive patients ($n = 661$)	126.6 (125.7, 127.4)		127.5 (126.7, 128.3)	
Normalized RWTT (ms)				
Healthy subjects ($n = 142$)	150.7 (146.5, 154.8)	0.0001	142.7 (138.3, 147.2)	0.005
Hypertensive patients ($n = 661$)	133.9 (131.9, 135.8)		135.5 (133.7, 137.4)	
Aortic PWV (m/s)				
Healthy subjects ($n = 142$)	10.0 (9.9, 10.2)	0.007	10.2 (10.0, 10.4)	0.410
Hypertensive patients ($n = 661$)	10.3 (10.2, 10.4)		10.3 (10.2, 10.4)	
Normalized aortic PWV (m/s)				
Healthy subjects ($n = 142$)	9.2 (8.7, 9.6)	0.025	9.5 (9.0, 10.1)	0.617
Hypertensive patients ($n = 661$)	9.8 (9.5, 10.0)		9.7 (9.5, 9.9)	
Peripheral AI (%)				
Healthy subjects ($n = 142$)	−40.7 (−45.1, −36.4)	0.0001	−20.0 (−23.6, −16.3)	0.005
Hypertensive patients ($n = 661$)	−9.7 (−11.7, −7.7)		−14.1 (−15.6, −12.6)	
Normalized peripheral AI (%)				
Healthy subjects ($n = 142$)	−46.8 (−51.8, −41.9)	0.0001	−31.5 (−36.3, −26.6)	0.015
Hypertensive patients ($n = 661$)	−21.3 (−23.6, −19.1)		−24.6 (−26.6, −22.6)	
Aortic AI (%)				
Healthy subjects ($n = 142$)	11.0 (8.5, 13.5)	0.0001	23.4 (21.3, 25.6)	0.252
Hypertensive patients ($n = 661$)	24.7 (23.5, 25.8)		22.0 (21.2, 22.9)	
Normalized aortic AI (%)				
Healthy subjects ($n = 142$)	8.6 (5.5, 11.6)	0.0001	19.7 (16.7, 22.7)	0.742
Hypertensive patients ($n = 661$)	21.5 (20.1, 22.9)		19.1 (17.9, 20.3)	
AASI				
Healthy subjects ($n = 142$)	0.27 (0.24, 0.29)	0.0001	0.38 (0.35, 0.41)	0.172
Hypertensive patients ($n = 661$)	0.42 (0.41, 0.44)		0.40 (0.39, 0.41)	

SBP: systolic blood pressure; DBP: diastolic blood pressure; RWTT: reflected wave transit time; PWV: pulse wave velocity; AI: augmentation index; AASI: ambulatory arterial stiffness index.
Data are shown as averages and 95% confidence intervals. The *P* values indicate the level of the statistical significance of the difference between the two study groups.

significantly different between the two groups for both the daytime and nighttime periods, with the exception of nighttime PWV (Figure 1(a)). After adjustment for confounding factors, only RWTT and central BP resulted systematically different between healthy subjects and hypertensive patients for both daytime and nighttime (Figure 1(b)). To note, all estimates of vascular health displayed a typical circadian rhythm: during night sleep RWTT and AI increased, while PWV and central BP decreased. Such a pattern was lost after correcting RWTT and aortic PWV by SBP and HR and peripheral AI by HR (normalized indices).

3.3. Correlation between Age, BP, and Arterial Stiffness Parameters. As shown in Table 3, for both healthy subjects and hypertensive patients the relation between age and BP or between age and the different indices of arterial stiffness was statistically significant: the only exception was peripheral SBP and AASI in controls. The magnitude of the correlation coefficient was the highest for AI, with no differences between controls and hypertensives.

As expected, peripheral BP and aortic BP were highly correlated with each other. Conversely, a weak relationship was observed between brachial BP and the different indices

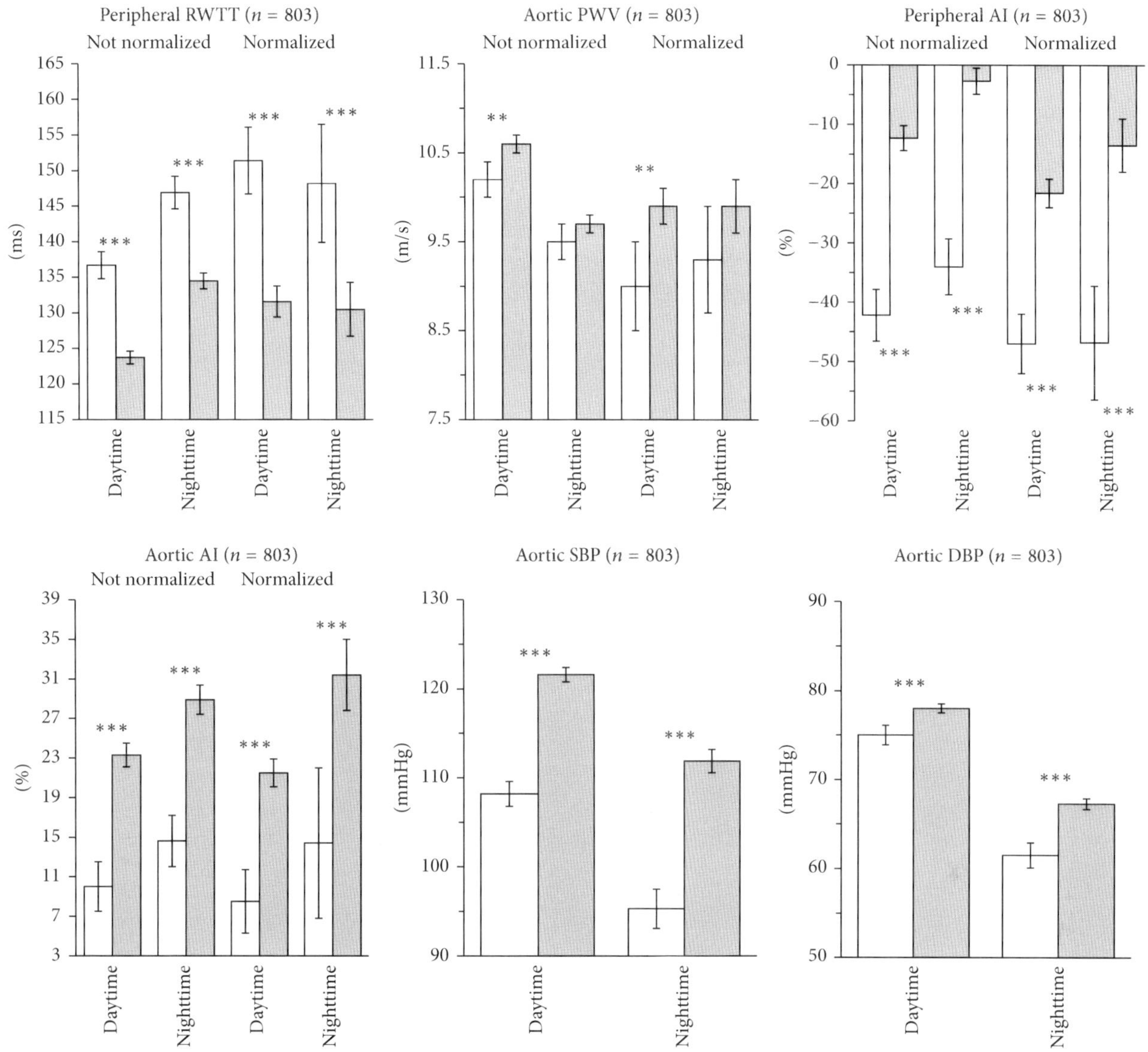

(a)

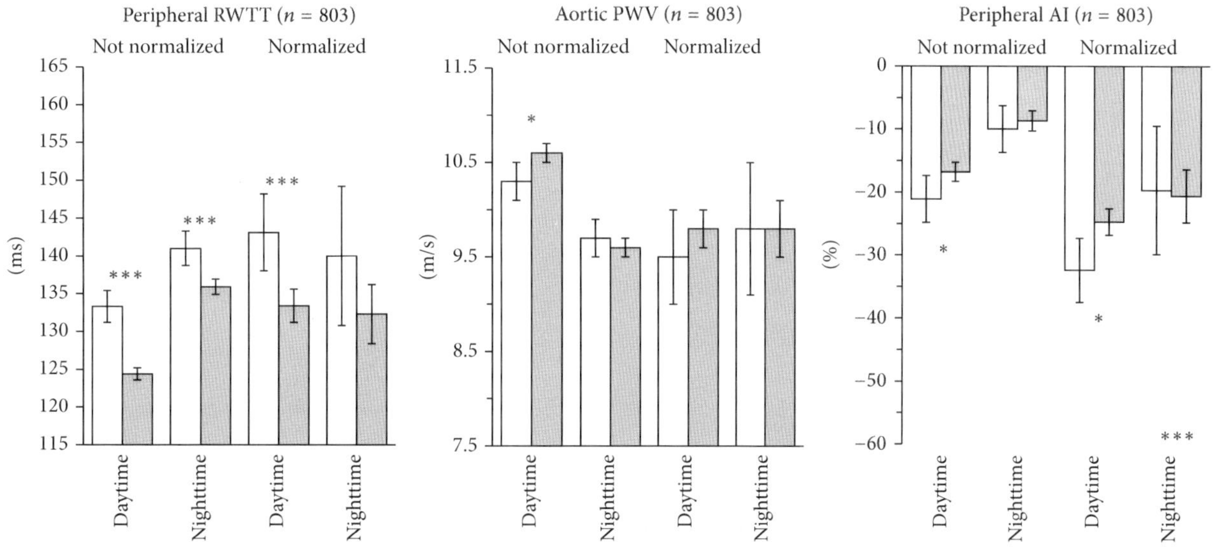

FIGURE 1: Continued.

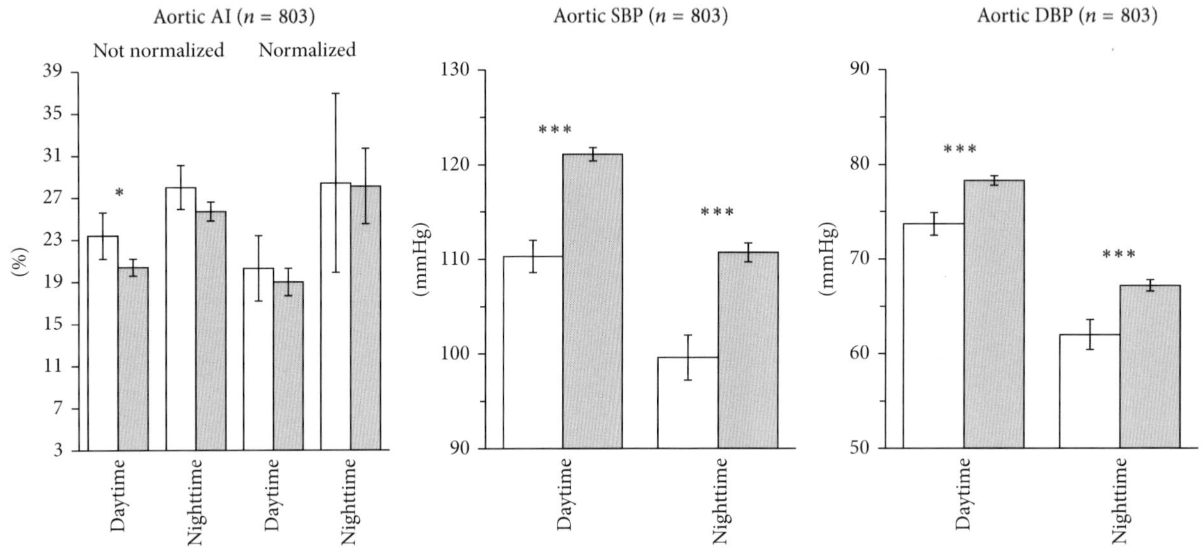

(b)

FIGURE 1: Daytime and nighttime reflected wave transit time (RWTT), aortic pulse wave velocity (PWV), peripheral and aortic augmentation index (AI), and central (aortic) systolic (SBP) and diastolic blood pressure (DBP) values in healthy controls (open bars) and hypertensive patients (gray bars). For RWTT, PWV, and AI not normalized and normalized data (corrected for SBP and/or heart rate) are represented. Data are shown as averages and 95% confidence intervals for crude estimates (a) and for adjusted estimates ((b) data adjusted by age, gender, body mass index, antihypertensive treatment, and 24-hour SBP and DBP). The asterisks indicate the level of the statistical significance of the difference between the two study groups ($^{***}P < 0.001$; $^{**}P < 0.01$; $^{*}P < 0.05$).

of arterial stiffness, though in some cases such a correlation was statistically significant, particularly in the hypertensive group (Table 3).

3.4. Correlation between Ambulatory Arterial Stiffness Indices. The different measures of arterial stiffness were variably correlated with each other (Table 4). Regarding central BP, the best correlation was found between peripheral or aortic AI and aortic SBP, with higher values in the hypertensive group. Aortic AI and brachial AI were highly correlated with each other, as was the case with RWTT versus PWV. A poor correlation was observed between PWV and AI and between all arterial stiffness indices and AASI, the only exception being represented by AI in hypertensive patients. In almost all cases correlation coefficients were better in healthy controls.

4. Discussion

In this study we report on the absolute levels and circadian pattern of arterial stiffness indices and central hemodynamics evaluated in dynamic conditions over the 24 hours in a large cohort of healthy volunteers and hypertensive subjects. Estimation was based on brachial pulse wave analysis of oscillograms obtained noninvasively by a validated cuff-based BP measuring device. We documented higher peripheral and central BP, higher PWV and AI, and lower RWTT in hypertensive than in normotensive subjects, suggesting that arterial indices derived from oscillometric ambulatory BP measures may help to detect differences in arterial function and to investigate vascular impairment in hypertension. When crude estimates were corrected by confounding factors (age, gender, BMI, and antihypertensive treatment ± 24-hour average BP levels), statistically significant between-group differences were still observed for central BP, RWTT, and AI, only. This suggests that these indices may be unaffected by intrinsic subjects' characteristics and/or BP levels and may thus represent a more sensitive index for evaluating arterial function, at least in ambulatory conditions.

Our paper also provides additional findings which are worth being discussed in detail.

The different indices displayed a typical circadian pattern, regardless of the normotensive or hypertensive status. In particular, central BP followed a diurnal course similar to that of peripheral brachial BP and thus decreased during nocturnal sleep. Conversely, AI increased overnight, likely because this index is inversely related to heart rate, which decreases at night, and it is strongly affected by the body posture, with absolute values increasing during recumbency [20, 21] and decreasing from supine to upright position, irrespective of age, due to a decrease in arterial wave reflection [22, 23].

Standardization of the AI to heart rate removed the diurnal profile, in case of being peripheral but not aortic AI. RWTT and PWV both depend on BP and were, respectively, higher and lower at night than at day. As in the case of peripheral AI, circadian pattern of RWTT and PWV both disappeared after correction for SBP and HR, suggesting that standardized parameters may be more robust as compared to uncorrected ones. All these findings are in line with and confirm those obtained in healthy volunteers or hypertensive patients with other oscillometric devices; although such studies were based on a different technology, they were carried out in smaller groups of subjects and

Table 3: Correlation coefficients of 24-hour BP and arterial stiffness measures with age and peripheral (brachial) SBP and DBP.

	Age (years)		Peripheral SBP (mmHg)		Peripheral DBP (mmHg)	
	Healthy subjects ($n = 142$)	Hypertensive patients ($n = 661$)	Healthy subjects ($n = 142$)	Hypertensive patients ($n = 661$)	Healthy subjects ($n = 142$)	Hypertensive patients ($n = 661$)
Peripheral SBP (mmHg)	0.02	0.22**	—	—	0.56**	0.21**
Peripheral DBP (mmHg)	0.27**	−0.13**	0.56**	0.21**	—	—
Aortic SBP (mmHg)	0.28*	0.35**	0.90**	0.96**	0.69**	0.27**
Aortic DBP (mmHg)	0.27**	−0.12**	0.55**	0.22*	0.99**	0.99**
RWTT (ms)	−0.25**	−0.35**	−0.08	−0.03	−0.11	−0.06
Normalized RWTT (ms)	−0.38**	−0.31**	0.10	−0.08*	0.14	0.03
Aortic PWV (m/s)	0.41**	0.26**	0.30**	0.02	0.31**	0.12**
Normalized aortic PWV (m/s)	0.44**	0.19**	0.04	0.08*	0.03	0.01
Peripheral AI (%)	0.56**	0.62**	−0.03	0.28**	0.16	−0.11**
Normalized peripheral AI (%)	0.39**	0.39**	−0.08	0.12**	0.08	−0.08
Aortic AI (%)	0.57**	0.60**	0.01	0.33**	0.22**	−0.11**
Normalized aortic AI (%)	0.41**	0.41**	−0.05	0.18**	0.13	−0.08**
AASI	−0.05	0.36**	0.28**	0.53**	0.03	−0.19**

SBP: systolic blood pressure; DBP: diastolic blood pressure; RWTT: reflected wave transit time; PWV: pulse wave velocity; AI: augmentation index; AASI: ambulatory arterial stiffness index.
Data are separately shown for healthy subjects and hypertensive patients. The asterisks refer to the statistical significance of the correlation coefficient (** $P < 0.01$; * $P < 0.05$).

Table 4: Correlation coefficients between reflected wave transit time (RWTT), pulse wave velocity (PWV), augmentation index (AI), ambulatory arterial stiffness index (AASI), and ambulatory blood pressure (BP) evaluated in the study.

	RWTT (ms)		Aortic PWV (m/s)		Peripheral AI (%)		Aortic AI (%)	
	Healthy subjects ($n = 142$)	Hypertensive patients ($n = 661$)	Healthy subjects ($n = 142$)	Hypertensive patients ($n = 661$)	Healthy subjects ($n = 142$)	Hypertensive patients ($n = 661$)	Healthy subjects ($n = 142$)	Hypertensive patients ($n = 661$)
Aortic SBP (mmHg)	−0.18*	−0.06	0.37**	0.02	0.34**	0.45**	0.37**	0.50**
Aortic DBP (mmHg)	−0.18*	−0.11**	0.31**	0.11**	0.20*	−0.07	0.26**	−0.07
Peripheral RWTT (ms)	—	—	−0.55**	−0.63**	−0.44**	−0.39**	−0.51**	−0.29**
Aortic PWV (ms/s)	−0.55**	−0.63**	—	—	0.25**	0.14**	0.29**	0.05
Peripheral AI (%)	−0.44**	−0.39**	0.25**	0.14**	—	—	0.92**	0.89**
Aortic AI (%)	−0.51**	−0.29**	0.29**	0.05	0.92**	0.89**	—	—
AASI	0.08	−0.06	−0.11	0.06	−0.05	0.39**	−0.03	0.41**

SBP: systolic blood pressure; DBP: diastolic blood pressure.
Data are separately shown for healthy subjects and hypertensive patients. The asterisks refer to the statistical significance of the correlation coefficient (** $P < 0.01$; * $P < 0.05$).

the majority of them evaluated central BP only [11, 24–26]. Our study also adds data to existing evidence collected in normotensive volunteers with the same technology [27]. Interestingly, regardless of the awake or asleep period and of the presence or absence of a circadian rhythm and with the only exception of nighttime PWV, average transit time was lower and PWV, AI, and central BP were higher in hypertensive than normotensive individuals.

We also examined the correlation between the different central and peripheral hemodynamic and arterial stiffness indices. A close relation was found between age and 24-hour arterial stiffness, in both healthy individuals and hypertensive patients, confirming previous evidence collected in resting conditions [28, 29]. ABP was weakly correlated with arterial stiffness indices suggesting that normalized pulse wave analysis may provide an estimate of arterial function involvement independently of BP levels. However, further studies are required in this sense. Though limited in size, the statistically significant correlation between the two main measures of arterial stiffness (PWV and AI) and between peripheral and central AI, found in our study, is consistent with results of published reports [28, 30–37]. However, our study is the first documenting such a relation in ambulatory conditions and in either apparently healthy subjects or hypertensive patients. Finally, PWV was poorly related to AASI, a finding which is in contrast with the results of a recent systematic review and meta-analysis of 51 cross-sectional and longitudinal studies in adults, which reported a good correlation between PWV and AASI [38]. However, unlike our study, in all the studies included in the meta-analysis, PWV was measured in resting and not in ambulatory conditions [38]. Conversely, our results support the evidence of another study which explored the relative importance of the different determinants of the AASI through a previously validated one-dimensional computer model of the arterial circulation applied to 10,000 ABPM simulations [39]. Outcomes of such study suggest that the AASI may not accurately reflect arterial stiffness in ambulatory conditions [39].

5. Limitations

The results of the present study must be interpreted also in the context of its limitations. First of all, we assessed arterial parameters noninvasively by applying transfer function analysis to an oscillometric reconstructed waveform rather than via a direct measurement. Indeed, several authors have questioned the goodness of the principle of one-site central BP, PWV, and AI measurements by oscillometry [7, 40, 41]. However, at present, oscillometry is a method that can be easily and conveniently employed for 24-hour monitoring of central hemodynamics, allowing obtaining repeated measurements in daily life conditions with hardly any discomfort to the patient. Additionally, the device used in our study has been properly validated versus alternative algorithms for computing arterial stiffness indexes and central hemodynamics, according to commonly accepted and standardized protocols. All these studies documented a good agreement between the oscillometric cuff-based estimates of central BP, PWV, and AI measured by the BPLab and the established radial tonometry methods [12, 14]. We must acknowledge that all these validation studies were conducted in resting laboratory conditions and not in ambulant subjects. Thus, we cannot exclude that values collected in dynamic conditions might be, at least in part, unrelated to those collected with other devices at rest. We can only rely on studies documenting that the feasibility and reproducibility of noninvasive assessment not only of BP but also of vascular biomarkers derived from the pulse wave analysis of oscillograms by the Vasotens technology are acceptable [10, 14]. Second, absolute data collected in this study may be useful as a reference for indices collected with the same device but may not be used for other ambulatory devices, which are based on different algorithms. Third, our hypertensive subjects were characterized by office DBP values that were on average slightly lower than those observed in healthy individuals, while SBP values were only marginally higher. Thus, our hypertensive population may not be fully representative of the category. Fourth, though based on a large sample of subjects, information provided by our study needs to be corroborated by data collected in future large cohort studies. We need to specifically address arterial stiffness indices and central hemodynamics in extended age ranges, in high-risk hypertensive patients, and in subjects with established target organ damage or comorbidities, such as diabetes. In this regard, a large database of patients evaluated at different centers has been recently established (Vasotens Registry).

6. Conclusions

Our results suggest that noninvasive assessment of ambulatory arterial stiffness and central hemodynamics may be feasible and help in assessing the degree of impairment of the arterial tree in hypertensive subjects in daily life dynamic conditions. Such an approach may help unraveling subclinical organ damage or functional changes, for instance, due to an increased sympathetic tone, which are typically associated with hypertension. However, further observations in diverse populations are required before ambulatory assessment of the central hemodynamic variables can make it to the clinical practice. Future studies should validate whether the assessment of noninvasive 24-hour central hemodynamics can provide further information regarding CV risk stratification and target organ damage beyond the 24-hour brachial BP. Additionally, reference values specifically obtained by the BPLab monitor, ideally in prospective studies, are needed. Nevertheless, our data may be used as preliminary diagnostic values of BPLab ABPM additional indices in adult healthy normotensive and hypertensive subjects.

Acknowledgments

The authors thank the following investigators for providing data for the study: Viktoria A. Korneva, Tatyana Y. Kuznetsova (Petrozavodsk State University, Petrozavodsk, Russia); Evgeniya N. Bryantseva, Vitaliy S. Barkan, Vladimir V. Gorbunov, Sergey A. Alekseev (the Hospital within the Russian Railroad Network, Chita, Russia).

References

[1] S. Laurent, J. Cockcroft, L. Van Bortel et al., "Expert consensus document on arterial stiffness: methodological issues and clinical applications," *European Heart Journal*, vol. 27, no. 21, pp. 2588–2605, 2006.

[2] C. Vlachopoulos, K. Aznaouridis, and C. Stefanadis, "Prediction of cardiovascular events and all-cause mortality with arterial stiffness: a systematic review and meta-analysis," *Journal of the American College of Cardiology*, vol. 55, no. 13, pp. 1318–1327, 2010.

[3] C. M. McEniery, J. R. Cockcroft, M. J. Roman, S. S. Franklin, and I. B. Wilkinson, "Central blood pressure: current evidence and clinical importance," *European Heart Journal*, vol. 35, no. 26, pp. 1719–1725, 2014.

[4] ESH/ESC Task Force for the Management of Arterial Hypertension, "2013 Practice guidelines for the management of arterial hypertension of the European Society of Hypertension (ESH) and the European Society of Cardiology (ESC)," *Journal of Hypertension*, vol. 31, pp. 1925–1938, 2013.

[5] M. F. O'Rourke and A. Adji, "Noninvasive studies of central aortic pressure," *Current Hypertension Reports*, vol. 14, no. 1, pp. 8–20, 2012.

[6] J. Baulmann, U. Schillings, S. Rickert et al., "A new oscillometric method for assessment of arterial stiffness: comparison with tonometric and piezo-electronic methods," *Journal of Hypertension*, vol. 26, no. 3, pp. 523–528, 2008.

[7] B. Trachet, P. Reymond, J. Kips et al., "Numerical validation of a new method to assess aortic pulse wave velocity from a single recording of a brachial artery waveform with an occluding cuff," *Annals of Biomedical Engineering*, vol. 38, no. 3, pp. 876–888, 2010.

[8] B. Hametner, S. Wassertheurer, J. Kropf, C. Mayer, B. Eber, and T. Weber, "Oscillometric estimation of aortic pulse wave velocity: comparison with intra-aortic catheter measurements," *Blood Pressure Monitoring*, vol. 18, no. 3, pp. 173–176, 2013.

[9] I. N. Posokhov, "Pulse wave velocity 24-hour monitoring with one-site measurements by oscillometry," *Medical Devices*, vol. 6, no. 1, pp. 11–15, 2013.

[10] O. A. Ageenkova and M. A. Purygina, "Central aortic blood pressure, augmentation index, and reflected wave transit time: reproducibility and repeatability of data obtained by oscillometry," *Vascular Health and Risk Management*, vol. 7, no. 1, pp. 649–656, 2011.

[11] L. Luzardo, I. Lujambio, M. Sottolano et al., "24-h ambulatory recording of aortic pulse wave velocity and central systolic augmentation: a feasibility study," *Hypertension Research*, vol. 35, no. 10, pp. 980–987, 2012.

[12] A. N. Rogoza and A. A. Kuznetsov, "Central aortic blood pressure and augmentation index: comparison between Vasotens and SphygmoCor technology," *Research Reports in Clinical Cardiology*, vol. 3, pp. 27–33, 2012.

[13] S. A. Koudryavtcev and V. M. Lazarev, "Validation of the BPLab 24-hour blood pressure monitoring system according to the European standard BS EN 1060-4:2004 and British Hypertension Society Protocol," *Medical Devices: Evidence and Research*, vol. 4, pp. 193–196, 2011.

[14] Y. V. Kotovskaya, Z. D. Kobalava, and A. V. Orlov, "Validation of the integration of technology that measures additional 'vascular' indices into an ambulatory blood pressure monitoring system," *Medical Devices: Evidence and Research*, vol. 7, no. 1, pp. 91–97, 2014.

[15] I. B. Wilkinson, C. M. McEniery, G. Schillaci et al., "ARTERY Society guidelines for validation of non-invasive haemodynamic measurement devices: part 1, arterial pulse wave velocity," *Artery Research*, vol. 4, no. 2, pp. 34–40, 2010.

[16] E. O'Brien, G. Parati, G. Stergiou et al., "European society of hypertension position paper on ambulatory blood pressure monitoring," *Journal of Hypertension*, vol. 31, no. 9, pp. 1731–1768, 2013.

[17] I. N. Posokhov, A. O. Konradi, E. V. Shlyakhto, O. V. Mamontov, A. V. Orlov, and A. N. Rogoza, "Day-to-day repeatability of the pulse time index of norm," *Medical Devices: Evidence and Research*, vol. 7, no. 1, pp. 29–33, 2014.

[18] E. Dolan, Y. Li, L. Thijs et al., "Ambulatory arterial stiffness index: rationale and methodology," *Blood Pressure Monitoring*, vol. 11, no. 2, pp. 103–105, 2006.

[19] G. Parati, S. Omboni, P. Palatini et al., "Italian society of hypertension guidelines for conventional and automated blood pressure measurement in the office, at home and over 24 hours," *High Blood Pressure and Cardiovascular Prevention*, vol. 15, no. 4, pp. 283–310, 2008.

[20] L. Stoner, J. Faulkner, A. Lowe et al., "Should the augmentation index be normalized to heart rate?" *Journal of Atherosclerosis and Thrombosis*, vol. 21, no. 1, pp. 11–16, 2014.

[21] D. Vrachatis, T. G. Papaioannou, A. Konstantopoulou et al., "Effect of supine versus sitting position on noninvasive assessment of aortic pressure waveform: a randomized cross-over study," *Journal of Human Hypertension*, vol. 28, no. 4, pp. 236–241, 2014.

[22] B. van den Bogaard, B. E. Westerhof, H. Best et al., "Arterial wave reflection decreases gradually from supine to upright," *Blood Pressure*, vol. 20, no. 6, pp. 370–375, 2011.

[23] S. C. A. T. Davis, B. E. Westerhof, B. van den Bogaard et al., "Active standing reduces wave reflection in the presence of increased peripheral resistance in young and old healthy individuals," *Journal of Hypertension*, vol. 29, no. 4, pp. 682–689, 2011.

[24] A. D. Protogerou, A. Argyris, E. Nasothimiou et al., "Feasibility and reproducibility of noninvasive 24-h ambulatory aortic blood pressure monitoring with a brachial cuff-based oscillometric device," *The American Journal of Hypertension*, vol. 25, no. 8, pp. 876–882, 2012.

[25] T. G. Papaioannou, A. Argyris, A. D. Protogerou et al., "Non-invasive 24 hour ambulatory monitoring of aortic wave reflection and arterial stiffness by a novel oscillometric device: the First Feasibility and Reproducibility Study," *International Journal of Cardiology*, vol. 169, no. 1, pp. 57–61, 2013.

[26] B. Williams, P. S. Lacy, F. Baschiera, P. Brunel, and R. Düsing, "Novel description of the 24-hour circadian rhythms of brachial versus central aortic blood pressure and the impact of blood pressure treatment in a randomized controlled clinical trial: the ambulatory central aortic pressure (AmCAP) Study," *Hypertension*, vol. 61, no. 6, pp. 1168–1176, 2013.

[27] T. Y. Kuznetsova, V. A. Korneva, E. N. Bryantseva et al., "The 24-hour pulse wave velocity, aortic augmentation index, and central blood pressure in normotensive volunteers," *Vascular Health and Risk Management*, vol. 10, pp. 247–251, 2014.

[28] M. J. Brown, "Similarities and differences between augmentation index and pulse wave velocity in the assessment of arterial stiffness," *QJM*, vol. 92, no. 10, pp. 595–600, 1999.

[29] G. F. Mitchell, H. Parise, E. J. Benjamin et al., "Changes in arterial stiffness and wave reflection with advancing age in healthy men and women: the Framingham Heart Study," *Hypertension*, vol. 43, no. 6, pp. 1239–1245, 2004.

[30] S. J. Marchais, A. P. Guerin, B. M. Pannier, B. I. Levy, M. E. Safar, and G. M. London, "Wave reflections and cardiac hypertrophy in chronic uremia: influence of body size," *Hypertension*, vol. 22, no. 6, pp. 876–883, 1993.

[31] U. I. Cieslik-Guerra, M. Kamiński, and M. Kurpesa, "Correlations of pulse wave velocity with augmentation index and ambulatory arterial stiffness index in the population of patients after acute coronary syndrome. Preliminary results of the FOREVER study," *Polskie Archiwum Medycyny Wewnętrznej*, vol. 123, pp. 327–329, 2013.

[32] S. C. Millasseau, S. J. Patel, S. R. Redwood, J. M. Ritter, and P. J. Chowienczyk, "Pressure wave reflection assessed from the peripheral pulse: is a transfer function necessary?" *Hypertension*, vol. 41, no. 5, pp. 1016–1020, 2003.

[33] S. A. Hope, I. T. Meredith, and J. D. Cameron, "Effect of non-invasive calibration of radial waveforms on error in transfer-function-derived central aortic waveform characteristics," *Clinical Science*, vol. 107, no. 2, pp. 205–211, 2004.

[34] P. Segers, E. Rietzschel, S. Heireman et al., "Carotid tonometry versus synthesized aorta pressure waves for the estimation of central systolic blood pressure and augmentation index," *The*

American Journal of Hypertension, vol. 18, no. 9, pp. 1168–1173, 2005.

[35] K. Kohara, Y. Tabara, A. Oshiumi, Y. Miyawaki, T. Kobayashi, and T. Miki, "Radial augmentation index: a useful and easily obtainable parameter for vascular aging," *American Journal of Hypertension*, vol. 18, supplement 1, pp. 11S–14S, 2005.

[36] J. Sugawara, H. Komine, K. Hayashi, S. Maeda, and M. Matsuda, "Relationship between augmentation index obtained from carotid and radial artery pressure waveforms," *Journal of Hypertension*, vol. 25, no. 2, pp. 375–381, 2007.

[37] K. Takazawa, H. Kobayashi, N. Shindo, N. Tanaka, and A. Yamashina, "Relationship between radial and central arterial pulse wave and evaluation of central aortic pressure using the radial arterial pulse wave," *Hypertension Research*, vol. 30, no. 3, pp. 219–228, 2007.

[38] A. Kollias, G. S. Stergiou, E. Dolan, and E. O'Brien, "Ambulatory arterial stiffness index: a systematic review and meta-analysis," *Atherosclerosis*, vol. 224, no. 2, pp. 291–301, 2012.

[39] J. G. Kips, S. J. Vermeersch, P. Reymond et al., "Ambulatory arterial stiffness index does not accurately assess arterial stiffness," *Journal of Hypertension*, vol. 30, no. 3, pp. 574–580, 2012.

[40] P. Boutouyrie, M. Revera, and G. Parati, "Obtaining arterial stiffness indices from simple arm cuff measurements: the holy grail?" *Journal of Hypertension*, vol. 27, no. 11, pp. 2159–2161, 2009.

[41] B. E. Westerhof, J. P. van den Wijngaard, J. P. Murgo, and N. Westerhof, "Location of a reflection site is elusive: consequences for the calculation of aortic pulse wave velocity," *Hypertension*, vol. 52, no. 3, pp. 478–483, 2008.

12

Excess of Aminopeptidase A in the Brain Elevates Blood Pressure via the Angiotensin II Type 1 and Bradykinin B2 Receptors without Dipsogenic Effect

Takuto Nakamura, Masanobu Yamazato, Akio Ishida, and Yusuke Ohya

Department of Cardiovascular Medicine, Nephrology and Neurology, Graduate School of Medicine, University of the Ryukyus, Okinawa Prefecture, Japan

Correspondence should be addressed to Masanobu Yamazato; mayamaz-ryk@umin.ac.jp

Academic Editor: Tomohiro Katsuya

Aminopeptidase A (APA) cleaves angiotensin (Ang) II, kallidin, and other related peptides. In the brain, it activates the renin angiotensin system and causes hypertension. Limited data are available on the dipsogenic effect of APA and pressor effect of degraded peptides of APA such as bradykinin. Wistar-Kyoto rats received intracerebroventricular (icv) APA in a conscious, unrestrained state after pretreatment with (i) vehicle, (ii) 80 μg of telmisartan, an Ang II type-1 (AT1) receptor blocker, (iii) 800 nmol of amastatin, an aminopeptidase inhibitor, and (iv) 1 nmol of HOE-140, a bradykinin B2 receptor blocker. Icv administration of 400 and 800 ng of APA increased blood pressure by 12.6 ± 3.0 and 19.0 ± 3.1 mmHg, respectively. APA did not evoke drinking behavior. Pressor response to APA was attenuated on pretreatment with telmisartan (vehicle: 22.1 ± 2.2 mmHg versus telmisartan: 10.4 ± 3.2 mmHg). Pressor response to APA was also attenuated with amastatin and HOE-140 (vehicle: 26.5 ± 1.1 mmHg, amastatin: 14.4 ± 4.2 mmHg, HOE-140: 16.4 ± 2.2 mmHg). In conclusion, APA increase in the brain evokes a pressor response via enzymatic activity without dipsogenic effect. AT1 receptors and B2 receptors in the brain may contribute to the APA-induced pressor response.

1. Introduction

Aminopeptidase A (APA) is an enzyme that hydrolyzes the N-terminal amino acid of peptides and expressed in both periphery and brain. Peripheral APA was reported to have potency to act as both protective [1, 2] and harmful [3, 4] agent on cardiovascular disease. Several studies reported that brain APA contributes to neurogenic hypertension. Brain APA activity was higher in spontaneously hypertensive rats (SHR) than in Wistar-Kyoto (WKY) rats [5]. Moreover, brain APA activity in SHR increased with the development of hypertension [6]. Intracerebroventricular (icv) administration of EC33, the specific APA activity inhibitor, decreased blood pressure in SHR [7]. Orally administered RB150, which is a prodrug of EC33, also decreased blood pressure in DOCA-salt rats [8] and SHR [9]. RB150 can cross the blood-brain barrier and gets degraded to EC33 in the brain; oral administration of RB150 inhibits brain APA activity [8]. This evidence suggests that increased brain APA activity participates in the maintenance of hypertension.

Research regarding the role of APA in the brain has focused on degradation of angiotensin (Ang) II to Ang III. Icv administration of EC33 and RB150 inhibited the degradation of Ang II to Ang III in the brains of Swiss mice [10], while that of EC33 abolished the pressor response of icv-administered Ang II. In contrast, icv administration of EC33 did not change the pressor response of icv-administered Ang III [7]. Therefore, conversion of Ang II to Ang III by APA may require elevated blood pressure in the brain [11–13]. However, little is known of the dipsogenic effect of APA. Icv administration of both Ang II and Ang III evokes pressor and dipsogenic responses via the Ang II type-1 (AT1) receptor [14], and Faber et al. reported that APA knock-out mice increase their water intake [15]. Therefore, systemic APA may participate in dipsogenic regulation. However, the dipsogenic effect of brain APA remains unclear.

Furthermore, the cardiovascular effect of brain APA activity has not been resolved beyond the degradation of Ang II to Ang III. It is important to note that APA is not specific to Ang II. Goto et al. reported that neurokinin B, cholecystokinin, and chromogranin A were efficiently cleaved by APA, and kallidin could also be cleaved by APA [16]. A role for the degradation of these peptides in cardiovascular regulation is unresolved. In the present study, we focused on kallidin, a precursor peptide of bradykinin. Bradykinin in the cerebrospinal fluid (CSF) [17] and bradykinin B1 and B2 receptors [18] increased in SHR. The pressor response evoked by icv-administered bradykinin was greater in SHR than in WKY [19] and increased with aging in SHR [18]. Both bradykinin B1 [20, 21] and B2 receptor were reported to contribute neurogenic hypertension; however, B2 receptor is constitutively expressed in physiological condition, whereas B1 receptor is induced by injury or inflammatory conditions [22]. Icv administration of the B2 receptor blocker HOE-140 blocked the pressor response of icv-administered bradykinin in WKY rats and SHR [18]. Microinjection of HOE-140 into the rostral ventrolateral medulla decreased blood pressure to a greater extent in SHR than in WKY rats [19, 23]. These results suggest that bradykinin in the brain plays a role in maintaining the blood pressure of hypertensive rats.

We anticipated that APA shifts the balance between substrates and degraded peptides via enzymatic activity to regulate cardiovascular control. We hypothesized that increased brain APA activity would evoke a pressor response and drinking behavior via AT1 receptor stimulation, and a decrease in kallidin and increase in bradykinin as a consequence of APA activity would increase B2 receptor contribution to the pressor response. To evaluate the role of excess brain APA, we measured the duration of drinking time after icv administration of APA and the pressor response evoked by APA under AT1 receptor or B2 receptor blockade.

2. Materials and Methods

2.1. Animals. Eleven- to 14-week-old male WKY/Izm rats were used for the experiments. WKY/Izm were provided from the Disease Model Cooperative Research Association, Kyoto, Japan, and were placed under artificial light (12 h light/12 h dark cycle) with a normal standard diet (CE-2; Japan CLEA) and water provided ad libitum. All procedures were in accordance with the National Institutes of Health Guidelines for the Care and Use of Laboratory Animals. The protocol was reviewed and approved by the Animal Care and Use Committee, University of the Ryukyus.

2.2. Histological Examination. Fixation and immunostaining procedures used in this study were previously described [24]. In brief, the rats were transcardially perfused with 70 ml of cold sodium phosphate buffered saline (PBS: 0.01 M phosphate buffer containing 0.9% sodium chloride, pH 7.2, 4°C) followed by 35 ml of 4% paraformaldehyde in PBS. The brain stem was removed, postfixed in 4% paraformaldehyde solution for 1 h, and transferred to a PBS containing 20% sucrose (pH 7.4). Frozen brain tissues were sectioned in the coronal plane (5 μm). Sections were first incubated with 0.3% H_2O_2 in methanol for 30 min, followed by incubation with 5% skim milk in tris-buffered saline (20 mM tris-HCl, 0.9% sodium chloride, 0.02% tween 20, pH 7.4) for 60 min. They were incubated with goat polyclonal anti-APA antibody (1 : 100, ab36122, abcam) for 120 min, biotinylated rabbit anti-goat immunoglobulin G for 120 min, and avidin-biotin-peroxidase complex reagents for 30 min and finally stained with diaminobenzidine solution for 8 min according to the manufacturer's instructions (Vector Laboratories). Each step was followed by washing the sections with PBS. Sections incubated without primary antibodies were used as negative controls.

2.3. Drugs. Telmisartan was kindly gifted by Boehringer Ingelheim. It was dissolved in dimethyl sulfoxide (DMSO). HOE-140 (Sigma-Aldrich Japan), amastatin (Santa Cruz Biotechnology), Ang II (Sigma-Aldrich Japan), and Ang III (Sigma-Aldrich Japan) were dissolved in artificial CSF (aCSF, 133.3 mM sodium chloride, 3.4 mM potassium chloride, 1.3 mM calcium chloride, 1.2 mM magnesium chloride, 0.6 mM sodium dihydrogen orthophosphate, 32.0 mM sodium bicarbonate, and 3.4 mM glucose) [15]. Mouse recombinant APA (Sino Biological) compound contains 1.28 mmol sodium chloride per 1 mg of APA. APA was dissolved and electrolyte concentration adjusted to match aCSF. For example, APA was dissolved to 0.1 mg/ml in a vehicle (5 mM sodium chloride, 3.4 mM potassium chloride, 1.3 mM calcium chloride, 1.2 mM magnesium chloride, 0.6 mM sodium dihydrogen orthophosphate, 32.0 mM sodium bicarbonate, and 3.4 mM glucose).

2.4. Surgical Procedure

2.4.1. Implantation of Arterial Catheter for Blood Pressure Measurement. Rats were anesthetized with an intraperitoneal injection of 50 mg/kg of pentobarbital sodium, and vascular catheters were inserted through the right femoral artery for blood pressure measurement. Catheters were exteriorized at the interscapular region through a subcutaneous tunnel.

2.4.2. Implantation of Guide Cannula for Icv Administration. Surgical procedures used in this study were previously described [25]. In brief, rats were placed on a stereotaxic frame (Narishige Scientific Instruments) in a prone position. A hole was drilled through the dorsal surface of the cranium 1.0 mm posterior to the bregma and 1.8 mm lateral to the midline. A 21-gauge stainless steel guide cannula was lowered 3 mm vertically from the skull surface toward the lateral ventricle. The cannula was anchored to the skull using cyanoacrylate. Before and after the surgery, each rat received an intramuscular injection of 10,000 U of penicillin G for prophylaxis.

2.5. Experiment Protocol. At least 2 days after arterial catheter implantation and icv cannula, the rats were placed in a plastic cage and freely allowed to move. The arterial catheter was

Table 1: Intracerebroventricular administration of aCSF, 400 ng of aminopeptidase A (APA), and 800 ng of APA.

	Change of MAP (mmHg)	Time to achieve peak pressor response (s)	Duration of pressor response (s)
Vehicle	0.3 ± 1.3	—	—
APA 400 ng	$12.6 \pm 3.0^{*}$	29 ± 5	263 ± 81
APA 800 ng	$19.0 \pm 3.1^{*}$	28 ± 17	$780 \pm 102^{**}$

Values are expressed as mean ± SE. Results were analyzed using ANOVA. $^{*}p < 0.05$ versus vehicle; $^{**}p < 0.05$ versus 400 ng of APA.

connected to a pressure transducer, and arterial pressure and heart rate were recorded using the powerlab system (AD Instrument) in a conscious, unrestrained state. Drugs were icv-administered by inserting a 27-gauge stainless steel needle into the guide cannula so that it extended 2 mm beyond the tip of the guide into the lateral ventricle.

Protocol 1 (Effect of Icv Administration of APA). Rats received icv administration of vehicle ($n = 4$), 400 ng/8 μl of APA ($n = 5$), or 800 ng/8 μl APA ($n = 4$). They were allowed free access to water. We recorded blood pressure, heart rate, and drinking time after icv administration of APA in a conscious, unrestrained state. Furthermore, a different set of rats received icv administration of 25 ng/2 μl of Ang II ($n = 4$) and 25 ng/2 μl of Ang III ($n = 4$) to establish a positive control for drinking time. This dose of Ang II and Ang III evoked similar pressor responses to icv-administered 800 ng of APA.

Protocol 2 (Icv Administration of APA under AT1 Receptor Blockade, Inhibition of Aminopeptidase Activity, or Bradykinin B2 Receptor Blockade). Rats received icv administration of DMSO as a vehicle ($n = 5$) or 80 μg/4 μl telmisartan ($n = 5$). This dose of telmisartan completely blocked the pressor response and drinking behavior induced by 25 ng of Ang II for at least 2 h. At least 30 min after the administration of telmisartan, rats received 800 ng/8 μl of APA. Finally, rats received 25 ng of Ang II to confirm AT1 receptor blockade. Furthermore, different groups of rats received icv administration of aCSF ($n = 6$), 800 nmol/8 μl of amastatin ($n = 6$), or 1 nmol/8 μl of HOE-140 ($n = 7$). The dose of amastatin was expected to block 97% of the activity of 800 ng of APA based on our preliminary in vitro experiment and the dose of HOE-140 was reported to inhibit the pressor response to icv administration of an equimolar dose of bradykinin [18]. At least 30 min after pretreatment with the drugs, rats received 800 ng/8 μl of APA.

At least 30 min after icv administration of APA, we administered 25 ng of Ang II to confirm the correct placement of icv cannula and the absence of nonspecific inhibition of pretreatment drugs. All icv administrations were performed over a period of 20 s. At the end of each experiment, the correct placement of the icv cannula was rechecked with postmortem icv administration of methylene blue.

2.6. Data and Statistical Analysis. Time dependent change and maximal change of mean arterial pressure (MAP) after icv administration of drugs were measured for each rat. Results were analyzed using ANOVA or Student's t-tests. Values are expressed as mean ± SE. A p value of < 0.05 was considered to be significant.

3. Results

3.1. Histological Examination. Figure 1 shows immunoreactivity of APA in the medulla oblongata. Immunoreactivity of APA was distributed in the rostral ventrolateral medulla and ambiguous nucleus and was observed in the cytoplasm of neurons and neuropils.

3.2. Effect of Icv Administration of APA. To evaluate cardiovascular and dipsogenic effects of brain APA, we performed icv administration of APA. Figure 2 shows representative traces of arterial pressure after icv administration of APA. Icv administration of APA rapidly increased arterial pressure (Table 1). The duration of pressor response persisted in a dose-dependent manner.

Icv administration of Ang II or Ang III immediately evoked a behavior of searching for a water bottle. After finding the bottle, the rats started drinking water. A continuous drinking behavior was observed, and the drinking time durations evoked by Ang II and Ang III were 256 ± 47 and 214 ± 51 s, respectively. Icv administration of Ang II and Ang III increased blood pressure by 17.8 ± 4.5 and 16.4 ± 3.3 mmHg, respectively. Both drinking time and pressor response were not different between icv-administered Ang II and Ang III. The drinking behavior and pressor response were abolished by icv administration of 80 μg of telmisartan. Contrary to icv administration of Ang II or Ang III, icv administration of APA did not evoke drinking behavior (Figure 3).

3.3. Icv Administration of APA under AT1 Receptor Blockade, Inhibition of Aminopeptidase Activity, or B2 Receptor Blockade. Figure 4 shows representative traces of arterial pressure after icv administration of APA following pretreatment with vehicle or telmisartan. Icv administration of 80 μg/4 μl of telmisartan or 4 μl of vehicle did not change the baseline arterial pressure (Table 2). Icv administration of telmisartan significantly attenuated the pressor response of APA (Figure 4, Table 2). The time dependent change of the pressor response to APA was not different with icv treatment (Table 2).

Figure 5 shows representative traces of arterial pressure of icv-administered APA following pretreatment with amastatin. Icv administration of 800 nmol of amastatin did not change the baseline blood pressure (Table 3). Icv administration of amastatin significantly attenuated the pressor response of APA (Figure 5, Table 3).

Figure 5 shows representative traces of arterial pressure for icv-administered APA following pretreatment with HOE-140. Icv administration of 1 nmol of HOE-140 did not change the baseline blood pressure (Table 3). Icv administration

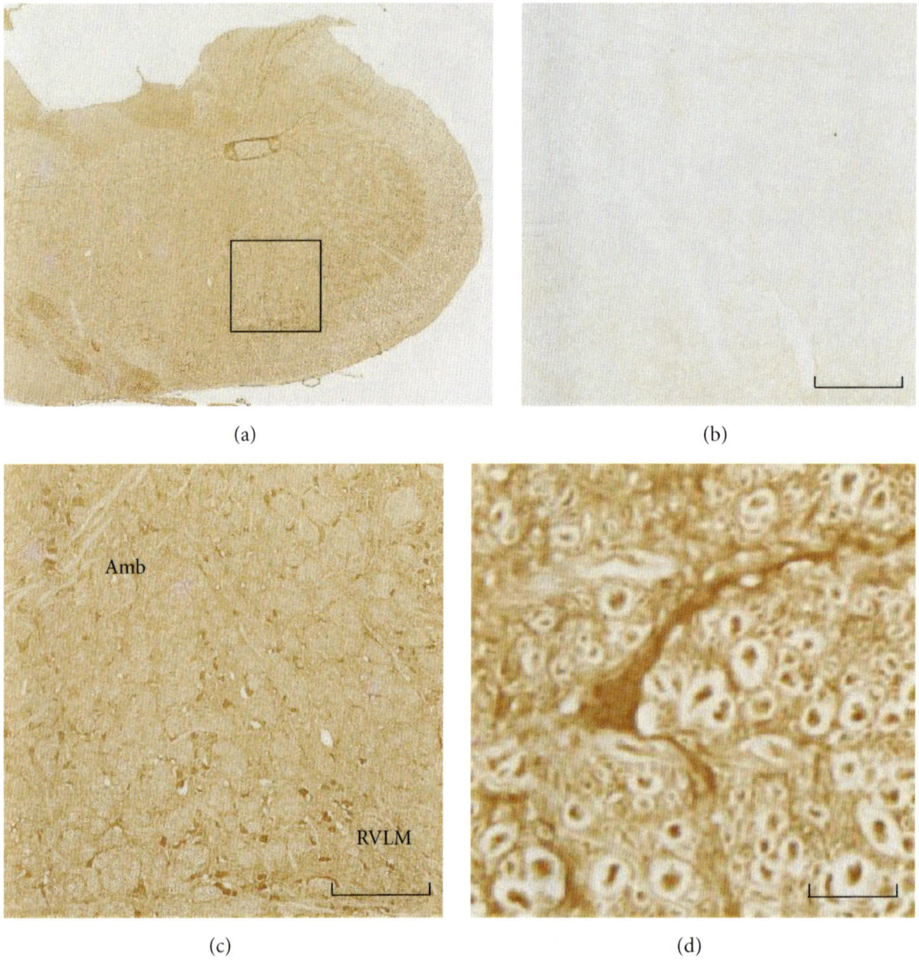

FIGURE 1: Immunoreactivity of the aminopeptidase A (APA) in the medulla oblongata of Wistar-Kyoto rats. Sections were immunostained with anti-APA antibody as described in the Materials and Methods. (a) The low-magnification photograph of medulla oblongata. APA immunoreactivity is diffusely distributed. The square in the photo indicates the area shown in (b) and (c). (b) Negative control. (c) APA immunoreactivities were observed in ambiguous nucleus (Amb) and rostral ventrolateral medulla (RVLM). (d) Higher magnification of APA-stained neuron. Neurons and neuropils were positive for APA immunoreactivity. The scale bar denotes 200 μm in (a) and (b) and 20 μm in (c).

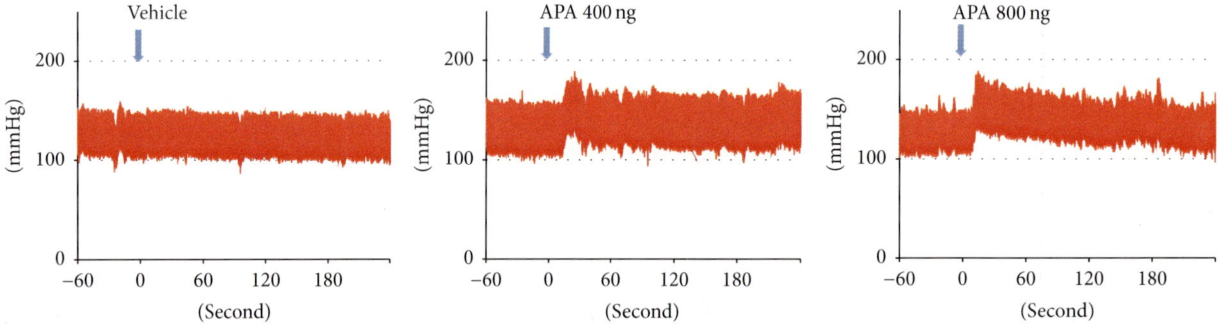

FIGURE 2: Representative traces of arterial pressure after intracerebroventricular (icv) administration of aminopeptidase A (APA). Wistar-Kyoto rats received icv administration of vehicle or APA in a conscious, unrestrained state. Icv of APA rapidly increased blood pressure. Then, blood pressure gradually decreased. The duration of pressor response was prolonged in a dose-dependent manner. Arrow: time for drug administration.

TABLE 2: Intracerebroventricular (icv) administration of 800 ng of aminopeptidase A (APA) after icv administration of vehicle or telmisartan.

Pretreatment drug	Baseline MAP change (mmHg)	MAP change after icv of APA (mmHg)	Time to achieve peak pressor response (s)	Duration of pressor response (s)
Vehicle	1.3 ± 3.2	22.1 ± 2.2	52 ± 22	662 ± 109
Telmisartan	−2.6 ± 1.9	10.4 ± 3.2*	41 ± 21	486 ± 153

Values are expressed as mean ± SE. Results were analyzed using Student's t-test. $^*p < 0.05$ versus vehicle.

TABLE 3: Intracerebroventricular (icv) administration of 800 ng of aminopeptidase A (APA) after icv administration of vehicle, amastatin, or HOE-140.

Pretreatment drug	Baseline MAP change (mmHg)	MAP change after icv of APA (mmHg)	Time to achieve peak pressor response (s)	Duration of pressor response (s)
Vehicle	−2.8 ± 3.2	26.5 ± 1.1	20 ± 3	399 ± 62
Amastatin	−3.6 ± 3.4	14.4 ± 4.2*	47 ± 18	618 ± 121
HOE-140	−0.3 ± 1.7	16.4 ± 2.2*	38 ± 9	469 ± 83

Values are expressed as mean ± SE. Results were analyzed using Student's t-test. $^*p < 0.05$ versus vehicle.

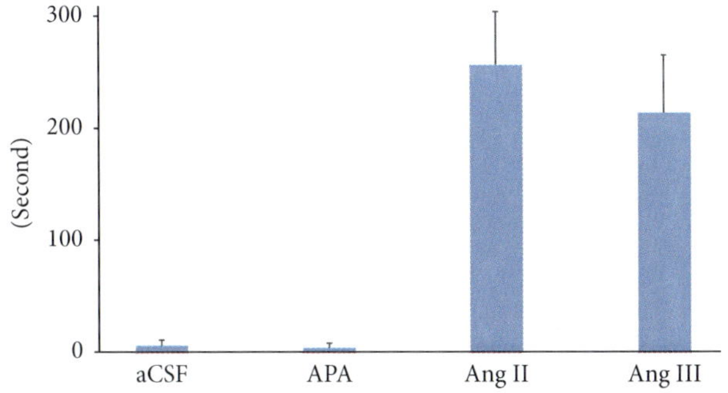

FIGURE 3: Duration of drinking time after intracerebroventricular (icv) administration of angiotensin (Ang) II, Ang III, or aminopeptidase A (APA). Duration of drinking time was measured after icv administration of aCSF, 25 ng of Ang II, 25 ng of Ang III, or 800 ng of APA. This dose of Ang II or Ang III evoked similar pressor response to 800 ng of APA. After icv administration of CSF, drinking behavior was not observed; after icv administration of Ang II and Ang III, continuous drinking behavior was observed; after icv administration of APA, drinking behavior was not observed. Values are expressed as mean ± SE.

of HOE-140 significantly attenuated the pressor response to APA (Figure 5, Table 3). Finally, administration of Ang II increased blood pressure by 31.9 ± 3.6 mmHg in pretreatment with aCSF, 32.3 ± 5.3 mmHg in pretreatment with amastatin, and 22.2 ± 4.7 mmHg in pretreatment with HOE-140. Magnitudes of pressor response were not significantly different between each group.

Furthermore, we performed icv administration of APA following icv coinjection of 80 μg of telmisartan and 1 nmol of HOE-140. Icv administration of APA after coinjection of telmisartan and HOE-140 increased blood pressure by 13.8 ± 2.6 mmHg ($n = 3$). There seems to be no additive effect of B2 receptor blockade to AT1 receptor blockade.

Finally, we performed additional experiment using lower dose of APA (200 ng) under inhibition of aminopeptidase activity, AT1 receptor blockade, or B2 receptor blockade using same dose of the blockers as protocol 2. Icv administration of 200 ng of APA increased blood pressure by 23.6 ± 2.3 mmHg in pretreatment with aCSF ($n = 4$). Pressor response of APA seemed to be smaller in amastatin (8.6 ± 4.5 mmHg, $n = 3$) than in telmisartan (16.5 ± 4.5 mmHg, $n = 2$) or HOE-140 (22.0 ± 5.9 mmHg, $n = 2$) (Figure 6). Two hundreds ng of APA did not induce drinking behavior (6.3 ± 6.3 s in pretreatment with aCSF, 5 ± 5 s in pretreatment with telmisartan).

4. Discussion

This study shows that (i) increase in brain APA elevates blood pressure via enzymatic activity in a dose-dependent manner, (ii) increase in brain APA did not evoke drinking behavior, and (iii) AT1 and B2 receptors contribute to the pressor response to brain APA. These results suggested that increased brain APA activity evokes a pressor response via the AT1 and B2 receptors without dipsogenic effect.

APA activity is diffusely distributed in the brain of rats [5]. Brain APA activity increased in SHR [5, 6]. In humans, APA activity and immunoreactivity are also diffusely distributed in the brain including the cardiovascular regulatory nuclei [26]. We also observed APA immunoreactivity diffusely in the medulla oblongata including cardiovascular regulatory areas. Our study intended to evaluate a role for brain APA in cardiovascular regulation.

Wright et al. showed that icv administration of placenta-derived APA increased blood pressure, and the pressor response was attenuated by icv administration of AT1 receptor blocker (ARB) under anesthesia in WKY rats and SHR [27]. In the present study, we supported their observation using conscious rats and recombinant APA. In the present study, inhibition of APA activity or AT1 receptor blockade attenuated the pressor response to icv-administered APA. As previously reported, inhibition of APA activity decreases blood pressure in hypertensive animals [7–9]. Therefore,

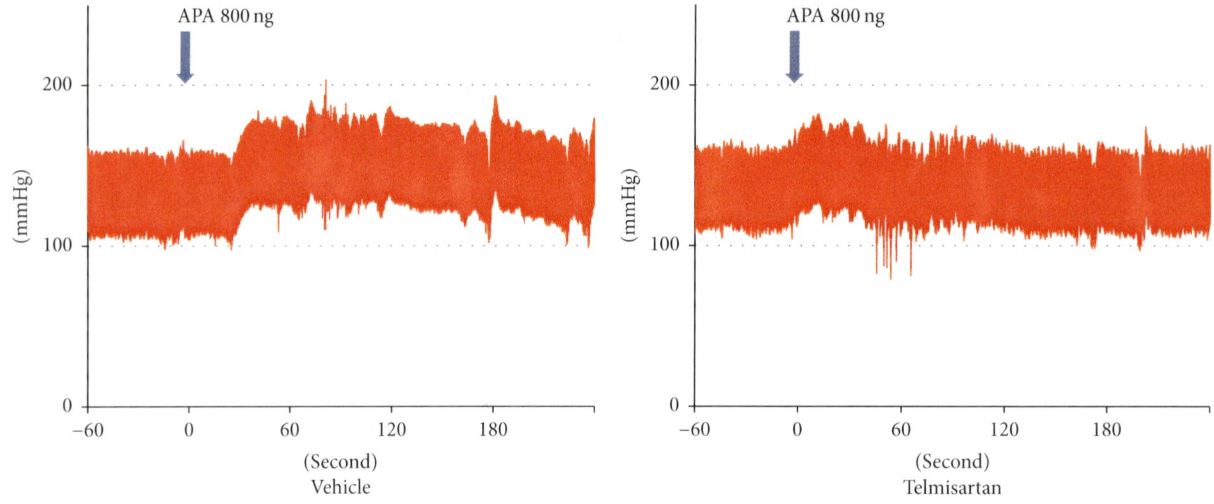

Figure 4: Representative traces of arterial pressure after intracerebroventricular (icv) administration of aminopeptidase A (APA) following pretreatment with telmisartan. Thirty minutes prior to the icv administration of 800 ng of APA, Wistar-Kyoto rats received icv administration of vehicle ($n = 5$) or 80 μg of telmisartan ($n = 5$) in a conscious, unrestrained state. Icv administration of telmisartan or vehicle did not change the baseline MAP. Pretreatment with telmisartan significantly attenuated the pressor response of APA. Arrow: time for APA administration.

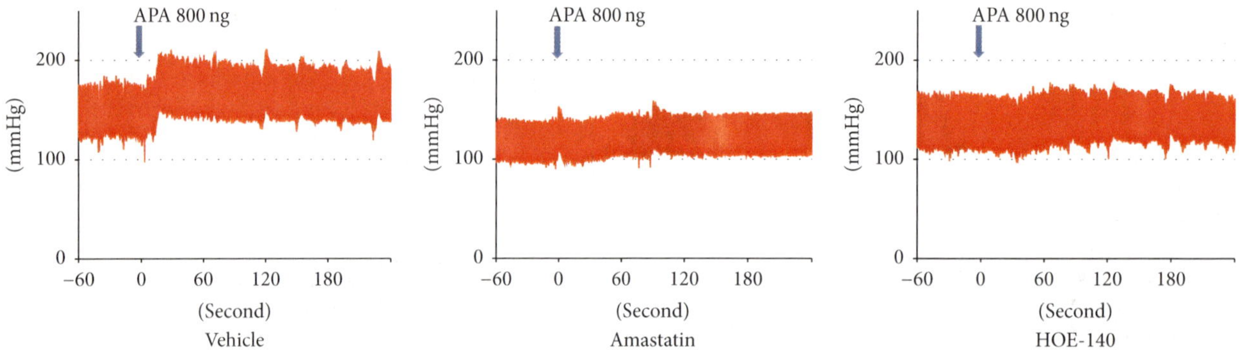

Figure 5: Representative traces of arterial pressure after intracerebroventricular (icv) administration of aminopeptidase A (APA) following pretreatment with amastatin or HOE-140. Thirty minutes prior to the icv administration of 800 ng of APA, Wistar-Kyoto rats received icv administration of the following drugs: vehicle ($n = 6$), 800 nmol of amastatin ($n = 6$), or 1 nmol of HOE-140 ($n = 7$). Icv administration of vehicle, amastatin, and HOE-140 did not change the baseline MAP. Pretreatment of amastatin and HOE-140 significantly attenuated the pressor response to APA. Arrow: time for APA administration.

brain APA is believed to act as a pressor agent via its enzymatic activity through the AT1 receptor.

Brain AT1 receptor stimulation induces blood pressure elevation and drinking behavior. However, present study showed that brain APA increased blood pressure elevation via the AT1 receptor, in contrast, did not induce drinking behavior. This discrepancy has not been fully understood. One possible explanation is that Ang II and Ang III have similar potent dipsogen; therefore, degradation of Ang II to Ang III did not evoke drinking behavior. Another possible explanation is that the response of icv-administered APA was sum of heterogeneous reactions of endogenous substrate and metabolites affecting many different cardiovascular regulatory areas in the brain simultaneously. This complex effect might be causing the difference in drinking behavior.

In the present study, amastatin had more potent effect than ARB on attenuation of the pressor response of APA. This result may suggest that the AT1 receptor mediated pressor response is a part of the pressor response of APA. In the present study, pressor response to APA was attenuated by not only ARB but also B2 receptor blocker. Excess APA is expected to convert kallidin to bradykinin even in the presence of Ca^{2+} which attenuates this process [16], such condition occurs in CSF. Both kallidin and bradykinin have a pressor potency in the brain. Bradykinin acts as a pressor peptide with longer duration than kallidin [28]. Therefore, degradation of kallidin to bradykinin is expected to increase blood pressure via prolonged pressor action and to function in the maintenance of hypertension. Further studies are needed to clarify the role of B2 receptor in the condition of increased APA.

In summary, increased brain APA may participate in the maintenance of hypertension. Brain APA is believed to modulate the renin-Ang system and to be a therapeutic target

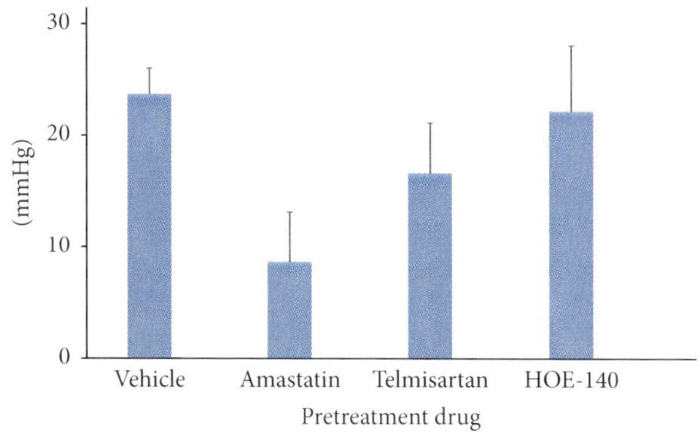

FIGURE 6: The pressor response of lower dose of aminopeptidase A (APA). Wistar-Kyoto rats received icv administration of 200 ng of APA following treatment of aCSF ($n = 4$) or each blocker. The pressor response of lower dose of APA seemed to be smaller in 800 nmol of amastatin ($n = 3$) than in 80 μg of telmisartan ($n = 2$) or 1 nmol of HOE-140 ($n = 2$).

in hypertension and cardiac dysfunction [29]. Phase I study of a centrally acting APA inhibitor prodrug has already been performed [30]. We believe that inhibition of brain APA may be a unique therapeutic target, which affects several cardiovascular peptides in the brain as shown in the B2 receptor. In addition, APA inhibition may be superior in the environment that is prone to dehydration. Further studies are needed to clarify the role of APA and its related peptides in the brain and periphery.

5. Conclusion

This study shows that excessive APA in the brain elevates blood pressure via its enzymatic activity through AT1 receptor and B2 receptor without dipsogenic effect. APA in the brain may be a unique therapeutic target for neurogenic hypertension that affects multireceptor mediated blood pressure regulation.

Acknowledgments

The authors thank Morihiro Ota and Masato Nohara for their excellent technical assistance.

References

[1] R. Kubota, Y. Numaguchi, M. Ishii et al., "Ischemia-induced angiogenesis is impaired in aminopeptidase A deficient mice via down-regulation of HIF-1α," *Biochemical and Biophysical Research Communications*, vol. 402, no. 2, pp. 396–401, 2010.

[2] S. Mizutani, J. Wright, and H. Kobayashi, "A new approach regarding the treatment of preeclampsia and preterm labor," *Life Sciences*, vol. 88, no. 1-2, pp. 17–23, 2011.

[3] H. X. Wang, Q. F. Zhang, X. J. Zeng, W. Wang, C. S. Tang, and L. K. Zhang, "Effects of angiotensin III on protein, DNA, and collagen synthesis of neonatal cardiomyocytes and cardiac fibroblasts in vitro," *Journal of Cardiovascular Pharmacology and Therapeutics*, vol. 15, no. 4, pp. 393–402, 2010.

[4] M. S. Alghamri, M. Morris, J. G. Meszaros, K. M. Elased, and N. Grobe, "Novel role of aminopeptidase-A in angiotensin-(1-7) metabolism post myocardial infarction," *American Journal of Physiology—Heart and Circulatory Physiology*, vol. 306, no. 7, pp. H1032–H1040, 2014.

[5] S. Zini, P. Masdehors, Z. Lenkei et al., "Aminopeptidase A: distribution in rat brain nuclei and increased activity in spontaneously hypertensive rats," *Neuroscience*, vol. 78, no. 4, pp. 1187–1193, 1997.

[6] D. P. Healy and L. Song, "Kidney aminopeptidase A and hypertension, part I: spontaneously hypertensive rats," *Hypertension*, vol. 33, no. 2, pp. 740–745, 1999.

[7] A. Reaux, M. C. Fournie-Zaluski, C. David et al., "Aminopeptidase A inhibitors as potential central antihypertensive agents," *Proceedings of the National Academy of Sciences of the United States of America*, vol. 96, no. 23, pp. 13415–13420, 1999.

[8] L. Bodineau, A. Frugière, Y. Marc et al., "Orally active aminopeptidase A inhibitors reduce blood pressure: a new strategy for treating hypertension," *Hypertension*, vol. 51, no. 5, pp. 1318–1325, 2008.

[9] Y. Marc, J. Gao, F. Balavoine, A. Michaud, B. P. Roques, and C. Llorens-Cortes, "Central antihypertensive effects of orally active aminopeptidase a inhibitors in spontaneously hypertensive rats," *Hypertension*, vol. 60, no. 2, pp. 411–418, 2012.

[10] M.-C. Fournie-Zaluski, C. Fassot, B. Valentin et al., "Brain renin-angiotensin system blockade by systemically active aminopeptidase A inhibitors: a potential treatment of salt-dependent hypertension," *Proceedings of the National Academy of Sciences of the United States of America*, vol. 101, no. 20, pp. 7775–7780, 2004.

[11] J. Gao, Y. Marc, X. Iturrioz, V. Leroux, F. Balavoine, and C. Llorens-Cortes, "A new strategy for treating hypertension by blocking the activity of the brain renin-angiotensin system with aminopeptidase A inhibitors," *Clinical Science*, vol. 127, no. 3, pp. 135–148, 2014.

[12] J. W. Wright, S. Mizutani, and J. W. Harding, "Focus on brain angiotensin III and aminopeptidase a in the control of hypertension," *International Journal of Hypertension*, vol. 2012, Article ID 124758, 12 pages, 2012.

[13] V. G. Yugandhar and M. A. Clark, "Angiotensin III: a physiological relevant peptide of the renin angiotensin system," *Peptides*, vol. 46, pp. 26–32, 2013.

[14] J. W. Wright, S. L. Morseth, R. H. Abhold, and J. W. Harding, "Pressor action and dipsogenicity induced by angiotensin II and III in rats," *The American Journal of Physiology*, vol. 249, part 2, no. 5, part 2, pp. R514–R521, 1985.

[15] F. Faber, F. Gembardt, X. Sun, S. Mizutani, W.-E. Siems, and T. Walther, "Lack of angiotensin II conversion to angiotensin III increases water but not alcohol consumption in aminopeptidase A-deficient mice," *Regulatory Peptides*, vol. 136, no. 1–3, pp. 130–137, 2006.

[16] Y. Goto, A. Hattori, Y. Ishii, S. Mizutani, and M. Tsujimoto, "Enzymatic properties of human aminopeptidase A: regulation of its enzymatic activity by calcium and angiotensin IV," *The Journal of Biological Chemistry*, vol. 281, no. 33, pp. 23503–23513, 2006.

[17] A. L. Alvarez, A. Delorenzi, D. Santajuliana, S. Finkielman, V. E. Nahmod, and C. J. Pirola, "Central bradykininergic system in normotensive and hypertensive rats," *Clinical Science*, vol. 82, no. 5, pp. 513–519, 1992.

[18] F. Cloutier, B. Ongali, M. M. Campos, G. Thibault, W. Neugebauer, and R. Couture, "Correlation between brain bradykinin receptor binding sites and cardiovascular function in young and adult spontaneously hypertensive rats," *British Journal of Pharmacology*, vol. 142, no. 2, pp. 285–296, 2004.

[19] P. J. Privitera, H. Thibodeaux, and P. Yates, "Rostral ventrolateral medulla as a site for the central hypertensive action of kinins," *Hypertension*, vol. 23, no. 1, pp. 52–58, 1994.

[20] C. Emanueli, J. Chao, D. Regoli, L. Chao, A. Ni, and P. Madeddu, "The bradykinin B1 receptor and the central regulation of blood pressure in spontaneously hypertensive rats," *British Journal of Pharmacology*, vol. 126, no. 8, pp. 1769–1776, 1999.

[21] H. De Brito Gariepy, P. Carayon, B. Ferrari, and R. Couture, "Contribution of the central dopaminergic system in the antihypertensive effect of kinin B1 receptor antagonists in two rat models of hypertension," *Neuropeptides*, vol. 44, no. 2, pp. 191–198, 2010.

[22] G. Naffah-Mazzacoratti Mda, T. L. Gouveia, P. S. Simões, and S. R. Perosa, "What have we learned about the kallikrein-kinin and renin-angiotensin systems in neurological disorders?" *World Journal of Biological Chemistry*, vol. 5, no. 2, pp. 130–140, 2014.

[23] P. J. Privitera and P. Yates, "Hypertensive effect of tissue kallikrein in rostral ventrolateral medulla is mediated by brain kinins," *Brain Research*, vol. 704, no. 1, pp. 103–106, 1995.

[24] M. Yamazato, C. Zukeran, H. Teruya et al., "Ouabain-like immunoreactivity in the medulla oblongata of rats," *Archives of Histology and Cytology*, vol. 61, no. 4, pp. 317–326, 1998.

[25] M. Yamazato, Y. Ohya, M. Nakamoto et al., "Sympathetic hyperreactivity to air-jet stress in the chromosome 1 blood pressure quantitative trait locus congenic rats," *American Journal of Physiology—Regulatory Integrative and Comparative Physiology*, vol. 290, no. 3, pp. R709–R714, 2006.

[26] N. de Mota, X. Iturrioz, C. Claperon et al., "Human brain aminopeptidase A: biochemical properties and distribution in brain nuclei," *Journal of Neurochemistry*, vol. 106, no. 1, pp. 416–428, 2008.

[27] J. W. Wright, S. Mizutani, C. E. Murray, H. Z. Amir, and J. W. Harding, "Aminopeptidase-induced elevations and reductions in blood pressure in the spontaneously hypertensive rat," *Journal of Hypertension*, vol. 8, no. 10, pp. 969–974, 1990.

[28] F. M. A. Corrêa and F. G. Graeff, "Central mechanisms of the hypertensive action of intraventricular bradykinin in the unanaesthetized rat," *Neuropharmacology*, vol. 13, no. 1, pp. 65–75, 1974.

[29] B. S. Huang, M. Ahmad, R. A. White, Y. Marc, C. Llorens-Cortes, and F. H. H. Leenen, "Inhibition of brain angiotensin III attenuates sympathetic hyperactivity and cardiac dysfunction in rats post-myocardial infarction," *Cardiovascular Research*, vol. 97, no. 3, pp. 424–431, 2013.

[30] F. Balavoine, M. Azizi, D. Bergerot et al., "Randomised, double-blind, placebo-controlled, dose-escalating phase I study of QGC001, a centrally acting aminopeptidase a inhibitor prodrug," *Clinical Pharmacokinetics*, vol. 53, no. 4, pp. 385–395, 2014.

13

Review of and Updates on Hypertension in Obstructive Sleep Apnea

Masood Ahmad,[1] Devan Makati,[1] and Sana Akbar[2]

[1]*Department of Medicine, West Virginia University School of Medicine, Morgantown, WV, USA*
[2]*Department of Medicine, Division of Nephrology, West Virginia University School of Medicine, Morgantown, WV, USA*

Correspondence should be addressed to Sana Akbar; sakbar@hsc.wvu.edu

Academic Editor: Markus P. Schlaich

Obstructive sleep apnea (OSA) is a prevalent sleep disorder as is hypertension (HTN) in the 21st century with the rising incidence of obesity. Numerous studies have shown a strong association of OSA with cardiovascular morbidity and mortality. There is overwhelming evidence supporting the relationship between OSA and hypertension (HTN). The pathophysiology of HTN in OSA is complex and dependent on various factors such as sympathetic tone, renin-angiotensin-aldosterone system, endothelial dysfunction, and altered baroreceptor reflexes. The treatment of OSA is multifactorial ranging from CPAP to oral appliances to lifestyle modifications to antihypertensive drugs. OSA and HTN both need prompt diagnosis and treatment to help address the growing cardiovascular morbidity and mortality due to these two entities.

1. Introduction

Obstructive sleep apnea (OSA) is a highly prevalent sleep disorder that affects 15 to 24% of all adults [1]. It is characterized by recurrent episodes of upper airway inspiratory collapse during sleep, causing breathing reduction (hypopnea) or cessation (apnea) that gives rise to transient hypoxemia and hypercapnia. Most apneic episodes are aborted by momentary arousal from sleep and a subsequent period of brief hyperventilation. This perpetual sleep fragmentation causes excessive daytime somnolence, fatigue, headaches, and decreased concentration. The severity of obstructive sleep apnea syndrome (OSAS) is classified based on the apnea-hypopnea index (number of apneic/hypopneic episodes per hour): 5–15, mild; 15–30, moderate; 30 or more, severe.

The major risk factors for OSA are obesity, male sex, and advancing age [1]. Since these conditions oftentimes predispose to and are concomitant with hypertension [2, 3] it can be confounding to determine the independent effects of OSA on the development of hypertension. However, there is increasing evidence that OSAS is independently associated with considerable cardiovascular morbidity and mortality, including ischemic heart disease, heart failure, arrhythmias, large vessel disease, and cerebrovascular disease [4–6]. There is also an increased frequency of nocturnal cardiovascular events such as angina, myocardial infarction, and sudden cardiac deaths most likely secondary to arrhythmias precipitated by nocturnal catecholamine surges [7, 8]. The acute autonomic and cardiopulmonary disturbances that are associated with repetitive nocturnal apneic episodes can lead to sustained diurnal hypertension, irrespective of other known risk factors for hypertension [9–12].

Numerous studies have shown the relation between elevated blood pressure and increased cardiovascular morbidity and mortality. However recent studies have implicated a stronger correlation of cardiovascular events with elevated ambulatory blood pressure monitor (ABPM) readings due to the elevated nocturnal readings and nondipping blood pressure patterns. Elevated nocturnal blood pressure as is noted with nocturnal catecholamine surges in patients with OSAS adds to poor outcomes. Findings from the MAPEC (Monitorizacion Ambulatoria para Prediccion de Eventos Cardiovasculares) study suggest that bedtime chronotherapy with $\geq$1 conventional hypertension medication to target sleep blood pressure significantly reduces cardiovascular disease risk [13]. The main acute physiological outcomes of OSAS are intermittent hypoxia, intrapleural pressure changes, and sleep fragmentation which induce endothelial dysfunction, sympathetic activation, renin-angiotensin-aldosterone system activation, and increased oxidative stress [14]. All these add to arterial stiffness and hence increased cardiovascular disease morbidity and mortality.

2. Prevalence

The prevalence of OSA continues to increase in developed countries in conjunction with the rise in obesity. Although its prevalence may vary across different populations and age groups, OSA has been ascertained to affect 24% to 26% of men and 17% to 28% of women between 30 and 70 years of age [15, 16]. Hypertension is also a highly prevalent disease, affecting 26.4% of all adults [17].

There is overwhelming epidemiologic evidence supporting the nexus between OSA and chronic hypertension which suggests a causal, bidirectional relationship between the two entities. Not only does OSA predispose patients to developing HTN, but also there is a greater incidence of OSA in hypertensive patients [18–20]. The prevalence of hypertension in OSA patients is estimated between 30 and 70% [21]. In patients with severe OSA, the prevalence of HTN was higher (53%) as compared to those with moderate OSA (46%) [20]. Likewise, the prevalence of OSA in hypertensive individuals is determined to be 30%–50%, which is probably an underestimate, since OSAS is markedly underdiagnosed [21–23]. The prevalence increases substantially to significant 83% if we consider just the subset of patients with resistant hypertension [24]. In fact, OSA was found to have the greatest association with resistant hypertension (64%), even more so than primary hyperaldosteronism (5.6%) [25]. Another study demonstrated a 2.5-fold elevated risk of OSA in patients with resistant hypertension relative to other hypertensives [26].

Over the years, numerous cross-sectional studies have established an association between OSA and hypertension, independently of age, weight, and other confounding factors [27–30], as a result of which OSA was listed as the most common cause of secondary hypertension in the JNC VII guidelines [31]. However, a temporal relationship between the two that implies causality is supported by two major longitudinal, prospective cohort studies, the Wisconsin Sleep Cohort Study (WSCS) [9] and the Sleep Heart Health Study (SHHS) [32]. Although both identified increased odds of developing HTN with increasing severity of OSA, the results of the SHHS that followed 2470 patients for 5 years were not statistically significant after accounting for the effect of BMI, whereas the WSCS reported a statistically significant association. This discrepancy can partly be explained by the fact that the SHHS cohort was much older than the WSCS one (average age of 60 versus 47). The strength of the association between OSAS severity and incident HTN appears to decline with age [33], a finding that is further corroborated by another study [34], where a cutoff age of 60 years was established, above which the correlation dwindles.

The WSCS found a dose-response relationship with increasing OSAS severity and incidence of HTN, independent of confounding risk factors such as age, sex, BMI, and initial BP. Those with AHI > 15 were reported to have a 3.2-fold greater odds of incident hypertension [9] and 4 times higher odds of developing nondipping nocturnal BP [35] compared to subjects with AHI < 5 at baseline. Further prospective analyses of the WSCS data suggest association of OSAS with the development of depression [36] and stroke [37]. An 18-year mortality follow-up on the WSCS sample [38] revealed that the rate of all-cause mortality was 3 times higher and the rate of cardiovascular mortality was 5.2 times higher for those with severe sleep disordered breathing (SDB), with AHI > 30 compared to those without SDB. The hazard ratio for all-cause mortality increased from 3.0 to 3.8 after excluding those who had been treated with CPAP.

Similarly, the Vitoria Sleep Cohort (VSC) [39] that observed a sample of 1180 subjects, aged 30–70 years for 7.5 years, described a positive correlation between incident hypertension and increasing SDB, but this association was attenuated and no longer statistically significant primarily after controlling for age. Adjustments for sex, BMI, neck circumference, fitness level, alcohol, tobacco, and coffee consumption further diminished the association between OSAS severity and HTN. The disparity observed among the WSCS, the SHHS, and the VSC might be attributable to the differences in the population sample and methods. The SHHS sample was older yet more obese (BMI = 28 versus 26 kg/m^2 in VSC); more hypertensive at baseline (51% versus 28% in WSCS and 24% in VSC); and more racially diverse than the other two. The WSCS cohort was also more obese (BMI = 29) with a higher male preponderance (56% men versus 48% in the VSC) and hailed from a working population instead of the general population. While the VSC and SHHS used unattended at-home polysomnography to diagnose SDB, the WSCS employed in-laboratory polysomnography. The WSCS used an AHI of 0 as their reference point, whereas SHHS used a range of 0–4.9. The VSC used 0–2.9th quartile for Respiratory Disturbance Index (RDI) as their reference range owing to the fact that very few patients truly have an AHI of 0.

In addition, a cross-sectional study in Canada demonstrated that an increase in the AHI by one event/h was associated with a 1% risk of having hypertension [20]. Data from a prospective study in Spain [11] that examined 1,889 subjects for an average of 10.1 years also revealed an elevated incidence of hypertension in participants who did not receive CPAP therapy, compared with those who did.

Population based studies employing 24 h ambulatory BP monitoring (ABPM) have demonstrated that participants with a drop in BP of <10% during the night (nondippers) and those who mount an increase in BP at night (risers) demonstrate a greater degree of end organ damage [40], higher risk of stroke [31], incident heart failure [41], and increased risk of renal disease progression [42] as compared to those hypertensives with preserved dipping, that is, a nocturnal decrease in BP of >10% [43, 44]. Studies with ABPM in OSA patients demonstrate a higher prevalence of diminished nocturnal BP dipping compared with those without OSA [45]. A study revealed an 84% prevalence of nondipping in a sample of untreated patients with mild to severe OSA [46]. Further analysis on a subset of the WSCS

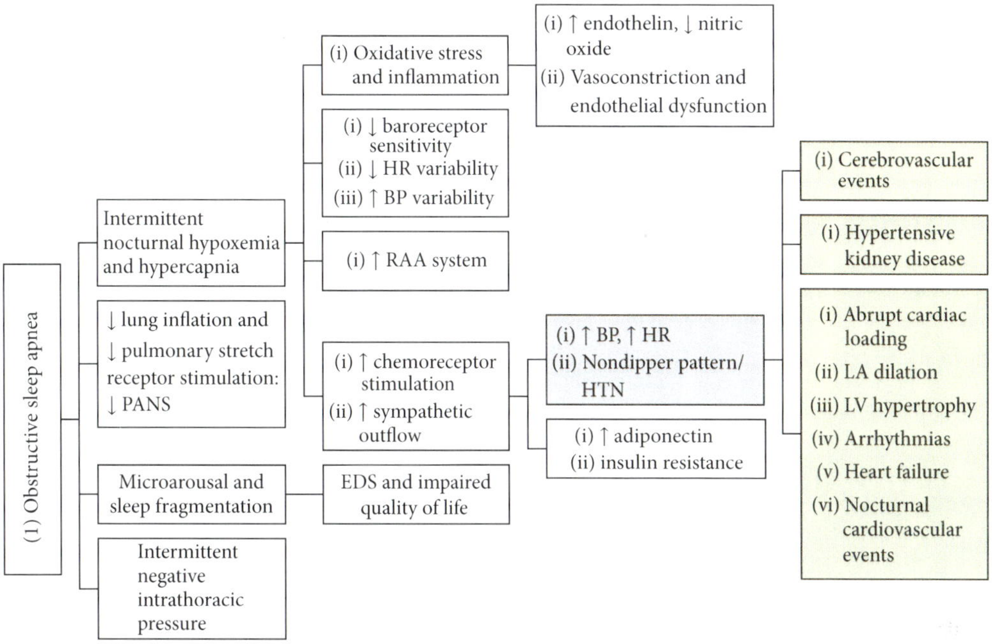

Figure 1: Mechanism of hypertension and end organ damage in obstructive sleep apnea. PANS, parasympathetic autonomic nervous system; RAA, renin-angiotensin-aldosterone; EDS, excessive daytime sleepiness; LV, left ventricular; LA, left atrial.

cohort depicted a positive correlation between an elevated risk of nondipping and the baseline severity of OSA [35]. In addition, nocturnal CPAP use among nondippers is more effective at lowering BP than antihypertensive drugs [47], suggesting the causal role of OSA in loss of dipping.

Sex appears to influence the prevalence of OSAS, which affects males 8–10 times more commonly than females [1, 48–50] in clinical studies and approximately 2-3 times higher in epidemiological studies. The reason for the heightened male predominance remains nebulous but could allegedly be explained by factors such as fat distribution [51], upper airway anatomy [52], craniofacial configuration [53], and hormonal variation across genders [54–56]. Females with OSA tend to depict typical symptoms such as snoring, apnea, and excessive daytime sleepiness (EDS) less commonly than atypical symptoms like fatigue, depression, and anxiety [57] and have a lower AHI, generally limited to REM sleep [58]. Thus, OSA may be grossly underdiagnosed in women owing to an altered presentation [48]. Despite the high prevalence of OSAS observed in males, the effect of sex on incident HTN in OSA has been relatively inconsistent [59]. Hedner et al. [60] investigated the confounders to the association between OSA and hypertension risk and found that the odds ratio for hypertension increased across AHI tertiles from 1.0 to 2.1 (95% CI: 0.9–4.5) and from 1.0 to 3.7 (95% CI: 1.7–8.2) in males but not in females where the OR increased from 1.0 to 1.8 (95% CI: 0.8–3.9) and 1.0 to 1.6 (95% CI: 0.7–3.5).

3. Pathophysiology of HTN in OSA

The pathophysiology of hypertension in OSA is complex and is dependent on various factors such as sympathetic tone, peripheral vasoconstriction, increased renin-angiotensin-aldosterone activity, and altered baroreceptor reflexes (Figure 1). The intermittent apneic episodes cause hypoxemia, which stimulates the carotid body chemoreceptors, causing reflex sympathetic stimulation of the medullary cardiorespiratory centers. The nocturnal catecholamine surges cause a resultant nocturnal increase in heart rate and blood pressure that is most prominent during the postapneic hyperventilation, soaring as high as 240/130 mmHg [61, 62]. The nocturnal BP surge manifests in many as failure of the normally observed "dipping" phenomenon [63] and in other cases precipitates cardiovascular events such as coronary spasm, angina, and arrhythmias.

Tamisier et al. [64] in their study found that intermittent hypoxia significantly increased daytime ambulatory blood pressure after a single night exposure (3 mm for mean diastolic) and further increased daytime pressures after 2 weeks of exposure (8 mm Hg systolic and 5 mm Hg diastolic) with no evident changes in either vascular reactivity or systemic inflammatory markers. The study also assessed muscle sympathetic nerve activity (MSNA) and found that MSNA increased across exposure also while baroreflex control of sympathetic outflow declined, thus suggesting that sympathoactivation induced by intermittent hypoxia likely contributes to blood pressure elevation and may derive from reduced baroreflex inhibition.

In addition to the increased sympathetic response to hypoxia, there is also a simultaneous reflex stimulation of the respiratory centers causing increased depth and frequency of breathing. Lung inflation reflexively stimulates the vagal stretch receptors, mitigating the increased sympathetic activity, hence maintaining autonomic homeostasis

[65–67]. In the absence of adequate lung inflation during apneic episodes, sympathetic outflow remains unchecked, resulting in an exaggerated sympathetic response to hypoxemia. This amplified chemoreflex sensitivity causes a baseline elevated sympathetic tone in OSA, which persists during the day even in the absence of hypoxia [68, 69]. In addition to impaired pulmonary stretch receptor and baroreceptor reflexes, blunted heart rate variability and increased BP variability are observed in OSAS [70], which is indicative of underlying autonomic dysfunction [71] and is a predictive marker for developing hypertension [72] and potential cardiovascular disease [73]. It is also associated with an increased risk of end organ damage in hypertensive individuals [74] and adverse outcomes in patients with preexisting cardiovascular disease [75].

OSAS causes intermittent negative intrathoracic pressure, which, coupled with transient nocturnal catecholamine surges, exerts profound mechanical stress on the heart, gradually causing left ventricular hypertrophy and atrial remodeling, thereby increasing the risk of heart failure and arrhythmias such as atrial fibrillation [76], even in the absence of sustained diurnal hypertension, as evaluated by 24 h ABPM.

Decreased sympathetic and increased parasympathetic activity during NREM sleep, which comprises the majority of sleep time, contributes to the normal circadian variation of blood pressure, causing "dipping" of both systolic and diastolic BP at night, approximately by 10–15% [77, 78]. NREM is intermittently punctuated by REM sleep, characterized by predominant sympathetic activity and transient nocturnal BP surges. The generalized skeletal muscle atonia in REM sleep predisposes the already susceptible airway in OSAS patients to collapse, exacerbating apneic episodes and further intensifying the nocturnal sympathetic hyperactivity.

Recurrent nocturnal hypoxemia with subsequent reoxygenation increases oxidative stress to the body, much like ischemia reperfusion injury, inducing release of reactive oxygen species, inflammatory cytokines, and vasoactive substances, thereby mediating endothelial damage [79–82]. OSAS patients demonstrated attenuated small vessel response to vasodilators such as acetylcholine in some studies [79, 83]. Carlson et al. [83] demonstrated in their study that forearm blood pressure flow after acetylcholine was reduced in OSA patients compared with that in controls, but there was no difference between hypertensive and normotensive subjects. However, this finding was not consistent with other studies [84]. OSAS patients were also found to have reduced levels of the vasodilator nitrogen monoxide, where the degree of decrease in levels is consistent with the severity of OSAS [85] and is also responsive to CPAP therapy [86].

Endothelin levels have been shown to increase in hypoxia in in vitro studies [87]. OSAS patients were found to have high nocturnal levels of endothelin-1 compared to controls [88], the magnitude of which corresponds to the degree of BP elevation and increasing AHI [89]. Furthermore, elevated endothelin levels were shown to decline following treatment with CPAP for 4 hours, implicating the role of endothelin in the pathogenesis of HTN in OSA patients [88, 89]. Elevated levels of C-reactive protein have also been observed in OSAS patients. Those with impaired nocturnal BP dipping were reported to have higher levels of CRP compared to those with relatively preserved dipping [90]. In addition, sleep deprivation can independently induce systemic inflammation [91, 92]. The synergistic combination of recurrent hypoxemia and sleep deprivation in OSAS patients may cause increased production of inflammatory mediators, upregulation of leucocyte adhesion molecules [93–95], serum amyloid A [96], CRP [97, 98], circulating angiogenic inhibitors [99, 100], and decreased cGMP [101], predisposing OSAS patients to endothelial injury and dysfunction, vasoconstriction, and subsequent vascular events, Figure 1.

Obesity is rampant in OSAS patients and is a well-known independent risk factor for glucose intolerance. Other mechanisms responsible for insulin resistance include enhanced resting sympathetic tone causing reduced levels of adiponectin [102], recurrent hypoxemia, and cumulative sleep debt. Several [103, 104] studies have endorsed an association of OSA with insulin resistance independent of obesity [105], which is further supported by trials that demonstrate mild reversal of glucose intolerance with CPAP use in OSA patients [106]. Seetho et al. [107] reported that patients with OSA with obesity have increased arterial stiffness that potentially influences cardiovascular risk independently of metabolic abnormalities. Arterial stiffness correlated with mean arterial blood pressure ($P = 0.003$) and obstructive sleep apnea severity (AHI; $P < 0.001$).

Another mechanism which potentially contributes to HTN in OSAS is increased activity of the renin-angiotensin-aldosterone system (RAAS). Periodic hypoxia has been shown to boost angiotensin I expression and angiotensin II receptor stimulation in the carotid body [108, 109] as well as increasing renin and aldosterone levels in animal studies [105–108]. A meta-analysis conducted on 13 studies observed increased Ang II levels in OSAS patients relative to controls, while elevated aldosterone levels were seen in OSAS patients with HTN compared to normotensive OSAS patients [110]. These elevated markers were seen to decline following CPAP therapy and subsequent BP reduction [111–114], thereby supporting the causal role of RAAS activation in OSA-mediated hypertension. Conversely, OSA was also found to be more prevalent in patients with hyperaldosteronism than those without (18% versus 8.8%), with hyperaldosteronism patients being 1.8 times more likely to have OSA after adjusting for confounding risk factors [115]. Excess aldosterone causes fluid retention, which, coupled with rostral fluid displacement during sleep, promotes accumulation of fluid within the neck, hence causing increased upper airway obstruction [115–127]. The fact that spironolactone helps reduce OSA severity by 50% in patients with resistant hypertension further testifies to the potential contribution of aldosterone in developing or exacerbating preexisting OSAS [128].

The nexus between OSA and HTN appears to be bidirectional according to epidemiological studies [18, 129]. The idea of reciprocal causality has been supported by experimental data in animals where acute BP surges have been shown to increase upper airway obstruction [130–132]. Accordingly, similar results have been demonstrated in humans where phenylephrine mediated rise in BP resulted in lower daytime genioglossus electromyographic activity [133]. Potential mechanisms that can contribute to upper airway collapsibility include inhibitory effect of baroreceptor activation on upper airway dilatory muscle or a change in brain perfusion by upsurge in mean arterial pressure [134].

4. Treatment

4.1. CPAP Therapy. While CPAP remains the mainstay therapy for OSAS, its effect on blood pressure reduction has been variable, most likely owing to the multifactorial nature of hypertension. CPAP therapy has been observed to attenuate the nocturnal sympathetic surge and mediate acute reduction in nocturnal BP in OSAS patients [68, 135–138]. However, results of several trials that evaluated the impact of long-term CPAP therapy on daytime blood pressure reduction in OSAS patients have been unremarkable [10, 139]. Numerous meta-analyses [10, 140–147] have demonstrated only a mild decrease in BP of about 1.3 to 3 mm Hg with CPAP. This modest BP lowering effect of CPAP, although not comparable to antihypertensive drugs, is significant nonetheless in improving cardiovascular and cerebrovascular sequelae by decreasing mortality by 6%–8% for stroke and 4%-5% for ischemic heart disease [148, 149].

The generalizability of the results of these trials however is limited owing to variability in factors affecting both the study population (such as age, sex, BMI, baseline severity of both hypertension and OSA, and concomitant use of antihypertensive drugs) and methodology (such as sample size, method of BP evaluation, e.g., office BP versus ABPM, use of placebo for control group, CPAP compliance, duration of CPAP used per night, and overall length of treatment and follow-up). The magnitude of the drop in BP is subject to various factors such as CPAP compliance [145, 146, 150, 151], duration of treatment with CPAP [145, 152] and its use during REM sleep [153], presence of EDS [146, 150], baseline BP [145, 147], and severity of OSAS with increased benefits seen in patients with baseline AHI > 30 [140, 146] and a high BMI [141, 154]. Patients who exhibited higher baseline BP, untreated hypertension, nocturnal hypertension/nondipper pattern, and resistant hypertension were found to benefit the most with CPAP therapy [141, 155–157]. CPAP therapy was observed to have a greater antihypertensive effect in patients with resistant hypertension than in those without [151, 156, 158–161], with a drop of −7.21 (95% CI, −9.04 to −5.35; $P < 0.001$; I^2, 58%) and −4.99 (95% CI, −6.01 to −3.96; $P < 0.001$; I^2, 31%) observed in SBP and DBP, respectively, according to a meta-analysis [162]. In nondippers, consistent use of CPAP led to the recovery of the nocturnal dipping pattern [156] which helps improve cardiovascular morbidity and mortality since those with nocturnal rising BP pattern have the greatest cardiovascular risk [163, 164]. These findings were corroborated by the HIPARCO Randomized Clinical Trial [151] conducted in Spain, which showed higher dipping patterns in patients who received CPAP therapy compared to those who did not (35.9% dipping in CPAP group versus 21.6% in control; adjusted OR = 2.4; $P = 0.02$). The BP lowering effect was also more pronounced in patients who used CPAP for at least 4 hours per night, with a drop of 1.3 mm Hg in BP detected per hour of CPAP therapy used.

A randomized controlled trial [152] was conducted, comparing the effect of therapeutic and subtherapeutic CPAP in patients with moderate to severe OSA. In the therapeutic CPAP group, treatment pressure was increased until apneas, hypopneas, and snoring were prevented during all sleep stages with the patient lying supine. Mean effective treatment pressure was 9.1 ± 2.3 cm H_2O (between 6 to 12 cm H_2O). In the subtherapeutic treatment group, pressure was left unchanged at the lowest possible value for the CPAP device used (3 or 4 cm H_2O). After an average treatment of 9 weeks, far substantial reductions in mean BP (9.9 ± 11.4 mm Hg) and both nocturnal and daytime systolic and diastolic BP (10 mm Hg approximately) were noted in the therapeutic CPAP group, most likely owing to the length of the trial and treatment pressure used (compared to 1.3–3 mm Hg in most trials lasting for about 4–6 weeks). The fact that, despite causing 50% reduction in AHI, subtherapeutic CPAP was not effective enough to cause any relevant change in BP ($P = 0.01$) further highlights the significance of highly effective therapy. Since OSA-mediated hypertension has a chronic etiology involving endothelial dysfunction and cardiovascular remodeling, it is very possible that short-term controlled studies may not entirely reveal the actual potentially far reaching consequences of scrupulous long-term CPAP therapy on hypertension and its cardiovascular sequelae.

Notwithstanding increased benefits of CPAP therapy in those patients who demonstrated more than 50% reduction in AHI following CPAP [152], this effect seems independent of normalization of oxygen saturation alone. A trial comparing CPAP versus oxygen therapy in OSAS patients demonstrated BP reductions in the CPAP group but not in the oxygen group, which, despite correcting the nocturnal hypoxia, did not lower BP [165].

CPAP mediated BP reduction is also contingent on the presence of daytime somnolence, with far lower efficacy observed in patients who did not report EDS, despite having severe OSA with AHI > 30/h [154, 166, 167]. Even those patients who experienced only modest subjective somnolence also reported some improvement in BP with CPAP therapy [168]. Additionally, those with fewer daytime symptoms are less likely to adhere to CPAP treatment, hence eliciting fewer benefits.

4.2. Lifestyle Modifications. Since obesity is the single most important risk factor for OSA, even modest reductions in weight help attenuate the severity of both OSA and OSA induced hypertension. In a study [169] that examined a sample of participants from the Wisconsin Sleep Cohort Study (WSCS) a 10% increase in weight predicted a 32% increase in the AHI and a 6-fold increase in the odds of developing moderate to severe SDB. Conversely, a 10% weight loss predicted a 26% decrease in the AHI.

Since both OSA and obesity have an independent causal relationship with hypertension, an integrated approach that includes lifestyle modifications such as weight loss should be recommended in OSA patients receiving treatment with

CPAP and antihypertensives. In a randomized control trial [170] assessing the impact of weight loss and CPAP on OSA, patients were assigned to receive treatment with CPAP alone, a weight-loss intervention, or combined CPAP and weight-loss intervention for 24 weeks. A greater reduction was observed in the combined-intervention group (14.1 mm Hg) than in either the weight-loss group (6.8 mm Hg) or the CPAP group (3.0 mm Hg). Combination therapy was also associated with a significantly greater drop in mean arterial pressure. These findings suggest the possibility of a synergistic interaction effect between lifestyle modifications and weight-loss and CPAP therapy in the management of hypertension in OSA patients.

4.3. Oral Appliances. Oral appliances are a recommended alternative treatment to CPAP in patients with mild to moderate OSA. There have been only limited clinical studies on this intervention, most of which were observational with small sample sizes and short durations. A meta-analysis of seven studies involving 399 OSAS patients [171] found a beneficial effect of oral appliances on BP comparable to that of CPAP. The average drop in SBP, DBP, and MAP was reported to be −2.7 mm Hg (95% CI: 0.8 to 4.6; $P = 0.04$), −2.7 mm Hg (95% CI: 0.9 to 4.6; $P = 0.004$), and −2.40 mm Hg (95% CI: 4.01 to 0.80; $P = 0.003$), respectively. Since most of the studies in this meta-analysis were also observational, the true effect of oral appliances on BP reduction in OSA remains nebulous. Andren et al. [172] in their study found that, in patients with OSA and hypertension, oral appliances therapy had a modest trend towards effect on reducing blood pressure. The trend was stronger towards treatment effect when patients with normal baseline ambulatory blood pressure were excluded. As per the systemic review by Okuno et al. [173] although oral appliances have demonstrated good efficacy in patients with mild to severe levels of OSA, they are not completely effective in all patients. Studies vary in the degree of bias and the definitions applied for treatment success. More recent data suggests that oral appliance therapy should be prescribed to patients with OSA who are intolerant to CPAP therapy or prefer alternate therapy as oral appliances are noninferior to CPAP on blood pressure and have better compliance and lastly CPAP and oral appliances lowered morning blood pressure [174].

4.4. Upper Airway Surgery. Surgical options such as tonsillectomy and uvulopalatopharyngoplasty (UPPP) have also been looked at for impact of blood pressure in patients with OSAS. The SKUP3 randomized controlled trial by Di Munro et al. [175] showed that modified UPPP significantly improved sleepiness, nocturnal respirations, and quality of life as well as lowering blood pressure significantly after surgery in a selected group of patients with moderate to severe OSA. Tonsillectomy and adenoidectomy are surgeries used to treat OSA in children. Gaddam et al. [128] from their care series inferred that, among children receiving tonsillectomy and adenoidectomy for OSA treatment, nonobese children improved more than obese children did in terms of blood pressure with a significantly decreased nocturnal DBP index (−12.0 to 18.8, $P = 0.18$) and morning SBP (111.1 to 105.8 mm Hg; $P = 0.014$), SBP index (−5.4 to −10.9, $P = 0.008$), and DBP (−12.0 to −18.7, $P = 0.023$).

4.5. Antihypertensive Drugs. Hypertensive patients with mild to moderate OSA who do not need CPAP are ideal candidates for hypertensive therapy, as are those with severe OSA who do not tolerate or are not compliant with CPAP. Due to lack of adequate evidence, there are no specific guidelines as to which class of antihypertensive medications should be used to treat hypertension in OSA patients. Hypothetically, however, owing to the pathophysiological mechanisms causing and maintaining HTN in OSA such as the sympathetic and RAAS overactivity, antihypertensive drugs that modulate the activity of these systems such as Β-blockers and aldosterone antagonists may be the best treatment options for hypertension in OSA patients. Aldosterone levels are generally normal in OSA except in patients with treatment resistant hypertension or severe OSA [175]. The aldosterone antagonist spironolactone has been very effective in decreasing the severity of OSA [128]. ACE inhibitors, angiotensin receptor blockers, and aldosterone antagonists have a moderate antihypertensive effect in moderate OSA. In severe OSA, aldosterone antagonists may be even more effective [176]. In a study [177] comparing Β-blockers and calcium channel blockers, 31 patients were treated for 6 weeks with either nebivolol ($n = 16$) or valsartan ($n = 15$). While both the drugs effectively reduced both systolic and diastolic BP, nebivolol had a significantly more marked impact on the decrease of heart rate compared to valsartan ($P < 0.001$), which may help in patients with nocturnal tachycardia. In a study by Kraiczi et al. [178], Β-blockers (atenolol) significantly reduced nocturnal diastolic and systolic BP more effectively compared to calcium channel blockers, ACE inhibitors, and angiotensin receptor blockers (but not hydrochlorothiazide). However, there was no difference noted in daytime BP and OSA severity across the different classes of antihypertensives.

According to most studies, antihypertensive drug mediated nocturnal blood pressure reduction has not been found to be associated with any significant decrease in the severity of sleep disordered breathing as measured by AHI, suggesting nocturnal high BP contributes only minimally to apneic events and OSA severity. The results have been observed across all the commonly used classes of antihypertensive drugs including Β-blockers, calcium channel blockers, angiotensin-converting enzyme (ACE) inhibitors, angiotensin receptor blockers (ARBs), hydrochlorothiazide, methyldopa, and clonidine [178–181]. However, one study [134] revealed a weak correlation between the influence of drug therapy on reduction of nocturnal BP and frequency of apneic episodes during REM sleep in hypertensive OSA patients despite no change in AHI during NREM sleep or for the overall sleep duration. This further supports the fact that any potential effect of elevated BP on upper airway collapse may be sleep stage dependent. Data from a few studies also demonstrated some resolution of apnea/hypopnea following antihypertensive drug therapy. Studies comparing Β-blockers and ACE inhibitors in hypertensive OSA patients [182–184] revealed that both Metoprolol and cilazapril caused a statistically significant decrease in both nocturnal BP and

AHI. However, according to one of the studies the effect of cilazapril was observed in all sleep phases and it was hence more favorable for the sleep disturbance pattern characteristic to OSA as compared to Metoprolol, which did not cause any changes during REM sleep [182]. Diuretics, particularly spironolactone, have been shown to be the most promising medication that relieves pharyngeal edema and secondary upper airway destabilization, hence improving both OSA severity and HTN [119, 128].

However, most of these studies had extremely limited samples (12–24 patients), variable populations, short duration of treatment and follow-ups, and lack of placebo effect and used noninvasive methods to measure BP. Since BP varies greatly during apneic cycles (between 150 and 300 mm Hg), invasive BP measurement is the most accurate technique to evaluate the mean nocturnal BP in patients with sleep disordered breathing. Hence there exists a lack of definitive recommendations regarding the use of antihypertensive agents for OSA treatment.

Conversely, there has been some incriminating evidence advising against the use of ACE inhibitors in hypertensive OSA patients. According to Cicolin et al. [185], enalapril induced a dry cough and increased upper airway inflammation (measured by exhaled nitric oxide, a marker of airway inflammation) subsequently causing OSA exacerbation, all of which resolved following cessation of enalapril. B-blockers have been shown to cause increased weight, which can aggravate OSA [185]. In addition, study on 186 OSA patients with HTN [186] reported significant sleep impairment associated with the use of calcium channel blockers with a reduction of 41 minutes in total sleep time ($P = 0.005$) and an 8% decrease in sleep efficiency ($P = 0.004$). On the other hand, no other antihypertensive drug, such as diuretics and beta-blockers, was found to have an adverse impact on sleep duration. Notwithstanding these results, it is worth mentioning that most of these adverse effects need a long time before they can be discernable. Hence, the limited duration of these studies is not adequate to assess the true impact that these medications have on OSA severity. Walia et al. [187] analyzed the data from the HeartBEAT (Heart Biomarker Evaluation in Apnea Treatment) trial and found that in patients at high cardiovascular risk or established cardiovascular disease there was a strong association of severe untreated OSA and resistant elevated blood pressure despite treatment with an aggressive antihypertensive medication regimen. Thus in these patients a combination of antihypertensive medications and other strategies such as CPAP should be used.

5. Conclusion

There are numerous mechanisms that can potentiate the development of hypertension in OSA, with wide variation in individual susceptibility. These include increased sympathetic tone, inflammation, endothelial dysfunction, peripheral vasoconstriction, increased RAAS, heightened chemoreflex, and blunted baroreflex sensitivity. Conversely, acute rise in BP may cause an inhibition of the upper airway muscles. This, coupled with volume overload due to increased activity of the RAAS and rostral fluid displacement during sleep, can cause pharyngeal edema and subsequent airway obstruction, thus causing OSA in hypertensive patients. Treatment options for OSA range from surgical options such as tonsillectomy and adenoidectomy in children to modified UPPP in adults, to noninvasive measures such as CPAP therapy, oral appliances, and lifestyle modifications to address obesity; and lastly use of antihypertensive drugs has been investigated. These measures help address the issues of resistant hypertension that are frequently found in patients with OSAS which is linked with cardiovascular morbidity and mortality. Hence OSA and HTN both need prompt diagnosis and treatment to help address the growing cardiovascular morbidity and mortality due to these two entities. Continued advancements in the field of medicine may lead to newer treatment modalities in the future.

References

[1] T. Young, P. E. Peppard, and D. J. Gottlieb, "Epidemiology of obstructive sleep apnea: a population health perspective," *The American Journal of Respiratory and Critical Care Medicine*, vol. 165, no. 9, pp. 1217–1239, 2002.

[2] P. W. Wilson, R. B. D'Agostino, L. Sullivan, H. Parise, and W. B. Kannel, "Overweight and obesity as determinants of cardiovascular risk; the Framingham experience," *Archives of Internal Medicine*, vol. 162, pp. 1867–1872, 2002.

[3] S. Sonne-Holm, T. I. A. Sorensen, G. Jensen, and P. Schnohr, "Independent effects of weight change and attained body weight on prevalence of arterial hypertension in obese and non-obese men," *British Medical Journal*, vol. 299, no. 6702, pp. 767–770, 1989.

[4] N. A. Shah, H. K. Yaggi, J. Concato, and V. Mohsenin, "Obstructive sleep apnea as a risk factor for coronary events or cardiovascular death," *Sleep and Breathing*, vol. 14, no. 2, pp. 131–136, 2010.

[5] D. J. Gottlieb, G. Yenokyan, A. B. Newman et al., "Prospective study of obstructive sleep apnea and incident coronary heart disease and heart failure: the sleep heart health study," *Circulation*, vol. 122, no. 4, pp. 352–360, 2010.

[6] H. K. Yaggi, J. Concato, W. N. Kernan, J. H. Lichtman, L. M. Brass, and V. Mohsenin, "Obstructive sleep apnea as a risk factor for stroke and death," *The New England Journal of Medicine*, vol. 353, no. 19, pp. 2034–2041, 2005.

[7] A. S. Gami, D. E. Howard, E. J. Olson, and V. K. Somers, "Day-night pattern of sudden death in obstructive sleep apnea," *The New England Journal of Medicine*, vol. 352, no. 12, pp. 1206–1279, 2005.

[8] F. H. Kuniyoshi, A. Garcia-Touchard, A. S. Gami et al., "Day-night variation of acute myocardial infarction in obstructive sleep apnea," *Journal of the American College of Cardiology*, vol. 52, no. 5, pp. 343–346, 2008.

[9] P. E. Peppard, T. Young, M. Palta, and J. Skatrud, "Prospective study of the association between sleep-disordered breathing and hypertension," *The New England Journal of Medicine*, vol. 342, no. 19, pp. 1378–1384, 2000.

[10] J. Durán-Cantolla, F. Aizpuru, C. Martínez-Null, and F. Barbé-Illa, "Obstructive sleep apnea/hypopnea and systemic hypertension," *Sleep Medicine Reviews*, vol. 13, no. 5, pp. 323–331, 2009.

[11] J. M. Marin, A. Agusti, I. Villar et al., "Association between treated and untreated obstructive sleep apnea and risk of hypertension," *The Journal of the American Medical Association*, vol. 307, no. 20, pp. 2169–2176, 2012.

[12] M. Guillot, E. Sforza, E. Achour-Crawford et al., "Association between severe obstructive sleep apnea and incident arterial hypertension in the older people population," *Sleep Medicine*, vol. 14, no. 9, pp. 838–842, 2013.

[13] R. C. Hermida, D. E. Ayala, M. H. Smolensky, J. R. Fernández, A. Mojón, and F. Portaluppi, "Sleep-time blood pressure: Unique sensitive prognostic marker of vascular risk and therapeutic target for prevention," *Sleep Medicine Reviews*, vol. 33, pp. 17–27, 2017.

[14] W. Zhang and L.-Y. Si, "Obstructive sleep apnea syndrome (OSAS) and hypertension: Pathogenic mechanisms and possible therapeutic approaches," *Upsala Journal of Medical Sciences*, vol. 117, no. 4, pp. 370–382, 2012.

[15] J. Durán, S. Esnaola, R. Rubio, and Á. Iztueta, "Obstructive sleep apnea-hypopnea and related clinical features in a population-based sample of subjects aged 30 to 70 yr," *American Journal of Respiratory and Critical Care Medicine*, vol. 163, no. 3, part 1, pp. 685–689, 2001.

[16] P. E. Peppard, T. Young, J. H. Barnet, M. Palta, E. W. Hagen, and K. M. Hla, "Increased prevalence of sleep-disordered breathing in adults," *The American Journal of Epidemiology*, vol. 177, no. 9, pp. 1006–1014, 2013.

[17] P. M. Kearney, M. Whelton, K. Reynolds, P. Muntner, P. K. Whelton, and J. He, "Global burden of hypertension: analysis of worldwide data," *The Lancet*, vol. 365, no. 9455, pp. 217–223, 2005.

[18] T. Young, P. Peppard, M. Palta et al., "Population-based study of sleep-disordered breathing as a risk factor for hypertension," *Archives of Internal Medicine*, vol. 157, no. 15, pp. 1746–1752, 1997.

[19] F. Javier Nieto, T. B. Young, B. K. Lind et al., "Association of sleep-disordered breathing sleep apnea, and hypertension in a large community-based study," *Journal of the American Medical Association*, vol. 283, no. 14, pp. 1829–1836, 2000.

[20] P. Lavie, P. Herer, and V. Hoffstein, "Obstructive sleep apnoea syndrome as a risk factor for hypertension: population study," *British Medical Journal*, vol. 320, no. 7233, pp. 479–482, 2000.

[21] E. C. Fletcher, R. D. DeBehnke, M. S. Lovoi, and A. B. Gorin, "Undiagnosed sleep apnea in patients with essential hypertension," *Annals of Internal Medicine*, vol. 103, no. 2, pp. 190–195, 1985.

[22] D. S. Silverberg and A. Oksenberg, "Are sleep-related breathing disorders important contributing factors to the production of essential hypertension?" *Current Hypertension Reports*, vol. 3, no. 3, pp. 209–215, 2001.

[23] A. J. Williams, D. Houston, S. Finberg, C. Lam, J. L. Kinney, and S. Santiago, "Sleep apnea syndrome and essential hypertension," *The American Journal of Cardiology*, vol. 55, no. 8, pp. 1019–1022, 1985.

[24] A. G. Logan, S. M. Perlikowski, A. Mente et al., "High prevalence of unrecognized sleep apnoea in drug-resistant hypertension," *Journal of Hypertension*, vol. 19, no. 12, pp. 2271–2277, 2001.

[25] R. P. Pedrosa, L. F. Drager, C. C. Gonzaga et al., "Obstructive sleep apnea: the most common secondary cause of hypertension associated with resistant hypertension," *Hypertension*, vol. 58, no. 5, pp. 811–817, 2011.

[26] M. Demede, A. Pandey, F. Zizi et al., "Resistant hypertension and obstructive sleep apnea in the primary-care setting," *International Journal of Hypertension*, vol. 2011, Article ID 340929, 2011.

[27] R. L. Verrier, J. E. Muller, and J. A. Hobson, "Sleep, dreams, and sudden death: The case for sleep as an autonomic stress test for the heart," *Cardiovascular Research*, vol. 31, no. 2, pp. 181–211, 1996.

[28] K. Spiegel, E. Tasali, P. Penev, and E. van Cauter, "Brief communication: sleep curtailment in healthy young men is associated with decreased leptin levels, elevated ghrelin levels, and increased hunger and appetite," *Annals of Internal Medicine*, vol. 141, no. 11, pp. 846–850, 2004.

[29] R. J. Kuczmarski, K. M. Flegal, S. M. Campbell, and C. L. Johnson, "Increasing Prevalence of Overweight Among US Adults: The National Health and Nutrition Examination Surveys, 1960 to 1991," *JAMA: The Journal of the American Medical Association*, vol. 272, no. 3, pp. 205–211, 1994.

[30] I. Hajjar and T. A. Kotchen, "Trends in prevalence, awareness, treatment, and control of hypertension in the United States, 1988–2000," *Journal of the American Medical Association*, vol. 290, no. 2, pp. 199–206, 2003.

[31] E. O'Brien, J. Sheridan, and K. O'Malley, "DIPPERS AND NON-DIPPERS," *The Lancet*, vol. 332, no. 8607, p. 397, 1988.

[32] G. T. O'Connor, B. Caffo, A. B. Newman et al., "Prospective study of sleep-disordered breathing and hypertension: The sleep heart health study," *American Journal of Respiratory and Critical Care Medicine*, vol. 179, no. 12, pp. 1159–1164, 2009.

[33] E. O. Bixler, A. N. Vgontzas, H.-M. Lin et al., "Association of hypertension and sleep-disordered breathing," *Archives of Internal Medicine*, vol. 160, no. 15, pp. 2289–2295, 2000.

[34] D. C. Haas, G. L. Foster, F. J. Nieto et al., "Age-dependent associations between sleep-disordered breathing and hypertension: importance of discriminating between systolic/diastolic hypertension and isolated systolic hypertension in the sleep heart health study," *Circulation*, vol. 111, no. 5, pp. 614–621, 2005.

[35] K. M. Hla, T. Young, L. Finn, P. E. Peppard, M. Szklo-Coxe, and M. Stubbs, "Longitudinal association of sleep-disordered breathing and nondipping of nocturnal blood pressure in the Wisconsin Sleep Cohort Study," *Sleep*, vol. 31, no. 6, pp. 795–800, 2008.

[36] P. E. Peppard, M. Szklo-Coxe, K. M. Hla, and T. Young, "Longitudinal association of sleep-related breathing disorder and depression," *Archives of Internal Medicine*, vol. 166, no. 16, pp. 1709–1715, 2006.

[37] M. Arzt, T. Young, L. Finn, J. B. Skatrud, and T. D. Bradley, "Association of sleep-disordered breathing and the occurrence of stroke," *The American Journal of Respiratory and Critical Care Medicine*, vol. 172, no. 11, pp. 1447–1451, 2005.

[38] T. Young, L. Finn, P. E. Peppard et al., "Sleep disordered breathing and mortality: eighteen-year follow-up of the wisconsin sleep cohort," *Sleep*, vol. 31, no. 8, pp. 1071–1078, 2008.

[39] I. Cano-Pumarega, J. Durán-Cantolla, F. Aizpuru et al., "Obstructive sleep apnea and systemic hypertension - Longitudinal study in the general population: The vitoria sleep cohort," *American Journal of Respiratory and Critical Care Medicine*, vol. 184, no. 11, pp. 1299–1304, 2011.

[40] ESH/ESC, "Force for the Management of Arterial Hypertension," *Journal of Hypertension*, vol. 31, no. 10, pp. 1925–1938, 2013.

[41] E. Ingelsson, K. Björklund-Bodegård, L. Lind, J. Ärnlöv, and J. Sundström, "Diurnal blood pressure pattern and risk of

congestive heart failure," *Journal of the American Medical Association*, vol. 295, no. 24, pp. 2859–2866, 2006.

[42] M. Timio, S. Venanzi, S. Lolli et al., "'Non-dipper' hypertensive patients and progressive renal insufficiency: A 3-year longitudinal study," *Clinical Nephrology*, vol. 43, no. 6, pp. 382–387, 1995.

[43] S. Hoshide, K. Kario, Y. Hoshide et al., "Associations between nondipping of nocturnal blood pressure decrease and cardiovascular target organ damage in strictly selected community-dwelling normotensives," *American Journal of Hypertension*, vol. 16, no. 6, pp. 434–438, 2003.

[44] J. Boggia, Y. Li, L. Thijs et al., "Prognostic accuracy of day versus night ambulatory blood pressure: a cohort study," *Lancet*, vol. 370, no. 9594, pp. 1219–1229, 2007.

[45] W. Pankow, B. Nabe, A. Lies et al., "Influence of sleep apnea on 24-hour blood pressure," *Chest*, vol. 112, no. 5, pp. 1253–1258, 1997.

[46] J. S. Loredo, S. Ancoli-Israel, and J. E. Dimsdale, "Sleep quality and blood pressure dipping in obstructive sleep apnea," *American Journal of Hypertension*, vol. 14, no. 9 I, pp. 887–892, 2001.

[47] H. M. Engleman, K. Gough, S. E. Martin, R. N. Kingshott, P. L. Padfield, and N. J. Douglas, "Ambulatory blood pressure on and off continuous positive airway pressure therapy for the sleep apnea/hypopnea syndrome: Effects in 'non-dippers'," *Sleep*, vol. 19, no. 5, pp. 378–381, 1996.

[48] E. Sforza, F. Chouchou, P. Collet, V. Pichot, J. C. Barthélémy, and F. Roche, "Sex differences in obstructive sleep apnoea in an elderly French population," *European Respiratory Journal*, vol. 37, no. 5, pp. 1137–1143, 2011.

[49] F. Kapsimalis and M. H. Kryger, "Gender and obstructive sleep apnea syndrome, part 2: Mechanisms," *Sleep*, vol. 25, no. 5, pp. 499–506, 2002.

[50] D. R. Dancey, P. J. Hanly, C. Soong, B. Lee, J. Shepard, and V. Hoffstein, "Gender Differences in Sleep Apnea," *Chest*, vol. 123, no. 5, pp. 1544–1550, 2003.

[51] R. P. Millman, C. C. Carlisle, S. T. McGarvey, S. E. Eveloff, and P. D. Levinson, "Body Fat Distribution and Sleep Apnea Severity in Women," *Chest*, vol. 107, no. 2, pp. 362–366, 1995.

[52] G. Pillar, A. Malhotra, R. Fogel, J. Beauregard, R. Schnall, and D. P. White, "Airway mechanics and ventilation in response to resistive loading during sleep: influence of gender," *American Journal of Respiratory and Critical Care Medicine*, vol. 162, no. 5, pp. 1627–1632, 2000.

[53] J. B. Schellenberg, G. Maislin, and R. J. Schwab, "Physical findings and the risk for obstructive sleep apnea: the importance of oropharyngeal structures," *The American Journal of Respiratory and Critical Care Medicine*, vol. 162, no. 2, pp. 740–748, 2000.

[54] D. R. Dancey, P. J. Hanly, C. Soong, B. Lee, and V. Hoffstein, "Impact of menopause on the prevalence and severity of sleep apnea," *Chest*, vol. 120, no. 1, pp. 151–155, 2001.

[55] P. V. Tishler, E. K. Larkin, M. D. Schluchter, and S. Redline, "Incidence of sleep-disordered breathing in an urban adult population: the relative importance of risk factors in the development of sleep-disordered breathing," *Journal of the American Medical Association*, vol. 289, no. 17, pp. 2230–2237, 2003.

[56] E. O. Bixler, A. N. Vgontzas, H. Lin et al., "Prevalence of sleep-disordered breathing in women: effects of gender," *The American Journal of Respiratory and Critical Care Medicine*, vol. 163, no. 3, pp. 608–613, 2001.

[57] T. Young, R. Hutton, L. Finn, S. Badr, and M. Palta, "The gender bias in sleep apnea diagnosis: are women missed because they have different symptoms?" *Archives of Internal Medicine*, vol. 156, no. 21, pp. 2445–2451, 1996.

[58] C. O'Connor, K. S. Thornley, and P. J. Hanly, "Gender differences in the polysomnographic features of obstructive sleep apnea," *American Journal of Respiratory and Critical Care Medicine*, vol. 161, no. 5, pp. 1465–1472, 2000.

[59] V. Mohsenin, "Obstructive sleep apnea and hypertension: a critical review," *Current hypertension reports*, vol. 16, no. 10, p. 482, 2014.

[60] J. Hedner, K. Bengtsson-Boström, Y. Peker, L. Grote, L. Råstam, and U. Lindblad, "Hypertension prevalence in obstructive sleep apnoea and sex: a population-based case—control study," *European Respiratory Journal*, vol. 27, no. 3, pp. 564–570, 2006.

[61] J. Hedner, H. Ejnell, J. Sellgren, T. Hedner, and G. Wallin, "Is high and fluctuating muscle nerve sympathetic activity in the sleep apnoea syndrome of pathogenetic importanee for the development of hypertension?" *Journal of Hypertension, Supplement*, vol. 6, no. 4, pp. S529–S531, 1988.

[62] V. K. Somers, M. E. Dyken, and J. L. Skinner, "Autonomic and hemodynamic responses and interactions during the Mueller maneuver in humans," *Journal of the Autonomic Nervous System*, vol. 44, no. 2-3, pp. 253–259, 1993.

[63] A. Okcay, V. K. Somers, and S. M. Caples, "Obstructive sleep apnea and hypertension," *Journal of Clinical Hypertension*, vol. 10, no. 7, pp. 549–555, 2008.

[64] R. Tamisier, J. L. Pépin, J. Rémy et al., "14 nights of intermittent hypoxia elevate daytime blood pressure and sympathetic activity in healthy humans," *The European Respiratory Journal*, vol. 37, no. 1, pp. 119–128, 2011.

[65] V. K. Somers, M. E. Dyken, A. L. Mark, and F. M. Abboud, "Sympathetic-nerve activity during sleep in normal subjects," *The New England Journal of Medicine*, vol. 328, no. 5, pp. 303–307, 1993.

[66] V. K. Somers, A. L. Mark, D. C. Zavala, and F. M. Abboud, "Influence of ventilation and hypocapnia on sympathetic nerve responses to hypoxia in normal humans," *Journal of Applied Physiology*, vol. 67, no. 5, pp. 2095–2100, 1989.

[67] M. L. Smith, O. N. W. Niedermaier, S. M. Hardy, M. J. Decker, and K. P. Strohl, "Role of hypoxemia in sleep apnea-induced sympathoexcitation," *Journal of the Autonomic Nervous System*, vol. 56, no. 3, pp. 184–190, 1996.

[68] V. K. Somers, M. E. Dyken, M. P. Clary, and F. M. Abboud, "Sympathetic neural mechanisms in obstructive sleep apnea," *Journal of Clinical Investigation*, vol. 96, no. 4, pp. 1897–1904, 1995.

[69] K. Narkiewicz, P. J. H. van de Borne, N. Montano, M. E. Dyken, B. G. Phillips, and V. K. Somers, "Contribution of tonic chemoreflex activation to sympathetic activity and blood pressure in patients with obstructive sleep apnea," *Circulation*, vol. 97, no. 10, pp. 943–945, 1998.

[70] K. Narkiewicz, P. J. H. Van De Borne, R. L. Cooley, M. E. Dyken, and V. K. Somers, "Sympathetic activity in obese subjects with and without obstructive sleep apnea," *Circulation*, vol. 98, no. 8, pp. 772–776, 1998.

[71] K. Narkiewicz, N. Montano, C. Cogliati, P. J. H. van de Borne, M. E. Dyken, and V. K. Somers, "Altered cardiovascular variability in obstructive sleep apnea," *Circulation*, vol. 98, no. 11, pp. 1071–1077, 1998.

[72] J. P. Singh, M. G. Larson, H. Tsuji, J. C. Evans, C. J. O'Donnell, and D. Levy, "Reduced heart rate variability and new-onset hypertension: Insights into pathogenesis of hypertension: The Framingham Heart Study," *Hypertension*, vol. 32, no. 2, pp. 293–297, 1998.

[73] H. Tsuji, M. G. Larson, F. J. Venditti Jr. et al., "Impact of reduced heart rate variability on risk for cardiac events: The Framingham Heart Study," *Circulation*, vol. 94, no. 11, pp. 2850–2855, 1996.

[74] A. Frattola, G. Parati, C. Cuspidi, F. Albini, and G. Mancia, "Prognostic value of 24-hour blood pressure variability," *Journal of Hypertension*, vol. 11, no. 10, pp. 1133–1137, 1993.

[75] X. Copie, K. Hnatkova, A. Staunton, L. Fei, J. A. Camm, and M. Malik, "Predictive Power of Increased Heart Rate Versus Depressed Left Ventricular Ejection Fraction and Heart Rate Variability for Risk Stratification after Myocardial Infarction: Results of a Two-Year Follow-Up Study," *Journal of the American College of Cardiology*, vol. 27, no. 2, pp. 270–276, 1996.

[76] T. D. Bradley and J. S. Floras, "Obstructive sleep apnoea and its cardiovascular consequences," *The Lancet*, vol. 373, no. 9657, pp. 82–93, 2009.

[77] J. Staessen, C. J. Bulpitt, E. O'Brien et al., "The diurnal blood pressure profile. A population study," *American Journal of Hypertension*, vol. 5, no. 6, pp. 386–392, 1992.

[78] J. A. Staessen, R. H. Fagard, P. J. Lijnen, L. Thijs, R. Van Hoof, and A. K. Amery, "Mean and range of the ambulatory pressure in normotensive subjects from a meta-analysis of 23 studies," *The American Journal of Cardiology*, vol. 67, no. 8, pp. 723–727, 1991.

[79] M. Kato, P. Roberts-Thomson, B. G. Phillips et al., "Impairment of endothelium-dependent vasodilation of resistance vessels in patients with obstructive sleep apnea," *Circulation*, vol. 102, no. 21, pp. 2607–2610, 2000.

[80] A. Atkeson, S. Y. Yeh, A. Malhotra, and S. Jelic, "Endothelial Function in Obstructive Sleep Apnea," *Progress in Cardiovascular Diseases*, vol. 51, no. 5, pp. 351–362, 2009.

[81] L. Lavie, "Oxidative stress-a unifying paradigm in obstructive sleep apnea and comorbidities," *Progress in Cardiovascular Diseases*, vol. 51, no. 4, pp. 303–312, 2009.

[82] W. T. McNicholas, "Obstructive sleep apnea and inflammation," *Progress in Cardiovascular Diseases*, vol. 51, no. 5, pp. 392–399, 2009.

[83] J. T. Carlson, C. Rångemark, and J. A. Hedner, "Attenuated endothelium-dependent vascular relaxation in patients with sleep apnoea," *Journal of Hypertension*, vol. 14, no. 5, pp. 577–584, 1996.

[84] H. Kraiczi, J. Hedner, Y. Peker, and J. Carlson, "Increased vasoconstrictor sensitivity in obstructive sleep apnea," *Journal of Applied Physiology*, vol. 89, no. 2, pp. 493–498, 2000.

[85] M. S. M. Ip, B. Lam, L.-Y. Chan et al., "Circulating nitric oxide is suppressed in obstructive sleep apnea and is reversed by nasal continuous positive airway pressure," *American Journal of Respiratory and Critical Care Medicine*, vol. 162, no. 6, pp. 2166–2171, 2000.

[86] A. Noda, S. Nakata, Y. Koike et al., "Continuous positive airway pressure improves daytime baroreflex sensitivity and nitric oxide production in patients with moderate to severe obstructive sleep apnea syndrome," *Hypertension Research*, vol. 30, no. 8, pp. 669–676, 2007.

[87] S. Kourembanas, P. A. Marsden, L. P. McQuillan, and D. V. Faller, "Hypoxia induces endothelin gene expression and secretion in cultured human endothelium," *The Journal of Clinical Investigation*, vol. 88, no. 3, pp. 1054–1057, 1991.

[88] B. G. Phillips, K. Narkiewicz, C. A. Pesek, W. G. Haynes, M. E. Dyken, and V. K. Somers, "Effects of obstructive sleep apnea on endothelin-1 and blood pressure," *Journal of Hypertension*, vol. 17, no. 1, pp. 61–66, 1999.

[89] P. H. Gjørup, L. Sadauskiene, J. Wessels, O. Nyvad, B. Strunge, and E. B. Pedersen, "Abnormally Increased Endothelin-1 in Plasma During the Night in Obstructive Sleep Apnea: Relation to Blood Pressure and Severity of Disease," *American Journal of Hypertension*, vol. 20, no. 1, pp. 44–52, 2007.

[90] J. Ishikawa, S. Hoshide, K. Eguchi et al., "Increased low-grade inflammation and plasminogen-activator inhibitor-1 level in nondippers with sleep apnea syndrome," *Journal of Hypertension*, vol. 26, no. 6, pp. 1181–1187, 2008.

[91] A. N. Vgontzas, D. A. Papanicolaou, E. O. Bixler, A. Kales, K. Tyson, and G. P. Chrousos, "Elevation of plasma cytokines in disorders of excessive daytime sleepiness: role of sleep disturbance and obesity," *Journal of Clinical Endocrinology and Metabolism*, vol. 82, no. 5, pp. 1313–1316, 1997.

[92] H. K. Meier-Ewert, P. M. Ridker, N. Rifai et al., "Effect of sleep loss on C-reactive protein, an inflammatory marker of cardiovascular risk," *Journal of the American College of Cardiology*, vol. 43, no. 4, pp. 678–683, 2004.

[93] E. Ohga, T. Tomita, H. Wada, H. Yamamoto, T. Nagase, and Y. Ouchi, "Effects of obstructive sleep apnea on circulating ICAM-1, IL-8, and MCP-1," *Journal of Applied Physiology*, vol. 94, no. 1, pp. 179–184, 2003.

[94] L. Lavie, "Sleep apnea syndrome, endothelial dysfunction, and cardiovascular morbidity," *Sleep*, vol. 27, no. 6, pp. 1053–1055, 2004.

[95] L. Dyugovskaya, P. Lavie, and L. Lavie, "Increased adhesion molecules expression and production of reactive oxygen species in leukocytes of sleep apnea patients," *The American Journal of Respiratory and Critical Care Medicine*, vol. 165, no. 7, pp. 934–939, 2002.

[96] A. Svatikova, R. Wolk, A. S. Shamsuzzaman, T. Kara, E. J. Olson, and V. K. Somers, "Serum amyloid a in obstructive sleep apnea," *Circulation*, vol. 108, no. 12, pp. 1451–1454, 2003.

[97] K. Minoguchi and M. Adachi, "The role of adrenomedullin in obstructive sleep apnea," *Hypertension Research*, vol. 30, no. 11, pp. 1007-1008, 2007.

[98] N. M. Punjabi and B. A. Beamer, "C-reactive protein is associated with sleep disordered breathing independent of adiposity," *Sleep*, vol. 30, no. 1, pp. 29–34, 2007.

[99] V. Mohsenin and F. Urbano, "Circulating antiangiogenic proteins in obstructive sleep apnea and hypertension," *Respiratory Medicine*, vol. 105, no. 5, pp. 801–807, 2011.

[100] B. Jafari and V. Mohsenin, "Endothelial dysfunction and hypertension in obstructive sleep apnea - Is it due to intermittent hypoxia?" *Journal of Cardiovascular Disease Research*, vol. 4, no. 2, pp. 87–91, 2013.

[101] B. Jafari and V. Mohsenin, "Activation of heme oxygenase and suppression of cGMP are associated with impaired endothelial function in obstructive sleep apnea with hypertension," *American Journal of Hypertension*, vol. 25, no. 8, pp. 854–861, 2012.

[102] J. C. Lam, A. Xu, S. Tam et al., "Hypoadiponectinemia is related to sympathetic activation and severity of obstructive sleep apnea," *Sleep*, vol. 31, no. 12, pp. 1721–1727, 2008.

[103] N. M. Punjabi, J. D. Sorkin, L. I. Katzel, A. P. Goldberg, A. R. Schwartz, and P. L. Smith, "Sleep-disordered breathing and insulin resistance in middle-aged and overweight men," *The American Journal of Respiratory and Critical Care Medicine*, vol. 165, no. 5, pp. 677–682, 2002.

[104] M. S. M. Ip, B. Lam, M. M. T. Ng, W. K. Lam, K. W. T. Tsang, and K. S. L. Lam, "Obstructive sleep apnea is independently associated with insulin resistance," *American Journal of Respiratory and Critical Care Medicine*, vol. 165, no. 5, pp. 670–676, 2002.

[105] N. M. Punjabi, M. M. Ahmed, V. Y. Polotsky, B. A. Beamer, and C. P. O'Donnell, "Sleep-disordered breathing, glucose intolerance, and insulin resistance," *Respiratory Physiology and Neurobiology*, vol. 136, no. 2-3, pp. 167–178, 2003.

[106] ia. Harsch and sp. schahin, "Continuous positive airway pressure treatment rapidly improves insulin sensitivity in patients with obstructive sleep apnea syndrome," *Am J Respir Crit Care Med*, vol. 169, no. 2, pp. 156–162, 2004.

[107] I. W. Seetho, R. J. Parker, S. Craig, N. Duffy, K. J. Hardy, and J. P. H. Wilding, "Obstructive sleep apnea is associated with increased arterial stiffness in severe obesity," *Journal of Sleep Research*, vol. 23, no. 6, pp. 700–708, 2014.

[108] M. L. Fung, G. L. Tipoe, and P. S. Leung, "Mechanisms of maladaptive responses of peripheral chemoreceptors to intermittent hypoxia in sleep-disordered breathing," *Sheng li xue bao : [Acta physiologica Sinica]*, vol. 66, no. 1, pp. 23–29, 2014.

[109] S.-Y. Lam, Y. Liu, K.-M. Ng et al., "Upregulation of a local renin-angiotensin system in the rat carotid body during chronic intermittent hypoxia," *Experimental Physiology*, vol. 99, no. 1, pp. 220–231, 2014.

[110] Z.-N. Jin and Y.-X. Wei, "Meta-analysis of effects of obstructive sleep apnea on the renin-angiotensin-aldosterone system," *Journal of Geriatric Cardiology*, vol. 13, no. 4, pp. 333–343, 2016.

[111] P. Lloberes, G. Sampol, E. Espinel et al., "A randomized controlled study of CPAP effect on plasma aldosterone concentration in patients with resistant hypertension and obstructive sleep apnea," *Journal of Hypertension*, vol. 32, no. 8, pp. 1650–1657, 2014.

[112] D. D. M. Nicholl, P. J. Hanly, M. J. Poulin et al., "Evaluation of continuous positive airway pressure therapy on renin-angiotensin system activity in obstructive sleep apnea," *American Journal of Respiratory and Critical Care Medicine*, vol. 190, no. 5, pp. 572–580, 2014.

[113] P. Lloberes, G. Sampol, and E. Espinel, "Effect of 3-month CPAP treatment on blood pressure and serum aldosterone concentration in patients with resistant hypertension. Respir," in *Effect of 3-month CPAP treatment on blood pressure and serum aldosterone concentration in patients with resistant hypertension. Eur Respir J*, pp. 57–307, Suppl. 57, 307, 2013.

[114] X.-L. Zhang and Y.-Q. Li, "Efficacy of continuous positive airway pressure therapy upon resistant hypertension in patients with obstructive sleep apnea hypopnea syndrome," *Zhonghua yi xue za zhi*, vol. 89, no. 26, pp. 1811–1814, 2009.

[115] J. J. Sim, E. H. Yan, I. L. A. Liu et al., "Positive relationship of sleep apnea to hyperaldosteronism in an ethnically diverse population," *Journal of Hypertension*, vol. 29, no. 8, pp. 1553–1559, 2011.

[116] E. Pimenta, D. A. Calhoun, and S. Oparil, "Sleep Apnea, Aldosterone, and Resistant Hypertension," *Progress in Cardiovascular Diseases*, vol. 51, no. 5, pp. 371–380, 2009.

[117] E. Avrahami and M. Englender, "Relation between CT axial cross-sectional area of the oropharynx and obstructive sleep apnea syndrome in adults," *American Journal of Neuroradiology*, vol. 16, no. 1, pp. 135–140, 1995.

[118] A. Yucel, M. Unlu, A. Haktanir, M. Acar, and F. Fidan, "Evaluation of the upper airway cross-sectional area changes in different degrees of severity of obstructive sleep apnea syndrome: Cephalometric and dynamic CT study," *American Journal of Neuroradiology*, vol. 26, no. 10, pp. 2624–2629, 2005.

[119] C. B. Bucca, L. Brussino, A. Battisti et al., "Diuretics in obstructive sleep apnea with diastolic heart failure," *Chest*, vol. 132, no. 2, pp. 440–446, 2007.

[120] S. Shiota, C. M. Ryan, K.-L. Chiu et al., "Alterations in upper airway cross-sectional area in response to lower body positive pressure in healthy subjects," *Thorax*, vol. 62, no. 10, pp. 868–872, 2007.

[121] C. C. Gonzaga, K. K. Gaddam, and M. I. Ahmed, "Severity of obstructive sleep apnea is related to aldosterone status in subjects with resistant hypertension. Clin Sleep Med," in *Severity of obstructive sleep apnea is related to aldosterone status in subjects with resistant hypertension. J Clin Sleep Med*, pp. 363–368, 4, 363–368, 2010.

[122] G. Parati, J. E. Ochoa, G. Bilo et al., "Obstructive sleep apnea syndrome as a cause of resistant hypertension," *Hypertension Research*, vol. 37, no. 7, pp. 601–613, 2014.

[123] D. A. Calhoun, "Obstructive sleep apnea and hypertension," *Current Hypertension Reports*, vol. 12, no. 3, pp. 189–195, 2010.

[124] T. Dudenbostel and D. A. Calhoun, "Resistant hypertension, obstructive sleep apnoea and aldosterone," *Journal of Human Hypertension*, vol. 26, no. 5, pp. 281–287, 2012.

[125] M. Jhamb and M. Unruh, "Bidirectional relationship of hypertension with obstructive sleep apnea," *Current Opinion in Pulmonary Medicine*, vol. 20, no. 6, pp. 558–564, 2014.

[126] O. Friedman, T. D. Bradley, C. T. Chan, R. Parkes, and A. G. Logan, "Relationship between overnight rostral fluid shift and obstructive sleep apnea in drug-resistant hypertension," *Hypertension*, vol. 56, no. 6, pp. 1077–1082, 2010.

[127] R. Wolk and V. K. Somers, "Obesity-related cardiovascular disease: implications of obstructive sleep apnea," *Diabetes, Obesity and Metabolism*, vol. 8, no. 3, pp. 250–260, 2006.

[128] K. Gaddam, E. Pimenta, S. J. Thomas et al., "Spironolactone reduces severity of obstructive sleep apnoea in patients with resistant hypertension: A preliminary report," *Journal of Human Hypertension*, vol. 24, no. 8, pp. 532–537, 2010.

[129] L. Grote, T. Ploch, J. Heitmann, L. Knaack, T. Penzel, and J. H. Peter, "Sleep-related breathing disorder is an independent risk factor for systemic hypertension," *American Journal of Respiratory and Critical Care Medicine*, vol. 160, no. 6, pp. 1875–1882, 1999.

[130] A. R. SCHWARTZ, J. A. ROWLEY, C. O'DONNELL, E. D. KING, A. MAYOR, and P. L. SMITH, "Effect of hypertension on upper airway function and sleep apnoea," *Journal of Sleep Research*, vol. 4, pp. 83–88, 1995.

[131] D. W. Carley, S. M. Trbovic, and M. Radulovacki, "Hydralazine reduces elevated sleep apnea index in spontaneously hypertensive (SHR) rats to equivalence with normotensive Wistar-Kyoto rats," *Sleep*, vol. 19, no. 5, pp. 363–366, 1996.

[132] D. W. Carley, S. Trbovic, and M. Radulovacki, "Effect of REM sleep deprivation on sleep apneas in rats," *Experimental Neurology*, vol. 137, no. 2, pp. 291–293, 1996.

[133] E. Garpestad, R. C. Basner, J. Ringler et al., "Phenylephrine-induced hypertension acutely decreases genioglossus EMG activity in awake humans," *Journal of Applied Physiology*, vol. 72, no. 1, pp. 110–115, 1992.

[134] L. Grote, K. Wutkewicz, L. Knaack, T. Ploch, J. Hedner, and J. H. Peter, "Association between blood pressure reduction with antihypertensive treatment and sleep apnea activity," *American Journal of Hypertension*, vol. 13, no. 12, pp. 1280–1287, 2000.

[135] N. J. Ali, R. J. O. Davies, J. A. Fleetham, and J. R. Stradling, "The acute effects of continuous positive airway pressure and oxygen administration on blood pressure during obstructive sleep apnea," *Chest*, vol. 101, no. 6, pp. 1526–1532, 1992.

[136] J. E. Dimsdale, J. S. Loredo, and J. Profant, "Effect of continuous positive airway pressure on blood pressure: A placebo trial," *Hypertension*, vol. 35, no. 1 I, pp. 144–147, 2000.

[137] O. Shirasaki, S. Yamashita, S.-I. Kawara et al., "A new technique for detecting sleep apnea-related "midnight" surge of blood pressure," *Hypertension Research*, vol. 29, no. 9, pp. 695–702, 2006.

[138] K. Kario, "Obstructive sleep apnea syndrome and hypertension: Ambulatory blood pressure," *Hypertension Research*, vol. 32, no. 6, pp. 428–432, 2009.

[139] T. L. Giles, T. J. Lasserson, B. J. Smith, J. White, J. Wright, and C. J. Cates, "Continuous positive airways pressure for obstructive sleep apnoea in adults," *Cochrane Database of Systematic Reviews*, no. 1, Article ID CD001106, 2006.

[140] P. Haentjens, A. van Meerhaeghe, A. Moscariello et al., "The impact of continuous positive airway pressure on blood pressure in patients with obstructive sleep apnea syndrome: evidence from a meta-analysis of placebo-controlled randomized trials," *Archives of Internal Medicine*, vol. 167, no. 8, pp. 757–764, 2007.

[141] L. A. Bazzano, Z. Khan, K. Reynolds, and J. He, "Effect of nocturnal nasal continuous positive airway pressure on blood pressure in obstructive sleep apnea," *Hypertension*, vol. 50, no. 2, pp. 417–423, 2007.

[142] F. Barbé, J. Durán-Cantolla, F. Capote et al., "Long-term effect of continuous positive airway pressure in hypertensive patients with sleep apnea," *American Journal of Respiratory and Critical Care Medicine*, vol. 181, no. 7, pp. 718–726, 2010.

[143] M. Alajmi, A. T. Mulgrew, J. Fox et al., "Impact of continuous positive airway pressure therapy on blood pressure in patients with obstructive sleep apnea hypopnea: a meta-analysis of randomized controlled trials," *Lung*, vol. 185, no. 2, pp. 67–72, 2007.

[144] L. Mo and Q. He, "Effect of long-term continuous positive airway pressure ventilation on blood pressure in patients with obstructive sleep apnea hypopnea syndrome: A meta-analysis of clinical trials," *National Medical Journal of China*, vol. 87, no. 17, pp. 1177–1180, 2007.

[145] S. B. Montesi, B. A. Edwards, A. Malhotra, and J. P. Bakker, "Effect of continuous positive airway pressure treatment on blood pressure: a systematic review and meta-analysis of randomized controlled trials," *Journal of Clinical Sleep Medicine*, vol. 8, no. 5, pp. 587–596, 2012.

[146] C. Fava, S. Dorigoni, F. Dalle Vedove et al., "Effect of CPAP on blood pressure in patients with OSA/hypopnea: A systematic review and meta-analysis," *Chest*, vol. 145, no. 4, pp. 762–771, 2014.

[147] J. P. Bakker, B. A. Edwards, S. P. Gautam et al., "Blood Pressure Improvement with Continuous Positive Airway Pressure is Independent of Obstructive Sleep Apnea Severity," *Journal of Clinical Sleep Medicine*.

[148] A. V. Chobanian, G. L. Bakris, H. R. Black et al., "The seventh report of the joint national committee on prevention, detection, evaluation, and treatment of high blood pressure: the JNC 7 report," *The Journal of the American Medical Association*, vol. 289, no. 19, pp. 2560–2572, 2003.

[149] F. Turnbull, "Effects of different blood-pressure-lowering regimens on major cardiovascular events: results of prospectively-designed overviews of randomised trials," *The Lancet*, vol. 362, no. 9395, pp. 1527–1535, 2003.

[150] D. J. Bratton, J. R. Stradling, F. Barbé, and M. Kohler, "Effect of CPAP on blood pressure in patients with minimally symptomatic obstructive sleep apnoea: A meta-analysis using individual patient data from four randomised controlled trials," *Thorax*, vol. 69, no. 12, pp. 1128–1135, 2014.

[151] M. A. Martínez-García, F. Capote, and F. Campos-Rodríguez, "Spanish Sleep Network . Effect of CPAP on blood pressure in patients with obstructive sleep apnea and resistant hypertension: the HIPARCO randomized clinical trial," *JAMA ., , 310*, vol. 22, pp. 2407–2415, 2013.

[152] H. F. Becker, A. Jerrentrup, T. Ploch et al., "Effect of nasal continuous positive airway pressure treatment on blood pressure in patients with obstructive sleep apnea," *Circulation*, vol. 107, no. 1, pp. 68–73, 2003.

[153] B. Mokhlesi, L. A. Finn, E. W. Hagen et al., "Obstructive sleep apnea during REM sleep and hypertension: Results of the Wisconsin sleep cohort," *American Journal of Respiratory and Critical Care Medicine*, vol. 190, no. 10, pp. 1158–1167, 2014.

[154] G. V. Robinson, B. A. Langford, D. M. Smith, and J. R. Stradling, "Predictors of blood pressure fall with continuous positive airway pressure (CPAP) treatment of obstructive sleep apnoea (OSA)," *Thorax*, vol. 63, no. 10, pp. 855–859, 2008.

[155] J.-P. Baguet, G. Barone-Rochette, and J.-L. Pépin, "Hypertension and obstructive sleep apnoea syndrome: current perspectives," *Journal of Human Hypertension*, vol. 23, no. 7, pp. 431–443, 2009.

[156] A. G. Logan, R. Tkacova, S. M. Perlikowski et al., "Refractory hypertension and sleep apnoea: Effect of CPAP on blood pressure and baroreflex," *European Respiratory Journal*, vol. 21, no. 2, pp. 241–247, 2003.

[157] M. A. Martínez-García, R. Gomez-Aldaraví, J. Soler-Cataluña, T. G. Martinez, B. Bernácer-Alpera, and P. Roman-Sánchez, "Positive effect of CPAP treatment on the control of difficult-to-treat hypertension," *European Respiratory Journal*, vol. 29, no. 5, pp. 951–957, 2007.

[158] M. A. Martínez-García, R. Gómez-Aldaraví, J.-J. Soler-Cataluña, T. G. Martínez, B. Bernácer-Alpera, and P. Román-Sánchez, "Positive effect of CPAP treatment on the control of difficult-to-treat hypertension," *European Respiratory Journal*, vol. 29, no. 5, pp. 951–957, 2007.

[159] L. Lozano, J. L. Tovar, G. Sampol et al., "Continuous positive airway pressure treatment in sleep apnea patients with resistant hypertension: a randomized, controlled trial," *Journal of Hypertension*, vol. 28, no. 10, pp. 2161–2168, 2010.

[160] A. Y. Litvin, Z. N. Sukmarova, E. M. Elfimova et al., "Effects of CPAP on "vascular" risk factors in patients with obstructive sleep apnea and arterial hypertension.," *Vascular health and risk management*, vol. 9, pp. 229–235, 2013.

[161] R. P. Pedrosa, L. F. Drager, L. K. G. de Paula, A. C. S. Amaro, L. A. Bortolotto, and G. Lorenzi-Filho, "Effects of OSA treatment on BP in patients with resistant hypertension: a randomized trial," *Chest*, vol. 144, no. 5, pp. 1487–1494, 2013.

[162] I. H. Iftikhar, C. W. Valentine, L. R. A. Bittencourt et al., "Effects of continuous positive airway pressure on blood pressure in patients with resistant hypertension and obstructive sleep apnea: A meta-analysis," *Journal of Hypertension*, vol. 32, no. 12, pp. 2341–2350, 2014.

[163] I. Z. Ben-Dov, J. D. Kark, D. Ben-Ishay, J. Mekler, L. Ben-Arie, and M. Bursztyn, "Predictors of all-cause mortality in clinical ambulatory monitoring: Unique aspects of blood pressure during sleep," *Hypertension*, vol. 49, no. 6, pp. 1235–1241, 2007.

[164] P. Verdecchia, C. Porcellati, G. Schillaci et al., "Ambulatory blood pressure: An independent predictor of prognosis in essential hypertension," *Hypertension*, vol. 24, no. 6, pp. 793–801, 1994.

[165] D. Norman, J. S. Loredo, R. A. Nelesen et al., "Effects of continuous positive airway pressure versus supplemental oxygen on 24-hour ambulatory blood pressure," *Hypertension*, vol. 47, no. 5, pp. 840–845, 2006.

[166] G. V. Robinson, D. M. Smith, B. A. Langford, R. J. O. Davies, and J. R. Stradling, "Continuous positive airway pressure does not reduce blood pressure in nonsleepy hypertensive OSA patients," *European Respiratory Journal*, vol. 27, no. 6, pp. 1229–1235, 2006.

[167] F. Barbé, L. R. Mayoralas, J. Duran et al., "Treatment with continuous positive airway pressure is not effective in patients with sleep apnea but no daytime sleepiness: a randomized, controlled trial," *Annals of Internal Medicine*, vol. 134, no. 11, pp. 1015–1023, 2001.

[168] D. S. Hui, K. W. To, F. W. Ko et al., "Nasal CPAP reduces systemic blood pressure in patients with obstructive sleep apnoea and mild sleepiness," *Thorax*, vol. 61, no. 12, pp. 1083–1090, 2006.

[169] P. E. Peppard, T. Young, M. Palta, J. Dempsey, and J. Skatrud, "Longitudinal study of moderate weight change and sleep-disordered breathing," *The Journal of the American Medical Association*, vol. 284, no. 23, pp. 3015–3021, 2000.

[170] J. A. Chirinos, I. Gurubhagavatula, K. Teff et al., "CPAP, weight loss, or both for obstructive sleep apnea," *New England Journal of Medicine*, vol. 370, no. 24, pp. 2265–2275, 2014.

[171] I. H. Iftikhar, E. R. Hays, M.-A. Iverson, U. J. Magalang, and A. K. Maas, "Effect of oral appliances on blood pressure in obstructive sleep apnea: A systematic review and meta-analysis," *Journal of Clinical Sleep Medicine*, vol. 9, no. 2, pp. 165–174, 2013.

[172] A. Andren, P. Hedberg, P. Wahlen et al., "Effects of treatment with oral appliance on 24-h blood pressure in patients with obstructive sleep apnea and hypertension: A randomized clinical trial," *Sleep and Breathing*, vol. 17, no. 2, pp. 705–712, 2013.

[173] K. Okuno, B. T. Pliska, M. Hamoda, A. A. Lowe, and F. R. Almeida, "Prediction of oral appliance treatment outcomes in obstructive sleep apnea: A systematic review," *Sleep Medicine Reviews*, vol. 30, pp. 25–33, 2016.

[174] K. Ramar, L. C. Dort, S. G. Katz et al., "Clinical practice guideline for the treatment of obstructive sleep apnea and snoring with oral appliance therapy: An update for 2015," *Journal of Clinical Sleep Medicine*, vol. 11, no. 7, pp. 773–828, 2015.

[175] A. Di Munro, L. Petramala, D. Cotesta et al., "Renin-angiotensin-aldosterone system in patients with sleep apnoea: Prevalence of primary aldosteronism," *JRAAS - Journal of the Renin-Angiotensin-Aldosterone System*, vol. 11, no. 3, pp. 165–172, 2010.

[176] M. G. Ziegler, M. Milic, and H. Elayan, "Cardiovascular regulation in obstructive sleep apnea," *Drug Discovery Today: Disease Models*, vol. 8, no. 4, pp. 155–160, 2011.

[177] J. Heitmann, T. Greulich, C. Reinke et al., "Comparison of the effects of nebivolol and valsartan on BP reduction and sleep apnoea activity in patients with essential hypertension and OSA," *Current Medical Research and Opinion*, vol. 26, no. 8, pp. 1925–1932, 2010.

[178] H. Kraiczi, J. Hedner, Y. Peker, and L. Grote, "Comparison of atenolol, amlodipine, enalapril, hydrochlorothiazide, and losartan for antihypertensive treatment in patients with obstructive sleep apnea," *American Journal of Respiratory and Critical Care Medicine*, vol. 161, no. 5, pp. 1423–1428, 2000.

[179] P. R. Bartel, M. Loock, P. Becker, E. Robinson, C. Van Der Meyden, and S. Rossouw, "Short-term antihypertensive medication does not exacerbate sleep- disordered breathing in newly diagnosed hypertensive patients," *American Journal of Hypertension*, vol. 10, no. 6, pp. 640–645, 1997.

[180] L. H. Pelttari, E. K. Hietanen, T. T. Salo, M. J. Kataja, and I. M. Kantola, "Little effect of ordinary antihypertensive therapy on nocturnal high blood pressure in patients with sleep disordered breathing," *American Journal of Hypertension*, vol. 11, no. 3 I, pp. 272–279, 1998.

[181] F. G. Issa, "Effect of clonidine in obstructive sleep apnea," *American Review of Respiratory Disease*, vol. 145, no. 2, pp. 435–439, 1992.

[182] J. Mayer, U. Weichler, B. Herres-Mayer, H. Schneider, U. Marx, and J. H. Peter, "Influence of metoprolol and cilazapril on blood pressure and on sleep apnea activity," *Journal of Cardiovascular Pharmacology*, vol. 16, no. 6, pp. 952–961, 1990.

[183] J. H. Peter, W. Gassel, J. Mayer et al., "Effects of cilazapril on hypertension, sleep, and apnea," *The American Journal of Medicine*, vol. 87, no. 6, 1989.

[184] U. Weichler, B. Herres-Mayer, J. Mayer, K. Weber, R. Hoffmann, and J. H. Peter, "Influence of antihypertensive drug therapy on sleep pattern and sleep apnea activity," *Cardiology*, vol. 78, no. 2, pp. 124–130, 1991.

[185] A. Cicolin, L. Mangiardi, R. Mutani, and C. Bucca, "Angiotensin-converting enzyme inhibitors and obstructive sleep apnea," *Mayo Clinic Proceedings*, vol. 81, no. 1, pp. 53–55, 2006.

[186] F. B. Nerbass, R. P. Pedrosa, P. R. Genta, L. F. Drager, and G. Lorenzi-Filho, "Calcium channel blockers are independently associated with short sleep duration in hypertensive patients with obstructive sleep apnea," *Journal of Hypertension*, vol. 29, no. 6, pp. 1236–1241, 2011.

[187] H. K. Walia, H. Li, M. Rueschman et al., "Association of severe obstructive sleep apnea and elevated blood pressure despite antihypertensive medication use," *Journal of Clinical Sleep Medicine*, vol. 10, no. 8, pp. 835–843, 2014.

14

CYP17A1 and Blood Pressure Reactivity to Stress in Adolescence

Mariel Van Woudenberg,[1] Jean Shin,[1] Manon Bernard,[1] Catriona Syme,[1] Michal Abrahamowicz,[2] Gabriel Leonard,[3] Michel Perron,[4] Louis Richer,[4] Suzanna Veillette,[4] Daniel Gaudet,[5] Tomas Paus,[6] and Zdenka Pausova[1]

[1] *The Hospital for Sick Children, University of Toronto, Toronto, ON, Canada M5G 1X8*
[2] *Department of Epidemiology, Biostatistics and Occupational Health, McGill University, Montreal, QC, Canada H3A 0G4*
[3] *Montreal Neurological Institute and Hospital, McGill University, Montreal, QC, Canada H3A 2B4*
[4] *Université du Québec à Chicoutimi, Chicoutimi, QC, Canada G7H 2B1*
[5] *Community Genomic Centre, Chicoutimi Hospital, Université de Montréal, Montreal, QC, Canada G7H 5H6*
[6] *Rotman Research Institute, University of Toronto, Toronto, ON, Canada M6A 2E1*

Correspondence should be addressed to Zdenka Pausova; zdenka.pausova@sickkids.ca

Academic Editor: Hiromi Rakugi

Adolescents who exhibit exaggerated blood pressure (BP) reactivity to physical and mental challenges are at increased risk of developing hypertension in adulthood. BP at rest and in response to challenges is higher in males than females, beginning in early adolescence. *CYP17A1* is one of the well-established gene loci of adult hypertension. Here, we investigated whether this gene locus is associated with elevated BP at rest and in response to physical (active standing) and mental (math stress) challenges in adolescence. We studied 496 male and 532 female adolescents (age 12–18 years) who were recruited from a genetic founder population. Our results showed that the variant of *CYP17A1* rs10786718 was associated with enhanced BP reactivity to the mental but not physical challenge and in males but not females. In males, BP increase in response to math stress was higher in major versus minor allele homozygotes by 7.6 mm Hg ($P = 8.3 \times 10^{-6}$). Resting BP was not associated with the *CYP17A1* variant in either sex. These results suggest that, in adolescent males but not females, *CYP17A1* enhances BP reactivity to mental stress. Whether this effect contributes to the higher prevalence of hypertension in males than females later in life remains to be determined.

1. Introduction

A growing body of evidence suggests that preclinical features of hypertension emerge already during adolescence [1–3], which is a period of human development when adult blood pressure (BP) and body composition develop [4, 5]. Enhanced BP reactivity to a physical or mental stressor in childhood and adolescence predicts adult hypertension [6–8]. Marked sex differences exist in resting BP and BP reactivity as well as in the prevalence of hypertension, with all being higher in males than females during reproductive years [6, 9–13].

Susceptibility to hypertension is determined by both genetic and environmental factors. The estimated heritability of resting BP and hypertension is around 50% [14]. Similarly, the estimated heritability of BP response to math stress is around 50% [15]. The underlying genetic architecture involves multiple contributory genes. One of the well-established gene loci of hypertension is *CYP17A1* [16–22]. This gene encodes the enzyme cytochrome P-450c17 that mediates steroid 17α-hydroxylase and 17,20-lyase activities (Figure 1). The first enzymatic activity is key in the steroidogenic pathway that produces mineralocorticoids, which affect sodium and water handling in the kidney, and glucocorticoids, which control the body response to stress [23, 24]. The second enzymatic activity is involved in the biosynthesis of male and female sex hormones [24]. Thus, *CYP17A1* may influence BP reactivity in a sex-specific manner. While *CYP17A1* is associated with resting BP and hypertension in adults, whether the gene locus influences BP reactivity and

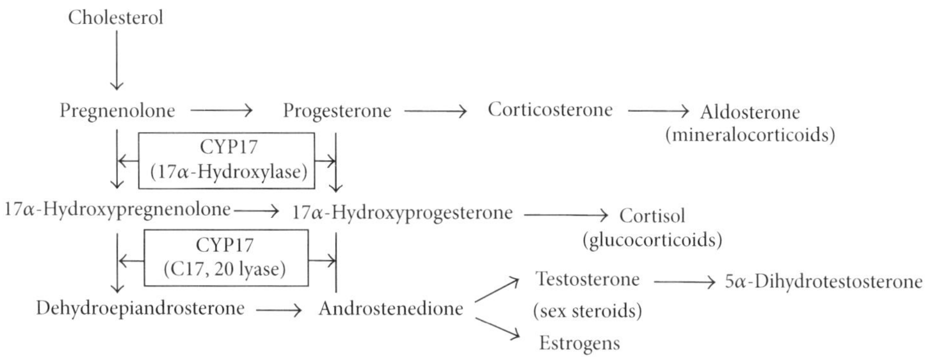

FIGURE 1: Simplified pathway of steroid hormone biosynthesis and the role of *CYP17A1*. *CYP17A1* encodes the enzyme cytochrome P-450c17α (CYP17) that catalyzes steroid 17α-hydroxylase and 17,20-lyase activities and is hence essential for the synthesis of glucocorticoids (17α-hydroxylase activity) and sex steroids (17,20 lyase activity). Adapted from Molina and Belldegrun, 2011 [28].

whether it plays a role in BP regulation already in adolescence have not been studied.

The aim of this study was to investigate whether *CYP17A1* is associated with BP at rest and in response to physical and mental challenges during adolescence. This investigation was carried out in a community-based sample of 1,028 adolescents recruited from a genetic founder population of Quebec, Canada [25–27].

2. Methods and Procedures

2.1. Study Population. White Caucasian adolescents (496 males, 532 females), aged 12 to 18 years, were recruited from a genetic founder population living in the Saguenay-Lac St. Jean region of Quebec, Canada, as part of the Saguenay Youth Study [29]. This is a community-based cohort investigating cardiometabolic and brain health in adolescence. Male and female participants were recruited via high schools; detailed recruitment and selection criteria are described elsewhere [29]. The Saguenay Youth Study is family based, focusing on collection of sib pairs.

The Saguenay-Lac St. Jean population is one of the largest founder populations in North America [25–27], originating from French ancestors who migrated to the region in the early 19th century. The population grew from 5,200 inhabitants in 1852 to 285,000 at present, due to high intrinsic growth and little emigration. Because of the founder effect, there is a higher prevalence of certain recessive disorders in the Saguenay-Lac St. Jean region compared with other populations [25], as well as limited allelic diversity among patients with these disorders [26, 27].

The current study sample consists of 496 male and 532 female adolescents recruited and tested between November 2003 and February 2012. The prevalence of hypertension (sitting SBP or DBP ≥95th age-, sex-, and height-specific percentile) in this sample was 7.1% in males and 3.3% in females, which is similar to that in the Canadian adolescent population at large (Canadian Health Measures Survey) [30]. Additional characteristics of the studied males and females are provided in Table 1. Written consent from the parents and assent from the adolescents were obtained before the commencement of data collection. The research ethics committees of the Chicoutimi Hospital and the Hospital for Sick Children in Toronto approved the study protocols.

2.2. Assessments. All adolescents underwent a 52-minute cardiovascular protocol, conducted in the Chicoutimi Hospital on Saturdays, commencing between 8:00 and 12:00 [29]. The protocol consisted of physical and mental challenges (Figure 2). The physical challenges were changes in posture: each participant was first supine for 10 min, then standing for 10 min, and finally sitting for 10 min. The mental challenge was a math-stress test, consisting of an explanation (<1 min), postexplanation waiting period (4 min), math stress (2 min), and math-stress recovery (10 min). The math stress was a sequence of 46 simple arithmetic problems of increasing difficulty (to ensure some failure in all participants) to be solved out loud.

Throughout the protocol, a noninvasive hemodynamic monitor, Finometer (FNS Finapres, Amsterdam, Netherlands), was used to record continuous finger blood flow. The Finometer derives beat-by-beat brachial systolic BP (SBP) and diastolic BP (DBP) by the reconstruction and level-correction of the finger blood-flow waveform. This method has been validated for tracking BP in adults and children over the age of six years [31]. One-minute averages of these data were calculated for the duration of the protocol and used to compute two BP reactivity parameters and two resting BPs for each SBP and DBP (Figure 2). The BP reactivity parameters were (1) *BP reactivity to standing*, which was a change in BP from the last minute of supine to the first minute of standing, and (2) *BP reactivity to math stress*, which was a change in BP from the last minute of the prestress period to the first minute of the math stress. The two resting BPs were (1) *poststanding resting BP*, which was the average BP during the last 5 minutes of the 10 min sitting period during the posture test, and (2) *postmath resting BP*, which was the average BP during the last 5 min of the 10-min period following the math stress. Resting BPs were intended to mimic "clinic" BP, defined by the Canadian Hypertension Society as repeated BP measurements taken after 5 minutes of rest while seated [32]. Sex-specific means and standard deviations of all initial and resting BPs for SBP and DBP are presented in Table 1.

Table 1: Basic characteristics and studied BP phenotypes.

	Males	Females	Estimated difference (95% CI)	*P* value
(A) Basic characteristics*				
Age (years)	14.4 ± 1.8	14.6 ± 1.9	0.2 (−0.1–0.4)	0.15
Height (cm)	166.8 ± 10.7	159.6 ± 6.7	7.6 (6.7–8.6)	<0.0001
Body weight (kg)	61.3 ± 16.9	56.0 ± 12.6	0.9 (−0.7–2.5)	0.29
BMI (kg/m^2)	21.8 ± 4.6	21.9 ± 4.4	0.02 (−0.5–0.6)	0.94
(B) SBP, mm Hg†				
Prestanding	118.7 ± 12.8	120.1 ± 11.3	1.4 (−0.2–3.1)	0.09
Standing	129.6 ± 15.4	129.0 ± 13.5	0.6 (−1.4–2.6)	0.53
Reactivity to standing	11.1 ± 9.8	8.8 ± 9.2	2.3 (1.0–3.6)	0.0007
Premath stress	122.6 ± 14.2	119.7 ± 13.0	2.9 (1.0–4.8)	0.002
Math stress	140.4 ± 16.3	136.2 ± 14.6	4.3 (2.2–6.4)	<0.0001
Reactivity to math stress	18.2 ± 10.6	16.7 ± 10.6	1.5 (0–3.0)	0.05
Poststanding resting[c]	123.2 ± 13.6	120.0 ± 11.8	3.1 (1.4–4.9)	0.0004
Postmath resting[c]	127.3 ± 13.1	124.8 ± 12.5	2.6 (0.8–4.3)	0.004
(C) DBP, mm Hg†				
Prestanding	70.3 ± 8.1	68.4 ± 7.4	1.9 (0.8–3.0)	0.0006
Standing	80.4 ± 11.1	78.8 ± 10.1	1.6 (0.1–3.1)	0.03
Reactivity to standing	10.4 ± 5.9	10.2 ± 5.8	0.2 (−0.7–1.0)	0.69
Premath stress	78.7 ± 9.6	76.1 ± 9.2	2.6 (1.3–3.9)	0.0001
Math stress	89.0 ± 11.4	86.6 ± 10.6	2.4 (0.8–3.9)	0.002
Reactivity to math stress	10.4 ± 5.8	10.6 ± 6.0	0.2 (−0.7–1.0)	0.67
Poststanding resting[c]	78.9 ± 9.6	76.1 ± 9.0	2.8 (1.5–4.1)	<0.0001
Postmath resting[c]	81.9 ± 9.7	79.8 ± 8.9	2.2 (0.9–3.5)	0.001

*Nonadjusted means ± standard deviations are shown. The differences between males and females are given, adjusted for age and, when appropriate, height.
†Means adjusted for age and height ± standard deviations are shown. The differences between males and females are given, adjusted for age and height.
[c]Resting SBP/DBP is a 5-minute average of SBP/DBP measured while seated after 5 minutes at rest.
CI = confidence interval.

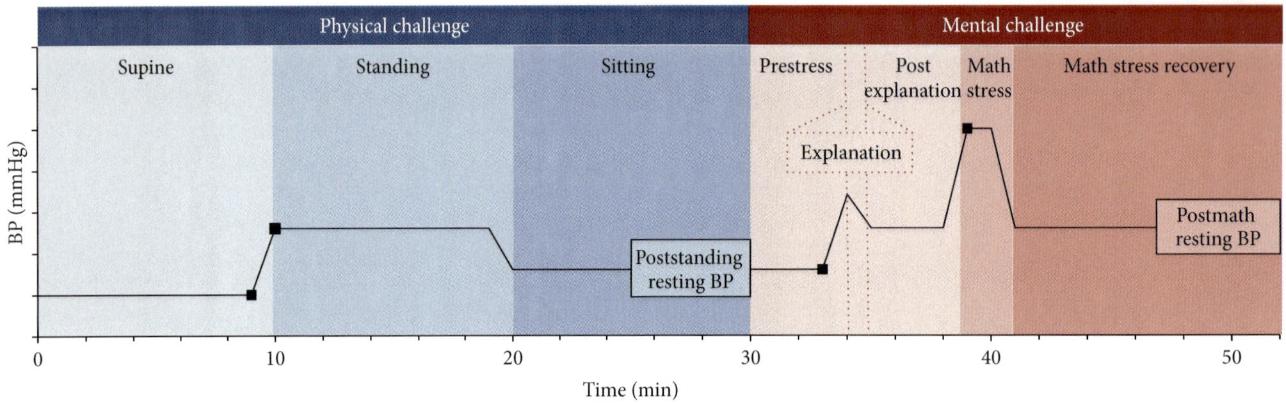

Figure 2: Schematic diagram of the cardiovascular protocol. The cardiovascular protocol consisted of one physical challenge and one mental challenge. The physical challenge was active posture test, which consisted of three periods during which the participant was first supine (10 minutes), then standing (10 minutes), and finally sitting (10 minutes). The mental challenge was a math-stress test, which consisted of a prestress (4 min), explanation (~1 min), postexplanation waiting (4 minutes), math-stress (2 minutes), and math-stress recovery (10 minutes) periods. Black squares indicate the initial and final BP values used to calculate BP reactivity to standing and math stress and the boxes show 5-minute averages of poststanding and postmath resting BPs.

2.3. Genotyping and Genotype Imputation. The study population ($n = 1,028$) was genotyped in two waves. The first wave, involving 601 participants of the SYS, was genotyped with the Illumina Human610-Quad BeadChip (Illumina, San Diego, CA; $n = 582,892$ SNPs) at the Centre National de Génotypage (Paris, France). The second wave, involving the remaining 427 participants of the SYS, was genotyped with the HumanOmniExpress BeadChip (Illumina, San Diego, CA; $n = 729,295$ SNPs) at the Genome Analysis Centre of Helmholtz Zentrum München (Munich, Germany). In both subsamples, SNPs with call rate <95% and minor allele frequency <0.01 and SNPs that were not in Hardy-Weinberg equilibrium ($P < 1 \times 10^{-6}$) were excluded. After this genotype quality control, 542,345 markers on the first SNP chip and 644,283 markers on the second chip were available for analysis.

Genotype imputation was used to equate the set of SNPs of the adolescents genotyped on each platform and to increase the SNP density. Haplotype phasing was performed with SHAPEIT [33] using an overlapping subset of 313,653 post-quality-control SNPs that were present on both genotyping platforms and the 1,000 Genomes SNPs in European reference panel (Phase 1, Release 3). Imputation was conducted on the phased data with IMPUTE2 [34]. Markers with low imputation quality (information score < 0.5) or low minor allele frequency (<0.01) were removed. After this imputation quality control, a total of 1,392 typed and imputed SNPs were available for a segment of human chromosome 10 that covered the entire previously reported *CYP17A1* locus of adult SBP, DBP, and hypertension (~400 kb from *CYP17A1* to *NT5C2* [17]) and its flanking sequences (90 kb upstream of *CYP17A1* and 147 kb downstream of *NT5C2*, Figure 3 and Figure S4; see Supplementary Material available online at http://dx.doi.org/10.1155/2015/734586).

2.4. Statistical Analyses. Genotype-phenotype association analyses were conducted with Merlin (version 1.1.2) [35, 36] under an additive model. They involved the above-selected 1,392 SNPs covering the previously reported *CYP17A1* locus [17] and the following SBP and DBP phenotypes: (1) BP reactivity to math, (2) BP reactivity to standing, (3) poststanding resting BP, and (4) postmath resting BP. With Merlin, a simple regression model is fitted to each trait, and a variance component approach is used to account for correlation between observed phenotypes within sibships. Analyses were done in males and females separately, with age, height, and, when appropriate, initial BP included as covariates. In supplementary analyses, body weight was added as an additional covariate to control for potentially confounding effects of obesity. BP values outside the mean ± three standard deviations were excluded prior to these analyses (n = 974–992 per variable). As we used a candidate-gene approach, $P < 0.05$ was deemed significant for one test. However, since we tested 4 blood pressure phenotypes in 2 sexes, our results were considered significant at $P < 0.05/8 \leq 6.3 \times 10^{-3}$ when Bonferroni's correction is applied. LocusZoom [37] was used to view the results of the above-described genotype-phenotype association analyses as plots showing both the magnitude of association for each SNP (1,392 SNPs within the *CYP17A1* locus) and the pairwise linkage disequilibrium (LD) pattern with the most strongly associated SNP (Figure 3). These plots were generated based on human genome hg19, and the LD was calculated based on the 1,000 Genomes Project (EUR reference panel, March 2012 version).

3. Results

The genotype-phenotype association analyses were carried out while adjusting for age, height, and initial BP when relevant. These analyses showed that, for both SBP and DBP, the *CYP17A1* locus was associated with enhanced BP reactivity to the mental but not physical challenge, and this was observed in males but not in females (Figure 3 and Table 2). The most significantly associated SNP was rs10786718 (Figure 3). SBP increase in response to math stress was higher in major versus minor allele homozygotes by 7.6 mm Hg ($P = 8.3 \times 10^{-6}$) in males. Likewise, DBP increase in response to math stress was higher in major versus minor allele homozygotes by 4.8 mm Hg ($P = 1.1 \times 10^{-5}$) in males (Figure S1). Neither poststanding nor postmath resting BPs were associated with the *CYP17A1* locus in either sex (Figure 3 and Table 2). All these results remained virtually unchanged when additionally adjusted for body weight (Figures S2 and S3), indicating that the *CYP17A1* locus impacts BP independently of obesity. Similar to the previous studies, the *CYP17A1* locus showed a long-range LD pattern, spreading over a region of ~400 kb [17]. In the present study, however, this locus contained a subregion of highly correlated SNPs that demonstrated a stronger association with the BP phenotype and was closer to *CYP17A1* (Figure 3); this observation provides further support for the possibility that *CYP17A1* may be the causal gene within this BP locus.

4. Discussion

The results of the current study show that a well-established gene locus of hypertension in adults [16–22], *CYP17A1*, may play a role in increasing BP reactivity to stress during adolescence. This effect, however, may be sex-specific and limited to mental stressors.

CYP17A1 has been identified as a gene locus of hypertension and resting blood pressure in several large-scale genome-wide and replication studies of adult European and Asian populations [16–20]. It encodes a key enzyme in the steroidogenic pathway that may influence BP through its effects on the production of mineralocorticoids, glucocorticoids, and sex hormones. The enzyme has both 17α-hydroxylase and 17,20-lyase activities that contribute to steroidogenesis in the adrenal gland and sex gonads [24]. During that process, pregnenolone derived from cholesterol is processed to (a) mineralocorticoids in the adrenal zona glomerulosa (neither enzyme activity present), (b) glucocorticoids in the adrenal zona fasciculata (17α-hydroxylase activity present), or (c) sex steroids in the adrenal zona reticularis and gonads (both enzyme activities present) [24]. Each of these steroid hormones plays a role in the regulation of BP. (a) Mineralocorticoids (e.g., aldosterone) can increase BP by augmenting renal sodium and water reabsorption and thus circulating blood volume [23]. (b) Glucocorticoids (e.g., cortisol) can increase BP by enhancing the vasoconstrictive effects of catecholamines, as well as by having some mineralocorticoid activity described above [23]. (c) Sex steroids impact BP mostly indirectly, via their influences on the autonomic and renin-angiotensin-aldosterone systems, endothelial function, and oxidative stress; in general, androgens are considered to be BP-increasing, while estrogens are thought to be BP-decreasing [12, 38]. Importantly, some of the above effects of steroid hormones underlie slower BP responses (e.g., blood

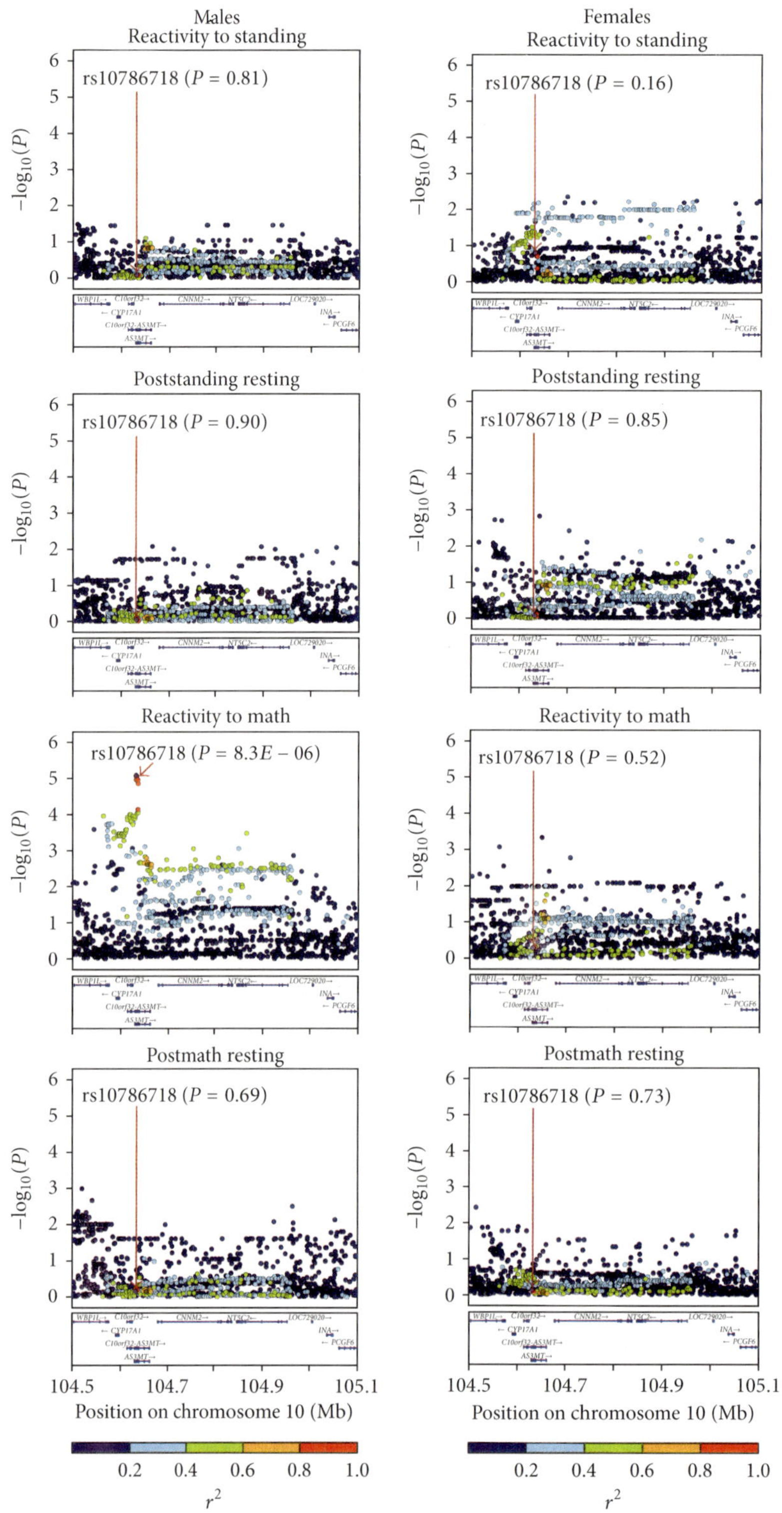

FIGURE 3: *CYP17A1* locus and SBP in response to physical and mental challenges and at rest. Individual points indicate $-\log_{10}$ (P values) for associations of SNPs within the *CYP17A1* locus and studied SBP phenotypes. Plots on the left and right show the results in males and females, respectively. Data were adjusted for age, height, and, when appropriate (SBP reactivity to standing and mental stress), initial SBP. The SNP, rs10786718, demonstrating the strongest association with SBP reactivity to math stress in males is indicated in purple and is the index SNP in all plots. The correlation (r^2) between this index SNP, rs10786718, and each of the other tested SNPs in the region is shown in red ($1 \geq r^2 \geq 0.8$), orange ($0.8 > r^2 \geq 0.6$), green ($0.6 > r^2 \geq 0.4$), light blue ($0.4 > r^2 \geq 0.2$), or dark blue ($0.2 > r^2 \geq 0$) colors. Gene positions are indicated at the bottom. The LD was calculated based on the 1,000 Genomes Project (EUR reference panel, March 2012 version); the chromosome positions are based on human genome hg19.

Table 2: Associations of the *CYP17A1* locus (rs10786718[#]) and studied BP phenotypes.

	Males					Females				
	Beta (SE)	AA Mean (SD)	GA Mean (SD)	GG Mean (SD)	*P* value	Beta (SE)	GG Mean (SD)	GA Mean (SD)	AA Mean (SD)	*P* value
(A) SBP										
Reactivity to standing	−0.17 (0.70)	8.5 (1.5)	11.8 (0.8)	10.1 (0.6)	0.81	0.92 (0.66)	9.5 (0.5)	9.4 (0.7)	7.6 (1.4)	0.16
Poststanding resting*	0.12 (0.98)	120.9 (2.0)	125.7 (1.0)	123.5 (0.8)	0.90	−0.17 (0.85)	118.7 (0.7)	119.8 (0.9)	117.9 (1.9)	0.85
Reactivity to math	3.40 (0.76)	12.4 (1.6)	17.3 (0.8)	20.0 (0.6)	$8.3E-06$	0.48 (0.75)	16.5 (0.6)	16.8 (0.8)	14.4 (1.6)	0.52
Postmath resting*	0.38 (0.95)	125.6 (2.0)	129.1 (1.0)	127.8 (0.8)	0.69	0.31 (0.90)	124.0 (0.7)	123.9 (1.0)	123.6 (2.0)	0.73
(B) DBP										
Reactivity to standing*	0.09 (0.42)	9.2 (0.9)	10.5 (0.5)	10.1 (0.4)	0.83	0.23 (0.42)	10.4 (0.4)	10.5 (0.5)	9.3 (0.9)	0.58
Poststanding resting	−0.07 (0.68)	77.3 (1.5)	80.6 (0.7)	78.9 (0.6)	0.92	0.44 (0.65)	75.3 (0.5)	76.5 (0.7)	72.5 (1.4)	0.50
Reactivity to math*	1.85 (0.42)	6.6 (0.9)	10.5 (0.4)	11.4 (0.4)	$1.1E-05$	0.24 (0.42)	10.5 (0.4)	10.5 (0.5)	9.4 (0.9)	0.57
Postmath resting	0.03 (0.69)	80.6 (1.5)	83.0 (0.7)	81.9 (0.6)	0.97	0.30 (0.66)	79.3 (0.5)	79.7 (0.7)	77.8 (1.5)	0.65

Beta (SE = standard error) is the effect size on BP in mm Hg, per 1 copy of the index allele (G) based on an additive model adjusted for age and height.

*Model was additionally adjusted for initial BP.

#Minor allele (A) frequencies in males and females are 0.27 and 0.26, respectively.

volume regulation) whereas other effects mediate faster BP responses (e.g., the enhancement of catecholamine-driven vasoconstriction). The latter ones are more likely to be relevant to the present study of acute BP reactivity.

The regulation of BP reactivity to mental stress involves the coordinated action of the hypothalamic-pituitary-adrenal (HPA) and autonomic nervous systems, whereas the regulation of BP reactivity to simple standing up engages only the autonomic system (baroreflex) [39, 40]. Our results show that the *CYP17A1* locus is associated with BP reactivity to mental stress but not to active standing up. This observation is consistent with mental stress (but not active standing up) involving the activation of the HPA axis and *CYP17A1* regulating the production of its final effector, cortisol [23]. Further, our results suggest that *CYP17A1* is involved in the regulation of BP reactivity to mental stress mainly in males. SBP increase in response to math stress was higher in major versus minor allele homozygotes by 6.3 mm Hg ($P = 8.3 \times 10^{-6}$) but only by 1.6 mm Hg ($P = 0.52$) in females. Although *CYP17A1* increases the production of both male and female sex hormones, androgens are expected to enhance BP reactivity, whereas estrogens are predicted to suppress BP reactivity [12, 38]. As such, sex hormones, through their opposing modulatory effects, may lead to the development of the observed sex dimorphism in the genotype-phenotype association. Taken together, *CYP17A1* may contribute to the regulation of BP reactivity to mental stress through its parallel effects on the production of cortisol and sex hormones.

Finally, our study did not observe significant association between *CYP17A1* and resting BP in either males or females. It is likely that, at this stage, the effect of the gene is detectable on BP reactivity but not yet on resting BP. Previous research suggests that enhanced BP reactivity increases risk for future hypertension [6–8]. Chronically exaggerated BP responses increase repeatedly pressure load on the vessels, heart, and kidneys, leading to their structural and functional adaptations, which in turn may increase resting BP and promote the development of hypertension over time. Given that *CYP17A1* may enhance BP reactivity to mental stress, it may be an early genetic marker of hypertension risk. Substantial overlap exists between genes influencing clinic BP and BP measured in an experimental setting. It has been estimated that up to 81% of the heritability of clinic SBP and 71% of the heritability of clinic DBP were attributed to genes that also influenced stress BP during a video game challenge and social stress interview [41]. Although this locus is a well-established locus of hypertension in adults [16–22], further studies in adolescents and young adults are needed to elucidate its potential age and sex dependence and phenotypic transition from enhanced reactivity to elevated resting blood pressure.

Our results remained virtually unchanged when adjusted, or not adjusted, for body weight (Figures S2 and S3), indicating that the *CYP17A1* locus impacts BP independently of obesity. As such, the locus may be relevant obesity-dissociated hypertension [42]. Although obesity is a leading risk factor of hypertension, obesity and hypertension do not have 1 : 1 correspondence; only about 50% of obese individuals are hypertensive and about 30% of hypertensive individuals are not obese [43].

The *CYP17A1* locus was discovered as a relatively wide locus, including several genes [17]. It was named the *CYP17A1* locus, as *CYP17A1* was considered the best physiological candidate within the association locus. Nevertheless, other genes within the identified locus cannot be entirely excluded. The two genes closest to *CYP17A1* are *C10orf32*, which encodes "chromosome 10 open reading frame 32" (a protein of unknown function), and *AS3MT*, which encodes an enzyme that catalyzes the transfer of a methyl group from S-adenosyl-L-methionine to trivalent arsenical and may play a role in arsenic metabolism [44]. However, the role of these two genes in blood pressure regulation is not clear.

In conclusion, our results suggest that, in adolescent males but not females, *CYP17A1* enhances BP reactivity to mental stress. Whether this effect contributes to the higher prevalence of hypertension in males than females later in life remains to be determined.

Perspectives

Adolescence is a period of human development when adult physiology develops and initial stages of cardiovascular disorders, including hypertension, may emerge. Our hope is that it is also a period when disease trajectories can still be altered and full-blown diseases (such as hypertension) prevented. Early vulnerability genes may represent useful tools in this effort.

Authors' Contribution

Mariel Van Woudenberg and Jean Shin contributed equally to this paper.

Acknowledgments

The authors thank the following individuals for their contributions in acquiring data: Manon Bernard (database architect, The Hospital for Sick Children) and Helene Simard and her team of research assistants (Cégep de Jonquière). The Saguenay Youth Study project is funded by the Canadian Institutes of Health Research (Zdenka Pausova and Tomas Paus); Heart and Stroke Foundation of Canada (Zdenka Pausova); the Canadian Foundation for Innovation (Zdenka Pausova). Dr. Abrahamowicz is a James McGill Professor of Biostatistics at McGill University. Mariel Van Woudenberg was supported by an Ontario Graduate Scholarship and Restracomp Studentship from the Hospital for Sick Children Research Institute.

References

[1] W. Bao, S. A. Threefoot, S. R. Srinivasan, and G. S. Berenson, "Essential hypertension predicted by tracking of elevated blood

pressure from childhood to adulthood: the Bogalusa heart study," *The American Journal of Hypertension*, vol. 8, no. 7, pp. 657–665, 1995.

[2] H. C. McGill Jr. and C. A. McMahan, "Starting earlier to prevent heart disease," *The Journal of the American Medical Association*, vol. 290, no. 17, pp. 2320–2322, 2003.

[3] G. S. Berenson, S. R. Srinivasan, W. Bao, W. P. Newman III, R. E. Tracy, and W. A. Wattigney, "Association between multiple cardiovascular risk factors and atherosclerosis in children and young adults," *The New England Journal of Medicine*, vol. 338, no. 23, pp. 1650–1656, 1998.

[4] G. Mercuro, M. Deidda, A. Piras, C. C. Dessalvi, S. Maffei, and G. M. C. Rosano, "Gender determinants of cardiovascular risk factors and diseases," *Journal of Cardiovascular Medicine*, vol. 11, no. 3, pp. 207–220, 2010.

[5] J. D. Veldhuis, J. N. Roemmich, E. J. Richmond et al., "Endocrine control of body composition in infancy, childhood, and puberty," *Endocrine Reviews*, vol. 26, no. 1, pp. 114–146, 2005.

[6] K. A. Matthews, C. R. Katholi, H. McCreath et al., "Blood pressure reactivity to psychological stress predicts hypertension in the CARDIA Study," *Circulation*, vol. 110, no. 1, pp. 74–78, 2004.

[7] B. Falkner, G. Onesti, E. T. Angelakos, M. Fernandes, and C. Langman, "Cardiovascular response to mental stress in normal adolescents with hypertensive parents. Hemodynamics and mental stress in adolescents.," *Hypertension*, vol. 1, no. 1, pp. 23–30, 1979.

[8] A. Steptoe and M. Marmot, "Impaired cardiovascular recovery following stress predicts 3-year increases in blood pressure," *Journal of Hypertension*, vol. 23, no. 3, pp. 529–536, 2005.

[9] K. Narkiewicz, B. G. Phillips, M. Kato, D. Hering, L. Bieniaszewski, and V. K. Somers, "Gender-selective interaction between aging, blood pressure, and sympathetic nerve activity," *Hypertension*, vol. 45, no. 4, pp. 522–525, 2005.

[10] K. Wolf-Maier, R. S. Cooper, J. R. Banegas et al., "Hypertension prevalence and blood pressure levels in 6 European countries, Canada, and the United States," *The Journal of the American Medical Association*, vol. 289, no. 18, pp. 2363–2369, 2003.

[11] J. B. Meigs, P. W. F. Wilson, D. M. Nathan, R. B. D'Agostino Sr., K. Williams, and S. M. Haffner, "Prevalence and characteristics of the metabolic syndrome in the San Antonio Heart and Framingham Offspring Studies," *Diabetes*, vol. 52, no. 8, pp. 2160–2167, 2003.

[12] K. M. Denton, L. M. Hilliard, and M. Tare, "Sex-related differences in hypertension: seek and ye shall find.," *Hypertension*, vol. 62, no. 4, pp. 674–677, 2013.

[13] W. Gerin and T. G. Pickering, "Association between delayed recovery of blood pressure after acute mental stress and parental history of hypertension," *Journal of Hypertension*, vol. 13, no. 6, pp. 603–610, 1995.

[14] K. Zhang, A. B. Weder, E. Eskin, and D. T. O'Connor, "Genome-wide case/control studies in hypertension: only the 'tip of the iceberg'," *Journal of Hypertension*, vol. 28, no. 6, pp. 1115–1123, 2010.

[15] M. Feinleib, R. J. Garrison, R. Fabsitz et al., "The NHLBI twin study of cardiovascular disease risk factors: methodology and summary of results," *American Journal of Epidemiology*, vol. 106, no. 4, pp. 284–295, 1977.

[16] D. Levy, G. B. Ehret, K. Rice et al., "Genome-wide association study of blood pressure and hypertension," *Nature Genetics*, vol. 41, 677, no. 6, p. 687, 2009.

[17] C. Newton-Cheh, T. Johnson, V. Gateva et al., "Genome-wide association study identifies eight loci associated with blood pressure," *Nature Genetics*, vol. 41, no. 6, pp. 666–676, 2009.

[18] F. Takeuchi, M. Isono, T. Katsuya et al., "Blood Pressure and hypertension are associated with 7 loci in the Japanese population," *Circulation*, vol. 121, no. 21, pp. 2302–2309, 2010.

[19] K.-W. Hong, H.-S. Jin, J.-E. Lim, S. Kim, M. J. Go, and B. Oh, "Recapitulation of two genomewide association studies on blood pressure and essential hypertension in the Korean population," *Journal of Human Genetics*, vol. 55, no. 6, pp. 336–341, 2010.

[20] C. Liu, H. Li, Q. Qi et al., "Common variants in or near *FGF5*, *CYP17A1* and *MTHFR* genes are associated with blood pressure and hypertension in Chinese Hans," *Journal of Hypertension*, vol. 29, no. 1, pp. 70–75, 2011.

[21] N. Kato, F. Takeuchi, Y. Tabara et al., "Meta-analysis of genome-wide association studies identifies common variants associated with blood pressure variation in east Asians," *Nature Genetics*, vol. 43, no. 6, pp. 531–538, 2011.

[22] T. N. Kelly, F. Takeuchi, Y. Tabara et al., "Genome-wide association study meta-analysis reveals transethnic replication of mean arterial and pulse pressure loci," *Hypertension*, vol. 62, no. 5, pp. 853–859, 2013.

[23] A. C. Guyton, *Textbook of Medical Physiology*, W. B. Saunders Company, Philadelphia, Pa, USA, 8th edition, 1991.

[24] W. L. Miller and R. J. Auchus, "The molecular biology, biochemistry, and physiology of human steroidogenesis and its disorders," *Endocrine Reviews*, vol. 32, no. 1, pp. 81–151, 2011.

[25] M. de Braekeleer, "Hereditary disorders in Saguenay-Lac-St-Jean (Quebec, Canada)," *Human Heredity*, vol. 41, no. 3, pp. 141–146, 1991.

[26] M. de Braekeleer, C. Mari, C. Verlingue et al., "Complete identification of cystic fibrosis transmembrane conductance regulator mutations in the CF population of Saguenay Lac-Saint-Jean (Quebec, Canada)," *Clinical Genetics*, vol. 53, no. 1, pp. 44–46, 1998.

[27] M. Grompe, M. St.-Louis, S. I. Demers, M. Al-Dhalimy, B. Leclerc, and R. M. Tanguay, "A single mutation of the fumarylacetoacetate hydrolase gene in French Canadians with hereditary tyrosinemia type I," *The New England Journal of Medicine*, vol. 331, no. 6, pp. 353–357, 1994.

[28] A. Molina and A. Belldegrun, "Novel therapeutic strategies for castration resistant prostate cancer: inhibition of persistent androgen production and androgen receptor mediated signaling," *Journal of Urology*, vol. 185, no. 3, pp. 787–794, 2011.

[29] Z. Pausova, T. Paus, M. Abrahamowicz et al., "Genes, maternal smoking, and the offspring brain and body during adolescence: design of the Saguenay Youth Study," *Human Brain Mapping*, vol. 28, no. 6, pp. 502–518, 2007.

[30] G. Paradis, M. S. Tremblay, I. Janssen, A. Chiolero, and T. Bushnik, "Blood pressure in Canadian children and adolescents," *Health Reports*, vol. 21, no. 2, pp. 15–22, 2010.

[31] H. Tanaka, O. Thulesius, H. Yamaguchi, M. Mino, and K. Konishi, "Continuous non-invasive finger blood pressure monitoring in children," *Acta Paediatrica*, vol. 83, no. 6, pp. 646–652, 1994.

[32] R. S. Padwal, B. R. Hemmelgarn, N. A. Khan et al., "The 2009 Canadian Hypertension Education Program recommendations for the management of hypertension: part 1—blood pressure measurement, diagnosis and assessment of risk," *Canadian Journal of Cardiology*, vol. 25, no. 5, pp. 279–286, 2009.

[33] O. Delaneau, J. F. Zagury, and J. Marchini, "Improved whole-chromosome phasing for disease and population genetic studies," *Nature Methods*, vol. 10, no. 1, pp. 5–6, 2013.

[34] B. N. Howie, P. Donnelly, and J. Marchini, "A flexible and accurate genotype imputation method for the next generation of genome-wide association studies," *PLoS Genetics*, vol. 5, no. 6, Article ID e1000529, 2009.

[35] G. R. Abecasis, S. S. Cherny, W. O. Cookson, and L. R. Cardon, "Merlin—rapid analysis of dense genetic maps using sparse gene flow trees," *Nature Genetics*, vol. 30, no. 1, pp. 97–101, 2002.

[36] W. M. Chen and G. R. Abecasis, "Family-based association tests for genomewide association scans," *The American Journal of Human Genetics*, vol. 81, no. 5, pp. 913–926, 2007.

[37] R. J. Pruim, R. P. Welch, S. Sanna et al., "LocusZoom: regional visualization of genome-wide association scan results," *Bioinformatics*, vol. 26, no. 18, pp. 2336–2337, 2010.

[38] J. F. Reckelhoff, "Sex steroids, cardiovascular disease, and hypertension: unanswered questions and some speculations," *Hypertension*, vol. 45, no. 2, pp. 170–174, 2005.

[39] P. Korner, "Psychosocial stress and hypertension," in *Essential Hypertension and Its Causes: Neural and Non-Neural Mechanisms*, pp. 317–358, Oxford University Press, New York, NY, USA, 2007.

[40] P. Korner, "Whole-organism baroreflexes," in *Essential Hypertension and Its Causes: Neural and Non-Neural Mechanisms*, pp. 241–283, Oxford University Press, New York, NY, USA, 2007.

[41] X. Wang, X. Ding, S. Su, G. Harshfield, F. Treiber, and H. Snieder, "Genetic influence on blood pressure measured in the office, under laboratory stress and during real life," *Hypertension Research*, vol. 34, no. 2, pp. 239–244, 2011.

[42] Z. Pausova, M. Jomphe, L. Houde et al., "A genealogical study of essential hypertension with and without obesity in French Canadians," *Obesity Research*, vol. 10, no. 6, pp. 463–470, 2002.

[43] R. P. Wildman, P. Muntner, K. Reynolds et al., "The obese without cardiometabolic risk factor clustering and the normal weight with cardiometabolic risk factor clustering: prevalence and correlates of 2 phenotypes among the US population (NHANES 1999–2004)," *Archives of Internal Medicine*, vol. 168, no. 15, pp. 1617–1624, 2008.

[44] M. Edwards, J. Hall, G. Gong, and S. E. O'Bryant, "Arsenic exposure, AS3MT polymorphism, and neuropsychological functioning among rural dwelling adults and elders: a cross-sectional study," *Environmental Health*, vol. 13, no. 1, article 15, 2014.

15

Determinants of Mean Blood Pressure and Hypertension among Workers in West Africa

William K. Bosu

Department of Epidemics and Disease Control, West African Health Organisation, 01 BP 153, Bobo-Dioulasso 01, Burkina Faso

Correspondence should be addressed to William K. Bosu; wbosu@wahooas.org

Academic Editor: Csaba Farsang

Background. This review was undertaken to estimate the mean blood pressure and evaluate its determinants as well as the determinants of hypertension among workers in West Africa. *Methods.* In a follow-up to an earlier study, a systematic search for articles published between 1980 and August 2015 was undertaken using major databases. *Results.* A total of 55 articles involving 34,919 different cadres of workers from six countries were retrieved. The mean systolic blood pressure (BP) ranged from 116.6 ± 1.3 mmHg to 151.7 ± 13.6 mmHg while the mean diastolic BP ranged from 69.6 ± 11.0 mmHg to 97.1 ± 9.1 mmHg. Population-wide prehypertension was common. The major determinants of mean BP and hypertension were similar and included male sex, older age group, higher socioeconomic status, obesity, alcohol consumption, plasma glucose, and sodium excretion. Ethnicity and educational level were inconsistently associated with hypertension. Workers at higher risk of cardiovascular event did not perceive themselves as such. *Conclusion.* The prevailing mean prehypertensive BP, low perception of risk, and clustering of risk factors call for interventions such as healthy diets, improved physical activity, and a favourable work environment. Successful models for improving the cardiovascular health of sedentary informal sector workers in Africa are urgently needed.

1. Introduction

The major modifiable risk factors for noncommunicable diseases (NCDs) are well known and have been the focus of the current WHO Plan of Action 2013–2020 under a 4-by-4 strategy [1]. Physical inactivity, unhealthy diet, smoking, and harmful alcohol use have been associated with increased all-cause, cancer- and cardiovascular-related mortality [2]. Consequently, the adherence to lifestyle factors is associated with as much as 66% reduction in all-cause mortality [3]. Applying such knowledge, often derived from studies in western countries, in policy and programmes for improved public health in resource-poor settings often requires customized approaches that take account of cultural appropriateness, cost-effectiveness, implementation capacity, and equity gaps [4].

The Sixtieth World Health Assembly, in endorsing the global plan of action 2008–2017 for workers' health, urged countries to institute workplace health programmes to promote health and to prevent NCDs, in particular through healthy dietary lifestyles and physical activity among workers [5]. Workers in West Africa deserve the best health and quality of lives during their productive working lives as well as in retirement. Concerted action should therefore be taken to adapt and implement the global plan of action for workers health. West African workers report multiple NCDs during their late working lives [6].

While the workplace health programmes are cost-effective in reducing NCDs [7], relatively little is known about the disease burden and existing programmes among workers in Africa. A recent systematic review among workers in West Africa reported a prevalence of hypertension of 12%–69% among workers [8]. This paper focuses on the factors and the determinants that are associated with blood pressure levels and hypertension among workers in the Economic Community of West African States (ECOWAS) Region. Knowledge of these determinants could enable better targeting of interventions to reduce elevated blood pressure among workers.

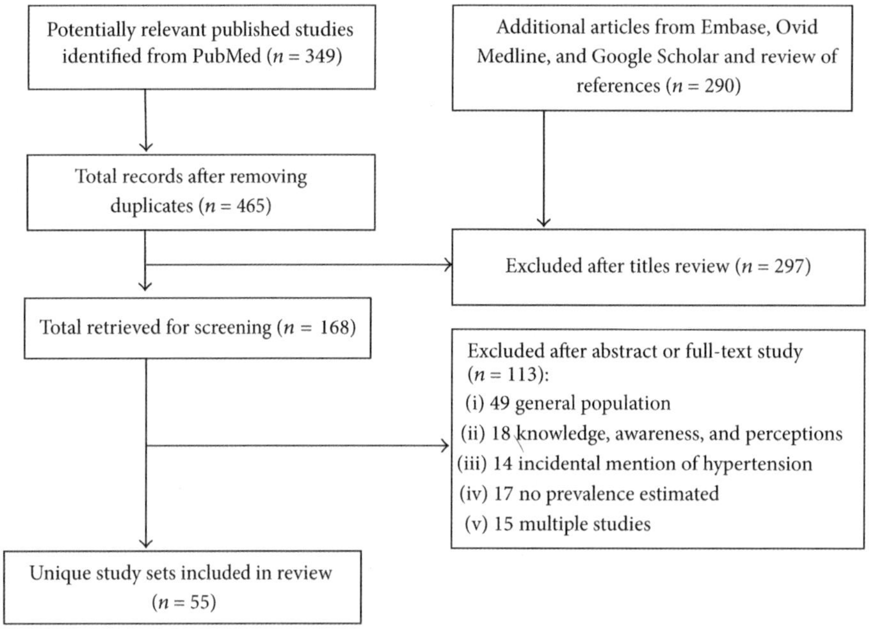

FIGURE 1: The process of selecting articles.

2. Methods

The study setting, detailed search strategy, data extraction, and definition of variables have been described elsewhere [8]. Briefly, the PubMed, Embase, and Google Scholar databases were systematically searched to identify articles estimating the prevalence of adult hypertension among workers in West Africa. In the original review, 45 papers published over the period from 1980 to September 2014 were retrieved. In this review, the publication date was extended to end of August 2015 using saved search items. The search terms were "hypertension" and "workers" combined in its various forms with the individual countries and collectively with West Africa. The bibliography of retrieved papers was screened manually to identify additional papers.

The inclusion criteria were that the total number of respondents was at least 75 and the minimum age of the workers 15 years. Population- or hospital-based studies on workers were excluded. Among the data extracted were the demographic characteristics of the workers, sampling technique, method of measuring the blood pressure (BP), prevalence of hypertension, mean systolic and diastolic BP (SBP and DBP), and the crude and adjusted factors associated with the mean BP or hypertension. Unlike the previous study that focussed on the prevalence, the present review focusses on factors and determinants associated with mean BP and hypertension.

3. Results

A total of 55 articles from six of the 15 ECOWAS countries satisfying the inclusion criteria were retrieved after screening 168 articles (Figure 1). Of the included articles, 41 (74.5%) were conducted in Nigeria, five conducted in Ghana, three each in Senegal and Togo, two in Cote d'Ivoire, and one in Liberia. The group of workers who were most frequently studied were civil servants [9–19], university workers [20–26], health care workers [27–32], traders [33–37], factory workers [38–40], farmers [41, 42], bankers [43–46], and office workers [47–52]. There were also studies on garage workers [53], music dealers [54], mill operators [55], port workers [56], drivers [57], and motorcyclists [58]. Except for three studies, all the studies were undertaken in urban or mixed settings. Overall, 34,919 workers were studies across the studies with a median sample size of 380 (range 75–5,200). Eight studies were conducted exclusively among male [39, 53, 57, 59–61] or female workers [33, 35]. The mean age of the workers across the studies ranged from 23.1 years in commercial cyclists to 63.0 years in rural farmers. In 51 of the studies in which hypertension was defined based on the 140/90 mmHg threshold, 6,745 workers were diagnosed with hypertension.

3.1. Mean Blood Pressure. Among 27 studies with information, the mean SBP ranged from 116.6 ± 1.3 mmHg among traders in Ijebu Ode, Nigeria [37], to 151.7 ± 13.6 mmHg among workers of a private telecommunication company in Senegal [47]. In one (3.7%) of these studies, the mean SBP was ≥140.0 mmHg; in five (18.5%), it was 130.0–139.9 mmHg; in 18 (66.7%), it was 120.0–129.9 mmHg; and in three (11.1%), it was <120.0 mmHg. The mean DBP ranged from 69.6 ± 11.0 mmHg among male factory workers in Nigeria [39] to 97.1 ± 9.1 mmHg among telecommunication workers in Senegal [47]. In one (3.7%) of the studies, the mean DBP was ≥90.0 mmHg; in two (7.4%), it was 85.0–89.9 mmHg; in eleven (40.7%), it was 80.0–84.9 mmHg; and in thirteen (48.1%), it was <80.0 mmHg.

3.2. *Factors Associated with Hypertension and Mean Blood Pressure Level*

3.2.1. Biological Factors. Age was a ubiquitous risk factor present among the same group of workers such as civil servants [9–11, 17, 59], health workers [13, 15, 27, 29], or university workers [23, 26] or among different groups of workers [38, 49].

SBP, DBP, and hypertension increased with increasing age in both sexes in different geographical settings [9–12, 14, 29, 39, 42, 44, 49, 59, 62]. The change in the mean BP with increasing age was, however, minimal in two studies in Nigeria [39] and Liberia [41].

Hypertension was more frequent among males than among females in 22 of 27 studies in which they could be compared, using the 140/90 mmHg threshold definition. It was only in six studies that the prevalence was higher in females. In one study with results in both directions, the prevalence was higher among male bankers and female traffic wardens [46]. The prevalence of hypertension ranged from 11.2% to 68.9% in male workers compared with 0% to 43.5% in female workers. Similarly, SBP and DBP were consistently higher in men than in women in all age groups in most studies (Table 1) [9, 11, 38, 44, 49, 63].

The relationship between positive family history of hypertension and hypertension was rarely investigated. It was more common in nonhypertensives than in hypertensives [31, 46] with the difference being statistically significant in some studies [31]. After stratifying civil servants into two age groups (<40 years or ≥40 years), the prevalence of hypertension was found to be higher in those with a positive family history of hypertension than in those without, but the difference was not statistically significant [13].

Ethnicity was inconsistently associated with hypertension in some studies. Giles et al. [41], in a large study in rural Liberia, found statistically significant differences in age- and sex-adjusted SBP and DBP by ethnicity. The prevalence ranged from 5% among the Grebo ethnic group to 24% among the Mano ethnic group. However, there were no statistically significant differences in the prevalence of hypertension by ethnic origin in Nigeria [11].

In Calabar, the Efik ethnic group had a significantly higher SBP and DBP as well as a higher prevalence of hypertension than the other ethnic groups [12]. Male civil servants in Sokoto from the southern and eastern tribes of Nigeria were reported to have significantly higher diastolic BP than those from the northern tribes [10]. However, these differences in the DBP disappeared after adjusting for age and BMI. Similarly, in Dakar, male workers of the Peul ethnic group had significantly higher systolic blood pressure levels than those of the Serer group but the difference disappeared in multivariate analysis [38].

3.2.2. Obesity. The prevalence of obesity among the workers, as provided by 23 studies, ranged from 2.0% among automobile garage workers in Kumasi, Ghana [53], to 42.1% among health workers in Umuahia, Nigeria [29]. The prevalence of overweight or obesity, as reported by 16 studies, ranged from 25.6% among pharmaceutical industry workers [40] to 97.7% among Senegalese workers of an information technology (IT) company [51]. It was more than 50% among civil servants [9, 13], health workers [27, 31], traders [35, 37], medical school lecturers [22], traffic wardens [46], and IT company workers [51].

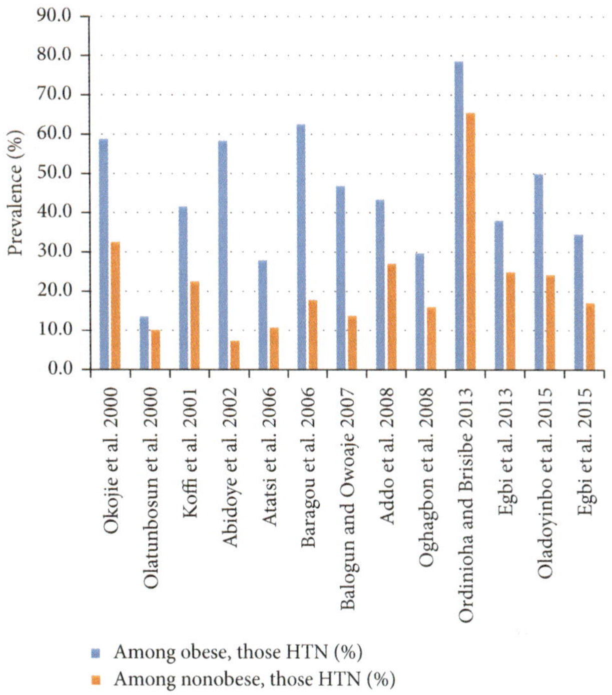

FIGURE 2: Prevalence of hypertension (HTN) in obese and nonobese workers.

Obesity was one of the strongest independent risk factors associated with hypertension. In 14 studies in which the prevalence of hypertension could be evaluated for obese and nonobese workers, the prevalence ratio ranged from 1.2 to 8.0. In most cases, the differences were statistically significant. The prevalence of hypertension ranged from 27.9% to 78.6% among obese subjects compared with 7.3% to 65.4% in nonobese subjects (Figure 2). Among health workers in a university teaching hospital, the odds ratio (OR) of the association between obesity and hypertension was 2.12, $p = 0.004$ [27]. Civil servants in Kaduna younger than 40 years and who were overweight or obese were five times as likely as those with healthy weight to have hypertension [13].

As with hypertension, fat-related variables such as BMI, waist circumference, and waist-to-hip ratio were frequently associated with BP [10]. The mean BP was positively correlated with BMI in all studies with available information [10, 15, 37–39, 44, 62, 64]. Ogunlesi et al. [39] found a correlation coefficient of 0.22 ($p < 0.01$) between BMI and BP. The correlation between BP and the BMI may not be linear. One study reported that, below the threshold of 21.5 kg/m^2, BP was not correlated with BMI [62].

Despite being a strong risk factor for hypertension and mean blood pressure, overweight and obesity were not well

TABLE 1: Age-specific mean blood pressure among workers in West Africa.

Study population	Location	15–24			25–34			35–44			45–54			55–64		
		M	F	T	M	F	T	M	F	T	M	F	T	M	F	T
Mean systolic blood pressure																
Bank workers [44]	Ibadan	118.2 ± 14.2	111.0 ± 11.4		114.8 ± 14.9	110.7 ± 15.7		118.9 ± 17.2	117.6 ± 17.8		131.7 ± 20.7	124.0 ± 20.4		144.2 ± 14.3	110	
Civil servants [9]	Accra				125	113.5	119.0	127.5	117.5	125.0	135.5	130.8	134.0	140.3	131.8	137.0
Civil servants [11]	Bendel State	NA	NA	NA	123.1	114.2	nr	127.7	117	nr	135.7	128.6	nr			
Civil servants [10]	Sokoto	121.6	116.5		122.0	122.5		127.5	129.2		138.6					
Health care workers [29]	Umuahia, Abia State									124.49			128.39			135.00
Male factory workers [39]	Ibadan	127.2 ± 9.3			128.2 ± 12.4			126.7 ± 13.2			132.8 ± 21.1					
Rubber plantation workers [41]	Rural	127.3	120.0		125.0	121.4		124.9	125.3		126.8	135.2		127.7	144.85	
Senior executives of industries and companies [49]	Benin City, Edo State	NA	NA	NA	122.7	121.5	122.3	125.6	123.6	125.3	137.2	133.9	136.4	142.0	140.0	141.5
Mean diastolic blood pressure																
Bank workers [44]	Ibadan	73.1 ± 9.8	69.4 ± 8.5		73.8 ± 10.6	70.0 ± 11.1		76.7 ± 11.2	76.6 ± 11.7		85.0 ± 12.0	76.2 ± 10.8		87.5 ± 11.3	70.0	
Civil servants [9]	Accra				72.5	69.0	71.3	77.5	76	76.5	84.5	83.5	84.0	85	79.8	84.5
Civil servants [11]	Bendel State	NA	NA	NA	79.1	74.8	nr	82.3	74.8	nr	86.6	83	nr			
Civil servants [10]	Sokoto	67.6	69.6		71.1	75.1		76.3	78.5		82.6					
Health care workers [29]	Umuahia, Abia State									78.06			80.77			84.87
Male factory workers [39]	Ibadan	63.8 ± 9.7			68.3 ± 10.0			72.6 ± 10.6				75.4 ± 14.0				
Rubber plantation workers [41]	Rural	71.0	69.5		71.8	72.0		72.2	73.5		75.0	75.7		73.8	78.8	
Senior executives of industries and companies [49]	Benin City, Edo State				75.7	76.5		90.2	77.8		88.6	83.7		91.7	90.3	

*Mean blood pressure ± standard deviation.

Bunker et al. 1996 [10]: lowest age groups 20–24 in both men and women. Only 3 age groups were reported for women; Giles: lowest age groups 20–24 in both men and women; last age group > 55 y; Uwanuruochi et al. 2013 [29]: lowest age groups 40–44.

Addo et al. 2008 [9]: median SBP and DBP values.

M: males; F: females; T: total sample.

appreciated among workers. Among university health workers in Ghana who did not consider themselves overweight, nearly half were actually obese (11%) or overweight (37%) actually [23]. Similarly, only 29.0% of university teaching hospital health workers who were overweight or obese considered themselves to be overweight [27].

3.2.3. Physical Activity. The prevalence of hypertension was significantly higher among those with low physical activity compared with those with moderate or intense physical activity [9]. Workers whose jobs were physically demanding such as automobile workers [53], mill operators [55], and plantation workers [41] appeared to have a lower prevalence of hypertension than those whose jobs were largely sedentary such as traders [35, 66], office executives [47, 49], and civil servants [9, 11, 16].

In Maiduguri, Nigeria, the mean SBP was significantly and inversely associated with four levels of physical activity [19]. Civil servants and health workers who were highly sedentary had a mean BP that was 19.1 mmHg higher than those who were highly physically active. The BP ranged from 123.8 ± 13.8 mmHg in highly active workers to 142.9 ± 18.7 mmHg in highly sedentary workers. Moderate-to-vigorous physical activity was significantly and negatively correlated with BMI and waist circumference, as well as SBP ($r = -0.224$, $p < 0.001$) and DBP ($r = -0.194$, $p < 0.001$).

3.2.4. Alcohol Consumption. Hypertension was significantly more frequent in alcohol drinkers than in abstainers [11]. Kadiri et al. [44] found that regular and moderate drinking and not just mere drinking was associated with hypertension. The prevalence was higher in medium and heavy drinkers than in nondrinkers and light drinkers [12]. It was also higher among medium and heavy smokers. University College of Health Sciences staff in Ghana who were hypertensive had six times the odds of consuming alcohol four or more times weekly compared with those who are not hypertensive (OR 6.0, 95% CI 1.5–23.8) [23]. In Dakar, neither alcohol nor tea consumption was significantly associated with blood pressure levels [38].

3.2.5. Sodium Excretion. Using the 140/90 mmHg threshold, sodium excretion was higher among female hypertensives than in normotensives but this was not the case in men [10]. However, using the higher 160/95 mmHg threshold, both sodium and potassium excretion were significantly higher in male and female hypertensives compared with normotensives.

The 24-hour urinary sodium excretion and the sodium : potassium ratio were weakly but significantly correlated with SBP and DBP among a combined group of railway workers, urban poor informal sector workers, and rural farmers aged 45 years and over in Oyo State [60]. Urinary potassium excretion was neither correlated with SBP nor DBP. Among the male rural farmers in this set, both the 24-hour sodium excretion and sodium : potassium ratio correlated strongly and significantly with both SBP and DBP ($r = 0.32$–0.51). In contrast, overnight urinary sodium, potassium or creatinine excretion, and sodium-potassium, sodium-creatinine, or potassium-creatinine ratio were not significantly correlated with SBP or DBP in men or women in Sokoto [10]. Neither SBP nor DBP was significantly correlated with serum creatinine or glomerular filtration rate in the civil servants of Bayelsa State [15].

3.2.6. Diabetes. The strongest risk factors associated with hypertension in telecommunication workers in Dakar were diabetes (OR 3.9, 95% CI 2.2–6.9), age ≥ 40 years compared with age <40 years (OR 2.8, 95% CI 2.2–3.6), overweight (OR 2.2, 95% CI 1.8–2.8), and male sex (OR 1.6, 95% CI 1.3–2.1) [38]. Diabetic bankers in Lagos, Nigeria, were 4.3 times as likely as those without diabetes to have diastolic hypertension [43].

Egbi et al. [15] observed that, unlike DBP, SBP was significantly correlated with random blood glucose (RBG) and serum urea in civil servants in Bayelsa State. However, the correlation was weak with coefficients of 0.13 and 0.18, respectively, unlike in civil servants where the same group of investigators found that DBP was also significantly correlated with RBG in health workers [31].

3.2.7. Socioeconomic Factors. Socioeconomic status was assessed using salary grades or, as a proxy, staff ranking or educational attainment. Hypertension was more common in workers with higher salary grades than in those with lower salary grades [12, 18]. It was more common in senior staff than in junior staff [9, 23, 24, 67], even after adjusting for age [10, 11]. The age-adjusted prevalence in senior and junior staff was 43% versus 23%, respectively, among male civil servants in Benin City [11]. The differential remained after controlling for BMI. The prevalence of hypertension among the male senior staff within the highest tertile band of BMI (23.8–42.2 kg/m^2) was significantly higher than that among the junior staff (61.4% versus 37.5%, $p = 0.005$).

In Sokoto, the age-adjusted prevalence of hypertension in senior (19.3%) and junior (19.8%) staff was similar [10]. However, senior staff were observed to have three times the prevalence of junior staff when the higher BP 160/95 mmHg cut-off limit was used (11.2% versus 3.6%).

Among civil servants in Accra in 2006, the differences in the prevalence of hypertension among the different employment grades were statistically significant, with senior staff more likely to be hypertensive than junior staff though the direction was not entirely uniform [9]. The prevalence was 20.8% among unskilled workers, 30.1% among clerical staff, and 37.4% among professional staff but only 11.7% among the directors. In Abidjan, the prevalence of hypertension in medical specialists was 2.5–3.5 times that among doctors, nurses, and nurse auxiliaries [28]. Consistent with these observations, Kaufman et al. [60] found that the prevalence increased across the socioeconomic gradient from rural farmer to urban poor to railway workers: 14.0%, 25.0%, and 29.0%, respectively, in Oyo State in 1994. However, Bunker et al. [10] observed similar age-adjusted prevalence of hypertension among senior and junior grade civil servants in Sokoto.

Generally, as with hypertension, the mean BP was higher in senior than in junior staff [11, 52]. An exception was in the Sokoto study in which junior civil servants had higher SBP but lower DBP after adjusting for age and BMI [10]. Unlike DBP, the mean SBP increased along the gradient from junior staff through senior staff to management among workers in a media organization in Ghana [52]. However, in a few studies, junior staff had significantly higher BP than senior staff [10, 38].

The association between educational level of workers and hypertension or mean BP levels was inconsistent. A higher prevalence of hypertension was reported in those with low level of education in some studies [13, 31, 38, 65] as well as in those with higher levels of education [11, 39]. The pattern at the different levels of education was downward [65], upward [39], or U-shaped with the highest prevalence in those with the lowest and highest levels of education [11]. In Dakar, the age-adjusted prevalence was three times as high in illiterates as in those with primary or secondary education, with the difference being statistically significant [38]. The prevalence of hypertension increased with increasing educational level among factory workers in Ibadan, Nigeria [39]. The pattern remained after adjustment for age, BMI, pulse rate, alcohol drinking, and antihypertensive treatment. Those with moderate and highest levels of education were 2.0 and 2.4 times as likely as those with the lowest levels of education to have hypertension, with the differences being statistically significant.

Among male factory workers in Ibadan in 1994, the mean age-adjusted SBP and DBP increased with increasing years of education [39]. In those with low level of education (0–9 years), the mean SBP and DBP were 125.8 mmHg and 67.9 mmHg, respectively, while, in those with high level of education (≥13 years), they were 130.1 mmHg and 71.7 mmHg, respectively. The pattern persisted after adjusting for age, BMI, pulse rate, alcohol drinking, and antihypertensive treatment. BP also correlated with years of education in male bank workers in Ibadan, but not in females [44]. Unlike the male factory workers, the age-adjusted SBP and DBP in male bankers were highest in those with secondary education. In women, the highest BP and lowest BP were in those with primary and secondary education, respectively. In Dakar, the age-adjusted SBP and DBP were highest in illiterates and lowest in those with primary education, with the difference being statistically significant [38].

3.2.8. Urban Residence. The prevalence of hypertension was higher in urban than in rural areas. The prevalence of hypertension in rural settings [41, 42, 60] ranged from 12.3% to 13.9% and was much lower than that in urban settings (12.0%–60.2%). Compared to other similarly aged workers in a broadly common environment, Kaufman et al. found that the prevalence of hypertension in urban poor informal sector workers was 1.8 times that of rural farmers [60].

As with hypertension, the mean SBP and DBP were higher in urban than in rural settings [14]. The mean SBP and DBP levels in men aged ≥45 years and older in Oyo State in Nigeria followed an urban-rural and socioeconomic gradient. They were highest among urban railway workers and lowest in rural farmers with the levels in the urban poor informal sector workers being intermediate [60]. The length of residence in urban area was, however, not associated with BP among workers in Dakar [38].

3.2.9. Occupational Exposures. In the earliest study covered by this review, rural office workers had a higher mean BP than rural field labourers in the Bendel State of Nigeria in 1976 [68]. Idahosa [59] observed that male civil servants were significantly more likely to have hypertension than the more physically active group of workers, policemen, in Benin City (33.6% versus 24.4%; $p < 0.001$). However, difference between the two groups ceased to be statistically significant when the higher BP cut-off point of 160/95 mmHg was used.

Female industry workers in Dakar exposed to noise levels that made it impossible to converse at the workplace were more likely than those not exposed to be hypertensive, but the difference was not statistically significant [38]. Similarly, Ebare et al. [54] found that, although mean SBP and DBP increased with increasing exposure across three categories of noise levels among music dealers in Benin City, the differences were not statistically significant. However, the prevalence of hypertension increased significantly with exposure to increasing noise levels (<85 dB = 14.3%, 85–90 dB = 39.5%, and >90 dB = 55.6%; $p = 0.003$).

Investigators in the study of civil servants in Benin City confirmed their hypothesis that hypertensives experience larger increases in BP during behavioural stress than normotensives [67]. They also found that, even when men and women occupied similar status jobs (senior staff or junior staff), men still had greater changes in their BP in response to stress than women. Similarly, Owolabi et al. [32] found that health workers who were classified as being exposed to high levels of work-related stress (based on a job-demand control questionnaire) were significantly more likely to have hypertension than others exposed to lower levels of stress (42.4% versus 12.1%, $p < 0.001$).

In terms of the relationship between working conditions and mean blood pressure, the age-adjusted SBP and DBP were higher among male shift workers in Dakar than in those with regular work schedule [38]. The age-adjusted BP did not differ between women exposed to occupational noise compared to those not exposed. The travel distance to work and occupational or recreational physical activity were not related to BP.

3.2.10. Other Factors. Hypertension was associated with obstructive sleep apnoea among the university staff in Ogbomosho, Oyo State, Nigeria (OR 3.2) [69]. Knowledge about risk factors associated with hypertension was not significantly associated with a lower prevalence. In a study comparing the knowledge of risk factors among bankers and traffic wardens in Ilorin, the former were more likely to know five risk factors. Yet, the bankers, being of a higher socioeconomic class and having a different risk factor profile, had a higher prevalence of hypertension than the traffic wardens (34.4% versus 22.2%; $p < 0.05$) [46]. Neither coffee consumption nor the daily smoking of two to five sticks of cigarettes was associated with hypertension among university workers in Ile Ife [26].

However, parity of 4 or more children was significantly associated with hypertension in these workers. In contrast, age-adjusted parity in women was not significantly related to BP in Dakar [38].

In Ghana, 31.7% of media workers self-reported having hypertension [52]. However, on screening, twice as many workers (60.2%) were found to have diastolic hypertension. The greatest gap was observed among junior staff in whom 3.6 times as many as those self-reporting hypertension were identified as having diastolic hypertension.

3.2.11. Clustering of Risk Factors. There was clustering of cardiovascular risk factors [25, 47, 51, 70]. Out of 1,229 telecommunication workers screened in Senegal, 341 (27.7%) had one cardiovascular risk factor, 632 (51.4%) had two risk factors, and 256 (20.8%) had three or more risk factors [47]. Seven percent of those diagnosed with hypertension had a moderate Framingham risk score while 18% were found to be at a high risk of a cardiovascular event. Nearly three-quarters of hypertensive telecommunication workers in Lome were assessed to have high (32.0%) or very high (41.8%) risk of cardiovascular event [71].

Among 525 university staff in Ibadan, Nigeria, 67.4% reported one risk behaviour, while 30.0% reported two or more risk behaviours (unhealthy diet, sedentary living, excessive alcohol use, and smoking) [25]. Remarkably, those with multiple risk factors did not perceive themselves to be at any greater risk of NCD morbidity than those without. Similarly, among the staff of another university in Ogbomosho, Nigeria, 96 male staff had average of 2.6 cardiovascular risk factors compared with 3.3 risk factors among 110 females [20]. The risk factors evaluated were smoking, hypertension, impaired glucose tolerance, obesity, elevated triglyceride level, elevated low-density lipoprotein- (LDL-) cholesterol, low level of high-density lipoprotein- (HDL-) cholesterol, elevated total cholesterol (TC), and presence of left ventricular hypertrophy (LVH) on electrocardiography (ECG).

3.2.12. Summary. In sum, risk factors that were positively associated with hypertension and increased BP in bivariate analysis included older age group, male sex, urban residence, higher socioeconomic class, physical inactivity, obesity, alcohol consumption, sodium excretion, and sodium-potassium ratio. High levels of work-related stress were also related to hypertension while shift work was related to mean BP. Unlike blood pressure, the exposure to high noise levels was associated with hypertension. The relationship between educational attainment and ethnicity and hypertension was inconsistent.

3.3. Determinants of Hypertension and Mean Blood Pressure. Seven studies evaluated the determinants of blood pressure levels while nine evaluated the determinants of hypertension among workers such as civil servants, health workers, and bank workers using logistic or multiple linear regression. Three studies examined determinants of both blood pressure and hypertension [10, 11, 18]. Generally, the studies rarely included more than five variables in their modelling (Tables 2 and 3).

Among male civil servants in Benin City in 1987-1988, age, BMI, alcohol drinking, and senior staff grade were independent risk factors for hypertension or BP [64]. In females, only BMI was independently associated with BP or hypertension (OR 13.2, comparing third tertile BMI with first tertile). Education was not independently associated with hypertension in men [11]. The strongest determinants of hypertension in men were staff grade, BMI, and alcohol consumption (Table 3).

In the 1990 Sokoto Civil Servants Study, the age- and BMI-adjusted DBP in male civil servants was significantly higher in senior staff than in junior staff (75.7 mmHg versus 73.3 mmHg, $p < 0.01$) [10]. In contrast, the adjusted SBP was lower in senior staff than in junior staff, but difference was not statistically significant. Age group (10-year intervals) and BMI tertile in men and sodium excretion in women were independently related to hypertension based on the 140/90 mmHg threshold [10]. Sodium excretion and senior staff grade became additional risk factors for hypertension in men when the model used the higher threshold 160/95 mmHg as the outcome.

In Ibadan, age, male sex, BMI, and plasma glucose were significantly associated with SBP in multivariate ANOVA model among 856 male and female civil servants [18]. Among only men, age, BMI, and glucose were highly significant while, in women, only age and BMI were significantly associated with SBP. In the model with DBP as outcome, age, sex, and BMI but not plasma glucose were significant factors in male and female civil servants combined. In the separate models for male and female civil servants, age and BMI were significant predictors of DBP.

Similarly, age, plasma glucose, and waist-to-hip ratio (WHR), as well as a family history of diabetes were the predictors of hypertension among the same group of civil servants in Ibadan [18]. The strongest predictor was WHR (OR 1.35). In a separate logistic regression model, height was found to be associated with abnormal glucose tolerance but not hypertension [72].

In addition to male sex, increasing age, and weight, marital status, number of children in the family, higher salary scale, and tobacco consumption were independently associated with SBP in a large study involving 5,200 civil servants and factory and plantation workers in Calabar [12]. Only the number of children in the family and salary scale were associated with DBP (Table 2). Occupation, educational level, support system and height were inversely associated with SBP.

Kaufman et al. [60], on the other hand, found that the number of children was significantly and strongly associated with a lower SBP among women in the Oyo State in 1994. Among rural farmers, pulse rate and sodium-potassium ratio were positively associated with SBP while BMI was positively associated with DBP. The strongest risk factor for increased SBP or DBP in either men or women was age ≥ 55 years while nonmigrant status (participants born in the same community in which they currently live) was significantly associated with lower BP.

Ogunlesi et al. [39] found that, among male factory workers, education level was significantly associated with BP, after controlling for age, body mass index, pulse, and alcohol

Table 2: Determinants of arterial blood pressure in workers in West Africa.

Study population	Location	Determinants of BP	Age	Sex	Physical activity	Obesity or adiposity	Alcohol	SES	Others	Variables in model	Analysis
Civil servants [11]	Benin City	Age, BMI, alcohol consumption, and senior staff grade independently and positively associated with BP in men. In women, only BMI independently associated with BP.	BP related to age in senior staff but not in junior staff in males. BP not significantly related to age in females.	—	—	Correlation with SBP and DBP, $r = 0.27$ and 0.29 in male senior staff. In male junior staff, $r = 0.25$ and 0.26, respectively.	Alcohol drinking positively associated with BP in men but not in women.	Staff grade (senior staff) positively associated with BP in men but not in women.		Age, BMI, alcohol drinking, and staff grade.	Multiple regression
Civil servants [10]	Sokoto	Age- and BMI-adjusted DBP in male civil servants in the 25–54 age group significantly higher in senior staff than in junior staff (75.7 versus 73.3 mmHg, $p < 0.01$). In contrast, the adjusted SBP was lower in senior staff than in junior staff, but difference was not statistically significant.								Age, BMI.	ANOVA, logistic regression
Civil servants [18]	Ibadan	In both sexes combined, age, sex, and BMI were highly significant for both SBP and DBP. Further, plasma glucose predicted SBP but not DBP. In men and women, age and BMI were significantly associated with BP.	Age determinant for SBP and DBP in both sexes separately and combined.	When both sexes combined, male sex is a determinant	—	BMI predicts both SBP and DBP.		—	Plasma glucose, family history of diabetes.	BMI, glucose, age, and sex.	Multivariate ANOVA model

Table 2: Continued.

Study population	Location	Determinants of BP	Age	Sex	Physical activity	Obesity or adiposity	Alcohol	SES	Others	Variables in model	Analysis
Civil servants, factory and plantation workers [12]	Calabar	Sex, age, marital status, number of children in the family, salary scale, tobacco consumption, and weight associated with SBP. Number of children in the family and salary scale associated with DBP. Occupation, educational level, support system, and height were protective of SBP.	Increasing age	Male sex		Weight		Salary scale for both SBP and DBP.	Marital status, parity, and tobacco use associated with SBP. Occupation, educational level, support system, and height were protective of SBP.	Sex, age, marital status, number of children, occupation, educational level, salary scale, social security, ethnicity, tobacco, alcohol, height, weight, SBP, and DBP.	Multiple linear regression
Retired railway workmen, rural farmers ≥ 45 years [60]	Idere village & Ibadan	BMI, waist circumference, radial pulse, and urinary sodium : potassium ratio were positively and significantly associated with blood pressure. Ambient temperature, nonmigrant status, and number of children were negatively associated with mean blood pressure.	Age ≥ 55 years strongly associated with SBP in men.		BMI positively and significantly associated with SBP and DBP in men, but not in women.				Nonmigrant status and ambient temperature are negative predictors while waist circumference, sodium : potassium ratio, and pulse were positive predictors.	Age, temperature, BMI, waist circumference, hip circumference, nonmigration status, number of children, sodium : potassium ratio, and ambient temperature.	Linear regression modelling
Bank workers [44]	Ibadan	BP correlated with income and education in men but not in women, after adjusting for age and BMI.						Higher income; educational level variable between men and women after adjusting for age and BMI.			Multiple linear regression; MANOVA

Table 2: Continued.

Study population	Location	Determinants of BP	Age	Sex	Physical activity	Obesity or adiposity	Alcohol	SES	Others	Variables in model	Analysis
Oil, printing, cotton mill, tobacco factory, canning factory, and hotel workers [38]	Dakar	SBP was associated with age, BMI, higher educational level, tea consumption, and ethnicity in men. DBP associated with age and BMI in men. In women, age and BMI were the only significant factors associated with both SBP and DBP.	Age statistically significant association with SBP and DBP in men and women.			BMI statistically significant association with both SBP and DBP in women and with DBP but not SBP in men.		Educational level with illiterates having highest levels of BP is associated with SBP but not DBP.	Tea consumption associated with SBP.	Age, BMI, shift work, tea consumption, occupational category, educational level, and ethnicity.	Multiple linear regression

BMI: body mass index; DBP: diastolic blood pressure; SBP: systolic blood pressure; SES: socioeconomic status.

TABLE 3: Determinants of hypertension in workers in West Africa.

Study population	Location	Determinants	Age	Sex	Physical activity	Obesity or adiposity	Alcohol	SES	Others	Variables in model	Type of analysis
Civil servants [11]	Benin City	BMI (OR 2.88 Tertile 3 versus Tertile 1), age (OR 10-year groups 1.42), alcohol drinking (OR 1.85), and high SES (OR 2.62) were all independent risk factors for HTN in men but not education. Only BMI (OR 13.2) related to HTN in women.	Age [OR 10-year groups 1.42, 95% CI 1.03–1.96] in men; not significant in women	—	—	BMI [OR 2.88 Tertile 3 versus Tertile 1, 95% CI 1.6–5.1 in men]; OR 13.2, 95% CI 1.5–113.0 in women	Alcohol drinking (OR 1.85, 95% CI 1.15–2.98) in men; not significant in women	Senior staff in men (OR 2.62, 95% CI 1.61–4.29); not significant in women	—	Staff grade, BMI, alcohol drinking, and age in 10-year intervals.	Logistic regression
Civil servants [10]	Sokoto	Only age group and BMI tertile in men and sodium excretion were statistically significant. No significant association with sodium excretion or SES in men or with age, BMI, or staff grade in women.	10-year age intervals OR = 2.4 (95% CI 1.8–3.4) in men			Tertile 3 OR = 2.9 (1.6–5.1) in men; OR = 13.2 (1.5–113.0) in women	Alcohol drinker OR = 1.9 (1.2–3.0) in men	Senior staff OR = 2.6 (1.6–4.3) in men	Potassium excretion not significant	Age group 10-year groups, BMI, sodium excretion, and staff status.	Logistic regression
Civil servants [18]	Ibadan	For both sexes, normalized WHR, plasma glucose, age, and family history of diabetes. Only age predicted HTN in women.	OR = 1.1	NS	—	WHR, OR = 1.35	—	—	Height not associated with BP or HTN	Age, family history of diabetes, sex, plasma glucose, and normalized WHR.	Logistic regression
Civil servants [9]	Accra	Age group > 35 years, male sex, and physical inactivity	Age group 35–44 years OR = 3.8 (2.0–7.4); 45–54 years OR = 11.3 (6.4–21.5); ≥55 years OR = 15.0 (8.2–29.8)	Female sex OR = 0.71 (0.50–0.99)	Moderate OR = 0.7 (0.5–1.0); intense OR = 0.6 (0.3–1.2)	NS	NS			Sex, age groups, BMI, physical activity, and alcohol use.	Logistic regression

Table 3: Continued.

Study population	Location	Determinants	Age	Sex	Physical activity	Obesity or adiposity	Alcohol	SES	Others	Variables in model	Type of analysis
Civil servants [65]	Accra	Positive graded association between staff grade and HTN and current wealth when adjusted for age and sex. Statistically significant associations are lost when BMI is controlled for.						NS		Age, sex, preadult and current wealth, employment grade, level of education, and BMI.	Logistic regression with age as continuous variable
Civil servants [13]	Kaduna City	Age group ≥ 40 years, family history (OR 1.5, 95% CI 1.1–2.1).	AOR ≥ 40 years = 6.7 (95% CI 4.1–11.0) compared with age group < 40 years						Marital status not significantly associated with HTN	Age, marital status, and family history	Logistic regression
Health workers in a Teaching Hospital [27]	Jos City	Alcohol (OR 2.58, $p = 0.03$) and obesity (OR 3.37, $p = 0.006$) were found to be independently associated with hypertension.				OR = 3.37, $p = 0.006$	OR = 2.58, $p = 0.03$			Age, sex, BMI, and alcohol	Logistic regression
Health workers [31]	Yenagoa	Age groups > 30 years.	AOR 30–45 years = 4.147 (95% CI 1.25–13.67), > 45 years = 5.45 (95% CI 1.46–22.80) compared with age group < 30 years	NS	—	Truncal obesity (WC > 102 cm in men, >88 cm in females) versus normal WC; AOR = 3.64 (95% CI 1.15–9.06). BMI and WHR = NS	—	Educational level: NS	Marital status: NS	Age, sex, marital status, level of education, family history of HTN, past history of diabetes, family history of diabetes, history of alcohol use, smoking, BMI, WC, and WHR.	Logistic regression

Table 3: Continued.

Study population	Location	Determinants	Age	Sex	Physical activity	Obesity or adiposity	Alcohol	SES	Others	Variables in model	Type of analysis
Male factory workers [39]	Ibadan	Education associated with BP, after adjusting for age, BMI, pulse, and alcohol consumption.								Age, BMI, pulse rate, and current alcohol drinking.	Multiple logistic analysis of covariance
Market workers (traders and artisans) [36]	Enugu	Age, BMI, and alcohol consumption predicted HTN.	Increasing age	Not significantly associated with HTN		Significant factor	Significant factor	—		Age, sex, smoking, snuff tobacco, alcohol, BMI, WHR, and educational status.	Multiple linear regression

HTN: hypertension; OR: odds ratio; SES: socioeconomic status.

consumption. The multivariable-adjusted mean SBP and DBP were each about 4 mmHg higher in those with the highest education level compared to those with the lowest educational level ($p < 0.05$). Male factory workers with 13 or more years of education were two and half times as likely to have hypertension as those with less than 10 years of education, after adjusting for age, body mass index, pulse, and alcohol consumption (OR 2.4, 95% CI 1.2–5.1) [39].

Among bank workers in Ibadan, age- and BMI-adjusted BP were correlated to years of education and income in men, but not in women [44]. However, there was no consistent association between the mean SBP and DBP and educational level in men and women. The highest mean SBP and DBP were not found among male or female subjects with tertiary education. Rather, in men, they were found in those with secondary education while, in women, they were found among those with primary education. Conversely, the lowest mean BP was found in men with and women with secondary education.

In multiple linear regression analyses, Lang et al. [38] found that, among 914 male industry and hotel workers in Dakar, increasing age, number of glasses of tea consumed daily, and illiteracy were significantly associated with SBP. However, only age and BMI were significantly associated with DBP. Shift work was associated with neither SBP nor DBP. Ethnicity was significantly associated with SBP ($p = 0.05$) but not with DBP.

The determinants of hypertension among civil servants in Kaduna in 2012 were older age and a positive family history of hypertension [13]. Those who were aged ≥ 40 years were 6.7 times (95% CI 4.1–11.0) as likely as those aged < 40 years to have hypertension. Those with a positive family history were 1.5 times (95% CI 1.1–2.1) as likely as those without a family history to have hypertension.

In the Accra Civil servants Study, Addo et al. [9] found that age groups older than 35 years, male sex, and obesity were the determinants of hypertension in a model adjusted for age and sex. However, after adjusting for additional variables (BMI, physical activity, and alcohol use), obesity lost its statistical significance. Alcohol intake was not related to hypertension in all the models while moderate and intense physical activities were protective. Multiple regression analyses showed that BMI, waist circumference, and SBP were inversely associated with physical activity among civil servants and health workers in Maiduguri, Nigeria [19].

Age, alcohol, and BMI were the predictors of hypertension among market workers in Enugu [36]. Sex, smoking, snuff tobacco, and WHR were not significantly associated with hypertension. Among health workers in a tertiary hospital in Jos City, Nigeria, alcohol (OR 2.58, $p = 0.03$) and obesity (OR 3.37, $p = 0.006$) were independently associated with hypertension [27]. However, among health workers in a tertiary hospital in Yenagoa, Nigeria, truncal obesity (as determined by waist circumference) but not general obesity was independently associated with hypertension after adjusting for age, gender, marital status, education, family history of diabetes or hypertension, and behavioural risk factors [31]. Health workers who had abdominal obesity were 3.2 times as likely as those with normal waist circumference to have hypertension (95% CI 1.15–9.06). Besides waist circumference, age was the only other variable that was independently associated with hypertension, using health workers younger than 30 years as the reference group (Table 3).

3.3.1. Summary. It can thus be concluded from these multivariate analyses that the major determinants of increased BP and hypertension among workers in West Africa were similar to the factors. They included older age group, male sex, higher income, senior staff grade, alcohol intake, BMI, general or truncal obesity, alcohol consumption, plasma glucose, sodium excretion, and sodium-potassium ratio. Nonmigrant status was associated with decreased BP while moderate-to-vigorous physical activity was protective against hypertension and BP. The number of children, educational level, and ethnicity were inconsistently associated with BP or hypertension.

4. Discussion

This is the first systematic review of the determinants of arterial blood pressure and hypertension among workers in West Africa. The review involved a large number of workers covering different groups of formal and informal sector workers, included articles in the French language, and covered a 35-year period. It showed that the mean BP levels among workers in West Africa are high. Twenty-three (85.1%) of the 27 studies reporting mean BP were in the prehypertension range. Nearly a fifth of the studies recorded mean populations' BP in the high-range prehypertension category. High mean BP is not unique to workers. A recent systematic review of 27 community-based studies in Nigeria including four covered by the current review estimated a pooled mean SBP of 128.6 mmHg (95% CI 125.5–130.8 mmHg) and a mean DBP of 80.6 mmHg (95% CI 78.5–82.7 mmHg) [73].

Prehypertension, particularly high-range grade, has been associated with increased risk of incident stroke and cardiovascular morbidity and mortality [74, 75]. Persons with prehypertension may have an increased risk of progressing to hypertension [76]. Consequently, the Seventh Joint National Committee recommended nonpharmacological measures in individuals such as weight management, reduced dietary intake of salt, physical activity, and moderation of salt intake to manage prehypertension [77]. Antihypertensives have also been shown to prevent the progression to hypertension in individuals with prehypertension [78]. There is a dearth of studies specifically evaluating the impact of population-based strategies on prehypertension. However, community-based interventions such as health education campaigns in the media, schools, and workplaces, nutritional advice, and worksite exercise breaks have been shown to reduce mean BP in low-income countries [79].

The factors and determinants associated with BP and hypertension were broadly similar. The most consistent biological factors were increasing age and male sex while the most consistent lifestyle factors were sodium excretion, alcohol consumption, and obesity. As in general population studies, workers in urban settings had higher BP than those in rural settings [73, 80, 81].

Among the lifestyle factors, dietary salt intake is one of the least studied in West Africa although reduction in dietary salt, fat, and sugar intake is one of the priority actions recommended by the expert Lancet NCD Group [82]. It is also one of the voluntary NCD targets in WHO's Global Action Plan [1]. In this review, urinary sodium excretion was one of the independent risk factors associated with hypertension. One-third of the relatively young population of bankers in Benin City reported that they added extra salt to their food [45]. In Nigeria, market workers spend most of their day at their market and have little options except to buy fast food or food from street vendors, which is typically high in salt content [36].

There are hardly any successful salt reduction programmes in Africa where, unlike in developed countries, salt tends to be added to the food during cooking and at serving and the consumption of processed foods is low [83]. In many countries, screening of food vendors is limited to microbiological safety with little interest in the nutritional quality of food that is sold to the general public including school children and workers. A community-based health promotion programme in 12 villages in Ghana led to modest declines in the BP after six months, although there was no significant change in the urinary sodium excretion. In the Iran Healthy Heart Program, an integrated set of interventions involving public education, healthy nutrition, physical activity, tobacco control, and stress management using the mass media, community participation was associated with statistically significant reductions in dietary salt intake, sodium excretion, and BP after a nine-year follow-up [84]. There are more concerted efforts by stakeholders including health professionals, regulatory agencies, industry, local government, social welfare, and the civil society to reduce dietary salt intake in West Africa.

Inadequate knowledge about hypertension in Africa is pervasive, with belief that it is due to fate, evil spirits, or excessive thinking and that it is curable [8, 20, 45, 85]. Some West African workers had a low perception of their risk of complications. Those who were obese or had multiple risk factors did not correctly identify themselves as such and so were little concerned about their risk profile. There was a significant gap between those who self-reported that they did not have hypertension and those who were found to have hypertension [52]. The misperceptions and the gaps in knowledge call for regular programmes to be instituted to educate formal and informal sector workers as well as the general public about cardiovascular health in the context of the current nutrition transition.

Over 90% of bankers in Nigeria felt that their work was stressful [45]. As with similar formal and sedentary jobs such as civil servants, bankers work long hours daily, up to six days weekly. Workers who constantly face this combination of sedentariness and stress should not simply be left to take care of themselves. As this review showed, there is often clustering of cardiovascular risk factors. Companies, therefore, have a responsibility to provide the enabling environment and programmes to encourage their workers to adopt healthy lifestyles within and without work hours. The example of an Employee Well-Being programme in Ghana involving eight private companies in partnership with the Ministry of Health and the German Cooperation is commendable [86]. The programme aims to improve the health, social protection, and financial wellness of employees and their immediate families. Worksite health programmes could improve cardiovascular health even at low attendance rates [87].

Obesity emerged as a strong predictor of BP and hypertension among workers. Successful models are needed for both formal and informal sector workers in resource-poor settings. In developing countries, community-based interventions have generally not been effective at reducing obesity. In a systematic review of community-based interventions [79], only one of four studies involving worksite interventions involving the integration of exercise breaks into organizational routine in Mexico was accompanied by reductions in BMI and waist circumference [88]. In western countries, successful worksite interventions for weight reduction combine diet, physical activity, and environmental changes [89]. Interventions such as price discounts for healthier foods from workplace canteens or vending machines and internet- or phone-based nutritional and exercise counselling, successful in western countries, may not be relevant or readily applicable in poor countries. On the other hand, health education to reduce fat, sugar, and alcohol and increase fruit and vegetable intake; small group sessions on increasing knowledge on weight management; newsletters, posters, and health promotional materials; and encouraging commuting to work, use of stairs, encouraging walking at lunch, environmental prompts to promote physical activity, and healthy eating and promoting group exercises could be useful.

The relationship between certain variables such as ethnicity and education among workers and hypertension in this review was not clear. Longitudinal studies are needed to better elucidate the determinants of incident cardiovascular disease in sub-Saharan Africa [90]. Studies are also needed to document what are the best delivery models to reduce chronic disease risks among sedentary workers in the informal sector with low literacy levels. Systematic reviews and meta-analysis to synthesize evidence on the prevalence or the determinants would help improve current understanding of the epidemiology of chronic diseases in Africa [73, 91–94].

Some limitations of this review should be noted. There was wide heterogeneity in the study population, definition of variables, methods of measurements, and analyses. These limit the generalizability of the findings to different types of workers in West Africa. Several studies adjusted for only a limited number of potential confounders and so may account for the differences in the effect sizes between studies. There was particular challenge in retrieving papers in this systematic review as 45% of the articles were published in less known African journals, some of which did not offer online full-text articles. The search strategy was meticulous and the database was comprehensive and so it is unlikely that significant studies among workers may have been missed. These limitations notwithstanding, the findings relating to factors and determinants were broadly consistent between studies conducted among workers and with studies conducted in the general population.

5. Conclusion

There are modifiable risk factors associated with BP and hypertension in workers in West Africa. Risk factors independently associated with mean BP include male sex, increasing age, marital status, higher income, senior staff grade, BMI, sodium excretion, and sodium-potassium ratio. The major determinants of hypertension among West African workers were similar to those of BP and included male sex, older age group, higher socioeconomic status, general or truncal obesity, alcohol consumption, plasma glucose, and sodium excretion. Measures to reduce mean BP and hypertension should include population-wide and worksite strategies to reduce dietary salt intake and other risk behaviours, reduce stress, improve physical activity, and increase knowledge of workers about cardiovascular health. More collaboration is needed between health sector, labour, local government, industry, nutrition and food societies, civil society, and workers' associations to prioritize the health of formal and informal sector workers in Africa.

Acknowledgments

The author would like to thank the management of the West African Health Organisation for the general support for programmes to prevent and control NCDs in the region. The author thanks all the authors who provided the full-text articles and clarified certain data in their papers.

References

[1] World Health Organization, *Global Action Plan for the Prevention and Control of Noncommunicable Diseases 2013–2020*, WHO, Geneva, Switzerland, 2013.

[2] R. M. van Dam, T. Li, D. Spiegelman, O. H. Franco, and F. B. Hu, "Combined impact of lifestyle factors on mortality: prospective cohort study in US women," *The BMJ*, vol. 337, article a1440, 2008.

[3] C. Heidemann, M. B. Schulze, O. H. Franco, R. M. van Dam, C. S. Mantzoros, and F. B. Hu, "Dietary patterns and risk of mortality from cardiovascular disease, cancer, and all causes in a prospective cohort of women," *Circulation*, vol. 118, no. 3, pp. 230–237, 2008.

[4] M. McKee, A. Haines, S. Ebrahim et al., "Towards a comprehensive global approach to prevention and control of NCDs," *Globalization and Health*, vol. 10, article 74, 2014.

[5] World Health Organization, "Workers' health: global plan of action 2008–2017. WHA60.26," in *Sixtieth World Health Assembly*, WHO, Geneva, Switzerland, 2007.

[6] J. U. Nwamarah and G. T. O. Otitoju, "Fruit and vegetable consumption pattern and health challenges of elderly (≥60 years) staff in the university of Nigeria, Nsukka and Enugu Campuses: a case study," *Pakistan Journal of Nutrition*, vol. 13, no. 11, pp. 626–630, 2014.

[7] World Health Organization, *A Global Brief on Hypertension: World Health Day 2013*, World Health Organization (WHO), Geneva, Switzerland, 2013.

[8] W. K. Bosu, "The prevalence, awareness, and control of hypertension among workers in West Africa: a systematic review," *Global Health Action*, vol. 8, Article ID 26227, 2015.

[9] J. Addo, L. Smeeth, and D. A. Leon, "Prevalence, detection, management, and control of hypertension in Ghanaian civil servants," *Ethnicity & Disease*, vol. 18, no. 4, pp. 505–511, 2008.

[10] C. H. Bunker, F. I. Okoro, N. Markovic et al., "Relationship of hypertension to socioeconomic status in a West African population," *Ethnicity and Health*, vol. 1, no. 1, pp. 33–45, 1996.

[11] C. H. Bunker, F. A. Ukoli, M. U. Nwankwo et al., "Factors associated with hypertension in Nigerian civil servants," *Preventive Medicine*, vol. 21, no. 6, pp. 710–722, 1992.

[12] E. B. Ekpo, O. Udofia, N. F. Eshiet, and J. J. Andy, "Demographic, life style and anthropometric correlates of blood pressure of Nigerian urban civil servants, factory and plantation workers," *Journal of Human Hypertension*, vol. 6, no. 4, pp. 275–280, 1992.

[13] A. M. Oladimeji, O. Fawole, P. Nguku, and P. Nsubuga, "Prevalence and factors associated with hypertension and obesity among civil servants in Kaduna, Kaduna State, June 2012," *Pan African Medical Journal*, vol. 18, supplement 1, article 18, 2014.

[14] V. O. Oviasu and F. E. Okupa, "Arterial blood pressure and hypertension in Benin in the equatorial forest zone of Nigeria," *Tropical and Geographical Medicine*, vol. 32, no. 3, pp. 241–244, 1980.

[15] O. G. Egbi, U. H. Okafor, K. E. Meibodei, O. E. Kunle-Olowu, and E. I. Unuigbe, "Prevalence of hypertension in an urban population in Bayelsa State, Nigeria," *Journal of Medical Research and Practice*, vol. 2, no. 1, pp. 11–15, 2013.

[16] K. Yayehd, F. Damorou, E. Ehlan et al., "Connaissances sur l'hypertension artérielle, attitudes et mode de vie parmi les employés d'un département ministériel à Lomé, Togo," *Angéiologie*, vol. 64, no. 3, pp. 63–70, 2013.

[17] S. L. Huston, C. H. Bunker, F. A. M. Ukoli, P. M. Rautaharju, and L. H. Kuller, "Electrocardiographic left ventricular hypertrophy by five criteria among civil servants in Benin City, Nigeria: prevalence and correlates," *International Journal of Cardiology*, vol. 70, no. 1, pp. 1–14, 1999.

[18] S. T. Olatunbosun, J. S. Kaufman, R. S. Cooper, and A. F. Bella, "Hypertension in a black population: prevalence and biosocial determinants of high blood pressure in a group of urban Nigerians," *Journal of Human Hypertension*, vol. 14, no. 4, pp. 249–257, 2000.

[19] A. L. Oyeyemi and O. Adeyemi, "Relationship of physical activity to cardiovascular risk factors in an urban population of Nigerian adults," *Archives of Public Health*, vol. 71, no. 1, p. 6, 2013.

[20] A. A. Akintunde, A. A. Salawu, and O. G. Opadijo, "Prevalence of traditional cardiovascular risk factors among staff of Ladoke Akintola University of Technology, Ogbomoso, Nigeria," *Nigerian Journal of Clinical Practice*, vol. 17, no. 6, pp. 750–755, 2014.

[21] A. Atatsi, M. Djibril, E. Goeh-Akue, A. Ephoevi-Ga, and L. Gayibor, "Aspects epidemiologiques de l'hypertension arterielle chez les travailleurs de l'universite de Lome," *Journal de la Recherche Scientifique de l'Universite de Lome*, vol. 8, no. 2, pp. 219–222, 2006.

[22] B. Ordinioha, "The prevalence of hypertension and its modifiable risk factors among lecturers of a medical school in Port Harcourt, south-south Nigeria: implications for control effort," *Nigerian Journal of Clinical Practice*, vol. 16, no. 1, pp. 1–11, 2013.

[23] R. Aryeetey and J. Ansong, "Overweight and hypertension among college of health sciences employees in Ghana," *African Journal of Food, Agriculture, Nutrition and Development*, vol. 11, no. 6, pp. 5444–5456, 2011.

[24] C. O. Emerole, E. N. Aguwa, C. N. Onwasigwe, and B. A. Nwakoby, "Cardiac risk indicess of staff of Federal Univesity of Technology Owerri, Imo state, Nigeria," *Tanzania Health Research Bulletin*, vol. 9, no. 2, pp. 132–135, 2007.

[25] O. K. Ige, E. T. Owoaje, and O. A. Adebiyi, "Non communicable disease and risky behaviour in an urban university community Nigeria," *African Health Sciences*, vol. 13, no. 1, pp. 62–67, 2013.

[26] W. O. Erhun, G. Olayiwola, E. O. Agbani, and N. S. Omotoso, "Prevalence of hypertension in a university community in South West Nigeria," *African Journal of Biomedical Research*, vol. 8, no. 1, pp. 15–19, 2005.

[27] O. Funke and K. S. Ibrahim, "Blood pressure and body mass index among Jos University Teaching Hospital staff," *Transnational Journal of Science and Technology*, vol. 3, no. 9, pp. 73–83, 2013.

[28] C. Konin, E. Kramoh, J. B. Anzouan-Kacou et al., "Approche diagnostique et prise en charge de l'hypertension artérielle chez le personnel soignant du district d'Abidjan (Côte d'Ivoire)," *Revue d'Epidémiologie et de Santé Publique*, vol. 60, no. 1, pp. 41–46, 2012.

[29] K. Uwanuruochi, O. J. Ukpabi, C. N. Onwuta, B. J. Onwubere, B. C. Anisiuba, and F. S. Michael, "Cardiovascular risk factors in adult staff of Federal Medical Centre, Umuahia: a comparison with other Nigerian studies," *West African Journal of Medicine*, vol. 32, no. 4, pp. 243–247, 2013.

[30] A. M. Adeoye, A. Adebiyi, and A. Falase, "PM247 Pre hypertension among apparently normal healthcare providers: an opportunity for workplace health promotion program," *Global Heart*, vol. 9, no. 1, supplement, p. e111, 2014.

[31] O. G. Egbi, S. Rotifa, and J. Jumbo, "Prevalence of hypertension and its correlates among employees of a tertiary hospital in Yenagoa, Nigeria," *Annals of African Medicine*, vol. 14, no. 1, pp. 8–17, 2015.

[32] A. O. Owolabi, M. O. Owolabi, A. D. OlaOlorun, and A. Olofin, "Work-related stress perception and hypertension amongst health workers of a mission hospital in Oyo State, south-western Nigeria," *African Journal of Primary Health Care and Family Medicine*, vol. 4, no. 1, pp. 1–7, 2012.

[33] M. O. Balogun and E. T. Owoaje, "Work conditions and health problems of female traders in Ibadan, Nigeria," *African Journal of Medicine and Medical Sciences*, vol. 36, no. 1, pp. 57–63, 2007.

[34] M. A. Charles-Davies, A. A. Fasanmade, J. A. Olaniyi et al., "Metabolic alterations in different stages of hypertension in an apparently healthy Nigerian population," *International Journal of Hypertension*, vol. 2013, Article ID 351357, 6 pages, 2013.

[35] T. O. Odugbemi, A. T. Onajole, and A. O. Osibogun, "Prevalence of cardiovascular risk factors amongst traders in an urban market in Lagos, Nigeria," *The Nigerian Postgraduate Medical Journal*, vol. 19, no. 1, pp. 1–6, 2012.

[36] I. I. Ulasi, C. K. Ijoma, B. J. C. Onwubere, E. Arodiwe, O. Onodugo, and C. Okafor, "High prevalence and low awareness of hypertension in a market population in Enugu, Nigeria," *International Journal of Hypertension*, vol. 2011, Article ID 869675, 5 pages, 2011.

[37] C. A. Oladoyinbo, N. N. Ekerette, and T. I. Ogunubi, "Obesity and hypertension amongst traders in Ijebu Ode, Nigeria," *African Journal of Biomedical Research*, vol. 18, no. 1, pp. 23–27, 2015.

[38] T. Lang, P. Pariente, G. Salem, and D. Tap, "Social, professional conditions and arterial hypertension: an epidemiological study in Dakar, Senegal," *Journal of Hypertension*, vol. 6, no. 4, pp. 271–276, 1988.

[39] A. Ogunlesi, B. Osotimehin, F. Abbiyessuku et al., "Blood pressure and educational level among factory workers in Ibadan, Nigeria," *Journal of Human Hypertension*, vol. 5, no. 5, pp. 375–380, 1991.

[40] R. O. Shittu, M. A. Sanni, L. O. Odeigah et al., "Medical examination findings among workers in a pharmaceutical industry in Nigeria, West Africa," *Research Journal of Pharmaceutical, Biological and Chemical Sciences*, vol. 5, no. 3, pp. 1660–1668, 2014.

[41] W. H. Giles, M. Pacqué, B. M. Greene et al., "Prevalence of hypertension in rural West Africa," *American Journal of the Medical Sciences*, vol. 308, no. 5, pp. 271–275, 1994.

[42] A. O. B. Olugbile and A. Oyemade, "Health and the environment—a comparative study of agricultural and industrial workers in Nigeria," *African Journal of Medicine and Medical Sciences*, vol. 10, no. 3-4, pp. 107–112, 1981.

[43] R. O. Abidoye, R. D. Izunwa, F. O. Akinkuade, and G. O. Abidoye, "Inter-relationships between lifestyle and diabetes mellitus, overweight/obesity and hypertension in Nigeria," *Nutrition and Health*, vol. 16, no. 3, pp. 203–213, 2002.

[44] S. Kadiri, O. Walker, B. L. Salako, and O. Akinkugbe, "Blood pressure, hypertension and correlates in urbanised workers in Ibadan, Nigeria: a revisit," *Journal of Human Hypertension*, vol. 13, no. 1, pp. 23–27, 1999.

[45] A. Ofili and V. Omuemu, "Knowledge and prevalence of risk factors for hypertension among workers in the banking industry in Benin-City, Edo State, Nigeria," *Tropical Journal of Health Sciences*, vol. 12, no. 1, pp. 26–30, 2005.

[46] A. G. Salaudeen, O. I. Musa, O. A. Babatunde, O. A. Atoyebi, K. A. Durowade, and L. O. Omokanye, "Knowledge and prevalence of risk factors for arterial hypertension and blood pressure pattern among bankers and traffic wardens in Ilorin, Nigeria," *African Health Sciences*, vol. 14, no. 3, pp. 593–599, 2014.

[47] A. Mbaye, M. B. Ndiaye, A. Kane et al., "Médecine du travail à travers le monde. Dépistage des facteurs de risque cardiovasculaire chez les travailleurs d'une société privée de télécommunications au Sénégal," *Archives des Maladies Professionnelles et de l'Environnement*, vol. 72, no. 1, pp. 96–99, 2011.

[48] E. K. Oghagbon, A. B. Okesina, and S. A. Biliaminu, "Prevalence of hypertension and associated variables in PATD workers in Ilorin, Nigeria," *Nigerian Journal of Clinical Practice*, vol. 11, no. 4, pp. 342–346, 2008.

[49] O. Okojie, E. Isah, and E. Okoro, "Assessment of health of senior executives in a developing country," *Public Health*, vol. 114, no. 4, pp. 273–275, 2000.

[50] R. O. Abidoye, L. A. Madueke, and G. O. Abidoye, "The relationship between dietary habits and body-mass index using the federal airport authority of Nigeria as the sample," *Nutrition and Health*, vol. 16, no. 3, pp. 215–227, 2002.

[51] S. M. Seck, S. Guéye, K. Tamba, and I. Ba, "Prevalence of chronic cardiovascular and metabolic diseases in senegalese workers: a cross-sectional study, 2010," *Preventing Chronic Disease*, vol. 10, no. 1, Article ID 110339, 2013.

[52] H. Aidoo, A. Essuman, P. Aidoo, A. O. Yawson, and A. E. Yawson, "Health of the corporate worker: health risk assessment among staff of a corporate organization in Ghana," *Journal of Occupational Medicine and Toxicology*, vol. 10, no. 1, article 30, 2015.

[53] N. Amidu, W. Owiredu, E. Mireku, and C. Agyemang, "Metabolic syndrome among garage workers in the automobile industry in Kumasi, Ghana," *Journal of Medical and Biomedical Sciences*, vol. 1, no. 3, pp. 29–36, 2012.

[54] M. N. Ebare, V. O. Omuemu, and E. C. Isah, "Assessment of noise levels generated by music shops in an urban city in Nigeria," *Public Health*, vol. 125, no. 9, pp. 660–664, 2011.

[55] F. O. Omokhodion and O. O. Kolude, "Health problems of mill operators in a tropical African population," *West African Journal of Medicine*, vol. 24, no. 3, pp. 256–258, 2005.

[56] N. M. Koffi, S. J. Sally, P. Kouame, K. Silue, and A. J. Diarra Nama, "Faciès de l'hypertension artérielle en milieu professionnel à Abidjan," *Médecine d'Afrique Noire*, vol. 48, no. 6, pp. 257–260, 2001.

[57] O. E. Amoran, A. A. Salako, and O. Jeminusi, "Screening for common occupational health diseases among long distance professional drivers in Sagamu, Ogun State, Nigeria," *International Journal of Preventive Medicine*, vol. 5, no. 4, pp. 516–521, 2014.

[58] Z. M. Ofuya, "The incidence of hypertension among a select population of adults in the Niger Delta region of Nigeria," *Southeast Asian Journal of Tropical Medicine and Public Health*, vol. 38, no. 5, pp. 947–949, 2007.

[59] P. E. Idahosa, "Hypertension: an ongoing health hazard in Nigerian workers," *American Journal of Epidemiology*, vol. 125, no. 1, pp. 85–91, 1987.

[60] J. S. Kaufman, E. E. Owoaje, S. A. James, C. N. Rotimi, and R. S. Cooper, "Determinants of hypertension in West Africa: contribution of anthropometric and dietary factors to urban-rural and socioeconomic gradients," *American Journal of Epidemiology*, vol. 143, no. 12, pp. 1203–1218, 1996.

[61] B. Ordinioha and S. Brisibe, "Prevalence of hypertension and its modifiable risk factors amongst traditional chiefs of an oil-bearing community in south-south Nigeria," *Sahel Medical Journal*, vol. 16, no. 1, pp. 24–27, 2013.

[62] C. H. Bunker, F. A. Ukoli, K. A. Matthews, A. M. Kriska, S. L. Huston, and L. H. Kuller, "Weight threshold and blood pressure in a lean black population," *Hypertension*, vol. 26, no. 4, pp. 616–623, 1995.

[63] A. M. Adeoye, A. Adebiyi, and A. Falase, "PM247 pre hypertension Among Apparently Normal Healthcare Providers: an opportunity for Workplace Health Promotion Program," *Global Heart*, vol. 9, no. 1, p. e111, 2014.

[64] C. H. Bunker, M. U. Nwankwo, F. A. Ukoli et al., "Factors related to blood pressure among urban Nigerian workers," *Journal of Human Hypertension*, vol. 4, no. 2, pp. 82–84, 1990.

[65] J. Addo, L. Smeeth, and D. A. Leon, "Socioeconomic position and hypertension: a study of urban civil servants in Ghana," *Journal of Epidemiology and Community Health*, vol. 63, no. 8, pp. 646–650, 2009.

[66] I. I. Ulasi, C. K. Ijoma, and O. D. Onodugo, "A community-based study of hypertension and cardio-metabolic syndrome in semi-urban and rural communities in Nigeria," *BMC Health Services Research*, vol. 10, article 71, 2010.

[67] N. Markovic, K. A. Matthews, S. L. Huston, E. Egbagbe, F. A. M. Ukoli, and C. H. Bunker, "Blood pressure reactivity to stress varies by hypertensive status and sex in Nigerians," *American Journal of Epidemiology*, vol. 142, no. 10, pp. 1020–1028, 1995.

[68] V. O. Oviasu and F. E. Okupa, "Occupational factors in hypertension in the Nigerian African," *Journal of Epidemiology and Community Health*, vol. 33, no. 4, pp. 274–278, 1979.

[69] A. A. Akintunde, A. A. Salawu, and O. G. Opadijo, "Assessment of Snoring and obstructive sleep apnoea in a Nigerian university: association with cardiovascular risk factors," *Nigerian Medical Journal: Journal of the Nigeria Medical Association*, vol. 55, no. 6, pp. 469–473, 2014.

[70] A. Edo and O. S. Adediran, "Dyslipidaemia among Nigerian oil workers with type 2 diabetes mellitus," *West African Journal of Medicine*, vol. 30, no. 3, pp. 206–209, 2011.

[71] S. Baragou, B. L. Soussou, E. Goeh-Akue, F. Damorou, A. Djato, and M. Pio, "Prevalence de l'hypertension arterielle et des principaux facteurs de risque cardiovasculaire en milieu professionnel a Lome," *Journal de la Recherche Scientifique de l'Universite de Lome*, vol. 8, no. 2, 2006.

[72] S. T. Olatunbosun and A. F. Bella, "Relationship between height, glucose intolerance, and hypertension in an urban African black adult population: a case for the 'thrifty phenotype' hypothesis?" *Journal of the National Medical Association*, vol. 92, no. 6, pp. 265–268, 2000.

[73] D. Adeloye, C. Basquill, A. V. Aderemi, J. Y. Thompson, and F. A. Obi, "An estimate of the prevalence of hypertension in Nigeria: a systematic review and meta-analysis," *Journal of Hypertension*, vol. 33, no. 2, pp. 230–242, 2015.

[74] Y. Huang, X. Cai, Y. Li et al., "Prehypertension and the risk of stroke. A meta-analysis," *Neurology*, vol. 82, no. 13, pp. 1153–1161, 2014.

[75] Y. Huang, L. Su, X. Cai et al., "Association of all-cause and cardiovascular mortality with prehypertension: a meta-analysis," *American Heart Journal*, vol. 167, no. 2, pp. 160.e1–168.e1, 2014.

[76] D. Conen, P. M. Ridker, J. E. Buring, and R. J. Glynn, "Risk of cardiovascular events among women with high normal blood pressure or blood pressure progression: prospective cohort study," *British Medical Journal*, vol. 335, no. 7617, pp. 432–436, 2007.

[77] A. V. Chobanian, G. L. Bakris, H. R. Black et al., "Seventh report of the joint national committee on prevention, detection, evaluation, and treatment of high blood pressure," *Hypertension*, vol. 42, no. 6, pp. 1206–1252, 2003.

[78] F. D. Fuchs, R. B. de Mello, and S. C. Fuchs, "Preventing the progression of prehypertension to hypertension: role of antihypertensives," *Current Hypertension Reports*, vol. 17, no. 1, pp. 1–6, 2015.

[79] S. van de Vijver, S. Oti, J. Addo, A. de Graft-Aikins, and C. Agyemang, "Review of community-based interventions for prevention of cardiovascular diseases in low- and middle-income countries," *Ethnicity and Health*, vol. 17, no. 6, pp. 651–676, 2012.

[80] J. Addo, L. Smeeth, and D. A. Leon, "Hypertension in sub-Saharan Africa: a systematic review," *Hypertension*, vol. 50, no. 6, pp. 1012–1018, 2007.

[81] W. K. Bosu, "A comprehensive review of the policy and programmatic response to chronic non-communicable disease in Ghana," *Ghana Medical Journal*, vol. 46, no. 2, pp. 69–78, 2012.

[82] R. Beaglehole, R. Bonita, R. Horton et al., "Priority actions for the non-communicable disease crisis," *The Lancet*, vol. 377, no. 9775, pp. 1438–1447, 2011.

[83] S. M. Kerry, L. Emmett, F. B. Micah et al., "Rural and semi-urban differences in salt intake, and its dietary sources, in Ashanti, West Africa," *Ethnicity & Disease*, vol. 15, no. 1, pp. 33–39, 2005.

[84] A. Khosravi, R. Kelishadi, N. Sarrafzadegan et al., "Impact of a community-based lifestyle intervention program on blood pressure and salt intake of normotensive adult population in a developing country," *Journal of Research in Medical Sciences*, vol. 17, no. 3, pp. 235–241, 2012.

[85] V. O. Adika, P. P. K. Joffa, and F. A. Apiyanteide, "Hypertension knowledge among non-academic employees of Niger delta university, Bayelsa state, Nigeria," *International Journal of Tropical Medicine*, vol. 6, no. 5, pp. 113–120, 2011.

[86] T. Holger and G. Newiger-Addy, *Building Effective Employee Wellbeing Programmes in Ghana: A Strategic Alliance for Health and Social Protection*, Deutsche Gesellschaft für Internationale Zusammenarbeit (GIZ) GmbH, Accra, Ghana, 2012.

[87] S. Z. Abbas, T. M. Pollard, P. Wynn, A. Learmonth, K. Joyce, and C. Bambra, "The effectiveness of using the workplace to identify and address modifiable health risk factors in deprived populations," *Occupational and Environmental Medicine*, vol. 72, no. 9, pp. 664–669, 2015.

[88] A. Lara, A. K. Yancey, R. Tapia-Conye et al., "Pausa para tu Salud: reduction of weight and waistlines by integrating exercise breaks into workplace organizational routine," *Preventing Chronic Disease*, vol. 5, no. 1, article A12, 2008.

[89] K. Gudzune, S. Hutfless, N. Maruthur, R. Wilson, and J. Segal, "Strategies to prevent weight gain in workplace and college settings: a systematic review," *Preventive Medicine*, vol. 57, no. 4, pp. 268–277, 2013.

[90] A. P. Kengne, L. M. Ntyintyane, and B. M. Mayosi, "A systematic overview of prospective cohort studies of cardiovascular disease in sub-Saharan Africa: review article," *Cardiovascular Journal of Africa*, vol. 23, no. 2, pp. 103–112, 2012.

[91] A. R. Abubakari, W. Lauder, C. Agyemang, M. Jones, A. Kirk, and R. S. Bhopal, "Prevalence and time trends in obesity among adult West African populations: a meta-analysis," *Obesity Reviews*, vol. 9, no. 4, pp. 297–311, 2008.

[92] O. Ekwunife and C. Aguwa, "PCV27 Increasing prevalence of hypertension in Nigeria: a systematic review from 1990 to 2009," *Value in Health*, vol. 13, no. 7, p. A345, 2010.

[93] M. Essouma, J. J. N. Noubiap, J. J. R. Bigna et al., "Hypertension prevalence, incidence and risk factors among children and adolescents in Africa: a systematic review and meta-analysis protocol," *BMJ Open*, vol. 5, no. 9, Article ID e008472, 2015.

[94] J. W. Stanifer, B. Jing, S. Tolan et al., "The epidemiology of chronic kidney disease in sub-Saharan Africa: a systematic review and meta-analysis," *The Lancet Global Health*, vol. 2, no. 3, pp. e174–e181, 2014.

16

The ACE2/Apelin Signaling, MicroRNAs, and Hypertension

Lai-Jiang Chen,[1,2,3] Ran Xu,[1,2] Hui-Min Yu,[4] Qing Chang,[1,2] and Jiu-Chang Zhong[1,2,3]

[1]*State Key Laboratory of Medical Genomics, Ruijin Hospital, School of Medicine, Shanghai Jiao Tong University, Shanghai 200025, China*
[2]*Shanghai Key Laboratory of Hypertension, Shanghai Institute of Hypertension, Shanghai 200025, China*
[3]*Institute of Health Sciences, Shanghai Institute for Biological Sciences, Chinese Academy of Sciences, Shanghai 200025, China*
[4]*Department of Cardiology, Guangdong General Hospital, Guangdong Academy of Medical Sciences, Guangzhou 510080, China*

Correspondence should be addressed to Jiu-Chang Zhong; jiuchangzhong@aliyun.com

Academic Editor: Markus Schlaich

The renin-angiotensin aldosterone system (RAAS) plays a pivotal role in the development of hypertension. Angiotensin converting enzyme 2 (ACE2), which primarily metabolises angiotensin (Ang) II to generate the beneficial heptapeptide Ang-(1-7), serves as a negative regulator of the RAAS. Apelin is a second catalytic substrate for ACE2 and functions as an inotropic and cardiovascular protective peptide. The physiological effects of Apelin are exerted through binding to its receptor APJ, a seven-transmembrane G protein-coupled receptor that shares significant homology with the Ang II type 1 receptor (AT1R). The deregulation of microRNAs, a class of short and small noncoding RNAs, has been shown to involve cardiovascular remodeling and pathogenesis of hypertension via the activation of the Ang II/AT1R pathway. MicroRNAs are linked with modulation of the ACE2/Apelin signaling, which exhibits beneficial effects in the cardiovascular system and hypertension. The ACE2-coupled crosstalk among the RAAS, the Apelin system, and microRNAs provides an important mechanistic insight into hypertension. This paper focuses on what is known about the ACE2/Apelin signaling and its biological roles, paying particular attention to interactions and crosstalk among the ACE2/Apelin signaling, microRNAs, and hypertension, aiming to facilitate the exploitation of new therapeutic medicine to control hypertension.

1. Introduction

Hypertension is a complex cardiovascular disease and contributes to worldwide morbidity and mortality, while its pathogenesis is closely related to abnormalities of the renin-angiotensin aldosterone system (RAAS) [1]. Angiotensin converting enzyme 2 (ACE2) serves as a negative regulator of RAAS and cleaves angiotensin (Ang) I to generate the inactive Ang-(1-9) peptide, which can then be converted to Ang-(1-7) by ACE [2, 3]. Meanwhile, ACE2 can directly metabolize Ang II to generate the beneficial heptapeptide Ang-(1-7), whose actions are often opposite to those attributed to the Ang II and its type 1 receptor (AT1R) signaling. Apelin, a second catalytic substrate for ACE2, has powerful positive inotropic actions and vasodilatation in an endothelium- and nitric oxide-(NO-) dependent way [4]. Intriguingly, recent studies have demonstrated that there is a link between the ACE2/Apelin signaling and microRNAs (miRNAs) in the pathogenesis of hypertension. The deregulation of miRNAs expression plays a pivotal role in the development of hypertension. The miRNAs are involved in the regulation of diverse biological processes determining cell proliferation, differentiation, migration, and apoptosis [5–7]. In this review, we focus on the relationship among the ACE2/Apelin signaling, miRNAs, and hypertension and aim to facilitate the exploitation of new therapeutic medicine to control hypertension.

2. miRNAs and Hypertension

The miRNAs are small double-stranded, noncoding RNAs that function as guide molecules in RNA silencing [5]. miRNAs may regulate gene expression by binding to the $3'$-untranslated region ($3'$-UTR) of target messenger RNA transcripts, leading to suppression of protein synthesis or mRNA degradation [5–7]. Previous studies have demonstrated that the majority of miRNAs generate from introns of protein-coding transcripts or noncoding genes in canonical pathways [8]. In general, miRNAs are transcribed by RNA polymerase

TABLE 1: The RAAS, Apelin/APJ signaling, and microRNAs in hypertension.

MicroRNAs	Targets	miRNA function	References
miR-143/145	Klf4; Klf5	Regulation of VSMCs proliferation	[7, 16, 17]
miR-365	Cyclin D1	Inhibition of VSMCs proliferation	[18]
miR-221/222	p27(Kip1); p57(Kip2)	Regulation of VSMCs differentiation and proliferation	[6, 7]
miR-126	VEGF; ICAM-1	Mediator of vascular dysfunction	[7, 18]
miR-221/222	Ets-1; VCAM-1; MCP-1	Regulation of inflammation and vascular remodeling	[7, 18]
miR-130a	GAX	Regulation of VSMCs proliferation	[11]
miR-145; -27a/27b;	ACE	Inhibition of ACE expression	[20–23]
miR-421; -143;	ACE2	Inhibition of ACE2 expression	[23, 32, 33]
miR-19b; -29; -132/212; -181b;	Ang II	Promotion of fibrosis and cardiovascular remodeling	[24–27, 29]
miR-146a	Ang-(1-7)	Inhibition of inflammation	[34]
miR-155	AT1R	Inhibition of VSMCs proliferation	[19, 30, 31]
miR-133a; -208; -1	Apelin/APJ	Regulation of cardiovascular hypertrophy and dysfunction	[47]
miR-424; -503	FGF2; FGFR1	Inhibition of VSMCs proliferation	[48]

RAAS: renin-angiotensin aldosterone system; Klf4: Krüppel-like factor4; Klf5: Krüppel-like factor5; p27(Kip1): cyclin-dependent kinase inhibitor 1B; p57(Kip2): cyclin-dependent kinase inhibitor 1B; VEGF: vascular endothelial growth factor; Ets-1: E26 transformation-specific sequence 1; VCAM-1: vascular cell adhesion molecule 1; MCP-1: monocyte chemoattractant protein 1; GAX: growth arrest-specific homeobox; ACE: angiotensin converting enzyme; ACE2: angiotensin converting enzyme 2; AT1R: Ang II type 1 receptor; FGF2: fibroblast growth factor 2; FGFR1: fibroblast growth factor receptor 1; VSMCs: vascular smooth muscle cells.

II as a pri-miRNA, which subsequently cleaved into mature miRNA by two RNase enzymes, Drosha and Dicer, in the nucleus and cytoplasm. miRNAs biogenesis is under stringently control and their deregulation links to various diseases [8]. The regulation of miRNAs occurs at multiple levels of their biogenesis. In the process of miRNAs transcription, miRNAs are controlled by RNA polymerase II-associated transcription factors and epigenetic regulators, such as DNA methylation and histone modifications, which are positively or negatively correlated with miRNAs expression, while in the posttranscriptional levels, the modification of miRNAs processing, including RNA editing, methylation, uridylation, adenylation, and RNA decay, contributes to miRNAs regulation. Several critical cell signaling systems have been linked with regulating miRNAs biogenesis at posttranscription levels, such as transforming growth factor-β/bone morphogenetic protein pathways and mitogen-activated protein kinases signaling pathways, indicating the diverse possibilities for the regulation of miRNAs biogenesis [8, 9].

miRNAs are abundant in all human cells, acting as critical regulators for major cellular functions and miRNAs deregulation associated with a variety of diseases [5, 6]. Recent studies have demonstrated that miRNAs are associated with the pathogenesis of hypertension [7]. In spontaneously hypertensive rats (SHR) model, the expressions of miR-155 and miR-208 were downregulated and negative correlated with blood pressure [10, 11]. Compared with healthy controls, the plasma levels of miR-126, miR-133, miR-143, and miR-145 were decreased in patients with essential hypertension, combined with enhanced expression of miR-1, miR-296-5p, and miR-let-7e [12–14]. Furthermore, expressions of miR-21, miR-143, and miR-145 were negatively correlated with blood pressure levels, while expressions of miR-9, miR-126, and miR-133 were positively correlated with blood pressure levels [5, 12–14].

It is well established that vascular smooth muscle cells (VSMCs) proliferation, differentiated phenotype, and migration are pivotal cellular events for the development of hypertension [15]. miRNAs are highly expressed in vasculature and modulate diverse vascular cell functions (Table 1) [5, 6]. Some specific miRNAs have been identified to be involved in VSMCs biology. MiR-143 and MiR-145 are highly expressed in VSMCs and promote VSMCs differentiation and phenotype transformation via the activation of Krüppel-like factor4 (Klf4) and Klf5 (Table 1) [7, 16, 17]. MiR-143 and miR-145 are important stimuli to maintain vascular smooth muscle contractile differentiation, while knockout of them would decrease the blood pressure levels [16]. In addition, miR-365 exerts an antiproliferative role in VSMCs proliferation via the cell cycle regulatory protein cyclin D1 (Table 1) [18]. p27(Kip1) and p57(Kip2) were 2 target genes that were involved in miR-221- and miR-222-mediated effect on VSMC growth and differentiation (Table 1) [6, 7]. These observations indicate that various miRNAs in vasculature may be linked with hypertension and provide novel pharmacologic implications for the prevention and treatment of hypertension.

3. The ACE/Ang II/AT1R Signaling and MicroRNAs in Hypertension

Activation of the ACE/Ang II/AT1R signaling promotes inflammation, oxidative stress, and fibrosis linked to hypertension, while inhibition of the ACE/Ang II/AT1R signaling

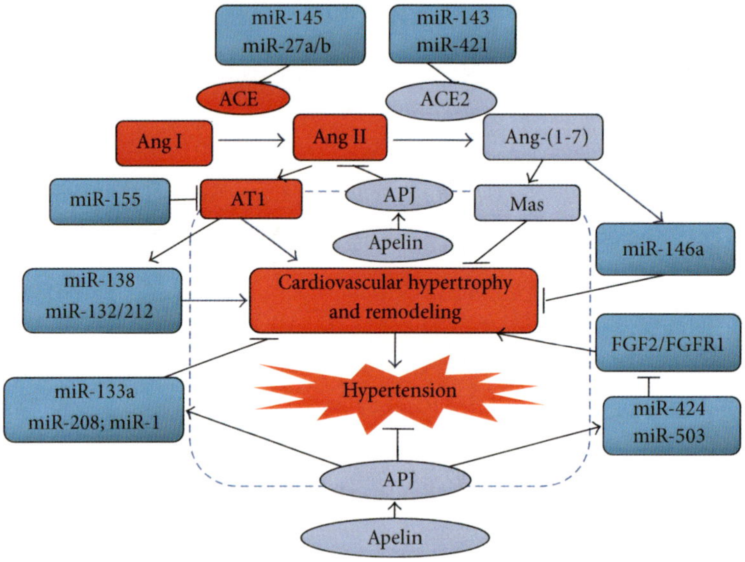

Figure 1: The crosstalk between ACE2/Apelin signaling and miRNAs in hypertension. On one hand, the miR-145 and miR-27a/b suppress the action of ACE/Ang II/AT1R, whereas miR-143 and miR-421 serve as negative regulators of ACE2 to modulate the balance between Ang II degradation and Ang-(1-7) generation. Overexpression of miR-155 inhibits the effects mediated by Ang II/AT1R signaling while Ang II regulates miR-138 and miR-132/212 expression via its receptor AT1R, contributing to cardiovascular hypertrophy and remodeling and elevated blood pressure. In contrast, Ang-(1-7) promotes the level of miR-146a, which blocks inflammation and cardiovascular remodeling. On the other hand, the Apelin/APJ signaling regulates the expression of miR-133a, miR-208, and miR-1, functioning as negative regulators for cardiac hypertrophy and contractile function. Moreover, the Apelin/APJ ameliorates cardiovascular hypertrophy and remodeling by modulating miR-424/-503-FGF signaling. ACE: angiotensin converting enzyme; ACE2: angiotensin converting enzyme 2; Ang II: angiotensin; AT1R: angiotensin II type 1 receptor; miRNAs: microRNAs; FGF2: fibroblast growth factor 2; FGFR1: fibroblast growth factor receptor 1.

has been regarded as important pharmacological tools to prevent and treat vascular diseases such as hypertension [1, 3, 19]. Recently, most researches have been focused on the interactions between the ACE/Ang II/AT1R axis and miRNAs in hypertension. The miR-145, miR-27a/27b, and miR-483-3p have been shown to inhibit ACE expression by directly targeting the putative binding sites in the 3′-UTR of ACE transcripts [20–23]. There exists a negative feedback loop between miR-145 and ACE expression, mediating the switch of VSMC phenotypic differentiation to dedifferentiation. The ACE/Ang II signaling mediates various miRNAs expression via the activation of AT1R and these miRNAs, thereby contributing to VSMCs proliferation, cardiovascular remodeling, and hypertension (Figure 1) [24, 25]. In hypertensive status, Ang II-induced miR-130a mediated VSMCs proliferation and vascular remodeling by preventing the expression of growth arrest-specific homeobox (GAX) [11]. In human microvascular endothelial cells, exposure to Ang II increased the stability of HIF1-α with consequent induction of miR-138, which attenuated the bioavailability of NO and mediated the proinflammatory signal transduction [26]. Eskildsen et al. [27] reported that chronic Ang II infusion enhanced the levels of miR-132/-212 in hypertensive rats, which were prevented by treatment with AT1R blocker. Moreover, they observed that miR-132/-212 fine-tune multiple targets in Ang II signaling led to cardiac hypertrophy and fibrosis [28]. Ang II-mediated miRNAs have been identified to involve hypertension, including miR-19b, miR-29, miR-129-3p, miR-181b, and miR-483-3p (Table 1) [22–25, 29]. Kemp et al. [23] investigated that the miR-483-3p could target some components of RAAS directly. In their study, miR-483-3p regulated homeostatic levels of ACE, ACE2, and AT2R, indicating that this miRNA might function as an important regulator of manipulating RAAS. The intrinsic regulation of Ang II-responsive miRNAs on RAS components suggests that the modulation between Ang II and miRNAs is complicated (Table 1). In another work [30], miR-155 was found as a potent regulator of Ang II-induced VSMCs proliferation by inhibiting AT1R (Figure 1). In hypertensive patients, AT1R expression was negatively correlated with miR-155 expression and the interplay between miR-155 and AT1R was associated with the polymorphism (+1166A/C single-nucleotide polymorphism) located in the 3′-UTR of the AT1R [31]. Although the specific downstream targets of AT1R remain unclear, these findings suggest that miR-155 involve the Ang II/AT1R signaling and relate to vascular diseases.

4. The ACE2/Ang-(1-7)/Mas Signaling and MicroRNAs in Hypertension

The classical pathway of the RAS involving the ACE-Ang II-AT1 receptor axis is now antagonized by the second arm constituted by the ACE2-Ang-(1-7)-Mas receptor axis, exerting protective effects via modulating the inflammation, fibrosis, and vascular remodeling in hypertension [1–3]. Recent studies have shown the link between the ACE2/Ang-(1-7)/Mas signaling and miRNAs in hypertension (Table 1 and Figure 1) [32–34]. miRNA-targeting prediction algorithms revealed pupative binding sites for a variety of miRNAs in the 3′-UTR of ACE2 transcript, while only several miRNAs have been identified as regulators in inhibiting ACE2 expression [23, 32, 33]. In SHR model [33], exercise training significantly decreased the blood pressure levels and miR-143 expression levels in aortas in association with a drastic augment in circulating ACE2 and Ang-(1-7) levels, indicating the regulatory roles of miR-143 in the ACE2/Ang-(1-7) signaling (Table 1 and Figure 1). By establishing luciferase report system containing ACE2 3′-UTR, both miR-421 and miR-483-3p strikingly decreased ACE2 protein levels while loss of the two miRNAs reversed these effects, implying that miR-421 and miR-483-3p modulated ACE2 expression via translational repression rather than degraded the transcripts (Table 1) [23, 32]. In human aortic endothelial cells (Table 1), Ang-(1-7) decreased glycated albumin-mediated vascular inflammation and improved the vascular function through modulating the expression of miR-146a [34]. In addition, treatment with telmisartan modulated the level of miR-146a/b, along with the improvement of the ACE2/Ang-(1-7) levels and attenuation of vascular remodeling in hypertension [35–38]. Satoh et al. [39] reported that blockade of RAAS in coronary artery disease patients decreased protein levels of TLR4 and upregulated TLR4-responsive miRNAs expression including miR-31, miR-181a, miR-16, and miR-145 compared to controls. Although the related mechanism has not been identified, these researches permit speculation that RAAS blockades may exert cardiovascular protective effects by modulating the ACE2/Ang-(1-7) signaling and miRNAs levels. Taken together, there are potential interactions between the ACE2/Ang-(1-7) signaling and miRNAs in hypertension.

5. The Apelin/APJ Signaling and MicroRNAs in Hypertension

Apelin is a second catalytic substrate for ACE2 and functions as an inotropic and cardioprotective peptide [4, 38, 40–43]. The physiological effects of Apelin are exerted through binding to its receptor APJ, a seven-transmembrane G protein-coupled receptor that shares significant homology with the AT1R. Intriguingly, there is 54% sequence homology of the transmembrane regions between the APJ and AT1R and the anatomical distribution of both receptors and peptides overlaps in the cardiovascular system [42]. However, the effects of Apelin is independent of AT1 receptor and Ang II cannot bind to the APJ, although both of Ang II and Apelin can be degraded by ACE2 [38, 43]. The Apelin/APJ system has been shown to be involved in a wide range of pathophysiology effects in cardiovascular system, which is a necessary process in the initiation and development of various cardiovascular diseases such as pulmonary hypertension and essential hypertension [40, 41, 43]. Apelin levels were reduced in patients with essential hypertension independent of left ventricular systolic and diastolic dysfunction [44]. Treatment with Apelin has been shown to lower systolic blood pressure levels in hypertensive rats via a NO-dependent signaling [45, 46]. miRNAs are involved in VSMCs proliferation, cardiovascular remodeling, and the pathogenesis of hypertension (Table 1) [7, 16–18]. Ceylan-Isik et al. [47] found that treatment with Apelin strikingly prevented high fat diet-induced cardiac hypertrophy and contractile dysfunction associated with increased levels of miR-1, miR-208, and miR-133a. In addition, Apelin treatment significantly reduced the expression of fibroblast growth factor 2 (FGF2) and FGF receptor 1 (FGFR1) by regulating miR-424 and miR-503, contributing to the attenuation of VSMCs proliferation (Table 1 and Figure 1). Conversely, Apelin deficiency resulted in a marked increase in FGF2 expression and a reduction in expression of miR-424 and miR-503 that worsen pulmonary arterial hypertension in experimental models, suggesting the regulatory roles of Apelin in maintaining vascular homeostasis via the miR-424/503-FGF signaling [48]. Intriguingly, Apelin upregulated ACE2 in the failing hearts, coupled with upregulation of miR-424 and miR-503, whereas Ang-(1-7) administration improved cardiovascular dysfunction of Apelin-deficient mice in vivo [40, 48]. Moreover, the Apelin-APJ increased ACE2 activity and improved cardiovascular remodeling independently of AT1R signaling [40]. Both ACE2 and Apelin exhibit beneficial effects in the cardiovascular system, and recombinant ACE2 has recently been shown as a candidate therapeutic for treating hypertension in animal models [38, 40, 41]. The crosstalk between the ACE2/Apelin signaling and miRNAs provides an important mechanistic insight into hypertension and may lead to the development of new therapeutic regimens.

6. Conclusions, Limitations, and Perspectives

The discovery of the interaction between the ACE2/Apelin signaling and miRNAs during hypertension is an exciting affair in hypertensive research. ACE2 is a pleiotropic monocarboxypeptidase responsible for the conversion of Ang II to Ang-(1-7), thereby functioning as a negative regulator of the RAAS in cardiovascular system [3, 19, 38]. Apelin, as the second substrate of ACE2, exerts a cardiovascular protective effect including lowering blood pressure and improving cardiac contractility [4, 38–41]. The ACE2/Apelin signaling exhibits beneficial effects in the cardiovascular system and hypertension [3, 4, 38, 40]. The ACE2-coupled crosstalk among the RAAS, the Apelin system, and miRNAs provides an important mechanistic insight into hypertension.

Although most researches indicate the interactions among RAAS, ACE2/Apelin, and miRNAs in hypertension, these correlations are just in statistic level. These researches just found the linkage between the ACE2/Apelin and miRNAs in patients with hypertension or animal models of hypertension or *in vitro* VSMCs. However, the ACE2/Apelin-related miRNAs are really big families which contain "good" or "bad" components and may have additional control mechanisms beyond our current understanding. Thus, the corresponding targets and functional roles of the ACE2/Apelin-related miRNAs still need to be identified. The investigation of the relationship between the ACE2/Apelin signaling and miRNAs is just a beginning; there is still a long way to go. Further studies will be needed to explore the interactions and precise mechanisms of the ACE2/Apelin signaling and evaluate the role of validated and predicted targets of miRNAs in hypertension. Targeting the ACE2/Apelin signaling and miRNAs could lead to the development of a novel therapeutic approach for patients with hypertension and other vascular diseases related to cardiovascular remodeling.

Authors' Contribution

Lai-Jiang Chen and Ran Xu contributed equally to this work.

Acknowledgments

This work was supported by the National Basic Research Program of China (973 Program; 2014CB542300), the Training Program of the National Major Research Plan (91339108), and General Program (81370362, 81273599, and 81170246) of the National Natural Science Foundation of China and Scientific Research Project of Health Bureau of Shanghai (201440368).

References

[1] J. Y. Moon, "Recent update of renin-angiotensin-aldosterone system in the pathogenesis of hypertension," *Electrolytes & Blood Pressure*, vol. 11, no. 2, pp. 41–45, 2013.

[2] V. B. Patel, J.-C. Zhong, D. Fan et al., "Angiotensin-converting enzyme 2 is a critical determinant of angiotensin II-induced loss of vascular smooth muscle cells and adverse vascular remodeling," *Hypertension*, vol. 64, no. 1, pp. 157–164, 2014.

[3] Z. Zhang, L. Chen, J. Zhong, P. Gao, and G. Y. Oudit, "ACE2/Ang-(1–7) signaling and vascular remodeling," *Science China Life Sciences*, vol. 57, no. 8, pp. 802–808, 2014.

[4] X.-H. Yu, Z.-B. Tang, L.-J. Liu et al., "Apelin and its receptor APJ in cardiovascular diseases," *Clinica Chimica Acta*, vol. 428, pp. 1–8, 2014.

[5] X. Song, D. Shan, J. Chen, and Q. Jing, "miRNAs and lncRNAs in vascular injury and remodeling," *Science China Life Sciences*, vol. 57, no. 8, pp. 826–835, 2014.

[6] E. Bronze-da-Rocha, "MicroRNAs expression profiles in cardiovascular diseases," *BioMed Research International*, vol. 2014, Article ID 985408, 23 pages, 2014.

[7] S. Bátkai and T. Thum, "MicroRNAs in hypertension: mechanisms and therapeutic targets," *Current Hypertension Reports*, vol. 14, no. 1, pp. 79–87, 2012.

[8] M. Ha and V. N. Kim, "Regulation of microRNA biogenesis," *Nature Reviews Molecular Cell Biology*, vol. 15, no. 8, pp. 509–524, 2014.

[9] A. Saj and E. C. Lai, "Control of microRNA biogenesis and transcription by cell signaling pathways," *Current Opinion in Genetics and Development*, vol. 21, no. 4, pp. 504–510, 2011.

[10] C. C. Xu, W. Q. Han, B. Xiao, N. N. Li, D. L. Zhu, and P. J. Gao, "Differential expression of microRNAs in the aorta of spontaneously hypertensive rats," *Sheng Li Xue Bao*, vol. 60, no. 4, pp. 553–560, 2008.

[11] W.-H. Wu, C.-P. Hu, X.-P. Chen et al., "MicroRNA-130a mediates proliferation of vascular smooth muscle cells in hypertension," *American Journal of Hypertension*, vol. 24, no. 10, pp. 1087–1093, 2011.

[12] J. E. Kontaraki, M. E. Marketou, E. A. Zacharis, F. I. Parthenakis, and P. E. Vardas, "Differential expression of vascular smooth muscle-modulating microRNAs in human peripheral blood mononuclear cells: novel targets in essential hypertension," *Journal of Human Hypertension*, vol. 28, no. 8, pp. 510–516, 2014.

[13] J. E. Kontaraki, M. E. Marketou, E. A. Zacharis, F. I. Parthenakis, and P. E. Vardas, "MicroRNA-9 and microRNA-126 expression levels in patients with essential hypertension: potential markers of target-organ damage," *Journal of the American Society of Hypertension*, vol. 8, no. 6, pp. 368–375, 2014.

[14] S. Li, J. Zhu, W. Zhang et al., "Signature microRNA expression profile of essential hypertension and its novel link to human cytomegalovirus infection," *Circulation*, vol. 124, no. 2, pp. 175–184, 2011.

[15] E. Schulz, T. Gori, and T. Münzel, "Oxidative stress and endothelial dysfunction in hypertension," *Hypertension Research*, vol. 34, no. 6, pp. 665–673, 2011.

[16] L. Elia, M. Quintavalle, J. Zhang et al., "The knockout of miR-143 and -145 alters smooth muscle cell maintenance and vascular homeostasis in mice: correlates with human disease," *Cell Death and Differentiation*, vol. 16, no. 12, pp. 1590–1598, 2009.

[17] T. Boettger, N. Beetz, S. Kostin et al., "Acquisition of the contractile phenotype by murine arterial smooth muscle cells depends on the Mir143/145 gene cluster," *The Journal of Clinical Investigation*, vol. 119, no. 9, pp. 2634–2647, 2009.

[18] M.-H. Kim, O. Ham, S.-Y. Lee et al., "MicroRNA-365 inhibits the proliferation of vascular smooth muscle cells by targeting cyclin D1," *Journal of Cellular Biochemistry*, vol. 115, no. 10, pp. 1752–1761, 2014.

[19] B. Song, Z.-Z. Zhang, J.-C. Zhong et al., "Loss of angiotensin-converting enzyme 2 exacerbates myocardial injury via activation of the CTGF-fractalkine signaling pathway," *Circulation Journal*, vol. 77, no. 12, pp. 2997–3006, 2013.

[20] B. Hu, J. T. Song, H. Y. Qu et al., "Mechanical stretch suppresses microRNA-145 expression by activating extracellular signal-regulated kinase 1/2 and upregulating angiotensin- converting enzyme to alter vascular smooth muscle cell phenotype," *PLoS ONE*, vol. 9, no. 5, Article ID e96338, 2014.

[21] K. Kohlstedt, C. Trouvain, T. Boettger, L. Shi, B. Fisslthaler, and I. Fleming, "AMP-activated protein kinase regulates endothelial cell angiotensin-converting enzyme expression via p53 and the post-transcriptional regulation of microRNA-143/145," *Circulation Research*, vol. 112, no. 8, pp. 1150–1158, 2013.

[22] R. Goyal, D. Goyal, A. Leitzke, C. P. Gheorghe, and L. D. Longo, "Brain renin-angiotensin system: fetal epigenetic programming by maternal protein restriction during pregnancy," *Reproductive Sciences*, vol. 17, no. 3, pp. 227–238, 2010.

[23] J. R. Kemp, H. Unal, R. Desnoyer, H. Yue, A. Bhatnagar, and S. S. Karnik, "Angiotensin II-regulated microRNA 483-3p directly targets multiple components of the rennin-angiotensin system," *Journal of Molecular and Cellular Cardiology*, vol. 75, pp. 25–39, 2014.

[24] X. Jiang, Q. Ning, and J. Wang, "Angiotensin II induced differentially expressed microRNAs in adult rat cardiac fibroblasts," *Journal of Physiological Sciences*, vol. 63, no. 1, pp. 31–38, 2013.

[25] P. L. Jeppesen, G. L. Christensen, M. Schneider et al., "Angiotensin II type 1 receptor signalling regulates microRNA

differentially in cardiac fibroblasts and myocytes," *British Journal of Pharmacology*, vol. 164, no. 2, pp. 394–404, 2011.

[26] A. Sen, P. Most, and K. Peppel, "Induction of microRNA-138 by pro-inflammatory cytokines causes endothelial cell dysfunction," *FEBS Letters*, vol. 588, no. 6, pp. 906–914, 2014.

[27] T. V. Eskildsen, P. L. Jeppesen, M. Schneider et al., "Angiotensin II regulates microRNA-132/-212 in hypertensive rats and humans," *International Journal of Molecular Sciences*, vol. 14, no. 6, pp. 11190–11207, 2013.

[28] T. V. Eskildsen, M. Schneider, M. B. Sandberg et al., "The microRNA-132/212 family fine-tunes multiple targets in Angiotensin II signalling in cardiac fibroblasts," *Journal of the Renin-Angiotensin-Aldosterone System*, 2014.

[29] S. Gao, T.-W. Liu, Z. Wang et al., "Downregulation of MicroRNA-19b contributes to angiotensin II-induced overexpression of connective tissue growth factor in cardiomyocytes," *Cardiology*, vol. 127, no. 2, pp. 114–120, 2014.

[30] L.-X. Yang, G. Liu, G.-F. Zhu et al., "MicroRNA-155 inhibits angiotensin II-induced vascular smooth muscle cell proliferation," *Journal of the Renin Angiotensin Aldosterone System*, vol. 15, no. 2, pp. 109–116, 2014.

[31] G. Ceolotto, I. Papparella, A. Bortoluzzi et al., "Interplay between miR-155, AT1R A1166C polymorphism, and AT1R expression in young untreated hypertensives," *The American Journal of Hypertension*, vol. 24, no. 2, pp. 241–246, 2011.

[32] D. W. Lambert, L. A. Lambert, N. E. Clarke, N. M. Hooper, K. E. Porter, and A. J. Turner, "Angiotensin-converting enzyme 2 is subject to post-transcriptional regulation by miR-421," *Clinical Science*, vol. 127, no. 4, pp. 243–249, 2014.

[33] Q. Gu, B. Wang, X.-F. Zhang, Y.-P. Ma, J.-D. Liu, and X.-Z. Wang, "Contribution of renin–angiotensin system to exercise-induced attenuation of aortic remodeling and improvement of endothelial function in spontaneously hypertensive rats," *Cardiovascular Pathology*, vol. 23, no. 5, pp. 298–305, 2014.

[34] H.-J. Wang, W.-Y. Lo, and L.-J. Lin, "Angiotensin-(1–7) decreases glycated albumin-induced endothelial interleukin-6 expression via modulation of miR-146a," *Biochemical and Biophysical Research Communications*, vol. 430, no. 3, pp. 1157–1163, 2013.

[35] Y. Takahashi, M. Satoh, Y. Minami, T. Tabuchi, T. Itoh, and M. Nakamura, "Expression of miR-146a/b is associated with the Toll-like receptor 4 signal in coronary artery disease: effect of renin-angiotensin system blockade and statins on miRNA-146a/b and Toll-like receptor 4 levels," *Clinical Science*, vol. 119, no. 9, pp. 395–405, 2010.

[36] C. M. Ferrario, J. Jessup, M. C. Chappell et al., "Effect of angiotensin-converting enzyme inhibition and angiotensin II receptor blockers on cardiac angiotensin-converting enzyme 2," *Circulation*, vol. 111, no. 20, pp. 2605–2610, 2005.

[37] J. C. Zhong, J. Y. Ye, H. Y. Jin et al., "Telmisartan attenuates aortic hypertrophy in hypertensive rats by the modulation of ACE2 and profilin-1 expression," *Regulatory Peptides*, vol. 166, no. 1-3, pp. 90–97, 2011.

[38] J. Zhong, R. Basu, D. Guo et al., "Angiotensin-converting enzyme 2 suppresses pathological hypertrophy, myocardial fibrosis, and cardiac dysfunction," *Circulation*, vol. 122, no. 7, pp. 717–728, 2010.

[39] M. Satoh, Y. Takahashi, T. Tabuchi et al., "Circulating Toll-like receptor 4-responsive microRNA panel in patients with coronary artery disease: results from prospective and randomized study of treatment with renin-angiotensin system blockades," *Clinical Science*, vol. 128, no. 8, pp. 483–491, 2015.

[40] T. Sato, T. Suzuki, H. Watanabe et al., "Apelin is a positive regulator of ACE2 in failing hearts," *Journal of Clinical Investigation*, vol. 123, no. 12, pp. 5203–5211, 2013.

[41] N. E. Clarke and A. J. Turner, "Angiotensin-converting enzyme 2: the first decade," *International Journal of Hypertension*, vol. 2012, Article ID 307315, 12 pages, 2012.

[42] K. Tatemoto, M. Hosoya, Y. Habata et al., "Isolation and characterization of a novel endogenous peptide ligand for the human APJ receptor," *Biochemical and Biophysical Research Communications*, vol. 251, no. 2, pp. 471–476, 1998.

[43] J. C. Zhong, X. Y. Yu, Y. Huang, L. M. Yung, C. W. Lau, and S. G. Lin, "Apelin modulates aortic vascular tone via endothelial nitric oxide synthase phosphorylation pathway in diabetic mice," *Cardiovascular Research*, vol. 74, no. 3, pp. 388–395, 2007.

[44] M. Przewlocka-Kosmala, T. Kotwica, A. Mysiak, and W. Kosmala, "Reduced circulating apelin in essential hypertension and its association with cardiac dysfunction," *Journal of Hypertension*, vol. 29, no. 5, pp. 971–979, 2011.

[45] H. Najafipour, A. Soltani Hekmat, A. A. Nekooian, and S. Esmaeili-Mahani, "Apelin receptor expression in ischemic and non- ischemic kidneys and cardiovascular responses to apelin in chronic two-kidney-one-clip hypertension in rats," *Regulatory Peptides*, vol. 178, no. 1–3, pp. 43–50, 2012.

[46] R. Akcilar, S. Turgut, V. Caner et al., "Apelin effects on blood pressure and RAS in DOCA-salt-induced hypertensive rats," *Clinical and Experimental Hypertension*, vol. 35, no. 7, pp. 550–557, 2013.

[47] A. F. Ceylan-Isik, M. R. Kandadi, X. Xu et al., "Apelin administration ameliorates high fat diet-induced cardiac hypertrophy and contractile dysfunction," *Journal of Molecular and Cellular Cardiology*, vol. 63, pp. 4–13, 2013.

[48] J. Kim, Y. Kang, Y. Kojima et al., "An endothelial apelin-FGF link mediated by miR-424 and miR-503 is disrupted in pulmonary arterial hypertension," *Nature Medicine*, vol. 19, no. 1, pp. 74–82, 2013.

17

Growing-Related Changes in Arterial Properties of Healthy Children, Adolescents, and Young Adults Nonexposed to Cardiovascular Risk Factors: Analysis of Gender-Related Differences

S. Curcio,[1] V. García-Espinosa,[1] M. Arana,[2] I. Farro,[1] P. Chiesa,[3] G. Giachetto,[2] Y. Zócalo,[1] and D. Bia[1]

[1] *Physiology Department, Faculty of Medicine, CUiiDARTE, University of the Republic, General Flores 2125, 11800 Montevideo, Uruguay*
[2] *Clínica Pediátrica "C", Pereira-Rossel Hospital Centre, Faculty of Medicine, University of the Republic, Bulevar Artigas 1550, 11600 Montevideo, Uruguay*
[3] *Pediatric Cardiology Service, Pereira-Rossell Hospital Centre, ASSE, Bulevar Artigas 1550, 11600 Montevideo, Uruguay*

Correspondence should be addressed to D. Bia; dbia@fmed.edu.uy

Academic Editor: Tomohiro Katsuya

The aims of our work were to determine normal aging rates for structural and functional arterial parameters in healthy children, adolescents, and young adults and to identify gender-related differences in these aging rates. *Methods.* 161 subjects (mean: 15 years (range: 4–28 years), 69 females) were studied. Subjects included had no congenital or chronic diseases, nor had they been previously exposed to traditional cardiovascular risk factors. Arterial parameters assessed were (1) central blood pressure (BP) and aortic pulse wave analysis, (2) arterial local (pressure-strain elastic modulus) and regional (pulse wave velocity, PWV) stiffness, and (3) arterial diameters and carotid intima-media thickness (CIMT). Simple linear regression models (age as the independent variable) were obtained for all the parameters and the resulting rates of change were compared between genders. *Results.* No gender-related differences were found in mean values of arterial structural and functional parameters in prepubertal ages (4–8 years), but they started to appear at ~15 years. Boys showed a greater rate of change for central systolic BP, central pulse pressure, CIMT, and carotid-femoral PWV. *Conclusion.* Gender-related differences in arterial characteristics of adults can be explained on the basis of different growing-related patterns between boys and girls, with no existing differences in prepubertal ages.

1. Introduction

In adults, age-related changes in structural and functional arterial properties have been well described and are jointly known as *vascular aging* (VA) [1]. These changes include arterial stiffening, luminal dilatation, and wall thickening [2] and are known to have a heterogeneous distribution between central and peripheral arteries [3]. As VA has been shown to accelerate in association with several pathological conditions and with cardiovascular risk factors (CRF) exposure (leading to target organ damage (TOD) and increased cardiovascular risk) [2, 4], the concept of *early vascular aging* (EVA) has been recently proposed and used in order to discriminate between normal and pathological VA [5]. The importance of EVA lies in its usefulness as an indicator of cumulative arterial damage and increased risk of cardiovascular events. Therefore, identifying subjects with a burden of components of the so-called EVA syndrome [5] in early stages could allow designing proper interventions to prevent and reduce vascular alterations, thus minimizing cardiovascular risk. Supported by the fact that the process of arterial impairment begins during childhood and by existing evidence of positive outcomes of intervention studies in pediatric populations [6–8], it has been suggested that preventing and controlling EVA should start in early life [9].

On the other hand, the existence of gender-related differences in arterial properties and cardiovascular risk is a well-known and described fact for adults [10–13]. At least in theory, sex-related differences in arterial behavior in adults could be explained on the basis of differences in growth-related vascular changes between boys and girls. However, whether these differences exist since birth or if they appear with growth in children and adolescents is still a controversial issue. In the latter case, information would also be lacking about the ages in which those differences can start being detected, for which parameters and in what magnitude. Moreover, information is lacking about normal VA in early ages. Describing normal VA patterns for these populations would allow distinguishing between normal VA and EVA and also determining those ages in which sex-distinction is needed for reference values utilization.

In this context, the aims of this work were (1) to determine normal growth-related changes for several vascular structural and functional parameters in a healthy and nonexposed to CRF population of children, adolescents, and young adults and (2) to identify the presence of gender-related differences in growth rates for different arterial properties.

2. Methods

2.1. Study Population. CUiiDARTE Center and Project is a Uruguayan Interdisciplinary University Program for Arterial Disease Early Diagnosis advocated in children and adults, supported by the Public Health Minister [14, 15]. Studied individuals were derived for arterial evaluation by CUiiDARTE Project medical staff. Subjects included had no congenital, chronic, or infectious diseases at the time of the study, nor had they been previously exposed to traditional CRF as hypertension, smoking, obesity, diabetes, dyslipidemia, physical inactivity, and premature family history of cardiovascular disease.

All studies were approved by the Institutional Ethics Committee, and written informed consent was obtained prior to the examination.

2.2. Medical Interview and Anthropometrics. Before vascular evaluation a clinical interview was conducted in order to assess CRF exposure. Subjects' weight and height were measured. Body mass index (BMI) was calculated as the weight-to-squared height ratio and, for underaged subjects, converted into percentiles/z-scores using the World Health Organization reference values. Children and adolescents with a BMI >97th percentile and/or a BMI z-score >2, for age and sex, and adults with a BMI >30 Kg/m^2 were excluded from the study. Children and adolescents with known arterial hypertension and/or with blood pressure (BP) levels >95th percentile for age, sex, and height were excluded. Adults with BP ≥ 140/90 mmHg were also excluded.

Finally, 161 healthy subjects nonexposed to cardiovascular risk factors (mean age: 15 years (range: 4–28 years), 69 females) were included in the present work.

2.3. Study Protocol. Prior to the study, all individuals had been for at least 4 hours fasting and took a 15-minute rest in supine position, in a calm environment with a controlled room temperature (21–23°C). During the examination, brachial BP and heart rate (HR) measurements were performed at fixed intervals of 8–10 minutes (HEM-433INT; Omron Healthcare Inc., Illinois, USA).

2.3.1. Arterial Stiffness. Pulse wave velocity (PWV) was measured to assess aortic (carotid-femoral PWV, cfPWV) and upper limb (carotid-radial PWV, crPWV) arterial stiffness, by applanation tonometry (SphygmoCor, AtCor Medical, Australia) [21]. Pulse wave travel distance was assessed using surface tape measurements. For cfPWV, the pulse wave path length was measured as the distance between carotid and femoral sampling sites, and for crPWV it was measured as the distance between radial sampling site and the sternal notch. In order to obtain "real" cfPWV [22], calculated cfPWV was multiplied by a scaling factor of 0.8. The resulting PWV values consisted of the mean of three different measurements and were only considered valid if standard deviation (SD) between measurements was <10%. Additionally, seeking to normalize cfPWV values by BP levels, βPWV Index was calculated as follows: $\mathrm{Ln(SBP/DBP)} \times 2.11 \times \mathrm{cfPWV2/PP}$, Ln being the natural logarithm and SBP, DBP, and PP the systolic, diastolic, and pulse pressure level [23].

Pressure-strain elastic modulus (EM) was calculated as follows: $\mathrm{EM} = \mathrm{PP}/((\mathrm{SD} - \mathrm{DD})/\mathrm{DD})$, where SD and DD are systolic and diastolic arterial diameters. Central PP was used to calculate common carotid artery (CCA) EM and peripheral PP to calculate common femoral artery (CFA) EM. Vascular ultrasound (6–13 MHz linear array probe, M-Turbo, SonoSite Inc., WA, USA) was used to obtain 30-second longitudinal image sequences of left and right CCA and CFA, which were stored for off-line analysis. Beat-to-beat diameter waveforms were obtained using automatic border detection software. SD and DD were quantified as the average of at least twenty beats [24]. Local stiffness was normalized by BP calculating β Index as follows: $\mathrm{Ln(SBP/DBP)}/((\mathrm{SD} - \mathrm{DD})/\mathrm{DD})$.

2.3.2. Intima-Media Thickness. CCA intima-media thickness (CIMT) was assessed in the proximal centimeter from the carotid bifurcation, using ultrasound system and specific software [25, 26]. CIMT was measured in the "posterior" wall at the moment corresponding to the end DD, and its value was the mean resulting from at least 10 measurements.

2.3.3. Central Aortic Pressure and Wave Reflection Parameters. In order to assess central aortic pressure and reflection parameters, radial artery pressure waveforms were recorded using applanation tonometry (SphygmoCor, AtCor Medical, Australia). After 20 seconds of recording, waveforms acquired were calibrated and averaged, and a generalized transfer function was used to synthesize the corresponding central aortic pressure waveform [27].

Augmentation index (AIx), augmented pressure (AP), and subendocardial viability ratio (SEVR) were derived from the aortic pressure waveform using pulse waveform analysis

(PWA). Considering that AIx is influenced by HR and height, an index normalized for a HR of 75 bpm was used (AIx@75) [28], and it was afterwards normalized by height calculating an AIx@75-to-height ratio.

2.4. Data Analysis and Statistics. Data are expressed as the mean ± standard deviation. Data analysis was performed using SPSS software (SPSS Inc., Illinois, USA). To study the relationship between age and arterial parameters, subjects were grouped by gender and classified in three age categories: <8, 8–14, and ≥15 years. Continuous variables were compared using tests according to their statistical distribution.

Reproducibility of the ultrasound technique and its derived variables was tested by analyzing intra- and interobserver variability (assessed as variation coefficient (VC) and intraclass correlation coefficient (ICC)). In this case, two trained observers (SC and VGE) were compared. Parameters analyzed were SD, DD, and CIMT. Overall intraobserver VC were as follows: SC (DD = 0.66%, SD = 0.55%, and IMT = 2.05%) and VGE (DD = 1.2%, SD = 0.56%, and IMT = 2.69%). Intraobserver ICC (95% confidence intervals expressed) between measurement times ($T1$ and $T2$) was 0.978 (0.910–0.994). Interobserver ICC was as follows: SD = 0.919 (0.811–0.965), DD = 0.917 (0.808–0.964), and IMT = 0.985 (0.944–0.996).

Age-related changes in arterial parameters were also explored by obtaining simple linear regression models for each gender. Gender-related differences in aging patterns were then investigated by comparison of the slopes of the corresponding models obtained, analyzing the interaction between age and sex as covariables (Table 2). An exception was made with the model obtained for AIx@75. As it was previously described that values for this parameter start to increase at ~20 years of age [29], to accomplish a good analysis in this case we limited the studied population to those ages.

The models for the parameters showing a significant correlation with age were used to calculate the predicted mean values at 4 and 18 years of age, and afterwards the average relative change expected with growing from 4 to 18 years was calculated (Table 3). The 95% confidence intervals (CI) expressed in Table 3 were calculated from the 95% CI obtained for the slope of each model. For every analysis performed, a p value < 0.05 was considered significant.

3. Results

No gender differences existed in age, height, and weight, except for the elder group (≥15 years), where the expected physiological differences determined that males were significantly heavier and taller than females (Table 1).

3.1. Peripheral and Central Arterial Pressure. No gender-related differences were found in peripheral diastolic BP (pDBP), with independence of the age group. The lower and middle age groups showed no difference in peripheral systolic BP (pSBP). As was expected, in the elder group pSBP was significantly higher in males than in females. Peripheral PP (pPP) did not show difference between genders in the lower age group but was statistically different for the elder group. For the middle age group it was higher in boys, but with no statistic significance.

Similar results were found for aortic pressure levels. Central systolic BP (cSBP) was significantly higher for boys in the elder age group (107 mmHg versus 99 mmHg, $p < 0.001$). Central PP (cPP) reached the significance in the middle age group, maintaining this difference for the elder group, being also higher in boys (42 mmHg versus 31 mmHg, $p < 0.001$; Table 1).

3.2. Wave Reflection Parameters. AIx@75 was significantly higher in females starting in the middle age group and maintained this difference for the elder group (2.6% versus −3.9%, $p < 0.001$), showing a greater influence of wave reflections in central BP in females since early ages (Table 1). This difference remained significant after adjusting AIx@75 by height. SEVR was found to be lower in girls for all the age groups, but this difference did not reach the statistic significance.

3.3. Arterial Diameters and CIMT. Arterial diameters were greater for males than for females. In the CCA, the difference was significant for the elder group, whereas in the CFA it was significant in the middle and elder age groups (Table 1). Mean values of CIMT were found to be higher in males, only reaching the statistic significance for the elder age group (0.497 mm versus 0.459 mm, $p = 0.04$; Table 1).

3.4. Local and Regional Arterial Stiffness. In the middle and elder age groups, males showed higher local arterial stiffness (EM) for CCA, whereas no gender-related differences were found for CFA. The differences in CCA EM were however found to be dependent on BP levels for the lower and middle age groups, since when β Index was calculated no gender-related differences in CCA stiffness were found (Table 1). However, for the elder group the difference was found to be only partially pressure-dependent, suggesting that boys have higher intrinsic wall stiffness than girls since ~15 years.

Regional arterial stiffness in the upper limb (crPWV) showed no gender-related difference for the different age groups, whereas cfPWV was found to be higher in males, reaching the statistic significance for the elder group (6.6 m/s versus 5.6 m/s, $p < 0.001$). This difference was still found when cfPWV levels were normalized by BP (βPWV Index). These results show that no gender-related differences exist in regional arterial stiffness for muscular arteries, but they can be found for elastic arteries, such as the aorta, starting at ~15 years.

3.5. Gender Differences in Growing-Related Changes in Arterial Structural and Functional Parameters. crPWV did not show a significant correlation with age. The remaining parameters showed a significant linear and positive correlation with age, except for AIx@75, which had an inverse correlation with age (Table 2).

cSBP was found to have a steeper increase with age in males than in females (1.614 mmHg/year versus

Table 1: Demographic, hemodynamic, and vascular parameters.

	Total			<8 years			8 to 14 years			≥15 years		
	Female VM ± DS	Male VM ± DS	P	Female VM ± DS	Male VM ± DS	P	Female VM ± DS	Male VM ± DS	P	Female VM ± DS	Male VM ± DS	P
Anthropometric data												
N	68	93		9	13		29	50		30	30	
Age (years)	16.2 ± 7.3	14.4 ± 6.2	0.08	6.8 ± 1.1	6.4 ± 0.9	0.38	11.8 ± 2.3	11.8 ± 1.9	0.93	23.4 ± 4.1	22.0 ± 3.8	0.20
Weight (kg)	46.3 ± 16.8	47.5 ± 20.8	0.69	23.2 ± 5.3	20.9 ± 2.4	0.18	40.3 ± 12.7	39.8 ± 12.1	0.85	59.4 ± 10.6	72.0 ± 9.2	**<0.001**
Height (m)	1.50 ± 0.18	1.53 ± 0.23	0.49	1.22 ± 0.08	1.17 ± 0.07	0.15	1.46 ± 0.14	1.47 ± 0.14	0.81	1.63 ± 0.07	1.77 ± 0.06	**<0.001**
Body mass index (Kg/m^2)	19.6 ± 3.9	19.1 ± 3.7	0.44	15.5 ± 2.0	15.2 ± 1.1	0.68	18.4 ± 3.0	18.0 ± 2.6	0.51	22.2 ± 3.5	22.9 ± 2.6	0.38
Hemodynamic parameters												
Heart rate	79 ± 11	74 ± 12	**0.03**	87 ± 3	85 ± 11	0.65	80 ± 12	74 ± 11	0.07	75 ± 10	68 ± 12	**0.04**
Peripheral blood pressure												
Brachial SBP (mmHg)	107 ± 10	110 ± 13	0.10	98 ± 5	97 ± 7	0.77	105 ± 7	106 ± 6	0.53	114 ± 11	125 ± 11	**<0.001**
Brachial DBP (mmHg)	61 ± 7	59 ± 8	0.20	60 ± 6	57 ± 7	0.44	59 ± 6	58 ± 6	0.39	64 ± 9	64 ± 7	0.74
Brachial PP (mmHg)	46 ± 7	51 ± 10	**<0.001**	39 ± 3	42 ± 6	0.22	46 ± 6	48 ± 6	0.07	49 ± 7	60 ± 10	**<0.001**
Central blood pressure												
Aortic SBP (mmHg)	92 ± 10	95 ± 12	0.26	82 ± 6	83 ± 6	0.85	89 ± 8	90 ± 8	0.50	99 ± 10	107 ± 9	**<0.001**
Aortic DBP (mmHg)	63 ± 7	61 ± 7	0.18	61 ± 5	59 ± 7	0.43	61 ± 7	59 ± 6	0.21	68 ± 10	65 ± 8	0.19
Aortic PP (mmHg)	28 ± 6	33 ± 10	**<0.001**	21 ± 2	23 ± 5	0.34	28 ± 5	31 ± 7	**0.04**	31 ± 6	42 ± 9	**<0.001**
Aortic pulse wave analysis												
Augmented pressure (mmHg)	2 ± 3	0 ± 3	**0.01**	2 ± 2	2 ± 2	0.32	1 ± 3	0 ± 3	0.35	2 ± 3	−1 ± 4	**<0.001**
Augmentation index 75 (%)	6 ± 11	1 ± 12	**0.00**	15 ± 9	15 ± 9	0.99	6 ± 9	1 ± 10	**0.04**	6 ± 8	−8 ± 5	**<0.001**
AIx-to-height ratio	4.6 ± 7.8	1.2 ± 8.4	**0.01**	12.4 ± 7.9	12.8 ± 8.5	0.92	4.5 ± 7.4	1.0 ± 6.8	**0.04**	2.6 ± 7.1	−3.9 ± 5.2	**<0.001**
SEVR	128 ± 33	140 ± 33	**0.02**	113 ± 20	126 ± 20	0.17	119 ± 26	133 ± 32	0.05	141 ± 37	158 ± 30	0.07
Mode B ultrasound												
Common carotid artery												
Diastolic diameter (mm)	5.6 ± 0.5	5.9 ± 0.7	**0.02**	5.0 ± 0.4	5.2 ± 0.6	0.27	5.6 ± 0.5	5.8 ± 0.7	0.12	5.9 ± 0.4	6.3 ± 0.5	**0.01**
IMT (mm)	0.442 ± 0.046	0.459 ± 0.061	0.08	0.405 ± 0.039	0.416 ± 0.048	0.58	0.433 ± 0.036	0.449 ± 0.054	0.16	0.459 ± 0.044	0.497 ± 0.069	**0.04**
Elastic modulus (mmHg)	252 ± 100	295 ± 138	**0.05**	134 ± 28	161 ± 40	0.11	220 ± 66	267 ± 101	**0.03**	349 ± 75	424 ± 137	**0.04**
β Index	1.64 ± 0.22	1.75 ± 0.30	**0.02**	1.46 ± 0.15	1.50 ± 0.29	0.74	1.63 ± 0.20	1.70 ± 0.25	0.21	1.74 ± 0.21	1.98 ± 0.24	**<0.001**
Common femoral artery												
Diastolic diameter (mm)	5.6 ± 1.1	6.3 ± 1.4	**<0.001**	4.5 ± 0.8	4.6 ± 0.4	0.63	5.4 ± 0.8	6.0 ± 1.0	**<0.001**	6.8 ± 0.7	7.8 ± 0.9	**<0.001**
Elastic modulus (mmHg)	803 ± 463	877 ± 599	0.45	484 ± 198	519 ± 194	0.70	725 ± 367	723 ± 366	0.98	1146 ± 547	1386 ± 803	0.32
β Index	2.25 ± 0.19	2.21 ± 0.18	0.26	2.33 ± 0.17	2.37 ± 0.17	0.66	2.27 ± 0.18	2.20 ± 0.17	0.09	2.09 ± 0.16	2.11 ± 0.16	0.86
Regional arterial stiffness												
Carotid-femoral PWV (m/s)	4.9 ± 0.9	5.3 ± 1.1	**0.05**	4.5 ± 0.7	4.4 ± 0.6	0.88	4.7 ± 0.6	4.8 ± 0.6	0.21	5.6 ± 0.9	6.6 ± 1.0	**<0.001**
βPWV Index	0.62 ± 0.17	0.72 ± 0.26	**0.01**	0.56 ± 0.15	0.58 ± 0.17	0.74	0.57 ± 0.12	0.63 ± 0.15	0.10	0.75 ± 0.21	1.01 ± 0.26	**0.01**
Carotid-radial PWV (m/s)	7.5 ± 1.1	7.8 ± 1.2	0.17	7.5 ± 1.1	7.8 ± 1.5	0.65	7.4 ± 1.2	7.6 ± 1.2	0.44	7.9 ± 1.0	8.7 ± 1.2	0.07

Data expressed as mean value (M) ± standard deviation (SD). SBP, systolic blood pressure; DBP, diastolic blood pressure; PP, pulse pressure; PWV, pulse wave velocity.

Table 2: Age-related changes. Simple linear regression models.

	Female Model	Female R	Female p	Male Model	Male R	Male p	Slope difference p
Central arterial pressure							
Aortic SBP	$0.902x + 77.51$	0.609	<0.001	$1.614x + 71.74$	0.827	<0.001	<0.001
Aortic DBP	$0.578x + 54.74$	0.469	<0.001	$0.508x + 53.84$	0.421	<0.001	0.692
Aortic PP	$0.285x + 23.23$	0.329	0.007	$1.135x + 17.35$	0.706	<0.001	<0.001
Augmentation index 75	$-0.937x + 18.7$	0.381	0.015	$-1.532x + 20.1$	0.555	<0.001	0.202
Mode B ultrasound							
Carotid diastolic diameter	$0.043x + 4.97$	0.548	<0.001	$0.055x + 5.16$	0.540	<0.001	0.373
Carotid IMT	$0.004x + 0.379$	0.608	<0.001	$0.006x + 0.378$	0.575	<0.001	0.04
Local arterial stiffness							
Carotid elastic modulus	$11.73x + 73.9$	0.816	<0.001	$16.08x + 75.38$	0.740	<0.001	0.010
Carotid β Index	$0.008x + 1.509$	0.350	0.009	$0.026x + 1.40$	0.549	<0.001	0.016
Femoral elastic modulus	$40.26x + 247.63$	0.538	<0.001	$58.89x + 70.89$	0.560	<0.001	0.178
Regional arterial stiffness							
Carotid-femoral PWV	$0.103x + 3.50$	0.722	<0.001	$0.147x + 3.22$	0.796	<0.001	0.018
βPWV Index	$0.016x + 0.39$	0.585	<0.001	$0.031x + 0.30$	0.482	<0.001	0.004
Carotid-radial PWV	$0.049x + 6.87$	0.236	0.118	$0.057x + 7.12$	0.192	0.119	0.855

SBP, systolic blood pressure; DBP, diastolic blood pressure; PP, pulse pressure; IMT, intima-media thickness; PWV, pulse wave velocity.

Table 3: Relative change (%) predicted in arterial parameters from 4 to 18 years.

	Female Model	Female Predicted value at 4 years	Female Predicted value at 18 years	Female Relative change% (95% CI)	Male Model	Male Predicted value at 4 years	Male Predicted value at 18 years	Male Relative change% (95% CI)
Central arterial pressure								
Aortic SBP	$0.902x + 77.51$	81	94	15.6 (10.7–20.35)	$1.614x + 71.74$	78	101	28.9 (25.0–32.7)
Aortic DBP	$0.578x + 54.74$	57	65	14.2 (7.7–20.5)	$0.508x + 53.84$	56	63	12.7 (7.1–18.2)
Aortic PP	$0.285x + 23.23$	24	28	16.4 (4.8–27.2)	$1.135x + 17.35$	22	38	72.6 (59.9–84.2)
Augmentation index 75	$-0.937x + 18.7$	15	2	88 (15–197)	$-1.532x + 20.1$	14	−7	153 (87–244)
Mode B ultrasound								
Carotid diastolic diameter	$0.043x + 4.97$	5.14	5.74	11.7 (7.2–16.1)	$0.055x + 5.16$	5.38	6.15	14.3 (9.5–18.7)
Carotid IMT	$0.004x + 0.379$	0.395	0.451	14.2 (10.7–20.8)	$0.006x + 0.378$	0.402	0.486	20.9 (14.2–27.3)
Local arterial stiffness								
Carotid β Index	$0.008x + 1.509$	1.54	1.65	7.3 (0.9–15.1)	$0.026x + 1.40$	1.50	1.87	24.2 (16.2–31.8)
Carotid elastic modulus	$11.73x + 73.9$	121	285	135.9 (116.3–152.5)	$16.08x + 75.38$	140	365	161.1 (139.8–178.5)
Femoral elastic modulus	$40.26x + 247.63$	409	972	137.9 (93.3–169.3)	$58.89x + 70.89$	306	1131	269 (241–286)
Regional arterial stiffness								
Carotid-femoral PWV	$0.103x + 3.50$	3.91	5.35	36.9 (27.9–45.6)	$0.147x + 3.22$	3.81	5.87	54.0 (46.4–61.6)
βPWV Index	$0.016x + 0.39$	0.45	0.68	49.3 (32.6–66.8)	$0.031x + 0.30$	0.45	0.98	102.4 (84.8–117.7)

SBP, systolic blood pressure; DBP, diastolic blood pressure; PP, pulse pressure; IMT, intima-media thickness; PWV, pulse wave velocity.

0.902 mmHg/year, $p < 0.001$). A greater difference was found for cPP (1.135 mmHg/year in males versus 0.285 mmHg/year in females, $p < 0.001$), indicating that in males cPP increases more rapidly with age. These results translate into a ~28.9% increase in cSBP for boys versus ~15.6% for girls from 4 to 18 years (Table 3), whereas for cPP the gender difference in relative increase was even greater (male: ~72.6% versus female: ~16.4%).

AIx@75 also showed more pronounced age-related changes in males (Figure 1(d)), but in this case with no statistic significance. However, the existing difference determines that for boys the relative decrease in AIx@75 from 4 to 18 years is almost twice than for girls (~153% versus ~88%, Table 3).

No significant gender-related differences were found in the rate of change for CCA diameters, whereas for CIMT a significant and higher rate of change was found for males (0.006 mm/year versus 0.004 mm/year, $p = 0.04$; Table 2).

Local arterial stiffness, evaluated through EM, showed significant gender differences in age-related changes only for the CCA, indicating that males have a greater rate of increase in CCA stiffness with age (Table 2, Figure 1(e)). Moreover, when normalized by BP levels (CCA β Index), this gender-related difference could still be found, suggesting that the most marked increases in CCA stiffness are independent of the higher levels of BP in males (Table 2). This determines an important difference in the predicted relative increase for local stiffness from 4 to 18 years (~24.2% versus ~7.3%, Table 3).

Males showed a steeper increase in aortic stiffness (0.147 m/s/year versus 0.103 m/s/year, $p = 0.018$; Table 2, Figure 1(h)). The βPWV Index also showed a greater changing rate for males (Table 2). These results indicate that boys present more pronounced age-related changes in intrinsic stiffness (pressure-independent) of the aortic wall, resulting in an average increase of ~54% versus ~36.9% for girls from 4 to 18 years.

4. Discussion

To our knowledge, this is the first study characterizing gender-related differences in arterial properties aging rates as an integrated approach (including both structural and functional parameters) in healthy children, adolescents, and young adults free of traditional CRF exposure. From the analysis of our results, five findings are of major relevance:

(1) During aging of healthy and nonexposed to CRF children, adolescents, and young adults, several changes can be found in both structural and functional arterial properties (Table 2). As the studied population was free of classic CRF exposure, our results suggest that these aging patterns could be explained on the basis of physiological changes due to development and growth in early ages.

(2) In prepubertal ages (4–8 years), no gender-related differences can be found for arterial characteristics (Table 1).

(3) The aging rates described determine that relative changes are lower for structural (arterial diameters and thickness) than functional and hemodynamic (aortic PP, arterial stiffness) parameters (Table 3).

(4) These growing-related changes occur at a higher rate for boys than for girls (Table 2), suggesting the existence of an accelerated aging rate for males.

(5) Jointly analyzed, the mentioned differences determine that (1) gender-related differences in pressure-dependent arterial stiffness can start being detected between 8 and 14 years and (2) since postpubertal ages gender-related differences in structural parameters can be evidenced, and arterial stiffness differences imply intrinsic wall changes, not only being determined by BP differences (Table 1).

4.1. Growing-Related Changes in Arterial Functional and Structural Parameters. Although several studies have characterized aging-related changes in vascular parameters for pediatric populations, little information is available about specific VA rates and the expected normal changes for these ages, even less utilizing an integrated approach as ours.

However, the tendencies shown by our results are similar to those found in other studies. For example, Hayward and Kelly [30] reported a marked age-related increase in central systolic and diastolic pressure and PP between the first two decades of life, as well as a decrease in AIx@75. This decrease in the influence of wave reflection on aortic augmentation is known to be highly dependent on the growth in height in early ages, as the wave reflection sites get progressively farther from the heart.

For structural parameters as luminal diameters and CIMT, several authors found significant increases with age in children and adolescents [20, 31–33]. Moreover, Engelen et al. [33] reported similar changing rates in CIMT for males (0.0052 mm/year) and females (0.0049 mm/year) to the ones we found in our population (0.006 mm/year and 0.004 mm/year, resp.). Whereas Ishizu et al. [32] reported a greater changing rate in CIMT (0.009 mm/year), their study included subjects with ages ranged between 5 and 14 years, and when we adjusted our regression models to a population limited to these ages a more similar rate of change could be found (0.008 mm/year, $r = 0.463$, $p < 0.001$). A possible explanation of these findings is that growing-related changes are not necessarily lineal but have differential patterns between smaller age ranges.

Age-related changes in local and regional stiffness parameters are also widely described for the first decades of life [16, 20, 34, 35]. Senzaki et al. [35] performed invasive measurements of aortic EM, finding a similar changing rate of ~10 mmHg/year in contrast to an average 14 mmHg/year found for carotid EM in our population. Reusz et al. [16] reported a strong correlation between age and cfPWV in a large multicentric study including more than 1000 children and adolescents.

Although most of the authors reporting reference values for arterial properties in children, adolescents, and young adults did not report the respective regression models, we estimated and compared them with ours by using the mean values provided for each age (Table 4).

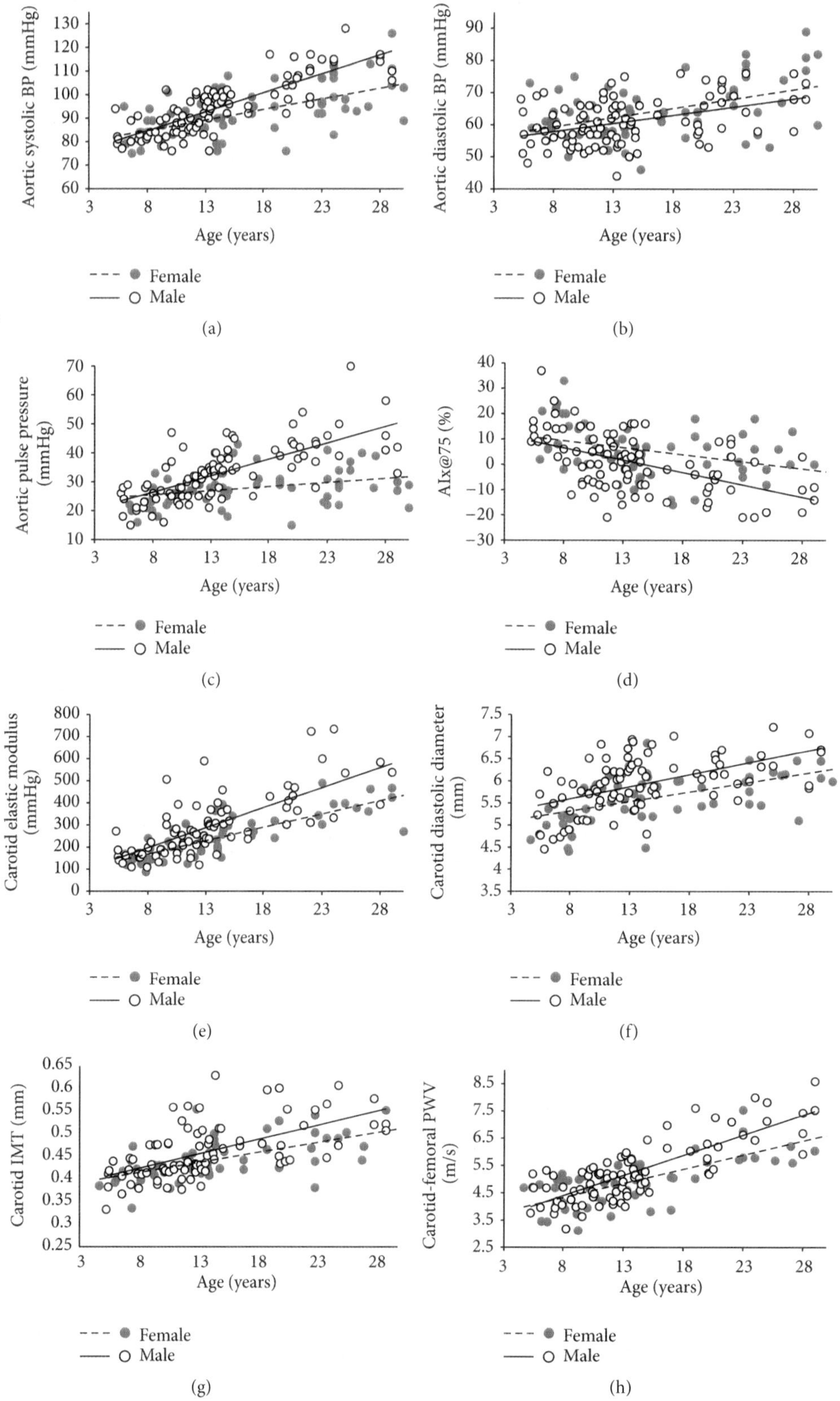

FIGURE 1: Regression plots for structural and functional arterial parameters. BP, blood pressure; AIx@75, augmentation index; IMT, intima-media thickness; PWV, pulse wave velocity.

Table 4: Regression models for cfPWV, CIMT, and cSBP (as a function of age) from other authors.

	Male	Female
cfPWV		
This paper	$0.147x + 3.22$	$0.103x + 3.50$
Reusz et al. [16]	$0.121x + 3.356$	$0.089x + 3.749$
Fischer et al. [17]	$0.133x + 3.108$	$0.080x + 3.468$
Elmenhorst et al. [18]	$0.088x + 3.588$	$0.051x + 3.936$
CIMT		
This paper	$0.006x + 0.378$	$0.004x + 0.379$
de Arriba Muñoz et al. [19]	$0.009x + 0.276$	$0.010x + 0.261$
Doyon et al. [20]	$0.003x + 0.347$	$0.001x + 0.357$
cSBP		
This paper	$1.614x + 71.74$	$0.902x + 77.51$
Elmenhorst et al. [18]	$2.206x + 72$	$1.456x + 80.1$

cfPWV, carotid-femoral pulse wave velocity; CIMT, carotid intima-media thickness; cSBP, central systolic blood pressure.

4.2. Gender-Related Differences in Vascular Aging. In males there is an accelerated rate of change for most of the vascular parameters studied. Even though previous studies did not analyze the integral (structural and functional) evolution of arterial changes, consistently with our findings, most of the authors investigating gender-related differences in arterial structural and functional parameters could not find them in ages below ~10 years but reported important differences since pubertal ages, thus suggesting the existence of differential aging patterns related to sex.

4.2.1. Differences in Hemodynamic Parameters. We found that boys present a greater rate of increase in cSBP and cPP. Since the presence of elevated central systolic pressure and PP determines an increase in cardiovascular risk, this phenomenon could be on the basis of the higher risk existing in males since early ages. In agreement with our findings, Hayward and Kelly [30] had similar results in their study, reporting a higher cPP in boys since the first decade of life. Recently, Elmenhorst et al. [18] studied gender-related differences in cSBP and found that girls underwent a minor increase in absolute cSBP with age compared to boys. In sight of their results they suggested that these could be reflecting gender differences in growing patterns, as we discuss in the present study.

McEniery et al. [29] also reported finding higher cPP in boys than in girls with ages below 20 years, but they found a steeper increase in cPP for women. However, their results were probably influenced by including subjects with ages ranged until ~90 years (youngest ages representing a small proportion of the sample) and the existence of a marked change in VA for women with the onset of menopause is well known [36]. These results suggest that the aging rates in the youth could explain the higher cardiovascular risk for middle-aged males, whereas the process of VA during adulthood would explain an increase in elderly female risk.

On the other side, the difference in changing rate for AIx@75 seems to be beneficial for males, as we could evidence a marked decrease in this parameter. This means that at least for the first two decades of life in healthy children, adolescents, and young adults there is not a great influence of wave reflections in central BP. Our results agree with those found by Hayward and Kelly [30], Stoner et al. [37], and Ayer et al. [38], as this difference could still be found after adjusting our results by height. Two important interpretations emerge from these results: the gender difference in AIx@75 is independent of body height, and the higher levels of central BP in boys are not explained by an earlier arrival of wave reflections.

4.2.2. Differences in Structural Parameters. Most of the studies investigating gender-related differences in CCA diameters and CIMT reported that boys have greater levels of CIMT, starting in postpubertal ages [20, 33]. Again, these findings together with those reporting greater CIMT levels for males in adult populations [39] determine that there must exist a gender-related difference in aging patterns to explain those differences. Engelen et al. found no gender difference in the increasing rate of CIMT, but their results could also be influenced by including individuals with a very wide range of ages. The higher increasing rate in CIMT for boys could be interpreted as an adaptative response to increasing cSBP and cPP. To test this hypothesis we calculated CCA wall stress (σ) for the total population and the different age groups [40]. As we could not find gender-related differences for this parameter, this result seems to back up our hypothesis.

4.2.3. Differences in Arterial Stiffness. Finally, gender differences in local and regional arterial stiffness parameters have also been previously described. Ayer et al. [38] found that boys present higher local stiffness (assessed as CCA distensibility) at ~8 years of age. Several authors found that boys have higher cfPWV levels than girls. Again, these differences could be found mostly for postpubertal or transitional ages [16, 34, 41]. Elmenhorst et al. [18] also suggested the existence of different gender-related growth patterns in cfPWV, reporting a more marked increase for boys.

We found that boys have a higher increasing rate in aortic regional stiffness than girls and that this difference was BP-independent, suggesting higher levels of intrinsic wall stiffness.

4.3. Physiological and Clinical Implications. The marked increase in CRF exposure in pediatric ages (mostly rising prevalence of obesity and physical inactivity) in the last decades, together with accumulating evidence showing the association of early development of arterial impairment with the presence of several CRF [41–43], determines the needs for designing a new approach in order to evaluate those children at risk of developing these alterations. Moreover, evidence showing positive outcomes when carrying out early interventions in pediatric patients who already present a burden or arterial alterations [6–8] enhances the importance of early detection of vascular impairment in young individuals.

This work contributes in determining the expected growing rates for several vascular parameters in healthy individuals, free of CRF exposure. Moreover, we provide the first approach in defining the expected relative changes in arterial properties during growing and development, as normal VA may be more accurately defined by a relative amount of change in a period than by a change in absolute values.

The integral approach carried out in our study allows a more comprehensive understanding of the normal process of aging in early ages and the interaction of structural and functional parameters during this process in the same population that could be underlying the existence of a higher cardiovascular risk in adult males.

Finally, the integral description of age-related changes in arterial properties in young populations of our work could be useful for distinguishing those subjects with abnormal rates of aging in whom it would be of benefit to design proper intervention strategies.

4.4. Limitations. The sample size of our study was relatively small, and although several findings were statistically significant, some real differences could have been missed.

Second, for the comparison between age groups we did not determine the pubertal stage of each participant. However, the main goal of our work was to determine gender-related differences in changing rates, and the group division was made seeking to preserve at least two groups with mostly prepubertal (<8 years) and mostly postpubertal (>15 years) individuals [44].

Third, to calculate the elastic modulus, ideally the local pressure (at CCA and CFA) should be used. As the difference between aortic and CCA pressure was smaller than 2 mmHg in adults [45] central aortic pressure may be a good surrogate for CCA pressure. Local CFA pressure is in general less easy to estimate and although in this case we use brachial pressure, its values may not be the same.

Fourth, the SphygmoCor technique for the assessment of central arterial pressure uses a population-based generalized transfer function that despite being used in several studies working with children and adolescents has not yet validated for pediatric populations. Additionally, we used brachial pressure to calibrate the radial waveforms and this could lead to ignoring the potential brachial-to-radial amplification. However, we calibrate our signals utilizing brachial DBP and calculated MAP, thus minimizing possible errors. Moreover, recently Picone et al. [46] found that especially in the younger subjects (<40 years) this remains a valid way of calibrating.

Fifth, the major changes found in hemodynamic parameters could be explained on the basis of different growing-related changes in cardiac function, but parameters regarding this aspect were not assessed in the present work as this matter exceeded our main aims.

Finally, we used simple linear regression models in order to simplify our comparisons. Future works will determine the utility of using nonlinear models to describe age-related changes in arterial properties and allow determining, for example, moments of steeper changes and their differences between genders and/or with CRF exposure.

5. Conclusions

Gender-related differences in arterial properties found for adults can be explained on the basis of different growing-related changes between boys and girls, with no existing differences for prepubertal children. Males showed an accelerated rate of change in vascular properties (faster VA), with respect to females. Finally, we determined that the relative changes in hemodynamic parameters are higher than in structural parameters, the latter possibly being a consequence of the former.

Acknowledgments

This work was supported by the Agencia Nacional de Investigación e Innovación (ANII) and Espacio Interdisciplinario (EI) and Comisión Sectorial de Investigación Científica (CSIC-Udelar) of the University of the Republic, Uruguay. Additionally, this work was supported by extrabudgetary funds generated by CUiiDARTE Centre and Project. Professor Dr. Yanina Zócalo and Professor Dr. Daniel Bia are the Clinical Director and General Director (resp.) of CUiiDARTE Centre and Project. The authors would also like to thank Eugenia del Palacio and Fiorella Cavalleri, for their support during the analysis process.

References

[1] W. W. Nichols, M. F. O'Rourke, and C. Vlachlopoulos, *Mcdonald's Blood Flow in Arteries*, Hodder Arnold, London, UK, 2011.

[2] P. M. Nilsson, P. Boutouyrie, P. Cunha et al., "Early vascular ageing in translation: from laboratory investigations to clinical applications in cardiovascular prevention," *Journal of Hypertension*, vol. 31, no. 8, pp. 1517–1526, 2013.

[3] J. J. Van der Heijden-Spek, J. A. Staessen, R. H. Fagard, A. P. Hoeks, H. A. Boudier, and L. M. van Bortel, "Effect of age on brachial artery wall properties differs from the aorta and is gender dependent: a population study," *Hypertension*, vol. 35, no. 2, pp. 637–642, 2000.

[4] J. D. Cameron, C. J. Bulpitt, E. S. Pinto, and C. Rajkumar, "The aging of elastic and muscular arteries: a comparison of diabetic and nondiabetic subjects," *Diabetes Care*, vol. 26, no. 7, pp. 2133–2138, 2003.

[5] P. M. Nilsson, E. Lurbe, and S. Laurent, "The early life origins of vascular ageing and cardiovascular risk: the EVA syndrome," *Journal of Hypertension*, vol. 26, no. 6, pp. 1049–1057, 2008.

[6] M. Ridha, S. E. Nourse, and E. S. Selamet Tierney, "Pediatric interventions using noninvasive vascular health indices," *Hypertension*, vol. 65, no. 5, pp. 949–955, 2015.

[7] A. A. Meyer, G. Kundt, U. Lenschow, P. Schuff-Werner, and W. Kienast, "Improvement of early vascular changes and cardiovascular risk factors in obese children after a six-month exercise program," *Journal of the American College of Cardiology*, vol. 48, no. 9, pp. 1865–1870, 2006.

[8] N. J. Farpour-Lambert, Y. Aggoun, L. M. Marchand, X. E. Martin, F. R. Herrmann, and M. Beghetti, "Physical activity reduces systemic blood pressure and improves early markers of atherosclerosis in pre-pubertal obese children," *Journal of the*

American College of Cardiology, vol. 54, no. 25, pp. 2396–2406, 2009.

[9] C. Delles, A. F. Dominiczak, U. Kingdom et al., "Hypertension management in the 21st century: major advances and achievements," *Medicographia*, vol. 34, no. 1, pp. 11–16, 2012.

[10] S. J. Vermeersch, E. R. Rietzschel, M. L. De Buyzere et al., "Age and gender related patterns in carotid-femoral PWV and carotid and femoral stiffness in a large healthy, middle-aged population," *Journal of Hypertension*, vol. 26, no. 7, pp. 1411–1419, 2008.

[11] P. G. Cunha, J. Cotter, P. Oliveira et al., "Pulse wave velocity distribution in a cohort study," *Journal of Hypertension*, vol. 33, no. 7, pp. 1438–1445, 2015.

[12] F. Yao, Y. Liu, D. Liu et al., "Sex differences between vascular endothelial function and carotid intima-media thickness by Framingham Risk Score," *Journal of Ultrasound in Medicine*, vol. 33, no. 2, pp. 281–286, 2014.

[13] M. Juonala, M. Kähönen, T. Laitinen et al., "Effect of age and sex on carotid intima-media thickness, elasticity and brachial endothelial function in healthy adults: the Cardiovascular Risk in Young Finns study," *European Heart Journal*, vol. 29, no. 9, pp. 1198–1206, 2008.

[14] D. B. Santana, Y. A. Zócalo, I. F. Ventura et al., "Health informatics design for assisted diagnosis of subclinical atherosclerosis, structural, and functional arterial age calculus and patient-specific cardiovascular risk evaluation," *IEEE Transactions on Information Technology in Biomedicine*, vol. 16, no. 5, pp. 943–951, 2012.

[15] D. B. Santana, Y. A. Zócalo, and R. L. Armentano, "Integrated e-health approach based on vascular ultrasound and pulse wave analysis for asymptomatic atherosclerosis detection and cardiovascular risk stratification in the community," *IEEE Transactions on Information Technology in Biomedicine*, vol. 16, no. 2, pp. 287–294, 2012.

[16] G. S. Reusz, O. Cseprekal, M. Temmar et al., "Reference values of pulse wave velocity in healthy children and teenagers," *Hypertension*, vol. 56, no. 2, pp. 217–224, 2010.

[17] D.-C. Fischer, C. Schreiver, M. Heimhalt, A. Noerenberg, and D. Haffner, "Pediatric reference values of carotid-femoral pulse wave velocity determined with an oscillometric device," *Journal of Hypertension*, vol. 30, no. 11, pp. 2159–2167, 2012.

[18] J. Elmenhorst, M. Hulpke-Wette, C. Barta, R. Dalla Pozza, S. Springer, and R. Oberhoffer, "Percentiles for central blood pressure and pulse wave velocity in children and adolescents recorded with an oscillometric device," *Atherosclerosis*, vol. 238, no. 1, pp. 9–16, 2015.

[19] A. de Arriba Muñoz, M. M. Domínguez Cajal, J. I. Labarta Aizpún, M. Domínguez Cunchillos, E. Mayayo Dehesa, and Á. Ferrández Longás, "Índice íntima-media carotídeo; valores de normalidad desde los 4 años," *Nutricion Hospitalaria*, vol. 28, no. 4, pp. 1171–1176, 2013.

[20] A. Doyon, D. Kracht, A. K. Bayazit et al., "Carotid artery intima-media thickness and distensibility in children and adolescents: reference values and role of body dimensions," *Hypertension*, vol. 62, no. 3, pp. 550–556, 2013.

[21] S. Laurent, J. Cockcroft, L. Van Bortel et al., "Expert consensus document on arterial stiffness: methodological issues and clinical applications," *European Heart Journal*, vol. 27, no. 21, pp. 2588–2605, 2006.

[22] L. M. Van Bortel, S. Laurent, P. Boutouyrie et al., "Expert consensus document on the measurement of aortic stiffness in daily practice using carotid-femoral pulse wave velocity," *Journal of Hypertension*, vol. 30, no. 3, pp. 445–448, 2012.

[23] K. Shirai, J. Utino, K. Otsuka, and M. Takata, "A novel blood pressure-independent arterial wall stiffness parameter; Cardio-Ankle Vascular Index (CAVI)," *Journal of Atherosclerosis and Thrombosis*, vol. 13, no. 2, pp. 101–107, 2006.

[24] D. Bia, Y. Zócalo, I. Farro et al., "Integrated evaluation of age-related changes in structural and functional vascular parameters used to assess arterial aging, subclinical atherosclerosis, and cardiovascular risk in uruguayan adults: CUiiDARTE project," *International Journal of Hypertension*, vol. 2011, Article ID 587303, 12 pages, 2011.

[25] J. H. Stein, C. E. Korcarz, R. T. Hurst et al., "Use of carotid ultrasound to identify subclinical vascular disease and evaluate cardiovascular disease risk: a consensus statement from the american society of echocardiography carotid intima-media thickness task force endorsed by the society for vascular," *Journal of the American Society of Echocardiography*, vol. 21, no. 2, pp. 93–111, 2008.

[26] E. S. Selamet Tierney, K. Gauvreau, M. R. Jaff et al., "Carotid artery intima-media thickness measurements in the youth: reproducibility and technical considerations," *Journal of the American Society of Echocardiography*, vol. 28, no. 3, pp. 309–316, 2015.

[27] C.-H. Chen, E. Nevo, B. Fetics et al., "Estimation of central aortic pressure waveform by mathematical transformation of radial tonometry pressure. Validation of generalized transfer function," *Circulation*, vol. 95, no. 7, pp. 1827–1836, 1997.

[28] I. B. Wilkinson, H. MacCallum, L. Flint, J. R. Cockcroft, D. E. Newby, and D. J. Webb, "The influence of heart rate on augmentation index and central arterial pressure in humans," *Journal of Physiology*, vol. 525, no. 1, pp. 263–270, 2000.

[29] C. M. McEniery, Yasmin, I. R. Hall, A. Qasem, I. B. Wilkinson, and J. R. Cockcroft, "Normal vascular aging: differential effects on wave reflection and aortic pulse wave velocity—the Anglo-Cardiff Collaborative Trial (ACCT)," *Journal of the American College of Cardiology*, vol. 46, no. 9, pp. 1753–1760, 2005.

[30] C. S. Hayward and R. P. Kelly, "Gender-related differences in the central arterial pressure waveform," *Journal of the American College of Cardiology*, vol. 30, no. 7, pp. 1863–1871, 1997.

[31] B. Böhm, K. Hartmann, M. Buck, and R. Oberhoffer, "Sex differences of carotid intima-media thickness in healthy children and adolescents," *Atherosclerosis*, vol. 206, no. 2, pp. 458–463, 2009.

[32] T. Ishizu, T. Ishimitsu, H. Yanagi et al., "Effect of age on carotid arterial intima-media thickness in childhood," *Heart and Vessels*, vol. 19, no. 4, pp. 189–195, 2004.

[33] L. Engelen, I. Ferreira, C. D. Stehouwer, P. Boutouyrie, and S. Laurent, "Reference intervals for common carotid intima-medi thickness measured with echotracking: relation with risk factors," *European Heart Journal*, vol. 34, no. 30, pp. 2368–2380, 2013.

[34] E. V. Hidvégi, M. Illyés, B. Benczúr et al., "Reference values of aortic pulse wave velocity in a large healthy population aged between 3 and 18 years," *Journal of Hypertension*, vol. 30, no. 12, pp. 2314–2321, 2012.

[35] H. Senzaki, M. Akagi, T. Hishi et al., "Age-associated changes in arterial elastic properties in children," *European Journal of Pediatrics*, vol. 161, no. 10, pp. 547–551, 2002.

[36] J. A. Staessen, J. J. van der Heijden-Spek, M. E. Safar et al., "Menopause and the characteristics of the large arteries in a

population study," *Journal of Human Hypertension*, vol. 15, no. 8, pp. 511–518, 2001.

[37] L. Stoner, J. Faulkner, N. Westrupp, and D. Lambrick, "Sexual differences in central arterial wave reflection are evident in prepubescent children," *Journal of Hypertension*, vol. 33, no. 2, pp. 304–307, 2015.

[38] J. G. Ayer, J. A. Harmer, G. B. Marks, A. Avolio, and D. S. Celermajer, "Central arterial pulse wave augmentation is greater in girls than boys, independent of height," *Journal of Hypertension*, vol. 28, no. 2, pp. 306–313, 2010.

[39] J. H. Stein, P. S. Douglas, S. R. Srinivasan et al., "Distribution and cross-sectional age-related increases of carotid artery intima-media thickness in young adults: the Bogalusa Heart study," *Stroke*, vol. 35, no. 12, pp. 2782–2787, 2004.

[40] D. B. Santana, J. G. Barra, J. C. Grignola, F. F. Ginés, and R. L. Armentano, "Pulmonary artery smooth muscle activation attenuates arterial dysfunction during acute pulmonary hypertension," *Journal of Applied Physiology*, vol. 98, no. 2, pp. 605–613, 2005.

[41] M. Charakida, A. Jones, E. Falaschetti et al., "Childhood obesity and vascular phenotypes: a population study," *Journal of the American College of Cardiology*, vol. 60, no. 25, pp. 2643–2650, 2012.

[42] A. T. Cote, K. C. Harris, C. Panagiotopoulos, G. G. S. Sandor, and A. M. Devlin, "Childhood obesity and cardiovascular dysfunction," *Journal of the American College of Cardiology*, vol. 62, no. 15, pp. 1309–1319, 2013.

[43] D. S. Freedman, D. A. Patel, S. R. Srinivasan et al., "The contribution of childhood obesity to adult carotid intima-media thickness: the Bogalusa Heart Study," *International Journal of Obesity*, vol. 32, no. 5, pp. 749–756, 2008.

[44] C. S. Tam, F. De Zegher, S. P. Garnett, L. A. Baur, and C. T. Cowell, "Opposing influences of prenatal and postnatal growth on the timing of menarche," *The Journal of Clinical Endocrinology & Metabolism*, vol. 91, no. 11, pp. 4369–4373, 2006.

[45] L. M. Van Bortel, E. J. Balkestein, J. J. van der Heijden-Spek et al., "Non-invasive assessment of local arterial pulse pressure: comparison of applanation tonometry and echo-tracking," *Journal of Hypertension*, vol. 19, no. 6, pp. 1037–1044, 2001.

[46] D. S. Picone, R. E. Climie, K. D. Ahuja, M. A. Keske, and J. E. Sharman, "Brachial-to-radial SBP amplification: implications of age and estimated central blood pressure from radial tonometry," *Journal of Hypertension*, vol. 33, no. 9, pp. 1876–1883, 2015.

18

Carotid Intima Media Thickness Reference Intervals for a Healthy Argentinean Population Aged 11–81 Years

Alejandro Diaz ,[1] Daniel Bia,[2] Yanina Zócalo ,[2] Hugo Manterola,[3] Ignacio Larrabide,[3] Lucas Lo Vercio,[3] Mariana Del Fresno,[3] and Edmundo Cabrera Fischer[4]

[1]*Instituto de Investigación en Ciencias de la Salud, UNICEN, CONICET, Tandil, Argentina*
[2]*Physiology Department, School of Medicine, Centro Universitario de Investigación, Innovación y Diagnóstico Arterial (CUiiDARTE), Republic University, General Flores 2125, 11800 Montevideo, Uruguay*
[3]*PLADEMA, Facultad de Ciencias Exactas, Universidad Nacional del Centro de la Provincia de Buenos Aires, Tandil, Argentina*
[4]*Instituto de Medicina Traslacional, Trasplante y Bioingeniería (IMETTyB), Universidad Favaloro-CONICET, Buenos Aires, Argentina*

Correspondence should be addressed to Alejandro Diaz; alejandrounicen@gmail.com

Academic Editor: Franco Veglio

Reference intervals (RIs) of carotid intima media thickness (CIMT) from large healthy population are still lacking in Latin America. The aim of this study was to determine CIMT RIs in a cohort of 1012 healthy subjects from Argentina. We evaluated if RIs for males and females and for left and right carotids were necessary. Second, mean and standard deviation (SD) age-related equations were obtained for left, right, and average (left + right)/2) CIMT using parametric regression methods based on fractional polynomials, in order to obtain age-specific percentiles curves. Age-specific percentile curves were obtained. Males showed higher A-CIMT (0.577 ± 0.003 mm versus 0.566 ± 0.004 mm, $P = 0.039$) in comparison with females. For males, the equations were as follows: A-CIMT mean $= 0.42 + 8.14 \times 10^{-5} * \text{Age}^2$; A-CIMT SD $= 5.9 \times 10^{-2} + 1.09 \times 10^{-5} * \text{Age}^2$. For females, they were as follows: A-CIMT mean $= 0.40 + 8.20 \times 10^{-5} * \text{Age}^2$; A-CIMT SD $= 4.67 \times 10^{-2} + 1.63 \times 10^{-5} * \text{Age}^2$. Our study provides the largest database concerning RIs of CIMT in healthy people in Argentina. Specific RIs and percentiles of CIMT for children, adolescents, and adults are now available according to age and gender, for right and left common carotid arteries.

1. Introduction

The early detection of subclinical arterial damage is of value for individual cardiovascular risk assessment and identification of subjects with increased risk (vulnerable subjects) who could benefit from specific preventive strategies [1].

In 1986, common carotid intima media thickness (CIMT) was firstly measured in in vitro studies of arteries from cadaveric donors and noninvasively in ambulatory healthy subjects [2]. Since then, arterial structure characterization through CIMT assessment was introduced in clinical practice and epidemiological investigations demonstrated the prognostic value of this noninvasive study. Common CIMT higher than 0.9 mm has been considered as a factor influencing cardiovascular prognosis by the 2013 ESH/ESC Guidelines for the management of arterial hypertension [3]. Recently, Amato et al. reported that CIMT is an independent predictor of vascular events and should be included in cardiovascular risk models destined to population stratification and preventive strategies [4]. Interestingly, a CIMT score improved the Framingham risk score to predict coronary heart diseases events [4–6]. Also, a recent European consensus reported that increase of CIMT has shown to be marker of hypertension vascular damage and increased cardiovascular risk [5]. Since CIMT is relatively easy to evaluate, the clinical use allows the risk stratification and target organ damage assessment [5, 6].

Age and gender specific percentiles for common CIMT were defined in large populations of healthy subjects and the influence of cardiovascular risk factors (CRFs) was quantified allowing comparative studies among groups with differentiated risk profiles [7]. Epidemiological studies also included pediatric research to characterize age-related CIMT changes in children and adolescent populations for the prediction of cardiovascular events [8].

Ethnicity has demonstrated being an independent predictor of CIMT [9], while intergeographic variations have been observed when comparing data from urban populations from Latin America [10]. Those findings point out that a direct extrapolation and use of CIMT reference intervals (RIs) defined for healthy subjects from European, Asian, or North American populations could not be appropriate and this would be even risky at the time of using CIMT in clinical practice.

Linked to what is mentioned above about factors influencing CIMT, it is noteworthy that left common carotid artery directly originates from the aortic arch, while in the right side the same vessel is a branch of the brachiocephalic trunk. The different origins led to the hypothesis that age, gender, CRFs, and hemodynamic factors would have differential effects on CIMT, depending on the artery analyzed [11]. On the other hand, it has been demonstrated that technical and methodological issues should be considered at the time of CIMT assessment, as well as when analyzing and comparing CIMT data. Then, the development of guidelines and recommendations for standardized CIMT assessment was considered necessary. In this regard, reports from the *Reference Values for Arterial Measurements Collaboration* group (Europe) [7] highlighted the relevance of standardizing both methods and statistical approaches used for vascular evaluation and analysis of large databases.

To the best of our knowledge, there are no works characterizing the CIMT levels and RIs for an urban-rural Argentinean healthy population nonexposed to CRFs, considering a wide age range.

In this context, the purpose of our research was to determine RIs values and age-related CIMT percentile curves in a healthy Argentinean population that included children, adolescents, and adults nonexposed to CRFs. Our data analysis took into account similar methodological considerations to those established by the European group *"Reference Values for Arterial Measurements Collaboration"* [7, 12].

2. Materials and Methods

2.1. Study Population. This study is part of a project started in 2010 aimed at investigating the prevalence of CRFs. Preliminary data have been previously published [13–16]. The socioeconomic indicators of this population are similar to that of the Argentinean population and other countries of the Southern Cone of Latin America [17, 18].

The protocol of this research was evaluated and approved by the Institutional Ethics and Research Committee. The study was carried on in agreement with the Declaration of Helsinki and the Guidelines for Good Clinical Practice of the European Medicines Agency. Written informed consent was obtained from the participants or those responsible for them.

Asymptomatic subjects from the community were considered for enrollment in this study. Subjects were submitted to clinical interview, blood sampling evaluation, and anthropometric assessment, carried out in all cases by the same group of physicians. Blood samples were obtained after 9–12 hours of fasting. Glycaemia, lipid profile, and kidney functional parameters were determined. Anthropometric evaluation and a brief clinical interview allowed assessing CRFs exposure. Subjects included in the study met the following criteria: (1) normal blood pressure (BP) at the time of examination (being BP < 140/90 mmHg in adults and BP < 90th percentile in younger subjects) [19], (2) no history of cardiovascular, pulmonary, or renal disease; (3) not taking medications (antihyperlipidemic, antihypertensive, or antidiabetic drugs), and (4) all having glycaemia < 6.11 mmol/L (<110 mg/dl), total blood cholesterol levels < 5.17 mmol/L (<200 mg/dl) [3], and normal triglycerides (TG) levels < 1.69 mmol/L (<150 mg/dl) and ≤1.5 mmol/L (<130 mg/dl) for subjects older than 18 years and subjects between 10 to 17 years, respectively [19, 20].

Current and past smokers, diabetic, obese subjects defined by a body mass index (BMI) ≥ 30 kg/m^2 for adults or BMI ≥ 97th percentile for subjects < 18 years old, hypertensive subjects, or subjects with averaged high BP levels at the time of the study were excluded. To this end, BP measurements were obtained after 5 minutes of sitting rest [3, 19] using fully automatic sphygmomanometers, operating on oscillometric principle (705IT, Omron Healthcare Inc., USA). Adults' BP levels were classified following guidelines for the management of arterial hypertension [3]. Thus, hypertension was defined as systolic BP (SBP) ≥ 140 mmHg and/or diastolic blood pressure (DBP) ≥ 90 mmHg. BP levels in children and adolescents were categorized, considering gender, age, and body height, according to criteria from the American Pediatrics Association and the European Society of Hypertension [19]. Subjects with atherosclerotic plaques in common, internal and/or external carotids, identified during the ultrasonographic study (see below) were excluded.

Based on inclusion and exclusion criteria we defined a population that included 1012 subjects (age range: 11–81 years, males: 61.3%) used to define CIMT RIs (Table 1).

2.2. CIMT Measurements. All examinations were performed by a single physician with certified skills in duplex scan diagnostic procedures. All measurements were done in a quiet room with stable temperature (22 ± 1°C) with the patient in supine position, after at least 10 minutes of rest. Studies were done using an Esaote MyLab 40 ultrasound system (Esaote, Genoa, Italy), using a 4–13 MHz linear transducer (LA523).

Left and right CCA and internal and external carotid arteries were scanned and analyzed to verify normal blood flow patterns. Next, sequences of images (videos including at least 5 beats cine-loops), obtained from CCA longitudinal views, were obtained, together with the ECG signal, and stored for offline analysis. Images were obtained in apnea and without swallowing movements. Using specific semiautomatic border detection software (CIMT-tool, Buenos Aires, Argentina), far wall CIMT was measured at end of diastole (peak R wave) selecting the best end diastolic frame out of the loop in the centimeter proximal to carotid bifurcation [21, 22]. CIMT was quantified for right and left common carotid arteries (R-CIMT and L-CIMT, resp.). Additionally, we calculated the averaged CIMT (A-CIMT) as follows: A-CIMT = (R-CIMT + L-CIMT)/2. Readers who did CIMT

Table 1: Subjects characteristics.

	All (n = 1012) MV ± SD	*Female* (n = 391) MV ± SD	*Males* (n = 621) MV ± SD	P value
Age [years]	42 ± 15	43 ± 14	41 ± 15	0.026
Body weight [Kg.]	66.5 ± 12.0	57.5 ± 11.0	72.5 ± 12.0	<0.001
Body height [cm]	166.0 ± 10.7	160.0 ± 10.0	170.0 ± 11.0	<0.001
BMI [Kg./m^2]	24.1 ± 3.1	22.6 ± 2.7	25.1 ± 2.9	<0.001
Total cholesterol [mg/dl]	155.5 ± 23.9	155.2 ± 23.9	155.7 ± 24.0	0.765
Triglycerides [mg/dl]	74.0 ± 22.4	73.7 ± 23.1	74.1 ± 21.9	0.789
Glycemia [mg/dl]	82.1 ± 8.8	82.1 ± 8.8	82.1 ± 8.8	0.986
Creatinine [mg/dl]	0.9 ± 2.5	0.8 ± 0.1	1.0 ± 3.1	0.417
Hematocrit [%]	41.7 ± 2.1	41.7 ± 2.1	41.7 ± 2.1	0.824
SBP [mmHg]	119 ± 11	115 ± 12	122 ± 10	<0.001
MBP [mmHg]	92 ± 9	89 ± 10	93 ± 8	<0.001
DBP [mmHg]	73 ± 8	72 ± 9	74 ± 8	0.002
PP [mmHg]	46 ± 8	43 ± 8	48 ± 7	<0.001
HR [beats/minute]	65 ± 10	66 ± 10	65 ± 9	0.205
A-CIMT [mm]	0.573 ± 0.885	0.574 ± 0.132	0.572 ± 0.128	0.753
A-CCA mean diameter [mm]	6.45 ± 0.88	6.26 ± 0.89	6.57 ± 0.86	<0.001

MV: mean value. SD: standard deviation. SBP, MBP, DBP, and PP: systolic pulse pressure, mean pulse pressure, diastolic pulse pressure, and pulse pressure. HR: heart rate. A-CIMT: common carotid artery intima media thickness average value. A-CCA: common carotid artery diameter average value. Average values are the mean of left and right measurements. Statistics: t-test (unpaired, two-tailed) analyzed differences between males and females. $P < 0.05$ was considered statistically significant.

offline measurements were blinded to participants' identity, age, and sex [10].

2.3. Data Analysis. Continuous and categorical data are expressed as mean value ± standard deviation (SD) or percentage, respectively. Data analysis was done using MedCalc Statistical Software (version 14.8.1., MedCalc Inc., Ostend, Belgium) and IBM SPSS 20.0 Software (SPSS Inc., Illinois, USA). A $P < 0.05$ was considered statistically significant.

A stepwise data analysis was done.

First, aiming at determining if RIs for R-CIMT and L-CIMT were necessary, we analyzed the degree of equivalence (agreement) between R-CIMT and L-CIMT data by assessing (potential) mean and/or proportional differences (errors) between data and constructing limits of agreement (correlation and Bland-Altman analysis). As a result, specific RIs for R-CIMT and L-CIMT were defined as necessary (Table 2). RIs for A-CIMT values were also defined, allowing analyzing our findings taking into account data from other groups [10, 21].

Second, we evaluated whether RIs for males and females were necessary. To this end, bivariate simple and point-biserial correlations between CIMT and subjects' demographic, anthropometric, and blood characteristics were analyzed (Table 3). That analysis enabled identifying variables that should be considered as cofactors in covariate analysis (ANCOVA). Then, sex influence was examined before and after adjustment for cofactors (i.e., age, BP, and total cholesterol) (Table 4). As a result, specific CIMT RIs for males and females were considered necessary (Table 4).

Third, age-specific mean and SD equations (for males and females) were obtained for L-CIMT, R-CIMT, and A-CIMT. To this end, parametric regression methods based on fractional polynomials (FPs), as described by Royston and Wright [23], were implemented in MedCalc Software (MedCalc, Ostend, Belgium). Briefly, fitting FPs for age-specific CIMT (right, left, and average) and SD regression curves were defined using iterative procedure (generalized least squares, GLS). The obtained results enabled estimating age-specific mean and SD for CIMT. For instance, CIMT = $a + b * \text{age}^p + c * \text{age}^q + \cdots$, where $a, b, c, \ldots$ are the coefficients and $p, q, \ldots$ are the powers, with numbers selected from the set $[-2, -1, -0.5, 0, 0.5, 1, 2, 3]$ estimated from the regression for the mean CIMT curve and likewise from the regression for the SD CIMT curve. Continuing the example, FPs with powers $[1, 2]$, that is, with $p = 1$ and $q = 2$, illustrate an equation with the form $a + b * \text{age} + c * \text{age}^2$ [23]. The residuals were used to assess the model fit, which was deemed appropriate if the residuals were normally distributed, with a mean of 0 and a SD of 1, randomly scattered above and below 0 when plotted against age. The best fitted curves, considering visual and mathematical criteria (Kurtosis and Skewness coefficients), were selected. Then, using the equations obtained for mean and SD, age-specific percentiles were defined using the standard normal distribution (Z) (Tables 5, 6, and 7). Age-specific 1st, 2.5th, 5th, 10th, 25th, 50th, 75th, 90th, 95th, 97.5th, and 99th percentile curves were calculated as mean CIMT + Zp $*$ SD, where Zp assumed the values of −2.3263, −1.9599, −1.6448, −1.2815, −0.6755, 0, 0.6755,

TABLE 2: Comparative study of left and right common carotid intima media thickness (CIMT).

(a) Regression analysis (left CIMT: y-axis, right CIMT: x-axis)

R^2	0.4856
Regression equation	$y = 0.1694 + 0.7601x$
Intercept	
Coefficient	0.1694
SE	0.02339
95% CI	0.1234 to 0.2154
P	<0.0001
Slope	
Coefficient	0.7601
SE	0.03902
95% CI	0.6834 to 0.8368
P	<0.0001

SE: standard error. CI: confidence interval.

(b) Differences (Bland & Altman)

	Left CIMT − right CIMT [mm]	Left − right CIMT/mean of left and right CIMT [%]
Arithmetic mean	0.029	4.641
95% CI	0.01899 to 0.03933	2.9958 to 6.2852
P (H_0: mean = 0)	<0.0001	<0.0001
SD	0.104	16.816
Lower limit	−0.175	−28.319
95% CI	−0.1920 to −0.1572	−31.1321 to −25.5058
Upper limit	0.233	37.600
95% CI	0.2156 to 0.2503	34.7867 to 40.4130
Regression equation	$y = -0.02913 + 0.09710x$	$y = -0.5378 + 8.6262x$
Intercept		
Coefficient	−0.029	−0.538
SE	0.026	4.170
t-value	−1.135	−0.129
P	0.257	0.897
95% CI	−0.07958 to 0.02132	−8.7351 to 7.6595
Slope		
Coefficient	0.097	8.626
SE	0.042	6.805
t-value	2.318	1.268
P	0.0209	0.206
95% CI	0.01476 to 0.1794	−4.7520 to 22.0044

SE and SD: standard error and standard deviation. Ho: null hypothesis. CI: confidence interval.

1.2815, 1.6448, 1.9599, and 2.3263, respectively. The obtained equations were as follows.

TABLE 3: Correlations between A-CIMT and subjects demographic, anthropometric, and blood characteristics.

	A-CIMT [mm]
Age [years]	
R	0.76
P value	**0.00**
Sex (1: male; 0: female)	
R	−0.01
P value	**0.75**
BMI [Kg./m^2]	
R	0.32
P value	**0.00**
SBP [mmHg]	
R	0.23
P value	**0.00**
DBP [mmHg]	
R	0.39
P value	**0.00**
MBP [mmHg]	
R	0.34
P value	**0.00**
Glycemia [mg/dl]	
R	0.06
P value	**0.05**
Total cholesterol [mg/dl]	
R	−0.13
P value	**0.00**
Triglycerides [mg/dl]	
R	0.07
P value	**0.02**

A-CIMT: average between left and right common carotid intima media thickness values. SBP, MBP, DBP, and PP: systolic pulse pressure, mean pulse pressure, diastolic pulse pressure, and pulse pressure. $P < 0.05$ was considered statistically significant.

(i) For males,

$$\begin{aligned}
\text{A-CIMT Mean} &= 0.415946945 + 0.000081403 * \text{Age}^2,\\
\text{A-CIMT SD} &= 0.059010065 + 0.000010936 * \text{Age}^2,\\
\text{L-CIMT Mean} &= 0.45081531 + 0.000078505 * \text{Age}^2,\\
\text{L-CIMT SD} &= 0.056001529 + 0.000024467 * \text{Age}^2,\\
\text{R-CIMT Mean} &= 0.442337809 + 0.000066517 * \text{Age}^2,\\
\text{R-CIMT SD} &= 0.069658789 + 0.000015017 * \text{Age}^2.
\end{aligned} \tag{1}$$

TABLE 4: Sex-related common carotid intima media thickness (A-CIMT) comparison: analysis of covariance (ANCOVA) adjusting by age and other cardiovascular risk factors.

	CIMT before adjustment		*CIMT after adjustment*				*Covariates appearing in the model are evaluated at the following values*						
	MV ± SE	*P* value	MV ± SE	*P* value	95% CI Lower limit	95% CI Upper limit	Age [years]	Total cholesterol [mg/dl]	Glycemia [mg/dl]	Triglycerides [mg/dl]	BMI [Kg./m^2]	SBP [mmHg]	DBP [mmHg]
Male	0.572 ± 0.128	0.753	0.577 ± 0.003	0.037	0.570	0.584	**41.91**	-----	-----	-----	-----	-----	-----
Female	0.574 ± 0.132		0.566 ± 0.004		0.557	0.574							
Male	0.572 ± 0.128	0.753	0.577 ± 0.003	0.039	0.570	0.584	**41.91**	**155.49**	**82.131**	**73.96**	-----	-----	-----
Female	0.574 ± 0.132		0.566 ± 0.004		0.557	0.574							
Male	0.572 ± 0.128	0.753	0.575 ± 0.004	0.322	0.568	0.582	**41.91**	-----	-----	-----	**24.1218**	-----	-----
Female	0.574 ± 0.132		0.569 ± 0.005		0.560	0.578							
Male	0.572 ± 0.128	0.753	0.570 ± 0.003	0.402	0.568	0.581	**41.91**	-----	-----	-----	-----	**119.23**	**73.21**
Female	0.574 ± 0.132		0.575 ± 0.004		0.561	0.578							

A-CIMT: average between left and right common carotid intima media thickness values. BMI: body mass index. SBP and DBP: systolic blood pressure and diastolic blood pressure. MV: mean value. SD: standard deviation. SE: standard error. CI: confidence interval. $P < 0.05$ was considered statistically significant.

TABLE 5: Common carotid intima media thickness [mm] percentiles for healthy male subjects (average of right and left arterial measurements).

Age [years]	1st	2.5th	5th	10th	25th	50th	75th	90th	95th	97.5th	99th
15	0.2913	0.3138	0.3332	0.3555	0.3927	0.4343	0.4758	0.5130	0.5354	0.5547	0.5773
20	0.3011	0.3243	0.3442	0.3673	0.4057	0.4485	0.4913	0.5297	0.5528	0.5727	0.5960
25	0.3136	0.3378	0.3585	0.3824	0.4223	0.4668	0.5113	0.5512	0.5751	0.5959	0.6200
30	0.3290	0.3543	0.3760	0.4010	0.4427	0.4892	0.5357	0.5774	0.6025	0.6242	0.6494
35	0.3472	0.3738	0.3966	0.4229	0.4668	0.5157	0.5646	0.6085	0.6348	0.6576	0.6841
40	0.3682	0.3962	0.4203	0.4481	0.4945	0.5462	0.5979	0.6442	0.6720	0.6961	0.7242
45	0.3920	0.4217	0.4473	0.4768	0.5260	0.5808	0.6356	0.6848	0.7143	0.7398	0.7696
50	0.4186	0.4502	0.4774	0.5088	0.5611	0.6195	0.6778	0.7301	0.7615	0.7887	0.8203
55	0.4480	0.4817	0.5107	0.5442	0.6000	0.6622	0.7244	0.7802	0.8137	0.8427	0.8764
60	0.4801	0.5162	0.5472	0.5829	0.6425	0.7090	0.7755	0.8351	0.8708	0.9018	0.9379
65	0.5151	0.5537	0.5868	0.6250	0.6888	0.7599	0.8309	0.8947	0.9329	0.9661	1.0046
70	0.5529	0.5941	0.6296	0.6705	0.7388	0.8148	0.8909	0.9591	1.0000	1.0355	1.0768
75	0.5935	0.6376	0.6756	0.7194	0.7924	0.8738	0.9553	1.0283	1.0721	1.1101	1.1542
80	0.6368	0.6841	0.7247	0.7716	0.8498	0.9369	1.0241	1.1022	1.1491	1.1898	1.2370

TABLE 6: Common carotid intima media thickness [mm] percentiles for healthy female subjects (average of right and left arterial measurements).

Age [years]	1st	2.5th	5th	10th	25th	50th	75th	90th	95th	97.5th	99th
15	0.3053	0.3238	0.3396	0.3579	0.3885	0.4225	0.4565	0.4870	0.5053	0.5212	0.5397
20	0.3130	0.3325	0.3493	0.3686	0.4009	0.4368	0.4728	0.5050	0.5244	0.5411	0.5606
25	0.3230	0.3438	0.3617	0.3824	0.4169	0.4553	0.4937	0.5282	0.5489	0.5668	0.5876
30	0.3351	0.3576	0.3769	0.3992	0.4364	0.4779	0.5193	0.5565	0.5788	0.5981	0.6206
35	0.3494	0.3739	0.3949	0.4191	0.4595	0.5045	0.5495	0.5899	0.6142	0.6352	0.6596
40	0.3660	0.3926	0.4156	0.4420	0.4861	0.5353	0.5844	0.6285	0.6550	0.6779	0.7046
45	0.3847	0.4139	0.4390	0.4680	0.5163	0.5701	0.6240	0.6723	0.7012	0.7263	0.7555
50	0.4057	0.4377	0.4653	0.4970	0.5500	0.6091	0.6682	0.7212	0.7529	0.7805	0.8125
55	0.4289	0.4640	0.4943	0.5292	0.5873	0.6522	0.7170	0.7752	0.8101	0.8403	0.8755
60	0.4542	0.4928	0.5260	0.5643	0.6282	0.6993	0.7705	0.8344	0.8726	0.9058	0.9444
65	0.4818	0.5241	0.5606	0.6025	0.6726	0.7506	0.8287	0.8987	0.9407	0.9771	1.0194
70	0.5116	0.5580	0.5978	0.6438	0.7205	0.8060	0.8915	0.9681	1.0141	1.0540	1.1003
75	0.5436	0.5943	0.6379	0.6881	0.7720	0.8654	0.9589	1.0428	1.0930	1.1366	1.1873

(ii) For females,

$$\begin{aligned}
\text{A-CIMT Mean} &= 0.404023579 + 0.000082031 * \text{Age}^2,\\
\text{A-CIMT SD} &= 0.046702325 + 0.000016293 * \text{Age}^2,\\
\text{L-CIMT Mean} &= 0.404650458 + 0.000093708 * \text{Age}^2,\\
\text{L-CIMT SD} &= 0.054233452 + 0.00002113 * \text{Age}^2,\\
\text{R-CIMT Mean} &= 0.403946979 + 0.000083633 * \text{Age}^2,\\
\text{R-CIMT SD} &= 0.046333378 + 0.000020631 * \text{Age}^2.
\end{aligned} \quad (2)$$

In the equations, CIMT and age were always expressed in mm and years, respectively.

Considering an 80% and a 95% reference limit and confidence interval (two-sided), respectively, and a 95% and 10% reference range and relative margin of error, respectively, and considering an equally distributed (in three groups at the midpoint and extreme ranges) covariate (age) in the sample, the minimum required sample size was 136 subjects [24].

Finally, the mathematical difference between specific percentiles (75th or 90th) obtained for L-CIMT and R-CIMT was quantified (i.e., 75th percentile for L-CIMT minus 75th percentile for R-CIMT) and analyzed according to age and sex. The analysis (graphic) allowed visualizing how the differences between similar percentiles obtained for left and right CCA were modified with aging, for both males and females.

3. Results

3.1. General Characteristics of the Analyzed Population. One thousand and twelve healthy subjects were included. Table 1

Table 7: Right common carotid intima media thickness [mm] percentiles for healthy male subjects.

Age [years]	1st	2.5th	5th	10th	25th	50th	75th	90th	95th	97.5th	99th
20	0.2929	0.3206	0.3445	0.3720	0.4178	0.4689	0.5201	0.5659	0.5934	0.6172	0.6450
25	0.3000	0.3290	0.3539	0.3826	0.4305	0.4839	0.5373	0.5852	0.6139	0.6388	0.6678
30	0.3087	0.3392	0.3654	0.3956	0.4460	0.5022	0.5584	0.6088	0.6390	0.6652	0.6957
35	0.3190	0.3512	0.3790	0.4110	0.4643	0.5238	0.5833	0.6367	0.6687	0.6964	0.7287
40	0.3308	0.3651	0.3947	0.4287	0.4855	0.5488	0.6120	0.6688	0.7029	0.7324	0.7667
45	0.3442	0.3809	0.4124	0.4488	0.5094	0.5770	0.6446	0.7053	0.7416	0.7732	0.8098
50	0.3592	0.3985	0.4323	0.4712	0.5362	0.6086	0.6810	0.7460	0.7850	0.8187	0.8580
55	0.3758	0.4180	0.4543	0.4961	0.5658	0.6436	0.7213	0.7910	0.8329	0.8691	0.9113
60	0.3940	0.4393	0.4783	0.5232	0.5982	0.6818	0.7654	0.8404	0.8853	0.9243	0.9696
65	0.4137	0.4625	0.5044	0.5528	0.6335	0.7234	0.8133	0.8940	0.9423	0.9843	1.0330
70	0.4350	0.4875	0.5327	0.5847	0.6715	0.7683	0.8650	0.9518	1.0039	1.0490	1.1015

Table 8: Right common carotid intima media thickness [mm] percentiles for healthy female subjects.

Age [years]	1st	2.5th	5th	10th	25th	50th	75th	90th	95th	97.5th	99th
25	0.3184	0.3401	0.3588	0.3803	0.4162	0.4562	0.4962	0.5321	0.5536	0.5723	0.5940
30	0.3282	0.3520	0.3725	0.3960	0.4354	0.4792	0.5231	0.5624	0.5860	0.6064	0.6302
35	0.3398	0.3661	0.3886	0.4146	0.4580	0.5064	0.5548	0.5982	0.6242	0.6467	0.6730
40	0.3532	0.3823	0.4073	0.4361	0.4842	0.5378	0.5914	0.6394	0.6683	0.6933	0.7223
45	0.3683	0.4006	0.4284	0.4604	0.5138	0.5733	0.6328	0.6862	0.7182	0.7460	0.7783
50	0.3853	0.4211	0.4520	0.4876	0.5469	0.6130	0.6792	0.7385	0.7741	0.8049	0.8408
55	0.4040	0.4438	0.4781	0.5176	0.5835	0.6569	0.7304	0.7963	0.8358	0.8701	0.9099
60	0.4245	0.4686	0.5066	0.5505	0.6236	0.7050	0.7865	0.8596	0.9034	0.9414	0.9856
65	0.4467	0.4956	0.5377	0.5862	0.6671	0.7573	0.8475	0.9284	0.9769	1.0190	1.0679
70	0.4708	0.5248	0.5713	0.6248	0.7142	0.8137	0.9133	1.0027	1.0562	1.1027	1.1567
75	0.4966	0.5561	0.6073	0.6663	0.7647	0.8744	0.9841	1.0825	1.1415	1.1926	1.2521

summarizes data from the entire population and shows findings for males and females. Compared to males, females were (slightly) older and showed lower weight, height, BMI, SBP, MAP, and PP levels ($P < 0.05$) (Table 1). L-CIMT values were higher ($P < 0.05$) than those obtained for R-CIMT. Those differences were observed in the entire population, in males and in females (Figure 1).

A-CIMT value for the entire group was 0.573 ± 0.88 mm, being slightly higher in females (PNS).

3.2. CIMT Reference Intervals: Need for Right and Left Specific Determinations. Table 2 and Figure 2(a) show L-CIMT and R-CIMT correlation and the Bland and Altman analysis done to identify potential differences between measurements (Figure 2(b)). As was expected, both determinations showed a significant positive correlation ($P < 0.0001$). In addition, in absolute and relative (percentage) terms, L-CIMT values were higher than R-CIMT (mean or systematic error = 0.029 mm or 4.64%, $P < 0.0001$) (see Figure 2(c)).

There was a proportional error (net slope = 0.097; $P = 0.0209$) between left and right CIMT values. The mentioned differences support the need for specific RIs in analysis of L-CIMT and R-CIMT.

3.3. Analysis of CIMT Reference Intervals: Need for Determinations Differentiated by Sex. As can be seen in Table 3, A-CIMT was positively associated with age ($r = 0.76$, $P = 0.0001$), BMI, BP (SBP, DBP, and MAP), glycaemia, cholesterol, and TG levels. It is noteworthy that there were no differences in A-CIMT between males and females (Table 3) before adjusting for covariates (Table 4). However, after adjusting (ANCOVA analysis) for age, total cholesterol, TG, and glycaemia, there were sex-related differences in A-CIMT (Table 4). Compared to females, males showed higher A-CIMT values (0.577 ± 0.003 mm versus. 0.566 ± 0.004 mm, $P = 0.039$). The sex-related differences in A-CIMT supported the need for RIs differentiated by gender.

As can be seen in Table 4 differences in A-CIMT between males and females could be explained considering the physiological differences in BMI and/or BP, since when the model was adjusted by those cofactors, the sex-related differences in A-CIMT disappeared.

3.4. CIMT Reference Intervals (Percentile Analysis). Age-specific (5-year intervals, RIs) percentile analyses for A-CIMT corresponding to males and females are shown in Tables 5 and 6, respectively. Similarly, in the Supplementary Materials, Tables A and B (for males and females, resp.) show the RIs for A-CIMT defined for each year of age.

Age-specific (5-year RIs) percentile analyses of R-CIMT corresponding to males and females are shown in Tables 7 and 8, respectively. In the Supplementary Materials, Tables C

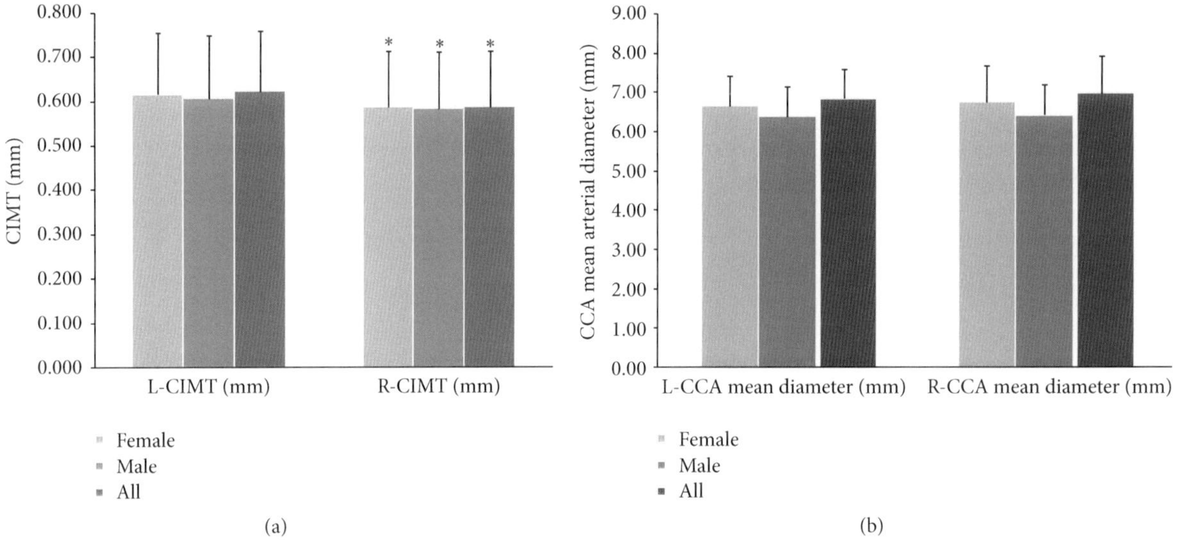

FIGURE 1: Left and right CIMT (a) and carotid diameter (b) in males, females, and all subject. CIMT: carotid intima media thickness. *Statistically significant difference.

and D show data for year of age in both males and females, respectively.

The age-specific (5-years RIs) percentile analysis of L-CIMT corresponding to males and females are shown in Tables 9 and 10, respectively. In the Supplementary Materials, Tables E and F, show data for year of age both, in males and females, respectively.

Figures 3, 4, and 5 show age and sex-specific A-CIMT percentile lines superimposed on the raw data (part (a) of each figure) and the residual distribution for A-CIMT values according to age (part (b) of each figure), for the whole population, males and females, respectively.

Percentile differences (75th and 90th) between L-CIMT and R-CIMT increased with age in both, males and females (Figure 6). The increase was more pronounced in males than in females. However, while percentile 75th and 90th showed an age-related increase in females, in males there was an inverse relationship before and after a given age (between 35 and 40 y.). As can be seen in Figure 6, 90th percentile showed the lowest values in younger males, while in older males exhibiting the highest differences between L-CIMT and R-CIMT.

4. Discussion

Most of the studies in which RIs for CIMT were defined included data obtained from retrospective analysis of patients evaluated in different specialized centers [4, 7, 9, 25]. On the other hand, differences in inclusion/exclusion criteria and/or in the methodological approaches make it difficult to carry out comparative analyses among studies and/or to extrapolate data to other populations.

Despite the recognized value of CIMT for predicting cardiovascular risk, in the Southern Cone of Latin America there is a scarcity of RIs. To the best of our knowledge, three research groups published reference values for CIMT in Latina America. CARMELA study reported normal CIMT values obtained from the study of 3071 subjects (25–64 years), from 7 cities of urban Latin America [10]. On the other hand, RIs for CIMT based on urban population screening have only been reported from Uruguay [26] and Peru [27].

In this context, the present research shows RIs for CIMT with respect to age, providing relevant clinical information in terms of carotid wall structure. About this, changes in CIMT have been described in association with aging, which should be taken into account when using CIMT in clinical practice. About this, the clinician should know expected mean and deviations values, so as to adequately interpret CIMT data obtained in a given subject and to orientate both diagnosis and preventive strategies.

Our work has methodological strengths and relevant findings that should be remarked.

First, this work represents the first rural-urban Argentine population based study aiming at determining CIMT reference values in a large number of normotensive and healthy subjects nonexposed to CRFs. It should be noted that demographic and sociocultural characteristics of the population from Tandil have similarities with the other populations from Argentina and South America [17]. About this, adequate interpretation and application of data obtained in this work require taking into account the studied population context and characteristics. In turn and in agreement with what is stated above, data could only be extrapolated to those communities with similar characteristics.

Second, the number of subjects included in our research is similar to that mentioned in the specialized literature (international databases) [28, 29], but in this work we considered a wider age range (11 to 81 years). CARMELA study included 3071 adults and healthy subjects between 25 and 64 years [10]. Therefore, no data about RIs for CIMT in the adolescents and elderly subjects were defined in the mentioned work. That would be considered an important issue, since it is known

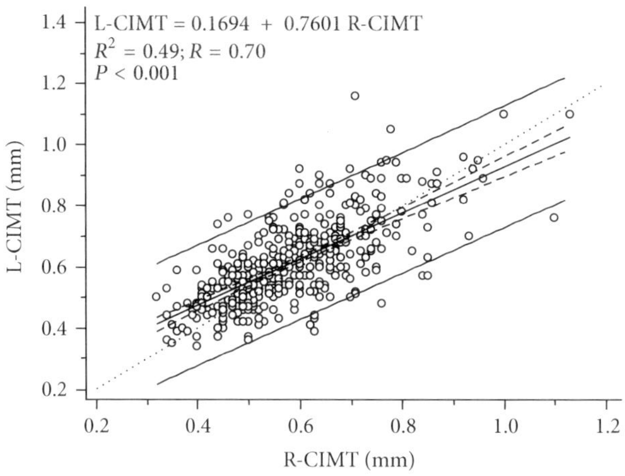

(a) Association between the left and right CIMT (simple regression analysis). CIMT: carotid intima media thickness

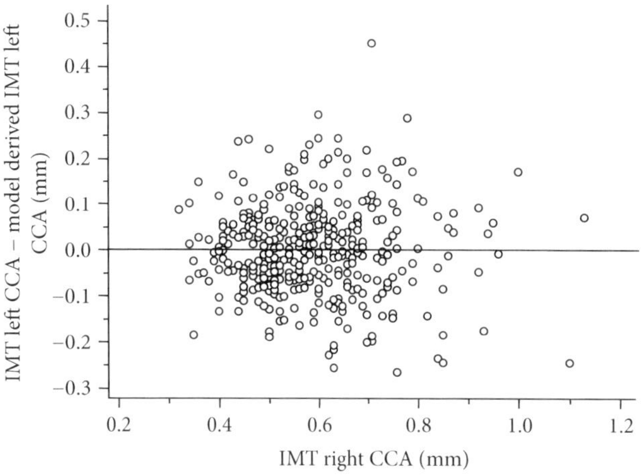

(b) Differences between the predicted L-CIMT values (model derived L-CIMT) and the observed L-CIMT values, when the regression equation shown in Figure 2(a) was applied. The residual plots allow the visual evaluation of the goodness of fit of the selected model. L: left. CIMT: carotid intima media thickness

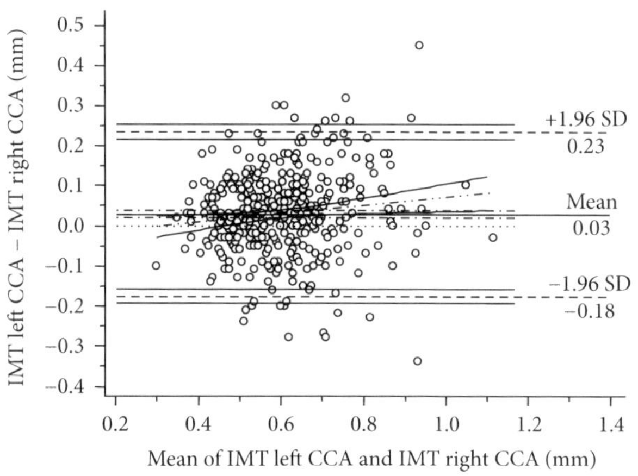

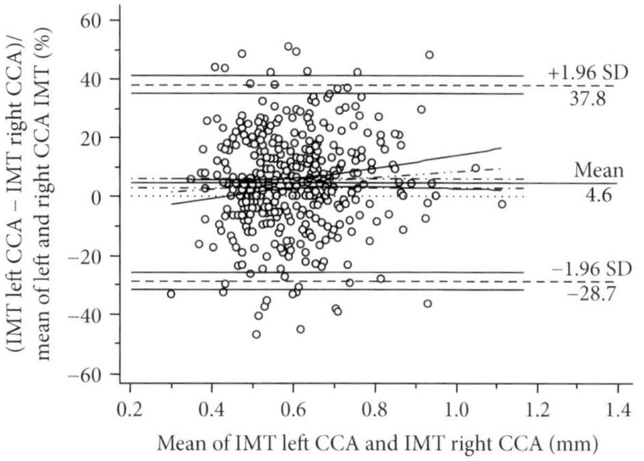

(c) Absolute (top) and relative difference (bottom) between left and right CIMT (Bland-Altman). CIMT: carotid intima media thickness

FIGURE 2

that elderly population would represent up to 15% of the total population of the Southern Cone countries [17]. On the other hand, the number of subjects included in other works is significantly smaller than that of this work. In Latin America Pastorius et al. reported CIMT RIs for adult males and females (20–80 years) based on 472 healthy subjects from Peru [27]. In Uruguay, Farro et al. reported RIs for CIMT in 367 subjects including adolescents selected from an urban population [26]. The European Registry of Reference Values for Arterial Measurements Collaboration reported normal

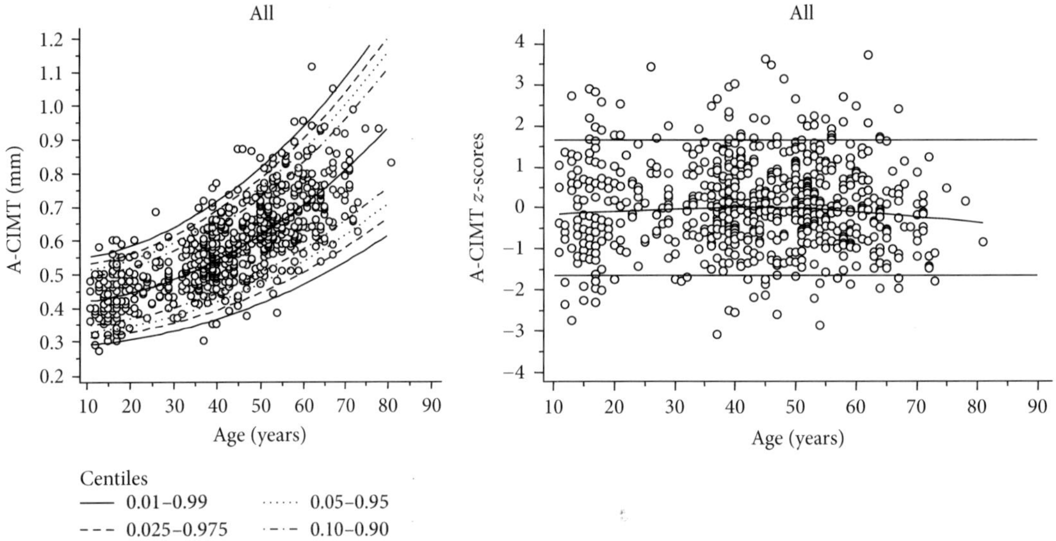

(a) Age-specific percentiles of the averaged CIMT for the entire population (n = 1,012). CIMT: carotid intima media thickness

(b) Residual distribution (z-scores) of the averaged CIMT-age analysis for the entire population. CIMT: carotid intima media thickness

FIGURE 3

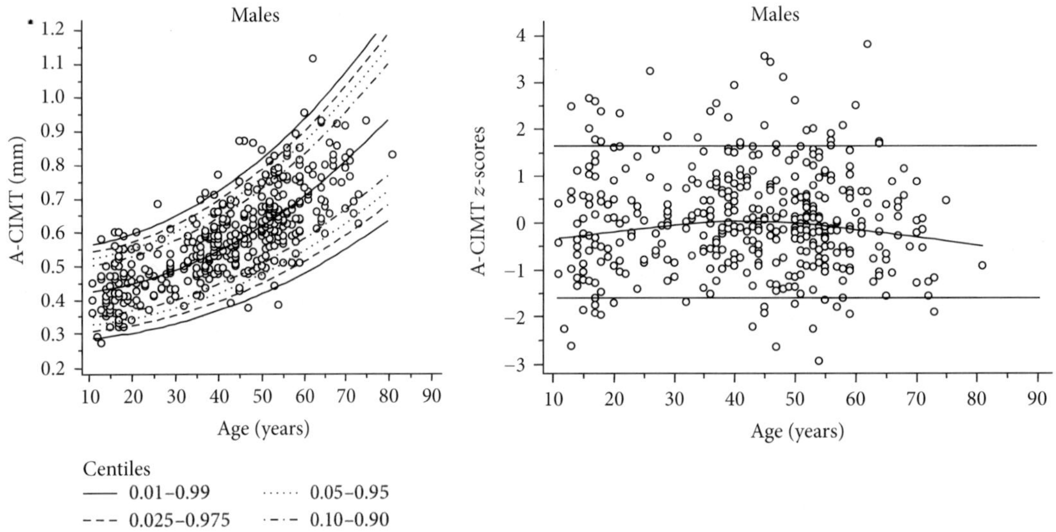

(a) Averaged CIMT percentiles according to age for males. CIMT: Carotid Intima Media Thickness

(b) Residual distribution (z-scores) for averaged CIMT-age in males. CIMT: carotid intima media thickness

FIGURE 4

values of CIMT based on 4234 records. Those values were obtained from a retrospective analysis of CIMT assessed with echotracking in 24 European centers of high complexity [7]. Then, the "normal population" was in fact a highly selected group of subjects whose characteristics would be quite different from those observed in a typical patient in daily clinical practice. Related to that, it is noteworthy that the *"normal population"* represented only 16.8% of the studied patients. The CAMP study by Ciccone et al. established that the percentiles for normal CIMT involved 1017 healthy subjects aged between 22 and 85 years from Italian centers. In this study CIMT was positively correlated with age and mean values were higher in men than in women [29]. This interesting report shows results in terms of CIMT RIs similar to those found in our research.

Third, we found sex-related differences in CIMT values. That finding is in agreement with data reported by other groups [7, 29]. The European "Reference Values of Arterial Measurements Collaboration Group" reported RIs and percentiles for each age group (from 15 to 85 years) separated by sex [7]. In CARMELA study mean CIMT and IC 95% were reported for males and females, separately [10]. Pastorius et

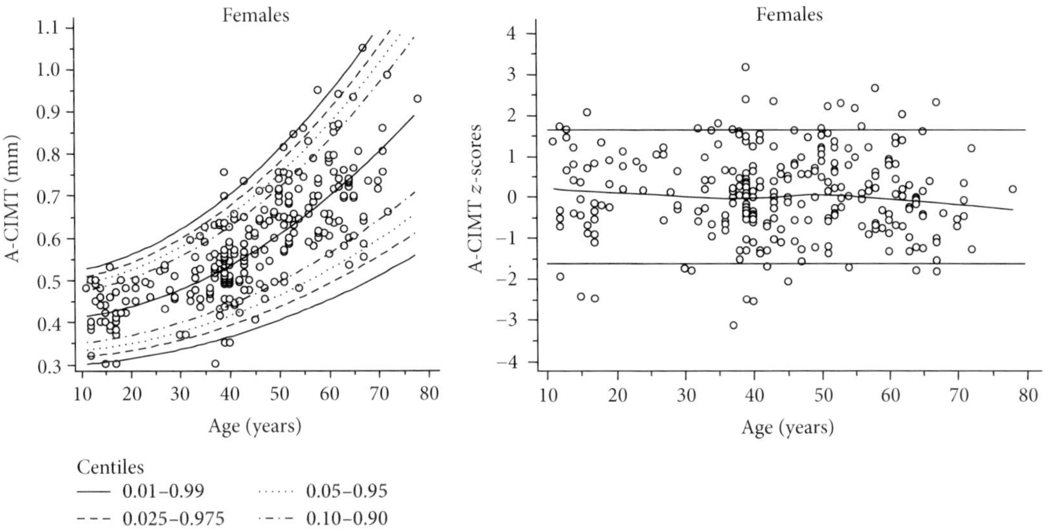

(a) Averaged CIMT percentiles according to age for females. CIMT: carotid intima media thickness

(b) Residual distribution (z-scores) for averaged CIMT-Age in females. CIMT: carotid intima media thickness

FIGURE 5

TABLE 9: Left common carotid intima media thickness [mm] percentiles for healthy male subjects.

Age [years]	1st	2.5th	5th	10th	25th	50th	75th	90th	95th	97.5th	99th
20	0.3292	0.3533	0.3740	0.3979	0.4378	0.4822	0.5267	0.5665	0.5904	0.6112	0.6353
25	0.3340	0.3601	0.3826	0.4085	0.4517	0.4999	0.5480	0.5912	0.6171	0.6396	0.6657
30	0.3400	0.3685	0.3931	0.4215	0.4688	0.5215	0.5742	0.6215	0.6498	0.6744	0.7030
35	0.3470	0.3785	0.4056	0.4368	0.4889	0.5470	0.6051	0.6572	0.6884	0.7155	0.7470
40	0.3551	0.3899	0.4199	0.4545	0.5122	0.5764	0.6407	0.6984	0.7329	0.7629	0.7978
45	0.3642	0.4029	0.4362	0.4745	0.5385	0.6098	0.6811	0.7451	0.7834	0.8167	0.8553
50	0.3745	0.4174	0.4544	0.4969	0.5679	0.6471	0.7262	0.7972	0.8398	0.8767	0.9197
55	0.3858	0.4335	0.4744	0.5217	0.6005	0.6883	0.7761	0.8549	0.9021	0.9431	0.9908
60	0.3982	0.4510	0.4964	0.5488	0.6361	0.7334	0.8308	0.9181	0.9704	1.0158	1.0686
65	0.4117	0.4701	0.5204	0.5783	0.6748	0.7825	0.8902	0.9867	1.0446	1.0949	1.1533
70	0.4263	0.4908	0.5462	0.6101	0.7167	0.8355	0.9543	1.0609	1.1248	1.1802	1.2447

TABLE 10: Left common carotid intima media thickness [mm] percentiles for healthy female subjects.

Age [years]	1st	2.5th	5th	10th	25th	50th	75th	90th	95th	97.5th	99th
25	0.3063	0.3310	0.3523	0.3768	0.4177	0.4632	0.5088	0.5496	0.5741	0.5954	0.6201
30	0.3186	0.3454	0.3685	0.3951	0.4395	0.4890	0.5385	0.5829	0.6095	0.6326	0.6594
35	0.3331	0.3624	0.3877	0.4168	0.4653	0.5194	0.5736	0.6221	0.6512	0.6765	0.7058
40	0.3498	0.3820	0.4098	0.4418	0.4951	0.5546	0.6141	0.6674	0.6994	0.7271	0.7594
45	0.3687	0.4043	0.4348	0.4701	0.5289	0.5944	0.6599	0.7187	0.7540	0.7846	0.8201
50	0.3899	0.4291	0.4628	0.5017	0.5666	0.6389	0.7112	0.7761	0.8150	0.8488	0.8880
55	0.4133	0.4565	0.4938	0.5367	0.6083	0.6881	0.7679	0.8395	0.8825	0.9197	0.9630
60	0.4389	0.4866	0.5277	0.5750	0.6540	0.7420	0.8300	0.9090	0.9563	0.9974	1.0451
65	0.4667	0.5193	0.5645	0.6167	0.7036	0.8006	0.8975	0.9845	1.0366	1.0818	1.1344
70	0.4968	0.5546	0.6043	0.6616	0.7572	0.8638	0.9704	1.0660	1.1233	1.1730	1.2308
75	0.5291	0.5925	0.6471	0.7099	0.8148	0.9318	1.0487	1.1536	1.2165	1.2710	1.3344

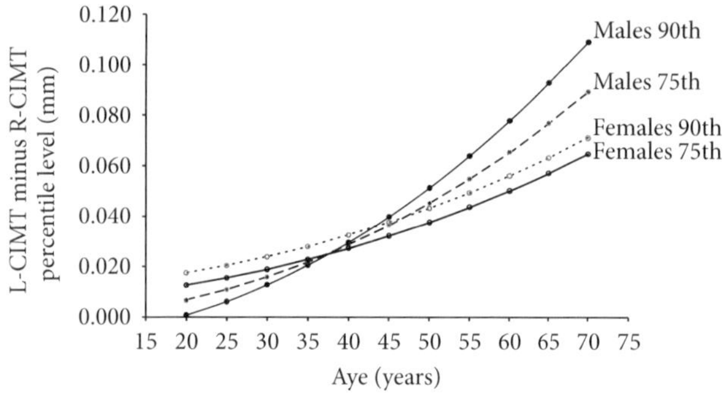

FIGURE 6: Percentile differences (75th and 90th) between L-CIMT and R-CIMT according to age and sex. L: left. R: right. CIMT: carotid intima media thickness.

al. reported RIs and specific percentile curve according to age and gender based on 207 males and 252 females [27].

Fourth, we found differences in the aging-related increase in CIMT when comparing left and right sides. As can be seen in Figure 6, the differences between right and left CIMT corresponding to percentiles 75th and 90th increased with age in both males and females. However, some issues should be analyzed considering the age-associated increases of the differences between L-CIMT and R-CIMT, which were not uniformly distributed:

(a) The finding of differences between L-CIMT and R-CIMT highlights the need for right and left CMIT evaluation.

(b) Left and right CIMT measurements are particularly necessary in older males, taking into account the fact that the differential behavior is more pronounced in men than in females.

(c) Despite percentiles 75th and 90th showed an age-associated increased in both sexes, in males in early ages (before 35–40 years) the 90th percentile showed the greatest increases.

Jointly considering what is stated above emphasizes the need for specific age-related left and right CIMT RIs for males and females.

4.1. Methodological Considerations. Recently, Dalla Pozza et al. commented on the lack of recommendations (universally accepted) on when and how the CIMT should be measured in a particular subject [8]. In addition, the authors emphasized that data analysis should be performed taken into account previous findings using a validated methodology. In this regard, we are convinced that this is an important issue and consequently in this research data analysis applied similar methodological approach to that used by the European group *"Reference Values for Arterial Measurements Collaboration"* [7, 12].

4.2. Limitations of This Research. This research used a cross-sectional design. Then, the age-associated increase in CIMT described would not represent aging-related changes in CIMT for a subject. An adequate data analysis, interpretation, and use in clinical practice should take into account what is stated above.

5. Conclusions

This study provides the largest database concerning RIs of CIMT in healthy rural-urban people in Argentina. CIMT RIs and percentiles were defined by age and sex considering a healthy population aged 11–81 years. In addition, specific RIs and percentiles of CIMT for right and left common carotid artery were reported.

References

[1] V. Fuster, "The Vulnerable Patient Providing a Lens Into the Interconnected Diseases of the Heart and Brain," *Journal of the American College of Cardiology*, vol. 66, no. 9, Article ID 21576, pp. 1077-1078, 2015.

[2] P. Pignoli, E. Tremoli, A. Poli, P. Oreste, and R. Paoletti, "Intimal plus medial thickness of the arterial wall: a direct measurement with ultrasound imaging," *Circulation*, vol. 74, no. 6, pp. 1399–1406, 1986.

[3] G. Mancia, R. Fagard, K. Narkiewicz et al., "2013 ESH/ESC Guidelines for the management of arterial hypertension: the Task Force for the management of arterial hypertension of the European Society of Hypertension (ESH) and of the European Society of Cardiology (ESC)," *Journal of Hypertension*, vol. 31, no. 7, pp. 1281–1357, 2013.

[4] M. Amato, F. Veglia, U. de Faire et al., "Carotid plaque-thickness and common carotid IMT show additive value in cardiovascular risk prediction and reclassification," *Atherosclerosis*, vol. 263, pp. 412–419, 2017.

[5] P. Perrone-Filardi, A. Coca, M. Galderisi et al., "Noninvasive cardiovascular imaging for evaluating subclinical target organ damage in hypertensive patients: A consensus article from the European Association of Cardiovascular Imaging, the European Society of Cardiology Council on Hypertension and the European Society of Hypertension," *Journal of Hypertension*, vol. 35, no. 9, pp. 1727–1741, 2017.

[6] J. F. Polak, M. Szklo, and D. H. O'Leary, "Carotid Intima-Media Thickness Score, Positive Coronary Artery Calcium Score, and Incident Coronary Heart Disease: The Multi-Ethnic Study of Atherosclerosis," *Journal of the American Heart Association*, vol. 6, no. 1, p. e004612, 2017.

[7] L. Engelen, I. Ferreira, C. D. Stehouwer, P. Boutouyrie, and S. Laurent, "Reference intervals for common carotid intima-medi thickness measured with echotracking: relation with risk factors," *European Heart Journal*, vol. 34, no. 30, pp. 2368–2380, 2013.

[8] R. Dalla Pozza, D. Ehringer-Schetitska, P. Fritsch, E. Jokinen, A. Petropoulos, and R. Oberhoffer, "Intima media thickness measurement in children: A statement from the Association for European Paediatric Cardiology (AEPC) Working Group on Cardiovascular Prevention endorsed by the Association for European Paediatric Cardiology," *Atherosclerosis*, vol. 238, no. 2, pp. 380–387, 2015.

[9] M. C. Tattersall, A. Gassett, C. E. Korcarz et al., "Predictors of carotid thickness and plaque progression during a decade: The multi-ethnic study of atherosclerosis," *Stroke*, vol. 45, no. 11, pp. 3257–3262, 2014.

[10] P. Touboul, E. Vicaut, J. Labreuche et al., "Common carotid artery intima-media thickness: the cardiovascular risk fac-

tor multiple evaluation in Latin America (CARMELA) study results," *Cerebrovascular Disease*, vol. 31, no. 1, pp. 43–50, 2011.

[11] X. Luo, Y. Yang, T. Cao, and Z. Li, "Differences in left and right carotid intima-media thickness and the associated risk factors," *Clinical Radiology*, vol. 66, no. 5, pp. 393–398, 2011.

[12] L. Engelen, J. Bossuyt, I. Ferreira et al., "Reference values for local arterial stiffness. Part a: carotid artery," *Journal of Hypertension*, vol. 33, no. 10, pp. 1981–1996, 2015.

[13] A. Díaz, M. Tringler, J. D. Molina et al., "Blood pressure control and arterial hypertension in children and adolescents from a rural population in Argentina. Preliminary data from Vela Proyect," *Archivos Argentinos de Pediatría*, vol. 108, no. 1, pp. 68–70, 2010.

[14] A. Díaz, C. Galli, M. Tringler, A. Ramírez, and E. I. Cabrera Fischer, "Reference Values of Pulse Wave Velocity in Healthy People from an Urban and Rural Argentinean Population," *International Journal of Hypertension*, vol. 2014, Article ID 653239, 2014.

[15] A. Diaz, M. Tringler, C. Galli, A. Ramirez, and E. I. C. Fischer, "Arterial Stiffness in a Rural Population of Argentina: Pilot Study," *High Blood Pressure & Cardiovascular Prevention*, vol. 22, no. 4, pp. 403–409, 2015.

[16] A. Diaz, M. Tringler, S. Wray, A. J. Ramirez, and E. I. Cabrera Fischer, "The effects of age on pulse wave velocity in untreated hypertension," *The Journal of Clinical Hypertension*, 2017.

[17] L. A. Sposato, M. L. Coppola, J. Altamirano et al., "Program for the epidemiological evaluation of stroke in Tandil, Argentina (PREVISTA) study: Rationale and design," *International Journal of Stroke*, vol. 8, no. 7, pp. 591–597, 2013.

[18] A. L. Rubinstein, V. E. Irazola, M. Calandrelli et al., "Multiple cardiometabolic risk factors in the Southern Cone of Latin America: A population-based study in Argentina, Chile, and Uruguay," *International Journal of Cardiology*, vol. 183, Article ID 19623, pp. 82–88, 2015.

[19] E. Lurbe, E. Agabiti-Rosei, J. K. Cruickshank et al., "2016 European Society ofHypertension guidelines for themanagement of high blood pressure in children and adolescents," *Journal of Hypertension*, vol. 34, no. 10, pp. 1887–1920, 2016.

[20] S. R. Srinivasan, M. G. Frontini, J. Xu, and G. S. Berenson, "Utility of childhood non-high-density lipoprotein cholesterol levels in predicting adult dyslipidemia and other cardiovascular risks: The Bogalusa Heart Study," *Pediatrics*, vol. 118, no. 1, pp. 201–206, 2006.

[21] P.-J. Touboul, M. G. Hennerici, and S. Meairs, "Mannheim carotid intima-media thickness and plaque consensus (2004–2006–2011). An update on behalf of the advisory board of the 3rd, 4th and 5th watching the risk symposia, at the 13th, 15th and 20th European Stroke Conferences, Mannheim, Germany, 2004, Brussels, Belgium, 2006, and Hamburg, Germany, 2011," *Cerebrovascular Disease*, vol. 34, no. 4, pp. 290–296, 2012.

[22] H. L. Manterola, L. Lo Vercio, A. Díaz, P. A. Pardini, M. W. Waks Serra et al., "Low-cost phantoms for validating measurements in ultrasound vascular images," in *Proc. SPIE 10160, 12th International Symposium on Medical Information Processing and Analysis*, 2017, http://dx.doi.org/10.1117/12.2255750.

[23] P. Royston and E. M. Wright, "A method for estimating age-specific reference intervals ('normal ranges') based on fractional polynomials and exponential transformation," *Journal of the Royal Statistical Society. Series A: Statistics in Society*, vol. 161, no. 1, pp. 79–101, 1998.

[24] C. A. Bellera and J. A. Hanley, "A method is presented to plan the required sample size when estimating regression-based reference limits," *Journal of Clinical Epidemiology*, vol. 60, no. 6, pp. 610–615, 2007.

[25] X. Liao, G. D. Norata, J. F. Polak et al., "Normative values for carotid intima media thickness and its progression: Are they transferrable outside of their cohort of origin?" *European Journal of Preventive Cardiology*, vol. 23, no. 11, pp. 1165–1173, 2016.

[26] I. Farro, D. Bia, Y. Zócalo et al., "Aging-related changes and reference values for the carotid intima-media thickness in a Uruguayan population.," *Conference proceedings: IEEE Engineering in Medicine and Biology Society*, pp. 5622–5625, 2012.

[27] C. A. Pastorius, J. Medina-Lezama, F. Corrales-Medina et al., "Normative values and correlates of carotid artery intima-media thickness and carotid atherosclerosis in Andean-Hispanics: The Prevencion Study," *Atherosclerosis*, vol. 211, no. 2, pp. 499–505, 2010.

[28] H. den Ruijter, S. Peters, and T. Anderson, "Common Carotid Intima-Media Thickness Measurements in Cardiovascular Risk Prediction: A Meta-Analysis," *Journal of Vascular Surgery*, vol. 56, no. 6, p. 1810, 2012.

[29] M. M. Ciccone, A. Balbarini, M. T. Porcelli et al., "Carotid artery intima-media thickness: normal and percentile values in the Italian population (camp study)," *European Journal of Cardiovascular Prevention and Rehabilitation*, vol. 18, no. 4, pp. 650–655, 2011.

19

Hypertension, an Emerging Problem in Rural Cameroon: Prevalence, Risk Factors, and Control

Walters Tabi Arrey,[1] Christian Akem Dimala,[2,3,4] Julius Atashili,[5] Josephine Mbuagbaw,[5,6] and Gottlieb Lobe Monekosso[5]

[1] *Ako District Hospital, North West Region, Cameroon*
[2] *Faculty of Epidemiology and Population Health, London School of Hygiene and Tropical Medicine, London, UK*
[3] *Orthopaedics Department, Southend University Hospital, Essex, UK*
[4] *Health and Human Development (2HD) Research Group, Douala, Cameroon*
[5] *Faculty of Health Sciences, University of Buea, Buea, Cameroon*
[6] *College of Medicine, Madonna University Nigeria, Rivers State, Nigeria*

Correspondence should be addressed to Christian Akem Dimala; christian.akem.dimala1@alumni.lshtm.ac.uk

Academic Editor: John M. Flack

Background. Despite the increasing trends suggesting that hypertension is a growing public health problem in developing countries, studies on its prevalence, associated risk factors, and extent of blood pressure control have been inequitably done in urban and rural communities in these countries. We therefore aimed to determine the prevalence of hypertension and extent of blood pressure control in rural Cameroon. *Methods.* This was a community-based cross-sectional study conducted in rural Cameroon (the Moliwe Health Area). Participants aged 21 years and above were recruited by a probability proportional to size multistage sampling method, using systematic sampling for household selection and random sampling for participant selection. Blood pressure, weight, and height were measured by standard methods. Hypertension was defined as BP ≥ 140/90 mmHg. *Results.* The prevalence of hypertension among the 733 participants recruited was 31.1% (95% CI: 27.8–34.6) and 71% (95% CI: 58.7–81.7) of these hypertensive patients were newly diagnosed. Only 21.2% (95% CI: 12.1–33.3) of known hypertensives had a well controlled BP. Age, obesity, low educational status, and being married were associated with HTN after adjusting for confounders. *Conclusions.* The high prevalence of hypertension and inadequate BP control among known hypertensives in rural Cameroon warrants greater sensitization and regular screening to reduce hypertension-related morbidity and mortality.

1. Background

It is predicted that by 2025, the prevalence of hypertension (HTN) will increase by 60% to a total of 1.56 billion worldwide [1] suggesting that HTN remains a major public health problem. HTN in Sub-Saharan Africa (SSA) has also been on the rise with reports indicating higher values in urban settings compared to rural settings [2–4]. The prevalence of HTN in SSA ranges between 14.5% in rural Eritrea [2], 32.9% in semiurban Ghana [3], and 40.1% in urban South Africa [4]. Likewise, adequate blood pressure (BP) control has been on the decline, ranging between 1.7% in rural Ghana [3], 4% in urban slum dwellers in Nigeria [5], and 21.5% in urban Kenya [6]. In Cameroon, the prevalence of HTN spans from 5.7% in rural settings [7] through 21.9% in semiurban [8] to 47.5% in urban milieu [9], with a national average survey of 31.0% [10]. Despite the relatively better BP control in urban over rural settings, levels of adequate BP control as low as 2% [11] to 27.5% (in men) and 38.7% (in women) [9] have been reported in urban settings.

Even though much has been done so far to reduce the incidence of hypertension in urban areas, this has not been the same in rural areas, with public health policies aimed at controlling hypertension mainly directed towards the large cities. Most of the studies done so far in these urban areas cannot therefore give a true estimate of the extent to which the rural population is affected by this major cardiovascular disease risk factor. An analysis of hypertension and its risk factors in rural Cameroon will therefore help guide health policy decisions and provide baseline data for future studies aimed at addressing this problem. We therefore had the following as objectives: determining the prevalence of hypertension in the adult population in the Moliwe Health Area in rural Cameroon; identifying the risk factors associated with HTN in this rural setting; determining the extent of BP control in known hypertensive patients in this locality.

2. Materials and Methods

2.1. Study Design, Period, and Setting. A community-based cross-sectional descriptive and analytical study was conducted over a 6-month period (June 20 to December 28, 2013) in the Moliwe Health Area (MHA). This principally rural health area is found in the Limbe Health District of the South West Region of Cameroon.

2.2. Participants and Sampling Method. A multistage sampling method was used to select participants from the 5 villages/settlements of the health area: Bonadikombo, Wotutu, Ewongo, Moliwe, and Tomatal. The sample selected was self-weighted through the probability proportional to size method used. The data of 2005 Cameroon census was used as a guide to the sampling frame with households considered as the primary sampling units. Using a random start, a systematic sample of households was then selected from a list of the approximate cumulative number of households of all the villages. This gave an estimate of the number of households to be selected from each village. As the secondary sampling units, two participants were then recruited from each selected household by simple random sampling from a list of eligible households occupants produced by the respective household heads. Three hundred and twenty-nine participants were thus recruited from Bonadikombo, 113 from Wotutu, 112 from Moliwe, 96 from Ewongo, and 83 from Tomatal.

The sample size was calculated using the formula: $n = z^2(p)(q)/d^2$. A combined estimate of the prevalence of HTN in rural Rwanda, Tanzania, and Malawi of 22% was used [12]. We recruited 733 participants by systematic and simple random sampling methods.

2.3. Study Procedures and Variables. At each selected household, a questionnaire was administered to each recruited participant to collect information on age, sex, level of education, marital status, status of HTN, treatment of HTN, smoking, quantity of alcohol intake, physical activity, diabetes status, and family history of HTN. Blood pressure measurements were also done at the home of the participants by a casually dressed clinician not in white coat. Two measurements (in mmHg) were taken on the right arm using an automated electronic BP machine (OMRON M3 HEM-7200-E Omron Matsusaka Co. Ltd., Kyoto, Japan) through the standard procedure (JNC 7 recommendations) [13]. Heights in meters (m) and weights in kilograms (kg) were measured using standard procedures and were used to determine the body mass index (BMI) as follows: BMI = weight (kg)/[height (m) $*$ height (m)]. WHO STEPS surveillance manual was used to assess sedentary lifestyle (physical inactivity) [14].

2.4. Data Analysis. The data was entered into Epi info statistical software, version 7.0 (CDC/WHO, Atlanta, USA). Quality control was done by double entry and checking. Frequencies and means were obtained for appropriate variables; Chi-square and Fischer's exact tests were used as appropriate to test for associations between binary and categorical variables. A logistic regression model was built to assess the effect of factors found to be significantly associated with hypertension while controlling for potential confounders. Statistical significance was considered at a P value < 0.05.

2.5. Ethical Considerations. An ethical clearance was obtained from the Institutional Review Board of the Faculty of Health Sciences, University of Buea. Administrative approvals were obtained from the Regional Delegate of Public Health as well as from the local Chiefs, Quarter heads, and camp presidents concerned. There were no associated risks since all procedures were noninvasive. Participants benefited from free screening for hypertension and counselling. All patients found to have elevated blood pressure values were advised and referred to the nearest health facility for proper management and follow-up.

3. Results and Discussion

3.1. Sociodemographic and Clinical Characteristics of the Study Population. Of the 733 participants, 479 (39.5%) were between 20 and 29 years. The male to female ratio was 1 : 1.2, 35.9% had primary education, and 50.5% were married. Less than half of the participants (47.3%) had normal BMI and 15% had sedentary life style. A small proportion, (2.9%) were known diabetics and 32.7% reported a family history of hypertension (Table 1).

3.2. Prevalence of Hypertension and BP Control. Of the 733 participants recruited, 228 were hypertensive, giving a prevalence of 31.1% (95% CI: 27.8–34.6). Sixty-six of the 228 hypertensive participants (28.9%, 95% CI: 23.2–35.3) knew their status prior to our study. Of these 66 known hypertensive participants already aware of their status, 14 of them (21.2%, 95% CI: 12.1–33.3) had their blood pressures well controlled even though as high as 47 of them (71%, 95% CI: 58.7–81.7) were on antihypertensive treatment at that moment (Figure 1).

Age 40 and above, obesity, smoking, alcohol consumption, diabetes, low educational level, and marriage were found to be associated with hypertension (Table 2). After adjusting for all significant factors using logistic regression, only age 40 and above, obesity, low educational level, and marriage were still strongly associated with hypertension (Table 3). There was a progressive increase in the prevalence of HTN with age when age below 40 was used as the reference: from 3 folds in the 40–59 years, through 8.3 folds in the 60–79 years, to 11.6 folds in 80^+ years age groups. People who were

TABLE 1: Participants' socio-demographic and clinical characteristics.

Characteristic	Categories	Participants (N = 733)	Percentage (%)
Age (years)	20–39	479	65.4
	40–59	167	22.8
	60–79	78	10.6
	80–99	9	1.2
Gender	Males	334	54.4
	Females	399	45.6
Level of education	None	74	10.1
	Primary	263	35.8
	Secondary	246	33.6
	High school or more	150	20.5
Marital status	Married	370	50.5
	Single	283	38.6
	Divorced	15	2.0
	Widowed	65	8.9
Body mass index	Normal	347	47.3
	Overweight	224	30.6
	Obese	162	22.1
Smoking	Yes	149	20.3
	No	584	79.7
Alcohol consumption	Yes	281	38.3
	No	452	61.7
Sedentary lifestyle	Yes	108	14.7
	No	625	85.3
Family history of HTN	Yes	240	32.7
	No	493	67.3
Diabetes mellitus	Yes	21	2.9
	No	722	97.1

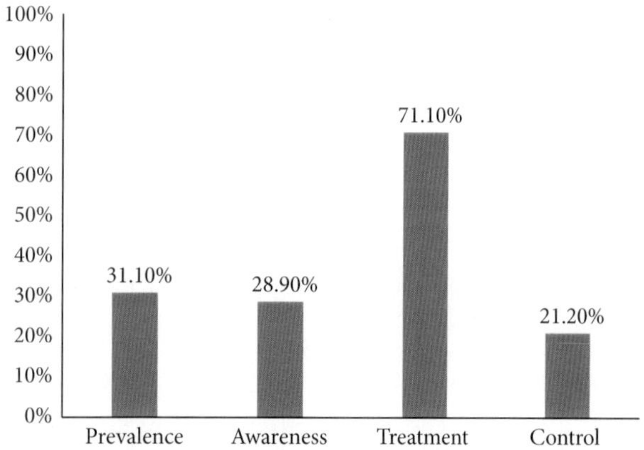

FIGURE 1: Descriptive characteristics of hypertension for the 733 participants in the Moliwe Health Area, Cameroon.

obese had 2.8 times the odds of being hypertensive compared to the nonobese. There was an inverse relationship between educational status and HTN. Those who never went to school had 6.7 times the odds of having HTN compared to those who had at least high school education (Table 3).

3.3. Discussion. Since the new recommendations for HTN diagnosis and management by JNC 7 in 2003 [13], no study had been done in rural Cameroon. The last published rural study on HTN was as far back as 1998 [7]. The 31.1% prevalence of HTN observed in the MHA is similar to the 31.0% reported in Cameroon by Kingue et al. [10] and the 32.9% reported by Amoah [15] in semiurban Ghana but higher than that reported elsewhere [3, 7, 8, 12, 16, 17]. The different settings and methodologies could account for this difference. However, our value was lower than 44.7% reported by Williams et al. [18] in rural Ghana and 40% reported by Chow et al. [19] in rural and urban high, middle, and low income countries.

Our study revealed low hypertension awareness similar to the 32.3% observed in rural Ghana by Addo et al. [20] and the 32.6% observed by Dzudie et al. [9] in Urban Cameroon. However, this value is higher than the 11% reported in rural Cameroon by Mbanya et al. [7] and 22% in rural and semiurban Ghana by Williams et al. [18]. This variation

TABLE 2: Association between clinical characteristics and hypertension of 733 participants in Moliwe Health Area, rural Cameroon.

Risk factors	Categories	Risk ratio (95% CI)	*P* value
Age (years)	<40	1.0	<0.001
	≥40	4.5 (3.0–6.8)	
Obesity	No	1.0	<0.001
	Yes	1.9 (1.5–2.3)	
Smoking	No	1.0	<0.001
	Yes	1.5 (1.2–1.9)	
Alcohol	No	1.0	<0.001
	Yes	1.6 (1.3–1.9)	
Diabetes	No	1.0	<0.001
	Yes	2.1 (1.4–2.9)	
Educational status	High (≥secondary)	1.0	<0.001
	Low (none and primary)	1.8 (1.4–2.3)	
Marital status	Unmarried	1.0	<0.001
	Married	1.6	

TABLE 3: Association between clinical characteristics and hypertension after adjusting for all the factors presented.

Risk factors	Categories	Odds ratio (95% CI)	*P* value
Age (years)	20–39	1.0	
	40–59	3.0 (2.0–4.6)	<0.001
	60–79	8.3 (4.4–15.7)	<0.001
	80 and above	11.6 (2.1–64.6)	<0.001
Educational status	High	1.0	
	None	6.7 (3.6–12.4)	<0.001
	Primary	2.0 (1.3–3.2)	<0.001
	Secondary	1.2 (0.7–2.0)	0.440
Body mass index	Normal	1.0	
	Overweight	1.0 (0.7–1.5)	0.850
	Obese	2.8 (1.9–4.2)	<0.001
Smoking	No	1.0	
	Yes	1.3 (0.8–2.0)	0.330
Alcohol	No	1.0	
	Yes	1.4 (0.9–2.1)	0.070
Diabetes	No	1.0	
	Yes	1.4 (0.5–3.9)	0.550
Marital status	Unmarried	1.0	
	Married	1.5 (1.1–2.2)	0.030

between rural and urban settings could be explained by poor knowledge of the disease, lesser access to health facilities, and poverty, in rural compared to urban communities.

Age was identified to be strongly associated with HTN, supporting the findings of other studies [9, 12, 21–23]. This is because as people get older, their blood vessels become harder and they are likely to have decreased baroreceptor sensitivity, increased responsiveness to sympathetic nervous system stimuli, altered renal and sodium metabolism, and an altered renin-aldosterone relationship thereby predisposing them to high blood pressure [24]. Obesity, which is one of the common pathways between diabetes and HTN [25], was also found to be strongly associated with HTN in our study, as earlier documented [8, 26]. Low educational status and being married were strongly linked with HTN in our study as reported in previous studies [21, 27, 28]. A poor understanding of the disease and its risk factors and the stress experienced my married couples, respectively, could put these groups at a higher risk. On the other hand, gender, family history of HTN, overweight, and physical inactivity were not statistically significant risk factors of HTN in this setting. Smoking, alcohol consumption, and diabetes mellitus which were associated with HTN on bivariate analysis were not significantly associated with hypertension on multivariate analysis by logistic regression.

The proportion of known hypertensives who were currently on antihypertensive treatment in our study was similar to the 64.9% reported [18] in Ghana but much higher than the 12.5% reported [7] in Cameroon. The high proportion on antihypertensives may be due to the increase in awareness of HTN and the availability and access to antihypertensive medications in Cameroon lately compared to 16 years ago [7]. Despite this considerable proportion of hypertensive patients being on treatment, only 21.8% of them had controlled blood pressures. Kishore et al. reported as low as 3% in rural Nigeria [23] and Yuvaraj et al. reported 12.5% in rural India [29]. However, higher proportions have been reported (33.1% [9] and 63.2% [8]) among hypertensives in urban and semiurban settings in Cameroon, respectively, 56.8% in Mexico [30], and 75.9% in urban India [31]. Noncompliance to treatment has been proposed as a possible explanation for this observation. And in this context noncompliance to treatment is multifactorial in aetiology with reasons such as inadequate knowledge of HTN, intolerance of side effects of medications, and low purchasing power.

This study was cross-sectional which means participants declared hypertensive may not necessarily be hypertensive clinically. Also, our study was done in a small rural area whose findings may not necessarily apply to all rural Cameroonian or Sub-Saharan African communities. Moreover, some known risk factors such as dyslipidaemia, salt intake, and psychosocial and socioeconomic status were not assessed in our study. Nevertheless, the large sample size, varied sampling method, and execution of standard measurement procedures make the findings of this study robust and accurate. Also, the white coat effect which could potentially produce an overestimation of the actual prevalence of hypertension in this setting was minimized since the casually dressed clinician without a white coat did the measurements from the participants' homes.

4. Conclusions

Our study revealed that about one out of three adults in the Moliwe Health Area could be hypertensive with only a quarter of them being aware of their status and a fifth of those on treatment having their blood pressure well controlled. This reveals how very much a cardiovascular risk the rural population may be exposed to. There is, therefore, need for massive improvement in awareness through education and repeated patient follow-up in these rural settings alongside the urban ones. Also, the importance of further research in other rural communities to assess trends and risk factors of hypertension and the extent of blood pressure control cannot be overemphasized.

Abbreviations

BP: Blood pressure
CDC: Centre for Disease Control and Prevention
CVD: Cardiovascular disease
HTN: Hypertension
JNC: Joint National Committee
MHA: Moliwe Health Area
SSA: Sub-Saharan Africa
USA: United States of America
WHO: World Health Organization.

Ethical Approval

Ethical approval was granted by the Institutional Review Board of the Faculty of Health Sciences, University of Buea. All participants provided their written consent to take in the study. All participants provided consent for publication. All information published is nonidentifying information.

Competing Interests

The authors declare that they have no competing interests.

Acknowledgments

The authors thank all study participants, chiefs, quarter heads, and camp presidents in the Moliwe Health Area. Further, they thank Mrs. Lucy Eyong Ngembus, Mr. Ncha Jonas Tataw, Mr. Arrey Giscard Awa, Finley Gisele Mankaa, and Mr. Ayuk Hastings for funding this project.

References

[1] P. M. Kearney, M. Whelton, K. Reynolds, P. Muntner, P. K. Whelton, and J. He, "Global burden of hypertension: analysis of worldwide data," *The Lancet*, vol. 365, no. 9455, pp. 217–223, 2005.

[2] J. Mufunda, G. Mebrahtu, A. Usman et al., "The prevalence of hypertension and its relationship with obesity: results from a national blood pressure survey in Eritrea," *Journal of Human Hypertension*, vol. 20, no. 1, pp. 59–65, 2006.

[3] F. P. Cappuccio, F. B. Micah, L. Emmett et al., "Prevalence, detection, management, and control of hypertension in Ashanti, West Africa," *Hypertension*, vol. 43, no. 5, pp. 1017–1022, 2004.

[4] R. Malhotra, T. Puone, C. Hoyo, and G. Hughes, "Prevalence and awareness of hypertension in an urban township of South Africa: compelling need for action," *Ethnicity and Disease*, vol. 18, pp. 401–402, 2008.

[5] O. J. Daniel, E. N. Adejumo, R. S. Owolabi, and R. W. Braimoh, "Prevalence of hypertension among urban slum dwellers in Lagos, Nigeria," *Journal of Health*, vol. 90, no. 6, pp. 1016–1025, 2013.

[6] S. J. M. Van De Vijver, S. O. Oti, C. Agyemang, G. B. Gomez, and C. Kyobutungi, "Prevalence, awareness, treatment and control of hypertension among slum dwellers in Nairobi, Kenya," *Journal of Hypertension*, vol. 31, no. 5, pp. 1018–1024, 2013.

[7] J. C. N. Mbanya, E. M. Minkoulou, J. N. Salah, and B. Balkau, "The prevalence of hypertension in rural and urban Cameroon," *International Journal of Epidemiology*, vol. 27, no. 2, pp. 181–185, 1998.

[8] J. Atashili, "Epidemiology of hypertension in the Fako Division, Cameroon (Hypertension in the Fako Division, Cameroon: Prevalence and risk factors)," 2010.

[9] A. Dzudie, A. P. Kengne, W. F. T. Muna et al., "Awareness, treatment, and control of Hypertension," *BMJ Open*, vol. 2, Article ID e001217, 2012.

[10] S. Kingue, C. NdongNgoe, A. Menanga, B. Fesuh, C. Nouedoui, and W. F. T. Muna, "Prevalence and risk factors of hypertension in urban areas of cameroon: a nationwide population-based cross-sectional study," *The Journal of Clinical Hypertension*, vol. 17, no. 10, pp. 819–824, 2015.

[11] R. M. Kamadjeu, R. Edwards, J. S. Atanga, N. Unwin, E. C. Kiawi, and J.-C. Mbanya, "Prevalence, awareness and management of hypertension in Cameroon: findings of the 2003 Cameroon Burden of Diabetes Baseline Survey," *Journal of Human Hypertension*, vol. 20, no. 1, pp. 91–92, 2006.

[12] S. Ramirez, D. Enquobahrie, G. Nyadzi et al., "Prevalence and correlates of hypertension in rural Africa," *Journal of Human Hypertension*, vol. 24, pp. 786–795, 2010.

[13] A. V. Chobanian, G. L. Bakris, H. R. Black et al., "Seventh report of the joint national committee on prevention, detection, evaluation, and treatment of high blood pressure," *Hypertension*, vol. 42, no. 6, pp. 1206–1252, 2003.

[14] WHO, STEPS surveillance manual: the WHO STEP wise approach to chronic disease risk factor surveillance, 2005, http://www.who.int/chp/steps/en/.

[15] A. G. B. Amoah, "Hypertension in Ghana: a cross-sectional community prevalence study in Greater Accra," *Ethnicity and Disease*, vol. 13, no. 3, pp. 310–315, 2003.

[16] R. A. Adebayo, M. O. Balogun, R. A. Adedoyin, O. A. Obashoro-John, L. A. Bisiriyu, and O. O. Abiodun, "Prevalence of hypertension in three rural communities of Ife North Local Government Area of Osun State, South West Nigeria," *International Journal of General Medicine*, vol. 6, pp. 863–868, 2013.

[17] R. Ratovoson, O. R. Rasetarinera, I. Andrianantenaina, C. Rogier, P. Piola, and P. Pacaud, "Hypertension, a neglected disease in rural and urban areas in Moramanga, Madagascar," *PLoS ONE*, vol. 10, no. 9, Article ID e0137408, 2015.

[18] E. A. Williams, K. E. Keenan, D. Ansong et al., "The burden and correlates of hypertension in rural Ghana: a cross-sectional study," *Diabetes & Metabolic Syndrome*, vol. 7, no. 3, pp. 123–128, 2013.

[19] C. K. Chow, K. K. Teo, S. Rangarajan et al., "Prevalence, awareness, treatment, and control of hypertension in rural and urban communities in high-, middle-, and low-income countries," *Journal of the American Medical Association*, vol. 310, no. 9, pp. 959–968, 2013.

[20] J. Addo, A. G. B. Amoah, and K. A. Kwadwo, "The changing patterns of hypertension in Ghana: a study of four rural communities in the Ga District," *Ethnicity and Disease*, vol. 16, no. 4, pp. 894–899, 2006.

[21] J. Chataut, R. K. Adhikari, and N. P. Sinha, "The prevalence of and risk factors for hypertension in adults living in central development region of Nepal," *Kathmandu University Medical Journal*, vol. 33, no. 1, pp. 13–18, 2011.

[22] I. M. Ismail, A. G. Kulkarni, A. D. Meundi, and M. Amruth, "A community-based comparative study of prevalence and risk factors of hypertension among urban and rural populations in a coastal town of South India," *Sifa Medical Journal*, vol. 3, no. 2, pp. 41–47, 2016.

[23] J. Kishore, N. Gupta, C. Kohli, and N. Kumar, "Prevalence of hypertension and determination of its risk factors in rural Delhi," *International Journal of Hypertension*, vol. 2016, Article ID 7962595, 6 pages, 2016.

[24] M. A. Weber, J. M. Neutel, and D. G. Cheung, "Hypertension in the aged: a pathophysiologic basis for treatment," *The American Journal of Cardiology*, vol. 63, no. 16, pp. 25–32, 1989.

[25] B. M. Y. Cheung and C. Li, "Diabetes and hypertension: is there a common metabolic pathway?" *Current Atherosclerosis Reports*, vol. 14, no. 2, pp. 160–166, 2012.

[26] M. E. Hendriks, F. W. N. M. Wit, M. T. L. Roos et al., "Hypertension in Sub-Saharan Africa: cross-sectional surveys in four rural and urban communities," *PLoS ONE*, vol. 7, no. 3, article e32638, 2012.

[27] C. A. Alikor, P. C. Emem-Chioma, and O. J. Odia, "Hypertension in a rural community in River States, Niger Delta Region of Nigeria: prevalence and risk factors," *The Nigerian Health Journal*, vol. 13, no. 1, pp. 18–25, 2013.

[28] P. Thawornchaisit, F. De Looze, M. C. Reid, S. Seubsman, and A. C. Sleigh, "Health risk factors and the incidence of Hypertension: 4-year prospective findings from a national cohort of 60,569 Thai Open University Students," *BMJ Open*, vol. 3, no. 6, Article ID e002826/1-6, 2013.

[29] B. Y. Yuvaraj, M. R. Nagendra Gowda, and A. G. Umakantha, "Prevalence, awareness, treatment, and control of hypertension in rural areas of Davanagere," *Indian Journal of Community Medicine*, vol. 35, no. 1, pp. 138–141, 2010.

[30] S. Barqora, I. Campos-Nondo, L. H. Barrera et al., "Hypertension in Mexican adults: results from the natural health and nutritional survey," *Salud Pública de México*, vol. 52, supplement 1, pp. 63–71, 2010.

[31] S. K. Bansal, V. Saxena, S. D. Kandpal, W. K. Gray, R. W. Walker, and D. Goel, "The prevalence of hypertension and hypertension risk factors in a rural Indian community: a prospective door-to-door study," *Journal of Cardiovascular Disease Research*, vol. 3, no. 2, pp. 117–123, 2012.

Prevalence, Awareness, Treatment, and Control of Hypertension and Its Risk Factors in (Central) Vietnam

Ho Anh Hien [1,2] **Nguyen Minh Tam,** [1] **Vo Tam,** [3] **Anselme Derese,** [4] **and Dirk Devroey** [2]

[1] *Department of Family Medicine, Hue University of Medicine and Pharmacy, Hue University, Hue, Vietnam*
[2] *Department of Family Medicine and Chronic Care, Faculty of Medicine and Pharmacy, Vrije Universiteit Brussel, Brussels, Belgium*
[3] *Department of Internal Medicine, Hue University of Medicine and Pharmacy, Hue University, Hue, Vietnam*
[4] *Department of Family Medicine and Primary Health Care, Faculty of Medicine and Health Sciences, Ghent University, Ghent, Belgium*

Correspondence should be addressed to Ho Anh Hien; hahien@huemed-univ.edu.vn

Academic Editor: Tomohiro Katsuya

Introduction. The objective of this study is to describe the prevalence, awareness, treatment, and control of hypertension and its associated risk factors in (Central) Vietnam. *Methods*. In this cross-sectional study, a multistage sampling was used to select 969 participants from the general population aged from 40 to 69 years. The cardiovascular risk factors were collected throughout the interviews with a standardized questionnaire. Multivariate logistic regression analysis was conducted to test the relationship between the prevalence, awareness, treatment, and control of hypertension and the prevalence of risk factors. *Results*. The prevalence of hypertension was 44.8%. It was higher in men than in women (51.3% versus 39.7%, $p < 0.001$). In total 67.3% (74.5% in women, 60.1% in men; $p = 0.001$) of the participants were aware of their hypertension, 33.2% (37.5% in women, 28.9% in men; $p = 0.01$) of the participants were treated, and 12.2% (16.7% in women, 7.8% in men; $p < 0.001$) of the hypertensive participants' hypertension was controlled. Age, gender, place of residence, body mass index, and diabetes were found to be independent risk factors for hypertension. *Conclusion*. The prevalence of hypertension in Vietnam is high, and the proportion of treated and controlled patients is rather low.

1. Introduction

Hypertension is one of the most important modifiable risk factors for cardiovascular diseases (CVD) worldwide. The complications of hypertension account for 9.4 million deaths worldwide every year [1]. Hypertension is responsible for at least 45% of the deaths from CVD and 51% of the deaths from stroke [2]. CVD accounted for more than 17.3 million deaths in 2013 which represented 31% of all global deaths and made it the world's leading cause of death and disability [1]. Especially in low- and middle-income countries, CVD accounts for around 70% of deaths [1]. In Vietnam, the prevalence of hypertension has rapidly increased over the last two decades from 16.9% over the period of 2001-2002 to 25.1% in 2008 [3]. In 2009, CVD was estimated to account for 33% of all deaths [4] and stroke was found to be the leading cause of death among them [5, 6]. At that time, the percentages of treatment and control of hypertension were rather low (29,6% and 10,7%, resp.) [3].

In other developing countries, the mean prevalence, awareness, treatment, and control of hypertension were 32.2, 40.6, 29.2, and 9.8 percent among men and 30.5, 52.7, 40.5, and 16.2 percent among women, respectively. In developed countries, these percentages in men were 40.8, 49.2, 29.1, and 10.8 percent, and in women they were 33.0, 61.7, 40.6, and 17.3 percent, respectively [7]. A successful hypertension detection and treatment program in Canada resulted in a large increase of the diagnosis of hypertension from 57% in 1992 to 84% in 2013 and a reduction in the national rates of death and hospitalization due to CVD. Several cross-sectional studies had been implemented to better understand the approach of hypertension in this country, resulting in a better prevention and treatment [8].

The impact of hypertension and CVD is influenced by a wide variety of risk factors such as tobacco use, excessive alcohol consumption, unhealthy diet, physical inactivity, overweight and obesity, elevated blood glucose, and abnormal blood lipids. The combination of a reduction of risk factors in the general population, primary prevention in high-risk groups, and intensive treatment in secondary prevention was claimed to be the best strategy to reduce CVD premature mortality [9]. Research from several countries has consistently shown that the treatment of risk factors such as hypertension has a higher impact on CVD than the treatment of established CVD [10, 11].

The prevalence of hypertension has significantly increased due to the rapid economic development, population aging, urbanization, and changes in dietary habits and lifestyle in Vietnam. From 2005 to 2011, few studies have attempted to explore the awareness, treatment, and control of hypertension in Vietnam [3, 12–14]. The increase in the prevalence of hypertension requires an improved approach of hypertension management; however, this kind of study was not conducted over the past 10 years in (Central) Vietnam or at least in Thua Thien Hue Province. There remained also little information on the influence of sociodemographic and risk factors on the awareness and control of hypertension. Therefore, the objectives of this study were to describe the prevalence, awareness, treatment, and control of hypertension and its risk factors in Thua Thien Hue Province in Central Vietnam. The findings of this study are expected to contribute to primary prevention and intervention strategies in the treatment of hypertension in Central Vietnam.

2. Methods

2.1. Study Design and Population. A cross-sectional study was designed to assess the characteristics and risk factors of patients with hypertension in (Central) Vietnam. The present study used data collected in a population-based survey that was carried out among residents of Thua Thien Hue Province in 2015 (population = 1,123,800, census 2013, Statistical Yearbook of Vietnam). Multistaged sampling methods were used to recruit a representative sample of the general population aged from 40 to 69 years. At first, one province, namely, Thua Thien Hue, was purposively selected to register the characteristics of Central Vietnam. Next, we selected one urban district, one low-lying district, and one mountainous district to obtain a sample representing the diversity of this province. Hue City was the only urban district in this province; Phu Loc District and Nam Dong District were selected as low-lying and mountainous districts, respectively. In each district, we randomly selected two communes, yielding a total of 6 selected communes in Thua Thien Hue Province. Finally, from those communes, we used the population list from the local government registers of household updated by 2013. We then selected those aged between 40 and 69 years from the list. After that, 200 persons aged 40 to 69 years were systematically selected from that population list per commune at an interval of every 10th unit. In total, there were 400 people selected in each district, resulting in 1200 selected participants in the whole province.

2.2. Data Collection. Twelve hundred randomly selected persons were invited to visit the six local community health centers in the morning on dates indicated in the invitation letters. In each letter, we informed the participants about the time, the site, and other dietary requirements. They were asked not to drink or eat and to bring accurate information about their blood pressure and blood glucose. First, the participants were asked some questions on their demographics and hypertension risk factors such as their current smoking status, alcohol consumption, and physical activity. At the second step, their blood pressure and capillary blood glucose were collected with anthropometric measurement. In total, 983 participants showed up in the local community health centers, resulting in a response rate of 81,9%. Fourteen participants were excluded because of lacking information in the risk factors. The survey teams consisted of medical doctors and medical students from Hue University of Medicine and Pharmacy, Hue University, along with local healthcare providers. All study investigators and staff members had successfully completed a training program that oriented them both on the aims of the study and the specific instruments and methodologies employed. Two trained medical students performed anthropometric measurements. A team of 15 doctors and medical students were in charge of the interviews and physical examinations using a standardized questionnaire based on the World Health Organization (WHO) stepwise approach [15]. The survey was conducted from April to October in 2015.

2.3. Study Variables. Demographic data (including age, gender, education, ethnicity, and occupation) were collected. The interviews included questions related to personal and family medical history of hypertension, CVD, smoking, alcohol consumption, physical activity, and fruit and vegetable consumption. Information on the awareness of and treatment for hypertension, body weight, height, waist and hip circumference, blood pressure, and glucose was also obtained. Anthropometric measurements were performed with the participants wearing light clothes without footwear. Body weight was measured to the nearest 0.1 kg using a digital scale (OMROM HN 283, Omron Healthcare, Tokyo, Japan) and height was recorded to the nearest 0.1 cm in the standing position using a Telescopic Measuring Rod (MZ10023-3, ADE, Germany). Waist circumference was recorded to the nearest 0.1 cm, using a tape measure (Hoechstmass tape 84.203, Sulzbach, Germany), directly over the skin, at the level of the midpoint between the inferior margin of the last rib and the iliac crest in the mid-axillary line. Hip circumference was also recorded to nearest 0.1 cm, using a tape measure directly over the skin, around the point with the maximum circumference over the buttocks.

Blood pressure was measured on at least two occasions with a minimum interval of 15 minutes in resting and sitting position, using automatic sphygmomanometers (OMRON HEM 7322, Omron Healthcare, Tokyo, Japan), with an appropriate sized cuff and a standard protocol. If the difference between the first two measurements was more than 10 mmHg, a third measurement was performed. The average of the last 2 measurements was calculated and used in the analysis. Fasting capillary blood glucose was measured by means of a glucometer (OneTouch Ultra 2, LifeScan, US) using the standard protocol, provided by the manufacturer.

The participants' occupational status was classified into three categories: (1) *experts and government staff*; (2) *manual worker* (farmers and building and production workers); and (3) *other jobs* such as small traders, housekeepers, housewives, and those unemployed. There were three educational levels: (1) *primary school or under* (<6 years of education), (2) *middle or high school* (≥6 years but ≤ 12 years), and (3) *college or university* (graduates of college or university). The vast majority of the respondents belonged to the ethnic majority of Vietnam, namely, "Kinh." The ethnic minorities included "Ta Oi," "Van Kieu," and "Co Tu." *Urban and rural residence* was identified on an administrative basis for each commune within each province. *Current smokers* were defined as those currently consuming tobacco products (cigarettes, cigars, and pipes) or having quit smoking for less than 12 months. The category *excessive alcohol consumption* included men who took more than 2 standard units per day or 14 standard units per week and women who took more than 1 standard unit of drink per day or 7 standard units of drink per week. Physical activity was categorized by metabolic equivalent tasks per minute per week (MET/min/week). *Physical inactivity (low level of physical activity)* referred to people with fewer than 600 MET/min/week of physical activity, moderate level of physical activity (601–3000 MET/min/week), and high level of physical activity (>3000 MET/min/week). Body mass index (BMI) was calculated as weight (kg) per height squared (m^2). At the time of our survey, underweight was defined by WHO Regional Office for Western Pacific as BMI < 18.5 kg/m^2; *normal weight* was defined as BMI from 18.5 to 22.9 kg/m^2; *overweight* was defined as BMI from 23 to 24.9 kg/m^2 and *obesity* was defined as BMI ≥ 25 kg/m^2 [16]. *Abdominal obesity* for the Asian population included those whose waist hip ratio was valued ≥0.9 for men or ≥0.8 for women [17].

Hypertension was defined as an average systolic blood pressure (SBP) ≥ 140 mmHg and/or average diastolic blood pressure (DBP) ≥ 90 mmHg and/or self-reported previous diagnosis of hypertension by a health professional [18]. *Awareness of hypertension* was defined as the self-report or any prior diagnosis of hypertension by a healthcare professional among the participants defined as having hypertension. *Treatment of hypertension* was defined as use of a prescriptive medication for management of the respondent's high blood pressure (BP) for at least 2 weeks at the time of the interview. Treatment was calculated among patients who were fully aware of their hypertension and among the whole hypertensive group (including those who were not aware). *Control of hypertension* was defined as pharmacological treatment of hypertension associated with an average SBP < 140 mmHg and an average DBP < 90 mmHg. The proportion of hypertension control was calculated as the hypertensive patients who were treated and among the whole hypertensive patients group (including those who were not treated). *Diabetes* was defined as having fasting capillary blood glucose ≥ 7.0 mmol/l on 2 different days or the use of insulin or oral hypoglycemic drugs at the time of our survey and prediabetes was defined from 6.1 to 6.9 mmol/l [19, 20].

2.4. Ethical Approval. The research proposal was approved by Hanoi Medical University and three local district health departments (Phu Loc, Nam Dong, and Hue City in Thua Thien Hue Province). The study was explained to all respondents willing to participate and all participants gave their consent before participating in the study. All participants had the right to withdraw from the study at any time. Patients with new diagnostics of hypertension and/or diabetes were advised to consult their community health center or district hospital for the follow-up.

2.5. Statistical Analysis. Statistical analyses were performed to estimate the prevalence of hypertension and the associated risk factors. All statistical results were based on two-sided tests and p value < 0.05 was considered to represent statistical significance. To compare the difference between continuous variables, a t-test for two independent samples was used, and for categorical variables a chi-square test was used. Multivariate logistic regression analysis was performed to examine predictors of prevalence, awareness, treatment, and control of hypertension. The independent variable entry included gender (man, woman), age group (40–49, 50–59, and 60–69), marriage (married, unmarried, and widow(er)), residence (urban versus rural), ethnicity (Kinh majority versus minority), occupation (manual work, governmental staff, other, or no occupation), educational level (primary school or under, secondary or high school, and college or university), current smoking (yes versus no), physical inactivity (yes versus no), excessive alcohol consumption (yes versus no), BMI (overweight or obesity, yes versus no), abdominal obesity (yes versus no), and diabetes (yes versus no). A stepwise conditional logistic regression analysis was performed in order to select variable adopted in the multivariate regression model. EpiData entry (version 3.1, EpiData Association, Denmark) was used to record the study data. Descriptive, analytical, and multivariate logistic regression statistical analyses were carried out using IBM SPSS (version 23.0; IBM Corp., Armonk, NY, USA).

3. Results

3.1. Population Characteristics. Of the 1200 invited people, 983 participated, resulting in a 81.9% response rate. After excluding 14 records with missing information on hypertension risk factors, 969 participants were included for analysis. They had a mean age of 55.5 years (standard deviation: 8.8); 43,9% were men (Table 1). Most participants were married (87.0%); most had an educational background of primary school or under (59,6%) and were manual workers (46.0%). The mean SBP and DBP were 129.6 and 81.9 mmHg, respectively; SBP increased with age in both genders; DBP increased from 40–49 years to 50–59 years but decreased again in the oldest age group. Blood pressure levels of men were significantly higher than those of women ($p < 0.001$).

The prevalence of current smoking and that of excessive alcohol consumption were 33% and 7.6% in the corresponding order. These proportions in men were significantly higher than in women (Table 1). Notwithstanding, the proportions of physical inactivity were similar in both genders. More than

TABLE 1: Characteristics of the study population aged 40–69 years by gender.

Characteristics [mean (SD) or *n* (%)]	Men	Women	Total
Age (in years)	56.2 (8.9)	55.0 (8.7)	55.5 (8.8)
BMI (kg/m^2)	21.6 (3.0)	22.3 (3.2)	22.0 (3.1)
Hip waist ratio	0.88 (0.06)	0.89 (0.07)	0.89 (0.07)
Blood pressure			
Systolic (mmHg)	135.0 (22.8)	125.3 (20.6)	129.6 (22.0)
40–49	128.6 (19.5)	118.1 (17.3)	122.7 (19.0)
50–59	134.5 (23.1)	125.3 (22.1)	128.8 (22.9)
60–69	139.2 (23.5)	131.1 (19.5)	135.2 (21.9)
Diastolic (mmHg)	85.6 (13.9)	79.0 (12.3)	81.9 (13.4)
40–49	84.5 (14.8)	77.1 (10.6)	80.3 (13.1)
50–59	87.4 (14.5)	80.5 (14.0)	83.1 (14.5)
60–69	85.1 (12.9)	78.8 (11.1)	82 (12.4)
Age groups			
40–49	111 (26.1)	146 (26.8)	257 (26.5)
50–59	131 (30.8)	215 (39.5)	346 (35.7)
60–69	183 (43.1)	183 (33.6)	366 (37.8)
Marital status			
Married	408 (96.0)	435 (80.0)	843 (87.0)
Unmarried, Widow(er)	17 (4.0)	109 (20.0)	126 (13.0)
Residence			
Urban	139 (32.7)	191 (35.1)	330 (34.1)
Rural	286 (67.3)	353 (64.9)	639 (65.9)
Ethnicity			
Ethnic majority (Kinh)	301 (70.8)	385 (70.8)	686 (70.8)
Ethnic minorities	124 (29.2)	159 (29.2)	283 (29.2)
Educational level			
Primary school or under	193 (45.4)	385 (70.8)	578 (59.6)
Middle or high school	201 (47.3)	141 (25.9)	342 (35.3)
College or university	31 (7.3)	18 (3.3)	49 (5.1)
Occupation			
Manual workers	217 (51.1)	217 (39.9)	434 (44.8)
Government staff	107 (25.2)	55 (10.1)	162 (16.7)
Other occupations	101 (23.8)	272 (50.0)	373 (38.5)
Current smoking status			
Yes	225 (52.9)	95 (17.5)	320 (33.0)
No	200 (57.1)	449 (82.5)	649 (67.0)
Excessive alcohol consumption			
Yes	69 (16.2)	5 (0.9)	74 (7.6)
No	356 (83.8)	539 (99.1)	895 (92.4)
Physical activity level			
Low	44 (10.4)	64 (11.8)	108 (11.1)
Moderate	73 (17.2)	85 (15.6)	158 (16.3)
High	308 (72.5)	398 (72.6)	703 (72.6)
Body mass index			
Underweight	68 (16.0)	56 (10.3)	124 (12.7)
Normal weight	219 (51.5)	272 (50.0)	491 (50.7)
Overweight, obesity	138 (32.5)	216 (39.7)	354 (36.5)
Abdominal obesity			
Yes	164 (38.6)	384 (70.6)	548 (56.6)
No	261 (61.4)	160 (29.4)	421 (43.3)
Blood glucose			
Diabetes	23 (5.4)	25 (4.6)	48 (5.0)
Prediabetes	43 (10.1)	39 (7.2)	82 (8.5)
No	359 (84,5)	480 (88.2)	839 (86.5)

BMI: body mass index, SD: standard deviation.

half of the participants had excessive abdominal fat and the proportion of overweight, including obesity, was one-third of the participants. These proportions were higher in women than in men. The prevalence of diabetes accounted for 5.0%; there was no significant difference between both genders.

As regards health-seeking behavior, the hypertensive patients mainly attended the local community health centers (61.3%) and much less a private clinic (15.1%), district hospital (11.3%), provincial hospital (5.3), or private pharmacy (6.5%).

3.2. Prevalence, Awareness, Treatment, and Control of Hypertension. Table 2 provides the prevalence of hypertension according to gender, age group, place of residence, and other social determinants. Overall, the prevalence of hypertension in the age group of 40–69 years in the Vietnamese population was 44.8%. It was significantly higher in men than in women (51.3% versus 39.7%, $p < 0.001$). Hypertension's prevalence progressively increased with age. There was no significant difference in the prevalence of hypertension between rural and urban residents or according to educational level. However, hypertension prevalence was higher in the ethnic minority groups than among those from the ethnic majority (52.6% versus 41.5%, $p < 0.001$).

Overall, two-thirds of the participants with hypertension were aware of their hypertension. This proportion increased with age and ranged from 37.3% at age of 40 to 49 years to 78.3% at age of 60 to 69 years. The proportion of hypertension treatment was less than 50% among participants who were aware of their hypertension and one-third among all participants with hypertension. These proportions were higher in women than in men (see Table 2). Among those who were aware of their hypertensive condition and were accordingly well treated, only one-third achieved control of hypertension. The proportion of treated women was significantly higher than that of treated men (44.4% versus 27.0%, $p = 0.03$). Among all participants with hypertension, the prevalence of controlled hypertension achieved 12.2% and was significantly higher in women than in men (16.7% versus 7.8%, $p < 0.001$). The proportion of participants with controlled hypertension also increased with age; however, there was no significant difference among the age groups.

The prevalence and awareness of hypertension are similar among participants from urban and rural areas. On the contrary, the proportions of treatment and control of hypertension were significantly higher in urban areas than in rural areas (46.4% versus 26.1% and 21.2% versus 7.4%, resp.). The prevalence of hypertension in ethnic minorities was higher than that in the Kinh majority of the population. On the contrary, the treatment and control of hypertension were not lower in ethnic minorities than in the majority. There were no significantly different prevalence, awareness, treatment, and control of hypertension according to the educational level.

The prevalence of hypertension in people with physical inactivity, overweight and obesity, abdominal obesity, and diabetes was higher than that in people without those risk factors. There was no significant difference in terms of the awareness, treatment, and control of hypertension between the groups with and without physical inactivity, overweight and obesity, abdominal obesity, or diabetes, respectively. On the other hand, the prevalence of hypertension was not higher in people who were currently smoking or admitted excessive alcohol consumption. The control of hypertension among current smokers or excessive alcohol users was significantly lower than that in the group without these characteristics (Table 2).

3.3. Prevalence, Awareness, Treatment, and Control of Hypertension and Associated Risk Factors. The results from the multivariate logistic regression analysis (Table 3) showed that gender, age, ethnicity, BMI, abdominal obesity, and diabetes were independently associated with hypertension. Gender, age, and excessive alcohol consumption were independently associated with awareness of hypertension. Ethnicity, age, and residence were independently associated with treatment among patients who were aware of their hypertension. Age, residence, and excessive alcohol consumption were independently associated with treatment among all hypertensive patients. Residence was independently associated with control among patients with treated hypertension. Gender, age, and residence were independently associated with control of hypertension among all hypertensive patients.

4. Discussion

4.1. Sociodemographic Characteristics and Hypertension. This study found a large gap between the prevalence, the awareness, the treatment, and the adequate control of hypertension in (Central) Vietnam. Nearly half of individuals were diagnosed with hypertension. However, more than one-third of the hypertensive patients did not know their blood pressure condition; only half of the aware (meaning one-third of all hypertensive patients) had received treatment. No more than one-third of the treated hypertensive (meaning one in eighth of all hypertensive patients) had been adequately controlled. This pattern was consistent with the results of national surveys previously reported in Vietnam and other low- and middle-income countries [3, 14, 21]. For example, the awareness, treatment, and control of hypertension in the low- and middle-income countries were 43,6%, 36,9%, and 9,9%, respectively, according to the PURE study [21]. Previously, poor access to medical facilities combined with limited availability of adequate treatment was shown to be correlated with hypertension in Vietnam and Southeast-Asian population. In addition to the population's lack of knowledge about hypertension, the relationship between physicians and patients, the adherence to medication, and health system characteristics were suggested to play an important role in the attitude of the population to the disease [22–24].

The prevalence of hypertension in our study was higher than that in previous studies in Vietnam (44.8% versus 25.1%). This could be explained by the previous studies sampled in a population aged 25 years or above and in different regions in Vietnam. During the last decades, there has been increasing prevalence of hypertension among Vietnamese citizens [3, 7, 13, 14]. However, reassuringly, the prevalence of hypertension in this study was rather similar to age-standardized prevalence reported in cross-sectional

TABLE 2: Prevalence, awareness, treatment, and control of hypertension of the adult population aged 40–69 years.

Characteristics	Number of participants (*N*)	Prevalence of hypertension *N*1 (*A*%) (*A* = *N*1/*N*)	Awareness of hypertension *N*2 (*B*%) (*B* = *N*2/*N*1)	Treated hypertension: Among awareness *N*3 (*C*%) (*C* = *N*3/*N*2)	Treated hypertension: Among All hypertensive *N*3 (*D*%) (*D* = *N*3/*N*1)	Controlled hypertension: Among treated *N*4 (*E*%) (*E* = *N*4/*N*3)	Controlled hypertension: Among All hypertensive *N*4 (*F*%) (*F* = *N*4/*N*1)
Total	969	434 (44.8)	292 (67.3)	144 (49.3)	144 (33.2)	53 (36.8)	53 (12.2)
Gender (p value)		<0.001	0.001	0.2	0.01	0.03	<0.001
Men	425	218 (51.3)	131 (60.1)	63 (48.1)	63 (28.9)	17 (27.0)	17 (7.8)
40–49	111	41 (36.9)	11 (26.8)	1 (9.1)	1 (2.4)	0	0
50–59	131	66 (50.4)	39 (59.1)	19 (48.7)	19 (28.8)	4 (21.1)	4 (6.0)
60–69	183	111 (60.7)	81 (73.0)	43 (53.1)	43 (38.7)	13 (30.2)	13 (11.7)
Women	544	216 (39.7)	161 (74.5)	81 (50.3)	81 (37.5)	36 (44.4)	36 (16.7)
40–49	146	33 (22.6)	17 (51.5)	7 (41.2)	7 (21.2)	3 (42.9)	3 (9.1)
50–59	215	91 (42.3)	66 (72.5)	29 (43.9)	29 (31.9)	14 (48.3)	14 (15.4)
60–69	183	92 (50.3)	78 (84.8)	45 (57.7)	45 (48.9)	19 (42.2)	19 (20.6)
Age group		<0.001	<0.001	0.06	<0.001	0.86	0.42
40–49	257	74 (28.8)	28 (37.3)	8 (28.6)	8 (10.8)	4 (44.4)	4 (5.3)
50–59	346	157 (45.4)	105 (66.9)	48 (45.7)	48 (30.6)	18 (37.5)	18 (11.5)
60–69	366	203 (55.5)	159 (78.3)	88 (55.3)	88 (43.3)	31 (35.6)	31 (15.3)
Ethnicity		0.001	0.3	<0.001	<0.001	0.06	0.001
Ethnic majority	686	285 (41.5)	187 (65.6)	110 (58.8)	110 (38.6)	45 (40.9)	45 (15.8)
Ethnic minority	283	149 (52.6)	105 (70.5)	34 (32.4)	34 (22.8)	8 (23.5)	8 (5.4)
Marital status		0.9	0.004	0.33	0.64	0.25	0.54
Married	843	378 (44.8)	245 (64.8)	123 (50.2)	123 (32.5)	47 (38.2)	47 (12.4)
Unmarried, Widow(er)	126	56 (44.4)	47 (83.9)	20 (42.6)	20 (35.7)	5 (25.0)	5 (8.9)
Residence		0.6	0.7	<0.001	<0.001	0.03	<0.001
Urban	330	151 (45.8)	103 (68.2)	70 (68.0)	70 (46.4)	32 (45.7)	32 (21.2)
Rural	639	283 (44.3)	189 (66.8)	74 (39.2)	74 (26.1)	21 (28.4)	21 (7.4)
Educational level		0.32	0.16	0.49	0.29	0.44	0.68
Primary school or under	578	254 (43.9)	180 (70.9)	84 (46.7)	84 (33.1)	33 (39.3)	33 (13.0)
Middle or high school	342	153 (44.7)	96 (62.7)	52 (54.2)	52 (34.0)	16 (30.8)	16 (10.5)
College or university	49	27 (55.1)	16 (59.3)	8 (50.0)	8 (47.1)	4 (50.0)	4 (14.8)
Occupation		<0.001	0.3	<0.001	<0.001	0.33	0.004
Manual worker	434	177 (39.4)	114 (64.3)	39 (35.4)	39 (22.8)	12 (28.2)	12 (6.4)
Government staff	162	98 (59.3)	64 (64.6)	36 (53.2)	36 (34.4)	12 (33.3)	12 (11.5)
Other occupations	348	159 (45.7)	114 (71.7)	69 (60.5)	69 (43.4)	29 (42.0)	29 (18.2)
Current smoking		0.7	0.5	0.39	0.65	0.03	0.04
Yes	320	146 (45.6)	101 (69.2)	46 (45.5)	46 (31.5)	11 (23.9)	11 (7.5)
No	649	288 (44.4)	191 (66.3)	98 (50.8)	98 (33.7)	42 (42.3)	42 (14.2)
Excessive alcohol consumption		0.154	<0.001	0.31	0.005		0.016
Yes	74	39 (52.7)	14 (5.9)	5 (35.7)	5 (12.8)	0	0
No	895	395 (44.1)	278 (70.4)	138 (49.6)	138 (34.9)	52 (37.7)	52 (13.2)

Table 2: Continued.

Characteristics	Number of participants (N)	Prevalence of hypertension $N1$ (A%) ($A = N1/N$)	Awareness of hypertension $N2$ (B%) ($B = N2/N1$)	Treated hypertension: Among awareness $N3$ (C%) ($C = N3/N2$)	Treated hypertension: Among All hypertensive $N3$ (D%) ($D = N3/N1$)	Controlled hypertension: Among treated $N4$ (E%) ($E = N4/N3$)	Controlled hypertension: Among All hypertensive $N4$ (F%) ($F = N4/N1$)
Physical inactivity		0.029	0.32	0.5	0.89	0.57	0.69
Yes	108	59 (54.6)	43 (72.9)	19 (44.2)	19 (32.2)	8 (42.1)	8 (13.6)
No	861	375 (43.6)	249 (66.4)	124 (49.8)	124 (33.1)	44 (35.5)	44 (17.2)
Overweight, obesity		<0.001	0.47	0.37	0.67	0.3	0.52
Yes	354	185 (52.3)	121 (65.4)	63 (52.1)	63 (34.1)	20 (31.7)	20 (10.8)
No	615	249 (40.5)	171 (68.7)	80 (46.8)	80 (32.1)	32 (40.0)	32 (12.9)
Abdominal obesity		0.011	0.068		0.025	0.44	0.5
Yes	548	265 (48.4)	187 (70.6)	98 (52.4)	98 (37.0)	34 (34.7)	18 (10.7)
No	421	169 (40.1)	105 (62.1)	45 (42.9)	45 (26.6)	18 (40.0)	34 (12.8)
Diabetes		0.001	0.025	0.28	0.96	0.19	0.25
Yes	48	33 (68.8)	28 (84.8)	11 (39.3)	11 (33.3)	6 (54.4)	6 (18.2)
No	921	401 (43.5)	264 (65.8)	132 (50.0)	132 (32.9)	46 (34.8)	46 (11.5)

Table 3: Multivariate logistic regression analysis demonstrating the relationship between the prevalence, awareness, treatment, and control of hypertension with several independent variables.

Risk factors	OR (95% CI)	*p* value
Prevalence of hypertension		
Gender (men versus women)	1.83 (1.37–2.44)	<0.001
Ethnicity (Kinh versus minority)	0.54 (0.40–0.73)	<0.001
Age group (per 10 years)	0.56 (0.47–0.67)	<0.001
BMI (overweight and obesity versus no)	1.82 (1.35–2.45)	<0.001
Abdominal obesity (yes versus no)	1.40 (1.03–1.91)	0.032
Diabetes (yes versus no)	2.18 (1.13–4.19)	0.019
Awareness of hypertension		
Gender (men versus women)	0.47 (0.29–0.77)	0.003
Age group (per 10 years)	0.42 (0.31–0.57)	<0.001
Excessive alcohol consumption (yes versus no)	0.33 (0.16–0.72)	0.005
Treatment among aware hypertensive patients		
Ethnicity (Kinh versus minority)	1.72 (0.95–3.12)	0.073
Age group (per 10 years)	0.62 (0.42–0.9)	0.013
Residence (urban versus rural)	2.6 (1.43–4.73)	0.002
Treatment among all hypertensive patients		
Age group (per 10 years)	0.47 (0.34–0.65)	<0.001
Residence (urban versus rural)	2.26 (1.43–3.58)	<0.001
Excessive alcohol consumption (yes versus no)	0.34 (0.13–7.93)	0.034
Control among treated hypertension		
Residence (urban versus rural)	2.14 (1.05–4.34)	0.035
Control among all hypertensive patients		
Gender (men versus women)	0.41 (0.21–0.79)	0.008
Age group (per 10 years)	0.49 (0.28–0.81)	0.005
Residence (urban versus rural)	3.49 (1.88–6.47)	<0.001

CI: confidence interval, BMI: body mass index.

national study [3]. The proportion of awareness with age-standardization in our study was higher than those in the other studies in Vietnam [3, 14]. Between those two sets of studies, there have been a lot of activities to raise the local people's awareness of hypertension. Health education campaigns have appeared on national as well as local television channels and in the newspapers [25, 26]. As a consequence, the population was sensitized about hypertension and hypertensive patients could be detected earlier. However, our proportion of treatment and control of hypertension was similar to the previous study in Vietnam and in other low- middle-income countries. There was no increase in the proportion of treatment or the control of hypertension either. These findings were far from optimal, a disturbing trend that has been observed in many other developing countries; for example, the proportion of awareness, treatment, and control in Canada in 2013 were 84.3%, 80%, and 68%, respectively [7, 8, 21]. Hypertension management is still a big challenge in Central Vietnam. In order to promote hypertension treatment and control, it is desirable to make people more aware of the risks of hypertension. Further, research should explore the barriers of optimal management of hypertension.

The overall mean SBP and DBP were significantly higher in men than in women and rose progressively with age in both genders. The prevalence of hypertension was also significantly higher in men than in women. However, the proportions of awareness, treatment, and control were higher in women than in men. Of particular concern is the proportion of awareness, treatment, and control of hypertension in young adults aged 40 to 49 years, which was substantially lower than in older adults. The early detection of hypertension in young adults should be conducted more regularly. This was consistent with other studies in Vietnam and in other low-, middle-, and high-income countries [3, 7, 11, 21]. In the multivariate logistic regression analysis, gender and age were independently associated with prevalence, awareness, and control of hypertension. Only age and not gender was found to be independently associated with the treatment of hypertension.

The prevalence and awareness of hypertension in urban and rural areas appeared to be similar (45.8% versus 44.3% and 68.2% versus 66.0%). These results were not consistent with the previous findings in Vietnam with much higher proportions in urban areas than in rural areas (32.7% versus 17.3% and 58.4% versus 28.8%) [3]. This situation might be related to economic development in rural areas, and associated lifestyle and diet changes lead to an increased prevalence and awareness of hypertension. However, the treatment and control were much higher in urban areas than in rural areas, and place of residence was an independent risk factor for treatment and control of hypertension. These findings were consistent with the results of the low- and middle-income countries such as China, Colombia, and Iran but were different from those of the high-income countries like Canada or Sweden [21]. In many developing countries, the treatment and control of hypertension were not only a burden for the health service in the rural areas, despite that their prevalence still remained lower than that in the urban areas [21]. In Vietnam, the prevalence of hypertension in rural areas has increased from 14.1% in 2005 to 22% in 2011, but the health services have not yet sufficiently developed to meet the population's needs [12, 13]. It was also suggested that the socioeconomic status gap had a strong influence on hypertension management. It requires improving the healthcare provision in rural areas to cope with the new challenges. Among the ethnic minority groups, there was high prevalence of hypertension, but the control and treatment were largely insufficient. Most of the ethnic minorities are living in the mountainous and remote rural areas, facing difficulties such as low income, poor health education, insufficient health facilities, difficult access to medical services, and lack of health resources [24, 27, 28]. There was no association between the level of education and prevalence, awareness, treatment, and control of hypertension in this study.

It was shown in our study that the community health centers were most frequently visited by hypertensive patients (61.3%) and that the other types of health facilities were much less popular. This does not necessarily indicate the differences in the quality of care; rather, it might have been because of the easier access to the community health centers and the fact that these centers were mainly in charge of providing primary healthcare, particularly hypertension treatment. Under any circumstances, the community health centers should therefore be considered an important stakeholder to increase the proportion of treatment and control of hypertension.

4.2. Health Behavior and Metabolic Risk Factors and Hypertension. One of the factors that could contribute to the high prevalence of hypertension in Vietnam was the increasing prevalence of overweight and obesity. The prevalence of overweight and obesity in adults increased from 2005 (standing at 19.8% in men and 21.9% in women) to 2008 (accounting for 18.4% in men and 22.7% in women) [3, 14]. Overweight including obesity and abdominal obesity has become highly prevalent in developed countries and has been rapidly reaching epidemic proportions in the developing ones. The high prevalence in our study, which was higher than the results of the previous research in Vietnam, could be related to the fact that the mean age in our sample was higher. The waist circumference is increasing with age in adults of both sexes up to the age of 70 years. The age-related differences in waist hip ratio were also reported in all BMI categories examined in both men and women. The increasing rate of obesity might as well be attributed to the fast urbanization, industrialization, and modernization [17, 18]. Also described in the present study was higher prevalence of hypertension in the overweight and obesity group as compared to those without overweight and obesity. In the multivariate logistic regression analysis, there was an independent association between obesity or abdominal obesity and hypertension. This finding was consistent with previous literature [9, 14, 29].

In this study, hypertension was more commonly diagnosed in the patients with diabetes type 2 as compared to the general population. High blood pressure was detected among over two-thirds of the patients with diabetes type 2, and its development coincided with the development of hyperglycemia. Diabetes was notified to be independently associated with hypertension like in previous studies [9, 30]. Simultaneously, a higher rate of hypertension was detected in the group with physical inactivity. As physical activity had a positive effect on many risk factors such as hypertension, obesity, and diabetes, regular physical exercise would reduce the risk of many adverse health outcomes (all-cause and CVD mortality) over a wide range of age [9]. Therefore, in order to reduce the risk of obesity, hypertension, and diabetes type 2, there should be a promotion of physical activities in the community.

In addition, according to our study, one-third of the study population, mostly men, had been currently smoking. The prevalence of hypertension in current smokers was not significantly higher than that in those without current smoking. There has been little if any association between the current smoking activity and the prevalence, awareness, treatment, and control of hypertension in the multivariate logistic regression analysis. However, among the treated hypertension patients, blood pressure was better controlled among noncurrent smokers than among current smokers. Therefore, the antismoking campaigns by the Ministry of Health, the Vietnamese Government, and the National Assembly's Policies should continue [24, 31]. In our study, men showed high prevalence of excessive alcohol consumption. People without excessive alcohol use were more likely to be aware of the risks related to hypertension. According the multivariate logistic regression analysis, excessive alcohol consumption was independently associated with diagnosed hypertension and treatment among all hypertensive patients. Previous studies also indicated that hypertension was higher in those with excessive alcohol consumption [13]. Hypertension awareness, treatment, and control should be integrated in the strategy of hypertension management for alcohol consumers.

4.3. Limitations and Strengths. According to the definition, the diagnosis of hypertension should have been based on two or more blood pressure readings taken at two or more visits after the initial screening [18]. In our study, blood pressure was measured in a single visit, so the prevalence of hypertension might have been overestimated and the control of hypertension underestimated. However, this common problem of large epidemiological study might have some effects on within sample comparisons, especially when a standard protocol and analysis were applied. The information collected through the interview may be inaccurate due to the education level and recall bias of the participants. Effective quality control procedures of blood pressure measurement and the interview were held by well-trained investigators to reduce the possibility of attrition bias.

In our study, there was a slight chance of misclassification of diabetes status, since it was determined by self-report or two hyperglycemic readings with a capillary glucometer. Fortunately, it was likely to be acceptable in such a setting with limited resources like ours [25, 26]. A comprehensive picture of hypertension and its risk factors among the Vietnamese population aged 40 and over in this research was then guaranteed.

5. Implication of Study

This study has several important implications for public health staff, clinicians, and health policy makers. It was shown from our findings that hypertension still remained a serious public health problem in Central Vietnam with high prevalence of hypertension and low level of awareness, treatment, and control. This result contributes to the ongoing policy debate with respect to the prevention and control of hypertension in Vietnam. In particular, it ascertained the necessity to improve the effectiveness of the current National Targeted Program for Prevention and Control of Hypertension. This program should focus more on the hypertensive patients in rural areas and the ethnical hypertensive groups because they showed high prevalence of hypertension and low proportion of treatment and control. This study also showed high prevalence of overweight and obesity, current smoking, and alcohol consumption. Therefore, clinicians should consider both nonmedication and medication approaches for treatment of hypertension. And such efforts might as well include the use of mass media to educate the general population, delivering brochures and leaflets to hypertensive patients and providing leadership from social and professional organizations to promote healthy lifestyles. Improving the capacity of the community health centers would be an important activity for enhancing the rate of early detection, treatment, and control of hypertension. Further studies could be conducted to explore the barriers of hypertension management from the healthcare provider and patient's perspective as well as the new community-based intervention approaches to find out the possible solutions to the present situation in (Central) Vietnam.

6. Conclusion

To summarize, the findings of this study indicated that hypertension remained an important public health problem in Central Vietnam. In spite of the increasing prevalence of hypertension over the past 10 years in (Central) Vietnam, the treatment and effective control of hypertension had remained unacceptably low. Nearly half of the adult Vietnamese population aged from 40 to 69 years was hypertensive, but only one-third of the hypertensive patients received due treatment, and not more than one in eighth of all hypertensive patients had been adequately controlled. Age, gender, place of residence, body mass index, and diabetes were found to be independent risk factors for hypertension. These findings suggested that early detection, raising awareness, and providing better treatment of hypertension could be very important to maintain and improve the quality of hypertension management, especially in rural areas to reduce the burden of hypertension. Moreover, the lifestyle modifications including the prevention of overweight and obesity, smoking, and alcohol consumption could help prevent hypertension.

Disclosure

The views presented in this paper present the view of the authors and not that of the organizations present. The funders had no role in study design, data collection and analysis, or decision to publish or preparation of the manuscript.

Authors' Contributions

Nguyen Minh Tam, Ho Anh Hien, Vo Tam, Dirk Devroey, and Anselme Derese contributed to conceiving and designing the experiments. Ho Anh Hien, Vo Tam, and Nguyen Minh Tam performed the experiments. Nguyen Minh Tam, Ho Anh Hien, Vo Tam, Dirk Devroey, and Anselme Derese contributed reagents, materials, and analysis tools. Ho Anh Hien, Dirk Devroey, Anselme Derese, Vo Tam, and Nguyen Minh Tam wrote the paper.

Acknowledgments

This work was supported by China Medical Board of New York, Inc. (Grant no. 05821) in the project "Family Medicine and Vietnamese Health Care Delivery System" and VLIR Inter-University Cooperation Programme VLIR-IUC with Hue University (ZIUC2016AP026 and ZIUC2017AP026). The authors are grateful to A/Professor Nguyen Phuong Hoa (Hanoi Medical University) and A/Professor Jeffrey Markuns (Boston University) for their dedicated support. They are also obliged to the study participants, investigators, and local healthcare providers.

References

[1] World Health Organization, "Causes of death 2008: Data sources and methods," Geneva. WHO. 2011, [Accessed 21th June, 2017], http://www.who.int/healthinfo/global_burden_disease/cod_2008_sources_methods.pdf.

[2] S. S. Lim, T. Vos, A. D. Flaxman et al., "A comparative risk assessment of burden of disease and injury attributable to 67 risk factors and risk factor clusters in 21 regions, 1990–2010: a systematic analysis for the Global Burden of Disease Study 2010," *The Lancet*, vol. 380, no. 9859, pp. 2224–2260, 2010.

[3] P. T. Son, N. N. Quang, N. L. Viet et al., "Prevalence, awareness, treatment and control of hypertension in Vietnam—results from a national survey," *Journal of Human Hypertension*, vol. 26, no. 4, pp. 268–280, 2012.

[4] World Health Organization, "Non communicable diseases country profiles 2014. Geneve. WHO," 2014, [Accessed October 17, 2017], http://www.who.int/nmh/publications/ncd-profiles-2014/en/.

[5] H. Van Minh, P. Byass, and S. Wall, "Mortality from cardiovascular diseases in Bavi District, Vietnam," *Scandinavian Journal of Public Health*, vol. 31, no. 62, pp. 26–31, 2003.

[6] N. P. Hoa, C. Rao, D. G. Hoy, N. Duc Hinh, N. T. K. Chuc, and D. A. Ngo, "Mortality measures from sample-based surveillance: Evidence of the epidemiological transition in Viet Nam," *Bulletin of the World Health Organization*, vol. 90, no. 10, pp. 764–772, 2012.

[7] M. Pereira, N. Lunet, A. Azevedo, and H. Barros, "Differences in prevalence, awareness, treatment and control of hypertension between developing and developed countries," *Journal of Hypertension*, vol. 27, no. 5, pp. 963–975, 2009.

[8] E. L. Schiffrin, N. R. C. Campbell, R. D. Feldman et al., "Hypertension in Canada: past, present, and future," *Annals of Global Health*, vol. 82, no. 2, pp. 288–299, 2016.

[9] M. F. Piepoli, A. W. Hoes, S. Agewall et al., "2016 European guidelines on cardiovascular disease prevention in clinical practice," *European Heart Journal*, vol. 37, no. 29, pp. 2315–2381, 2016.

[10] E. S. Ford, U. A. Ajani, J. B. Croft et al., "Explaining the decrease in U.S. deaths from coronary disease, 1980–2000," *The New England Journal of Medicine*, vol. 356, no. 23, pp. 2388–2398, 2007.

[11] E. Vartiainen, T. Laatikainen, M. Peltonen et al., "Thirty-five-year trends in cardiovascular risk factors in Finland," *International Journal of Epidemiology*, vol. 39, no. 2, Article ID dyp330, pp. 504–518, 2010.

[12] H. Van Minh, P. Byass, N. T. K. Chuc, and S. Wall, "Gender differences in prevalence and socioeconomic determinants of hypertension: Findings from the WHO STEPs survey in a rural community of Vietnam," *Journal of Human Hypertension*, vol. 20, no. 2, pp. 109–115, 2006.

[13] D. A. Ha, R. J. Goldberg, J. J. Allison, T. H. Chu, and H. L. Nguyen, "Prevalence, awareness, treatment, and control of high blood pressure: a population-based survey in Thai Nguyen, Vietnam," *PLoS ONE*, vol. 8, no. 6, Article ID e66792, 2013.

[14] H. T. P. Do, J. M. Geleijnse, M. B. Le, F. J. Kok, and E. J. M. Feskens, "National prevalence and associated risk factors of hypertension and prehypertension among vietnamese adults," *American Journal of Hypertension*, vol. 28, no. 1, pp. 89–97, 2015.

[15] World Health Organization, "WHO STEPS Surveillance Manual: The WHO STEP-wise Approach to Chronic Disease Risk Factors Surveillance, World Health Organization: Non-communicable Diseases and Mental health," Geneva, WHO, 2005, [accessed 15th January, 2015], http://www.who.int/ncds/surveillance/steps/en/.

[16] World Health Organization and International Obesity Task Force, "The Asia-Pacific Perspective: Redefining obesity and its treatment. Health Communications Australia. Melbourn," 2000, [accessed 20th July, 2015], http://www.wpro.who.int/nutrition/documents/docs/Redefiningobesity.pdf.

[17] World Health Organization, "Waist circumference and Waist-Hip ratio: Report of a WHO Expert Consultation, Geneva, World Health Organization," 2008, [accessed 20th July, 2015], http://apps.who.int/iris/bitstream/10665/44583/1/9789241501491_eng.pdf.

[18] G. Mancia, R. Fagard, and K. Narkiewicz, "2013 ESH/ESC guidelines for the management of arterial hypertension: the task force for the management of arterial hypertension of the european society of hypertension (ESH) and of the european society of cardiology (ESC)," *European Heart Journal*, vol. 34, no. 28, pp. 2159–2219, 2013.

[19] World Health Organization, "Definition and diagnosis of diabetes mellitus and intermediate hyperglycemia : report of a WHO/IDF consultation," WHO, 2006, [accessed 20th July, 2015], http://www.who.int/iris/handle/10665/43588.

[20] S. Somannavar, A. Ganesan, M. Deepa, M. Datta, and V. Mohan, "Random capillary blood glucose cut points for diabetes and pre-diabetes derived from community-based opportunistic screening in India," *Diabetes Care*, vol. 32, no. 4, pp. 641–643, 2009.

[21] C. K. Chow, K. K. Teo, S. Rangarajan et al., "Prevalence, awareness, treatment, and control of hypertension in rural and urban communities in high-, middle-, and low-income countries," *Journal of the American Medical Association*, vol. 310, no. 9, pp. 959–968, 2013.

[22] T.-P. Nguyen, C. C. M. Schuiling-Veninga, T. B. Y. Nguyen, T.-H. Vu, E. P. Wright, and M. J. Postma, "Adherence to hypertension medication: quantitative and qualitative investigations in a rural northern Vietnamese community," *PLoS ONE*, vol. 12, no. 2, Article ID e0171203, pp. 1–13, 2017.

[23] Q. N. Nguyen, S. T. Pham, V. L. Nguyen et al., "Implementing a hypertension management programme in a rural area: local approaches and experiences from Ba-Vi district, Vietnam," *BMC Public Health*, vol. 11, article 325, 2011.

[24] Vietnam Ministry of Health and Health Partnership Group, "Joint annual health review 2014: Strengthening prevention and control of non-communicable disease," Hanoi, 2015, http://www.jahr.org.vn/downloads/JAHR2014/JAHR%202014_EN_full.pdf.

[25] Government of Vietnam, "Ministerial Decision 172/2008/QĐ-TTg, National health target Program for prevention of social diseases, dangerous communicable diseases and HIV/AIDS from 2006 to 2010," [accessed 17th October, 2017], http://moj.gov.vn/vbpq/lists/vn%20bn%20php%20lut/view_detail.aspx?itemid=25287.

[26] Government of Vietnam, "Ministerial Decision 1208/2012/ QĐ-TTg, Approval of National health target Program from 2012 to 2015," [accessed 17th October, 2017], http://vanban.chinhphu.vn/portal/page/portal/chinhphu/hethongvanban?class_id=2&mode=detail&document_id=163367.

[27] H. Van Minh, T. T. Anh, J. Rocklöv et al., "Primary healthcare system capacities for responding to storm and flood-related health problems: a case study from a rural district in central Vietnam," *Global Health Action*, vol. 7, no. 1, Article ID 23007, pp. 1–11, 2014.

[28] Vietnam Ministry of Health and Health Partnership Group, "Joint Annual Health Review 2015: Strengthening primary health care at the grassroots toward universal health

coverage," Hanoi, 2016, http://jahr.org.vn/downloads/JAHR2015/JAHR2015_full_EN.pdf.

[29] Q. N. Nguyen, S. T. Pham, L. D. Do et al., "Cardiovascular disease risk factor patterns and their implications for intervention strategies in vietnam," *International Journal of Hypertension*, vol. 2012, Article ID 560397, 11 pages, 2012.

[30] E. Ferrannini and W. C. Cushman, "Diabetes and hypertension: the bad companions," *The Lancet*, vol. 380, no. 9841, pp. 601–610, 2012.

[31] Ministry of Health of Viet Nam, Hanoi Medical University, Centers for Disease Control and Prevention, and World Health Organization, "Global Adult Tobacco Survey. Hanoi," 2010, [Accessed 14th Decemder, 2017], http://www.who.int/tobacco/surveillance/en_tfi_gats_vietnam_report.pdf.

21

Hypertension Impact on Health-Related Quality of Life: A Cross-Sectional Survey among Middle-Aged Adults in Chongqing, China

Xianglong Xu,[1,2,3] Yunshuang Rao,[4] Zumin Shi,[5] Lingli Liu,[1,2,3] Cheng Chen,[1,2,3] and Yong Zhao[1,2,3]

[1] *School of Public Health and Management, Chongqing Medical University, Chongqing 400016, China*
[2] *Research Center for Medicine and Social Development, Chongqing Medical University, Chongqing 400016, China*
[3] *The Innovation Center for Social Risk Governance in Health, Chongqing Medical University, Chongqing 400016, China*
[4] *School of Nursing, Chongqing Medical University, Chongqing 400016, China*
[5] *School of Medicine, Faculty of Health Sciences, The University of Adelaide, North Terrace, Adelaide, SA 5005, Australia*

Correspondence should be addressed to Yong Zhao; zhaoyongzb@qq.com

Academic Editor: Tzi Bun Ng

Hypertension is a major risk factor of cardiovascular disease in China, and yet little is known about health-related quality of life (HRQOL) and its associations with demographic and social-economic characteristics in middle-aged patients with hypertension. A cross-sectional survey was undertaken in Chongqing, China, using a multistage stratified random sampling methodology. Data was collected on 1,224 eligible adults, aged between 45 and 53 years, including the Medical Outcomes Survey Short Form-36 to measure HRQOL. Hypertension was associated with poor state of physical functioning, role-physical, bodily pain, general health, vitality, and social function ($p < 0.05$ for all). In multivariable analyses, education level, job conditions, average monthly income, smoking status, sleep quality, perception of relationship with family, childhood breastfeeding history, and body mass index were associated with domains of SF36 among those with hypertension ($p < 0.05$ for all). Hypertensive respondents with high education, marital status, breastfeeding, higher incomes, good quality of sleep, positive relationship with family, and higher body mass index have better HRQOL in middle-aged people with hypertension. Those unemployed had a better state of general health and had a poorer state of social function. Nonsmokers had a poorer state of bodily pain than smokers. This study provides detailed information of the implications for health care providers to gain a more complete picture of their hypertension patients' health.

1. Introduction

Hypertension is a well-known independent risk factor for many chronic diseases including diabetes and cardiovascular diseases causing a significant burden to the society and families [1]. Hypertension has been identified as the second leading risk factor in China, which accounted for 12.0% of disability-adjusted life years and 24.6% of deaths in 2010 [2]. According to the 2015 Chinese Chronic Disease and Nutrition Report, the prevalence of hypertension among adults aged 45–59 years and over 60 was 35.7% and 58.9% in 2012, respectively [3]. The incidence of hypertension has increased from 2.9 per 100 person-years in 1991–1997 to 5.3 per 100 person-years in 2004–2009 [4]. A national survey conducted in 2011-2012 found that nearly 40% of Chinese people aged 45 years or older were hypertensive [5]. However, the prevalence of awareness, treatment, and control was low: 44.2%, 38.0%, and 13.1% among those aged 45–59 years, respectively and 53.7%, 48.8%, and 16.1%, among those aged 60 years and above, respectively [3].

Health-related quality of life (HRQOL) has become increasingly important in clinical research over the last 15 years [6]. It provides a multidimensional perspective encompassing a patient's emotional, physical, and social functioning [7]. HRQOL is related to an individual's perception of the position in life in the context of culture and value systems and is influenced in a complex way by the person's physical health, psychological state, level of independence, and social relationships [8]. Hypertension is closely related to psychological and emotional problems, particularly in severe life stresses [9]. Studies have found that people with hypertension had a poorer quality of life indicator than people without the condition [10–13]. By establishing a proven link between the disease and HRQOL, then developing interventions programs aiming at improving HRQOL will become a new relevant therapeutic objective in hypertensive subjects [11].

Middle age is a special stage of life. Just as Confucius said: "At thirty, I had planted my feet firm upon the ground. At forty, I no longer suffered from perplexities." Most of the middle-aged adults are leaders in every job and have increased family and job responsibilities. In China, middle age is the most stressful period of one's life because of job demands, caring for the older and younger generations, and paying for medical service and education. Studies on HRQOL among people with or without hypertension are limited in China. The aim of this study was to assess HRQOL as well as its sociodemographic and lifestyle determinants among middle-aged adults with or without hypertension.

2. Methods

2.1. Study Design. The study was conducted in Chongqing city in July 2009. This study used three-stage stratified random sampling method to recruit participants. Eligible participants were those born between 1956 and 1964 and were aged 45–53 years during time of the survey. At Stage 1, 10 districts and counties were randomly selected in Chongqing city. Stage 2 involved listing eligible villages within the selected districts and counties. In each selected district/count, about 8 to 10 villages were selected (Stage 2). About 10 to 15 participants were randomly selected in each village (Stage 3). In total, 1250 participated in the survey with a response rate of 98.4%. Of the 1250 participants, 6 were excluded in the analysis because of missing data.

2.2. Survey Administration. Face-to-face interview was conducted by senior medical school students. All of the participants were informed of the study's purpose, and their participation in the study was voluntary. The survey was conducted in compliance with the Ethical Committee of Chongqing Medical University. The questionnaire used in the study was divided into two sections. The first section collects information on sociodemographic and lifestyle factors and health conditions. Hypertension and other health conditions were assessed by the question "Have you ever been told by a doctor or other health professional that you have [disease or condition]?" Self-reported height and weight were collected to calculate body mass index (BMI). The second section was the short form (SF-36) survey. The questionnaire was piloted among 40 individuals in a hospital.

2.3. Outcome Measure: SF-36. A validated Chinese version of the SF-36 questionnaire is used in the study [14]. The questionnaire includes 36 questions; they were used to generate eight scales of HRQOL, namely, physical functioning (PF), role-physical (RP), bodily pain (BP), general health (GH), vitality (VT), social functioning (SF), role-emotional (RE), and mental health (MH). In the SF36 scoring system, the scales were assessed quantitatively, and a score is calculated based on the guidelines, with a higher score indicating a better state of health [15, 16].

2.4. Sociodemographic and Lifestyle Factors. Education was categorized into three groups: low (primary school), medium (junior school), and high (high school or above). Marital status was recorded as married and unmarried/divorced/widowed. Income was classified as low (<1600 Yuan/month) and high (>1600 Yuan/month). Job status was recorded as employed and unemployed/retired. Self-reported current living conditions were categorized as satisfactory and average/unsatisfactory. Smoking status and alcohol drinking were recorded into two categories (yes or no). Regular physical activity was categorized as usually and seldom/sometimes. Self-reported sleep quality was categorized as good and poor/average. Perception of family relationship and friend relationship was classified as harmony or poor/average. Childhood breastfeeding history was also assessed and categorized as yes or no.

2.5. Data Analysis. The data gathered from the questionnaires were carefully examined before inputting the data to the database using EpiData 3.1 software. The data were meticulously sorted, cleaned, and analyzed using Statistical Analysis System software (version 9.1, SAS Institute, Cary, NC). Chi-square test was used to compare differences between categorical variables, and t-test was conducted to compare differences in continuous variables between hypertensive and nonhypertensive groups. Multiple linear regression analyses were used to probe factors associated with domains of health-related quality of life among those with hypertension [17]. Sociodemographic and lifestyle factors included in the final multivariable regression models were based on findings from univariate analyses.

3. Results

Of the 1,224 participants, 150 (12.25%) reported having hypertension. Table 1 showed the sample characteristics by hypertension status. Men were more likely to have hypertension than women. Significant differences were found with respect to marital status ($p = 0.038$), smoking ($p = 0.0002$), sleep quality ($p = 0.049$), BMI ($p < 0.001$), and history of breast feeding ($p = 0.011$) between hypertensive and nonhypertensive groups.

Participants with hypertension had a lower score of physical functioning, role-physical, bodily pain, general health, vitality, and social function than those without the condition (Table 2). No difference of role-emotional and mental health was seen between hypertensive and nonhypertensive groups.

In multivariable analyses, several sociodemographic and lifestyle factors were associated with domains of SF36 among those with hypertension (Table 3). Compared with women, men had a lower score of role-physical. Low education was associated with a lower score of physical functioning

TABLE 1: Characteristics of participants in Chongqing, China.

Characteristic	Hypertensive ($n = 150$)	Nonhypertensive ($n = 1074$)	p value
Gender (%)			**<0.0001**
Male	75.3	53.5	
Female	24.7	46.6	
Educational level (%)			0.499
Low	16.7	15.1	
Medium	45.3	50.5	
High	38.0	34.5	
Marital status (%)			**0.038**
Unmarried/divorced or separated/widowed	12.0	7.2	
Married or cohabitation	88.0	92.83	
Job conditions (%)			0.678
Unemployed/retired at home	52.7	54.5	
Employed	47.3	45.5	
Average monthly income (%)			0.232
<1600 Yuan	52.7	57.8	
>1601 Yuan	47.3	42.2	
Smoking (%)			**0.0002**
Yes	52.7	36.7	
No	47.3	63.3	
Alcohol drinking (%)			**<0.001**
Yes	28.7	45.5	
No	71.3	54.5	
Regular physical activity (%)			0.614
Seldom/sometimes	78.7	76.8	
Usually	21.3	23.2	
Have a regular daily life (%)			0.525
Seldom/sometimes	94.7	93.3	
Usually	5.3	6.7	
Sleep quality (%)			**0.049**
Good	32.7	41.1	
Poor/average	67.3	58.9	
Perception of family relationships (%)			0.597
Harmonious	74.0	76.0	
Poor/average	26.0	24.0	
Perception of relationships with colleague or friends (%)			0.274
Harmonious	78.0	73.8	
Poor/average	22.0	26.2	
Current living conditions (%)			0.868
Satisfactory	53.3	52.6	
Unsatisfactory/average	46.7	47.4	
Body mass index (mean, SD)	24.792 ± 4.2638	23.112 ± 8.6582	**<0.001**
Childhood breastfeeding history (%)			**0.011**
Breastfeeding	73.3	82.0	
Nonbreastfeeding	26.7	18.0	

and bodily pain but not the others. Marital status was not significantly associated with the domains of HRQOL. Compared with those employed, those unemployed had higher score of general health and had a lower score of social function. Compared with those with higher incomes, those with low incomes had a lower score of bodily pain and vitality. Nonsmokers had a lower score of bodily pain than smokers. Those who had poor sleep had a lower score of physical functioning than those with good sleep. Compared with those with a good relationship with family, those who

TABLE 2: Descriptive statistics of each domain of the SF-36 among adults in Chongqing, China (mean, SD).

Domains	Hypertensive (n = 150)	Nonhypertensive (n = 1074)	p value
Physical functioning (PF)	80.2 (21.9)	88.2 (15.4)	**<0.001**
Role-physical (RP)	80.7 (19.5)	85.3 (17.7)	**0.004**
Bodily pain (BP)	76.7 (18.4)	81.7 (17.8)	**0.001**
General health (GH)	57.4 (15.3)	62.0 (14.5)	**0.000**
Vitality (VT)	61.1 (15.2)	65.9 (15.4)	**0.000**
Social function (SF)	80.3 (18.7)	84.8 (16.4)	**0.008**
Role-emotional (RE)	83.2 (14.7)	84.7 (17.0)	0.288
Mental health (MH)	66 (11.2)	67.0 (10.9)	0.310

Note: (1) values are mean and SD; (2) SD: standard deviation.

had a poor relationship with the family had a lower score of physical functioning, role-physical, social function, and role-emotional. Nonbreastfeeding had a lower score of bodily pain than breastfeeding. Those who had a higher body mass index had a higher score of role-physical and mental health.

4. Discussion

Our research shows that hypertension associated with physical functioning, role-physical, bodily pain, general health, vitality, and social function. In this study, middle-aged hypertensive adults reported significantly lower scores in most of the SF-36 dimensions, which were consistent with studies in other populations [18]. These findings further confirm that hypertension significantly affects health-related quality of life [19] among middle-aged hypertensive adults. Further longitudinal studies are required to test for the presence as well as the direction of associations between physical functioning, role-physical, bodily pain, general health, vitality, and social function and hypertension among hypertensive patients.

This study found that men had a poor state of role-physical. This study stressed the importance of gender on role-physical, among hypertensive patients. To understand the gender differences, biological factors may explain some of the differences but the main explanation is presumably gender disparities in work, economy, daily living, social life, and expectations between women and men [20]. More quantitative studies are needed to determine the association between gender and role-physical among hypertensive patients.

This study found that low education was associated with a lower score of physical functioning and bodily pain. Hypertensive patients with a low education level had a poorer state of lower score of physical functioning and bodily pain than those with a high education level. Educational attainment may influence the acquisition of knowledge about appropriate health practices, which may facilitate or constrain one's ability to maintain good physical function [21]. It may also due to the different social life and expectations. The link between education and HRQOL may be mediated by health literacy. Lifestyle intervention including weight reduction, physical activity, and healthy diet is beneficial for the management of hypertension [22, 23]. These healthy behaviors are often influenced by education.

This study found that among those with hypertension unemployment had a poorer social function and better state of general health than employment. This finding agrees with earlier research studies that unemployment and low socioeconomic status are associated with poor HRQOL [24, 25]. Previous study shows that job strain was significantly associated with vitality [26]. The results provide justification for further investigating the role of jobs as a risk factor for health-related quality of life among hypertensive patients.

Smoking has been associated with many adverse health outcomes including hypertension. Surprisingly, in our study we found that nonsmokers had a poor state of bodily pain than smokers, and we did not see a significant association between smoking and domains of SF36 except bodily pain among those with hypertension. Possible reasons are that quality of life rating is subjective and relative to a person's life expectations [27], influenced by a patient's strategies to cope with them [7]. Patients with hypertension who were smokers might feel contented and downscale their expectations for life and as long as they could stabilize their condition and be free from complications [28]. Further research is needed to assess whether quitting smoking may improve quality of life among those with hypertension in Chinese populations.

Previous studies have demonstrated that poor sleep was associated with poor health condition [28, 29]. We found that poor sleep quality was associated with poor state of physical functioning. Existing evidence suggests that there is a bidirectional association between obstructive sleep apnea and hypertension. Addressing sleep problems may improve quality of life among those with hypertension.

Our study stresses the importance of the relationship with family/colleagues/friends on health-related quality of life among hypertensive patients. This study found that those had a poor relationship with the family had a poorer state of physical functioning, role-physical, social function, and role-emotional than those with good relationship with family. It has been suggested that social support from family was strongly associated with hypertension treatment compliance [30] and better survival, lower depression, and higher compliance to medication [31]. Social support is the complex network of how a person gets and gives information and aid, as well as how they meet their emotional needs [32]. A good relationship with family and friends may enhance the social support and improve quality of life.

Table 3: Multiple linear regression analysis for the factors affecting health-related quality of life in hypertensive patients in Chongqing, China.

	PF		RP		BP		GH		VT		SF		RE		MH	
	B (s.e.)	*p*	*B* (s.e.)	*p*	*B* (s.e.)	*p*	*B* (s.e.)	*p*	*B* (s.e.)	*p*	*B* (s.e.)	*p*	*B* (s.e.)	*p*	*B* (s.e.)	*p*
Men versus women	−0.8 (5.4)	0.888	−10.8 (4.4)	**0.015**	−6.6 (4.5)	0.147	3.5 (4.1)	0.398	−4.4 (4.0)	0.277	−5.9 (4.34)	0.173	−1.9 (4.3)	0.664	0.8 (2.9)	0.779
Low education versus high education	−14.2 (6.2)	**0.023**	−6.5 (5.0)	0.194	−12.1 (5.4)	**0.028**	−4.8 (5.0)	0.345	1.3 (4.8)	0.781	−4.1 (5.3)	0.441	−4.5 (4.9)	0.353	−2.0 (3.5)	0.574
Medium education versus high education	2.2 (4.5)	0.621	0.4 (3.7)	0.922	−4.1 (4.0)	0.306	−2.3 (3.6)	0.529	5.9 (3.6)	0.100	5.7 (3.9)	0.145	0.0 (3.6)	0.993	2.0 (2.6)	0.457
Unmarried/divorced or separated/widowed versus married	−4.6 (5.5)	0.399	−4.8 (4.4)	0.283	−2.0 (4.8)	0.673	−3.9 (4.5)	0.387	−7.5 (4.2)	0.078	−8.7 (4.9)	0.079	−3.1 (4.3)	0.470	−1.9 (3.1)	0.539
Unemployed versus employed	−5.0 (3.7)	0.179	−7.3 (3.0)	0.017	−0.8 (3.2)	0.801	6.6 (2.9)	**0.025**	−0.1 (2.8)	0.960	−7.4 (3.1)	**0.018**	−3.9 (2.9)	0.191	−0.1 (2.1)	0.967
Low income versus high income	−5.0 (4.4)	0.254	−6.9 (3.5)	0.055	−7.8 (3.9)	**0.047**	−1.7 (3.5)	0.630	−9.4 (3.5)	**0.007**	−3.0 (3.8)	0.427	−5.5 (3.5)	0.119	−1.3 (2.5)	0.615
Nonsmokers versus smokers	−3.9 (4.3)	0.371	−3.4 (3.5)	0.338	−7.7 (3.8)	**0.044**	−0.5 (3.4)	0.883	−4.7 (3.3)	0.163	−3.3 (3.6)	0.361	1.0 (3.4)	0.758	0.8 (2.5)	0.760
Poor/average sleep quality versus good sleep quality	−8.8 (3.8)	**0.023**	−2.9 (3.0)	0.346	−1.6 (3.3)	0.634	−5.9 (3.0)	0.053	−3.0 (3.0)	0.306	−3.6 (3.2)	0.268	−5.8 (3.0)	0.056	−3.6 (2.2)	0.100
Poor/average versus good family relationship	−11.3 (4.7)	**0.018**	−7.8 (3.8)	**0.042**	−8.7 (4.2)	0.039	−7.3 (3.9)	0.061	−4.1 (3.7)	0.268	−14.5 (4.2)	**0.001**	−8.7 (3.7)	**0.021**	−4.3 (2.7)	0.117
Poor/average versus good relationship with colleague or friend	3.1 (5.4)	0.574	−2.6 (4.3)	0.543	4.0 (4.8)	0.408	3.7 (4.4)	0.406	0.6 (4.2)	0.880	7.8 (4.8)	0.110	1.0 (4.2)	0.822	1.4 (3.1)	0.652
Nonbreastfeeding versus breastfeeding	−7.1 (4.2)	0.097	−2.1 (3.4)	0.548	−7.7 (3.8)	**0.043**	0.6 (3.4)	0.859	−3.5 (3.3)	0.296	−5.9 (3.7)	0.114	−2.8 (3.4)	0.399	−0.9 (2.4)	0.706
Body mass index	0.5 (0.6)	0.364	1.1 (0.5)	**0.01**	0.4 (0.3)	0.264	0.2 (0.3)	0.47	0.5 (0.3)	0.147	1.1 (0.3)	0.00	0.8 (0.5)	0.107	0.6 (0.2)	**0.010**

Note: (1) PF: physical functioning; RH: role-physical; BP: bodily pain; GH: general health; VT: vitality; SF: social function; RE: role-emotional; MH: mental health; (2) potential independent variables for the multiple linear regression analysis include gender (1 = male; 2 = female (reference category)); educational level (1 = low; 2 = medium; 3 = high (reference category)); marital status (0 = unmarried/divorced or separated/widowed; 1 = married (reference category)); job conditions (0 = unemployed; 1 = employed (reference category)); average monthly income (0 = ≤1600 Yuan; 1 = >1601 Yuan (reference category)); smoking (0 = nonsmoker; 1 = smoker (reference category)); sleep quality (0 = poor or average sleep quality; 1 = good sleep quality (reference category)); condition of getting along with family (0 = poor or average condition of getting along with family; 1 = harmony condition of getting along with family (reference category)); condition of getting along with colleague or friend (0 = poor or average condition of getting along with colleague or friend; 1 = harmony condition of getting along with colleague or friend (reference category)); feeding procedure (0 = nonbreastfeeding; 1 = breast feeding (reference category)).

The beneficial effects of breastfeeding are well-known. Previous study showed that infant feeding patterns are associated with cardiovascular structures and function in childhood [33]. In this study, we found that hypertensive participants who were nonbreastfeeding had a poorer bodily pain among hypertensive patients than those who were breastfeeding. This study stressed the importance of breastfeeding on bodily pain among hypertensive patients.

This study found that body mass index was associated with role-physical and mental health among hypertensive patients. Hypertensive participants who have higher body mass index have a better state of role-physical and mental health. A previous study showed that the class I obese was significantly associated with better HRQL scores in the mental component summary than the normal weight in adults of the Chinese general population [34]. Some research presented that underweight was associated with poorer HRQL [35]. Previous studies showed the survival benefit or improved HRQL in the elderly or patients with existing chronic diseases who are overweight and moderately obese [36, 37]. This study stressed the importance of body mass index on role-physical and mental health among hypertensive patients.

This study has several limitations that should be noted. First, hypertension was based on self-reported doctor's diagnoses. According to the 2015 Chinese chronic disease and nutrition report, the prevalence of awareness was 44.2% among those aged 45–59 years [3]. In China, the prevalence of undiagnosed hypertension is high. Self-reported hypertension may not be accurate; many people with hypertension do not clearly know that they have hypertension in China. Hypertensive participants in this study may be relatively heavy, and this may lower the quality of life of hypertensive participants. And hypertensive patients with no obvious symptom may be mistaken for nonhypertensive patients. This may lower the quality of life of nonhypertensive participants. Second, we cannot establish any causation due to the cross-sectional design. Further longitudinal studies will be required to test for the presence of associations between demographics and the HRQOL and to fully interpret their clinical significance. Third, the study sample used in the investigation was relatively homogeneous regarding race/ethnicity. Future investigations with more heterogeneous samples are warranted. Fourth, the participants are middle-aged, and the findings may not apply to the younger or older individuals.

5. Conclusions

Hypertensive respondents with a high education, married, breastfeeding, and with higher incomes, good quality of sleep, positive relationship with family, and higher body mass index have better HRQOL in middle-aged people with hypertension. Respondents who currently do not smoke have poorer HRQOL in middle-aged people with hypertension. Those unemployed had a better state of general health and had a poorer state of social function. This study provides detailed information of the implications for health care providers to gain a more complete picture of their hypertension patients' health. What is more, to determine causal relationships, further longitudinal studies will be required to test for the presence of associations between sociodemographic and lifestyle and the HRQOL among hypertensive patients and to fully interpret their clinical and public health significance.

Disclosure

Xianglong Xu and Yunshuang Rao are to be considered as joint first authors.

Competing Interests

The authors declare that they have no competing interests.

Acknowledgments

The authors thank Yong-Hong Wang, Hong Wang, Ji-Bin Li, Yong Zhang, Yi Zhang, Yong-Fang Liu, Da-Mei Liu, Jing-Lin Yang, Ling-Li Han, Xiao-Qin Zong, and Ting-Yu Li in Chongqing Medical University for their active participation. They would also like to thank Eleonora Dal Grande at the University of Adelaide for proofreading. This study was supported by China Ministry of Education of Humanities and Social Science research of 2008 Youth Fund Projects, Grant no. 08JC840021 and Program of Science Committee at Yuzhong District in Chongqing (no. 20120301).

References

[1] J.-T. Zhang, K.-P. Chen, T. Guan, and S. Zhang, "Effect of aliskiren on cardiovascular outcomes in patients with prehypertension: a meta-analysis of randomized controlled trials," *Drug Design, Development and Therapy*, vol. 9, pp. 1963–1971, 2015.

[2] G. Yang, Y. Wang, Y. Zeng et al., "Rapid health transition in China, 1990–2010: findings from the Global Burden of disease study 2010," *The Lancet*, vol. 381, no. 9882, pp. 1987–2015, 2013.

[3] Bureau of Disease Prevention and Control (Office of the National Patriotic Health Campaign Committee), *2015 Report on Chinese Resident's Chronic Disease and Nutrition*, People's Medical Publishing House, Beijing, China, 2015.

[4] Y. Liang, R. Liu, S. Du, and C. Qiu, "Trends in incidence of hypertension in Chinese adults, 1991–2009: the China Health and Nutrition Survey," *International Journal of Cardiology*, vol. 175, no. 1, pp. 96–101, 2014.

[5] X. L. Feng, M. Pang, and J. Beard, "Health system strengthening and hypertension awareness, treatment and control: data from the China Health and Retirement Longitudinal Study," *Bulletin of the World Health Organization*, vol. 92, no. 1, pp. 29–41, 2014.

[6] A. Tchicaya, N. Lorentz, S. Demarest, J. Beissel, and D. R. Wagner, "Relationship between self-reported weight change, educational status, and health-related quality of life in patients with diabetes in Luxembourg," *Health and Quality of Life Outcomes*, vol. 13, article 149, 2015.

[7] L. Baladón, M. Rubio-Valera, A. Serrano-Blanco, D. J. Palao, and A. Fernández, "Gender differences in the impact of mental disorders and chronic physical conditions on health-related quality of life among non-demented primary care elderly patients," *Quality of Life Research*, vol. 25, no. 6, pp. 1461–1474, 2016.

[8] H. Halaweh, C. Willen, A. Grimby-Ekman, and U. Svantesson, “Physical activity and health-related quality of life among community dwelling elderly,” *Journal of Clinical Medicine Research*, vol. 7, no. 11, pp. 845–852, 2015.

[9] S. A. Everson, G. A. Kaplan, D. E. Goldberg, and J. T. Salonen, “Hypertension incidence is predicted by high levels of hopelessness in Finnish men,” *Hypertension*, vol. 35, no. 2, pp. 561–567, 2000.

[10] D. J. Trevisol, L. B. Moreira, A. Kerkhoff, S. C. Fuchs, and F. D. Fuchs, “Health-related quality of life and hypertension: a systematic review and meta-analysis of observational studies,” *Journal of Hypertension*, vol. 29, no. 2, pp. 179–188, 2011.

[11] W. Li, L. Liu, J. G. Puente et al., “Hypertension and health-related quality of life: an epidemiological study in patients attending hospital clinics in China,” *Journal of Hypertension*, vol. 23, no. 9, pp. 1667–1676, 2005.

[12] W. F. Lawrence, D. G. Fryback, P. A. Martin, R. Klein, and B. E. K. Klein, “Health status and hypertension: a population-based study,” *Journal of Clinical Epidemiology*, vol. 49, no. 11, pp. 1239–1245, 1996.

[13] J. G. Rabkin, E. Charles, and F. Kass, “Hypertension and DSM-III depression in psychiatric outpatients,” *American Journal of Psychiatry*, vol. 140, no. 8, pp. 1072–1074, 1983.

[14] L. Zhang, D.-Z. Xu, J.-Y. Huang, and L.-S. Li, “Study on the application of the Chinese version of SF-36 scales and selection of interceptive cents for its grade range,” *Zhonghua Liu Xing Bing Xue Za Zhi*, vol. 25, no. 1, pp. 69–73, 2004 (Chinese).

[15] J. E. Ware, *SF-36 Health Survey. Manual and Interpretation Guide*, The Health Institute, Boston, Mass, USA, 1993.

[16] J. Xu, M. Hu, Y. Yang, B. Wang, and Y. Xie, “The medical outcomes study 36-item short-form health survey,” *Chinese Journal of Behavioral Medical Science*, vol. 2, pp. 70–72, 1999 (Chinese).

[17] Regression with SAS, “Chapter 3—Regression with Categorical Predictors,” UCLA, Statistical Consulting Group, http://www.ats.ucla.edu/stat/sas/webbooks/reg/chapter3/sasreg3.htm.

[18] H.-M. Wang, M. Beyer, J. Gensichen, and F. M. Gerlach, “Health-related quality of life among general practice patients with differing chronic diseases in Germany: cross sectional survey,” *BMC Public Health*, vol. 8, article 246, 2008.

[19] L. Jiang, J. Beals, N. R. Whitesell, Y. Roubideaux, and S. M. Manson, “Health-related quality of life and help seeking among American Indians with diabetes and hypertension,” *Quality of Life Research*, vol. 18, no. 6, pp. 709–718, 2009.

[20] K. Bingefors and D. Isacson, “Epidemiology, co-morbidity, and impact on health-related quality of life of self-reported headache and musculoskeletal pain—a gender perspective,” *European Journal of Pain*, vol. 8, no. 5, pp. 435–450, 2004.

[21] S. L. Brennan and G. Turrell, “Neighborhood disadvantage, individual-level socioeconomic position, and self-reported chronic arthritis: a cross-sectional multilevel study,” *Arthritis Care & Research*, vol. 64, no. 5, pp. 721–728, 2012.

[22] L. J. Appel, “Effects of comprehensive lifestyle modification on blood pressure control: main results of the PREMIER clinical trial,” *The Journal of the American Medical Association*, vol. 289, no. 16, pp. 2083–2093, 2003.

[23] A. K. Ho, C. T. Thorpe, N. Pandhi, M. Palta, M. A. Smith, and H. M. Johnson, “Association of anxiety and depression with hypertension control: a US multidisciplinary group practice observational study,” *Journal of Hypertension*, vol. 33, no. 11, pp. 2215–2222, 2015.

[24] L. Cheng, S. Cumber, C. Dumas, R. Winter, K. M. Nguyen, and L. Z. Nieman, “Health related quality of life in pregeriatric patients with chronic diseases at urban, public supported clinics,” *Health and Quality of Life Outcomes*, vol. 1, article 63, 2003.

[25] A. L. Stewart and A. Nápoles-Springer, “Health-Related Quality-of-Life assessments in diverse population groups in the United States,” *Medical Care*, vol. 38, no. 9, pp. II102–II124, 2000.

[26] D. J. Lerner, S. Levine, S. Malspeis, and R. B. D'Agostino, “Job strain and health-related quality of life in a national sample,” *American Journal of Public Health*, vol. 84, no. 10, pp. 1580–1585, 1994.

[27] P. J. Allison, D. Locker, and J. S. Feine, “Quality of life: a dynamic construct,” *Social Science and Medicine*, vol. 45, no. 2, pp. 221–230, 1997.

[28] H.-X. Liu, J. Lin, X.-H. Lin et al., “Quality of sleep and health-related quality of life in renal transplant recipients,” *International Journal of Clinical and Experimental Medicine*, vol. 8, no. 9, pp. 16191–16198, 2015.

[29] T. R. Van Dyk, R. W. Thompson, and T. D. Nelson, “Daily bidirectional relationships between sleep and mental health symptoms in youth with emotional and behavioral problems,” *Journal of Pediatric Psychology*, 2016.

[30] P. E. Osamor, “Social support and management of hypertension in South-West Nigeria,” *Cardiovascular Journal of Africa*, vol. 26, no. 1, pp. 29–33, 2015.

[31] S. D. Cohen, T. Sharma, K. Acquaviva, R. A. Peterson, S. S. Patel, and P. L. Kimmel, “Social support and chronic kidney disease: an update,” *Advances in Chronic Kidney Disease*, vol. 14, no. 4, pp. 335–344, 2007.

[32] S. S. Patel, R. A. Peterson, and P. L. Kimmel, “The impact of social support on end-stage renal disease,” *Seminars in Dialysis*, vol. 18, no. 2, pp. 98–102, 2005.

[33] L. L. De Jonge, M. A. Langhout, R. Taal et al., “Infant feeding patterns are associated with cardiovascular structures and function in childhood,” *Journal of Nutrition*, vol. 143, no. 12, pp. 1959–1965, 2013.

[34] Y. Zhu, Q. Wang, G. Pang et al., “Association between body mass index and health-related quality of life: the ‘obesity paradox’ in 21,218 adults of the Chinese general population,” *PLoS ONE*, vol. 10, no. 6, Article ID e0130613, 2015.

[35] M. Dey, G. Gmel, and M. Mohler-Kuo, “Body mass index and health-related quality of life among young Swiss men,” *BMC Public Health*, vol. 13, no. 1, article 1028, 2013.

[36] M. R. Carnethon, P. J. D. De Chavez, M. L. Biggs et al., “Association of weight status with mortality in adults with incident diabetes,” *The Journal of the American Medical Association*, vol. 308, no. 6, pp. 581–590, 2012.

[37] A. Romero-Corral, V. M. Montori, V. K. Somers et al., “Association of bodyweight with total mortality and with cardiovascular events in coronary artery disease: a systematic review of cohort studies,” *The Lancet*, vol. 368, no. 9536, pp. 666–678, 2006.

22

Prevalence and Associated Risk Factors of Hypertension: A Cross-Sectional Study in Urban Varanasi

Shikha Singh,[1] Ravi Shankar,[1] and Gyan Prakash Singh[2]

[1]Department of Community Medicine, Institute of Medical Sciences, Banaras Hindu University, Varanasi 221005, India
[2]Division of Biostatistics, Department of Community Medicine, Institute of Medical Sciences, Banaras Hindu University, Varanasi 221005, India

Correspondence should be addressed to Shikha Singh; shikhasngh032@gmail.com

Academic Editor: Tomohiro Katsuya

Hypertension is a major public health problem and important area of research due to its high prevalence and being major risk factor for cardiovascular diseases and other complications. *Objectives.* (1) To assess the prevalence of hypertension and its associated factors and (2) to estimate awareness, treatment, and adequacy of control of hypertension among study subjects. *Methods and Materials.* A community based cross-sectional study with multistage sampling design was conducted among urban population of Varanasi. A modified WHO STEPS interview schedule on 640 study subjects aged 25–64 years was used. *Results.* The prevalence of hypertension was 32.9% (male: 40.9%, female: 26.0%). Mean systolic and diastolic BP were 124.25 ± 15.05 mmHg and 83.45 ± 9.49 mmHg, respectively. Higher odds of being hypertensive were found in male subjects, eldest age group, married subjects, subjects of upper socioeconomic status, illiterate subjects, and retired subjects. Tobacco and alcohol consumption, overweight, obesity, and abdominal obesity were also associated with hypertension. Out of the total hypertensive 211 subjects, only 81 (38.4%) were aware about their hypertension status; out of those, 57 (70.4%) were seeking treatment and 20 (35.08%) had their blood pressure adequately controlled. *Conclusion.* Around one-third of the subjects were hypertensive and half of the study subjects were prehypertensive in this area. The awareness, treatment, and control of high blood pressure were also very low.

1. Introduction

Hypertension is a major public health problem due to its high prevalence all around the globe [1–4]. Around 7.5 million deaths or 12.8% of the total of all annual deaths worldwide occur due to high blood pressure [5]. It is predicted to be increased to 1.56 billion adults with hypertension in 2025 [6].

Raised blood pressure is a major risk factor for chronic heart disease, stroke, and coronary heart disease. Elevated BP is positively correlated to the risk of stroke and coronary heart disease. Other than coronary heart disease and stroke, its complications include heart failure, peripheral vascular disease, renal impairment, retinal hemorrhage, and visual impairment [5].

Hypertension (or HTN) or high blood pressure is defined as abnormally high arterial blood pressure. According to the Joint National Committee 7 (JNC7), normal blood pressure is a systolic BP < 120 mmHg and diastolic BP < 80 mm Hg. Hypertension is defined as systolic BP level of ≥140 mmHg and/or diastolic BP level ≥ 90 mmHg. The grey area falling between 120–139 mmHg systolic BP and 80–89 mmHg diastolic BP is defined as "prehypertension" [7, 8]. Although prehypertension is not a medical condition in itself, prehypertensive subjects are at more risk of developing HTN [1].

It is a silent killer as very rarely any symptom can be seen in its early stages until a severe medical crisis takes place like heart attack, stroke, or chronic kidney disease [8–10]. Since people are unaware of excessive blood pressure, it is only through measurements that detection can be done. Although majority of patients with hypertension remain asymptomatic, some people with HTN report headaches, lightheadedness, vertigo, altered vision, or fainting episode [11].

There are several factors predisposing to hypertension. These factors vary from country to country and even there is difference between urban and rural regions of the same place [12]. Realizing the effect of urbanization on our collective health, World Health Organization has chosen "Urbanization and Health" as the theme for World Health Day 2010 [13]. Urbanization is considered a determinant of health and one of the key drivers of noncommunicable diseases (NCDs), especially in low- and middle-income countries (LMICs) [14]. Urban people are more at risk of these diseases as compared to their rural counterparts. As per the findings of National Family Health Survey (NFHS-4), the prevalence of hypertension, obesity, and blood glucose in urban area of Uttar Pradesh was 10.5%, 23.9, and 9.9%, respectively. However, the prevalence of the same phenomenon was 8.3%, 10.8%, and 8.2%, respectively in rural area [15]. It is clear that all the parameters are having higher prevalence in urban area as compared to rural area. Rapid urbanization, increasing elderly population, mechanization, sedentary life, and dietary changes act together as a web of risk factors which entangles people in it and leads to several chronic diseases. In order to take effective prevention measures, identification of the risk factors is an essential prerequisite. This study intends to generate information on prevalence of hypertension and their associated risk factors in urban area of Varanasi. In addition, it will also look into the awareness and control of hypertension among the study subjects.

2. Materials and Methods

2.1. Study Area. Varanasi is an Indian city on the bank of Ganges in Uttar Pradesh. It has total population of 3676841 as per Census 2011. As per Census 2011, out of total population, 52% people live in urban areas, while 48% live in the rural areas. There are 90 Census enumeration wards in Varanasi district. Out of these 90 wards, 5 wards were selected by using simple random sampling.

2.2. Study Design and Sample Size. A community based cross-sectional study was carried out among the people aged 25 to 64 years living in the selected study area. The sample size for the present study was calculated by taking most probable prevalence of hypertension as 50% and permissible error as 5% with 95% confidence interval. Fixing the permissible error as 50%, the minimum sample size was calculated as $n = 384$. Since sampling procedure was multistage, hence considering the design effect, the sample size was further increased by one and half times. Considering the nonresponse rate of 10% the final sample size in study was fixed as 640. In the present study, a prior written informed consent was also taken from the participants. Prior written informed consent was taken by the participants.

2.3. Sampling Methodology. A multistage sampling was used for this study. There were three stages and for each stage different sampling design was used.

At first, out of these 90 wards, 5 wards were selected by using simple random sampling. At second stage, from each selected ward the households were further selected by using systematic random sampling and probability proportional to size was done. At the third stage, one member of target age group was interviewed from selected household. If the selected family has more than one available eligible person then one was chosen randomly by using lottery method. In case of nonavailability of eligible person in a selected household, at the time of survey, the adjacent household was selected.

2.4. Selection of Study Subjects

2.4.1. Inclusion Criteria. Individuals aged 25–64 years in the selected study area who gave consent for participation were considered.

2.4.2. Exclusion Criteria. Individuals who are unable to give response due to serious physical or mental illness and with whom anthropometry measurements cannot be performed were excluded from the study.

2.5. Tools of the Study. Interview schedule [modified and pretested WHO stepwise approach to chronic disease risk factor surveillance (STEPS)], Libra weighing machine, steel anthropometry rod, measuring tape, and Omron BP Machine were used.

2.6. Techniques of the Study. In all study participants, a structured and pretested interview schedule was administered to obtain data on sociodemographic parameters.

2.6.1. Blood Pressure Measurement. Blood pressure was measured two times on the right arm of the selected subject using automatic electronic device (OMRON HEM-7261). The average of two readings was used.

2.6.2. Anthropometric Measurements. All the anthropometric measurements were done by the following standardized technique. Weight was measured by Libra weighing machine having an accuracy of 0.1 kg and height was measured by using a steel anthropometry rod with accuracy of 0.1 cm using standard techniques. Body Mass Index was calculated using the following formula: BMI = weight (kg)/height (mt)^2. Based on BMI obtained, the subjects were classified into different categories according to the WHO global classification [16]. Waist circumference (in cm) was measured using a nonstretchable measuring tape. Waist circumference was measured at the smallest horizontal girth between the costal margins and the iliac crest at the end of expiration. Hip circumference (in cm) was measured at the broadest part of the hips by using nonstretchable measuring tape. Waist-to-hip circumference (WHR) was calculated by dividing waist circumference by hip circumference [17].

2.7. Ethical Consideration. Ethical approval was obtained from the Institute Ethical Committee of the Institute of Medical Sciences, Banaras Hindu University Varanasi. Prior written consent was taken from the subjects who volunteered to participate in the study. Identified hypertensive subjects were referred to the nearby clinic for treatment.

2.8. Definitions Used

(i) Joint National Committee on Prevention, Detection, Evaluation, and Treatment of High Blood Pressure (JNC 7) classification was used for hypertension [8].

(ii) Hypertension is defined as systolic BP level of ≥140 mmHg and/or diastolic BP level of ≥90 mmHg or being previously diagnosed as hypertensive by any health professional. The area falling between 120–139 mmHg systolic BP and 80–89 mmHg diastolic BP is defined as "prehypertension" [8].

(iii) Isolated diastolic hypertension (IDH) having a systolic blood pressure ≤ 140 mmHg and diastolic blood pressure ≥ 90 mmHg and isolated systolic hypertension (ISH) having a systolic blood pressure ≥ 140 mmHg and diastolic blood pressure < 90 mmHg was used to diagnose IDH and ISH, respectively.

(iv) Awareness was defined as history of hypertension based on diagnosis by a healthcare provider. Treatment was defined as taking any medication or other treatment for hypertension in the last two weeks prior to the survey and control was defined as blood pressure < 140 and <90 mmHg in subjects who were taking medications

(v) WHO International BMI classification: BMI < 18.5 was classified as *"underweight"*; <16.00, *"severe thinness"*; 16.00–16.99, *"moderate thinness"*; 17.00–18.49, *"mild thinness"*; 18.50–24.99, *"normal range"*; BMI ≥ 25.00, *"overweight"*; 25.0–29.99, *"preobese"*; ≥30.00, *"obese"*; 30.00–34.99, *"obese class I"*; 35.00–39.99, *"obese class II"*; and >40.00, *"obese class III."*

(vi) Socioeconomic class categorization was done by using modified BG Prasad classification according to all India consumer price index (AICPI) for the month of January 2014 [18] (Table 1).

$$\text{Multiplication Factor} = \frac{\text{Value of price index} \times 4.93}{100}. \quad (1)$$

(vii) Current daily smokers are defined as those who were currently smoking cigarettes, bidis, or hookah daily. Current daily smokeless tobacco users are defined as those who were currently using chewable tobacco products, gutka, naswar, khaini, or zarda paan daily. Current alcohol drinkers are defined as those who reported to consuming alcohol within the past one year [17].

(viii) Physical activity was measured in three domains that is activity at work, to and from places, and recreational activities as well as time spent sitting. The interview schedule also covered type of activity (vigorous and moderate) at work and for recreational activities. Information was also collected on the number of days in a week spent on different activities and time spent in a day for each activity was also recorded [17]. Those who were not active in any domain were defined as "inactive," those who were vigorously active in any category were defined as "vigorously active," and the rest were "moderately active."

2.9. Data Processing. The information obtained from the survey was entered into a database developed for the study, using SPSS 16.0 program. Descriptive statistics (mean and standard deviation) were calculated for continuous variables and frequencies and percentages were calculated to summarize qualitative data. Other statistical tests like chi-square test and ANOVA were applied. Logistic regression was applied to identify the risk factors for hypertension. A significance level of 0.05 was used.

3. Results

A total of 640 study subjects were interviewed for the survey. Out of these, 301 (47%) were male subjects and 339 (53%) were female. The median age (±SD) of the study subjects was 39.0 (±11.9) years and for male and female it was 40.0 (±11.9) years and 38 (±11.8) years, respectively. Regarding religion and caste of the study subjects, around 96% subjects were Hindu and majority of the subjects were in general category, respectively. Majority of the study subjects were married and one-third of the subjects belonged to the upper socioeconomic class. Mean (±SD) BMI of the study subjects was $24.11 \pm 3.94\,kg/m^2$; for men it was $23.78 \pm 3.95\,kg/m^2$ and for women it was $24.41 \pm 3.92\,kg/m^2$. According to Body Mass Index (BMI), more than one-third of the study subjects were either overweight or obese. With regard to abdominal obesity as measured by waist circumference, 40% subjects were at risk (Table 2).

Table 3 depicts the mean values of systolic and diastolic BP according to age and gender. The mean systolic and diastolic BP of all the study subjects were 124.2 ± 15.0 mmHg and 83.4 ± 9.5 mmHg, respectively. In men, the highest mean systolic BP and mean diastolic BP were among the eldest age group and preceding eldest age group (45–54 years), respectively, while in female the highest mean value of systolic and diastolic BP both were among the 45–54-year age group. With regard to systolic BP, there was significant difference among all the age groups among both male and female study subjects and the same was with diastolic BP as well. The prevalence of isolated systolic BP was found to be 10.6% [95% CI: (8.27–13.37)] and isolated diastolic BP was 19.7% [95% CI: 16.6–23.18]. The proportion was higher in male (14.8%) as compared to female (6.8%). Among both groups (male and female), prevalence was higher among the eldest age group. The prevalence of isolated diastolic BP was higher among male subjects (28.1) against female subjects (12.2%). It was the highest among the second oldest age group among male and oldest age group in female subjects. With regard to systolic BP, age was associated with hypertension status among both genders, whereas diastolic BP was associated with age in male subjects only. There was no association between age and diastolic BP in female subjects.

The overall prevalence of hypertension was 32.96% [95% CI: (29.4–36.7)]. The sex specific prevalence was 40.9% [95% CI: 35.5–46.5] for male and 26.0% [95% CI: 21.6–30.9] for

Table 1: Revised modified BG Prasad socioeconomic classification scale, January 2014.

Socioeconomic class	Per capita monthly income	
	1961 (base year)	Revised income categories 2014
Upper class	100 and above	5357 and above
Upper middle class	50–99	2652–5356
Middle class	30–49	1570–2651
Lower middle class	15–29	812–1569
Lower class	<15	<811

female. Prehypertension was prevalent in 45.9% [95% CI: (40.3–51.5)] of men and 38.05% [95% CI: (33.0–43.2)] of women. In men, hypertension was significantly associated with age but in women, age does not have any effect on their hypertension status. History of hypertension or the prediagnosed cases of hypertension was more among female (6.7%) as compared to male (5.9%) subjects (Table 4).

Table 5 shows the associated factors of prehypertension and hypertension. Gender, age, marital status, occupation, education status, tobacco use, and physical activity were significantly associated with the hypertension status of the study subjects ($p < 0.05$). Both the rate of prehypertension and hypertension were higher among male. Hypertension was more prevalent in the 45–54 years, while prehypertension was more in the 35–44-year age group. Being married and government servant were found to be risk factors for both hypertension and prehypertension. Hypertension was found to be more among illiterate subjects, and with regard to prehypertension, primary educated subjects suffered more. Study subjects from lower and upper socioeconomic status were almost equal victims of hypertension. Tobacco use and alcohol use were found to be risk factors for being hypertensive in the study subjects. Although alcohol use was not significantly associated with hypertension status but rate of hypertension was higher among the alcohol users.

The binary logistic regression analysis showed that odds of being hypertensive were higher among the male subjects (OR: 1.97), eldest age group (OR: 6.49), married subjects (OR: 2.34), uneducated subjects (OR: 1.17), retired subjects (OR: 3.66), and those who were from upper socioeconomic status (1.31). With regard to anthropometric risk factors, being overweight (OR: 1.99), being obese (OR: 3.57), and having abdominal obesity (OR: 1.73) had higher odds of hypertension. Tobacco use (OR: 1.86), alcohol use (OR: 1.55), and nonvegetarian diet (OR: 1.10) also had higher odds of being hypertensive. Gender, age, marital status, occupation, BMI, abdominal obesity, and tobacco use were significantly associated with hypertension. Education, socioeconomic status, and alcohol use were not statistically associated with hypertension. Being female, younger in age, unmarried, highly educated, and staying away from any kind of addiction could serve as protective factors against hypertension (Table 6).

Out of the total subjects with hypertension, around one-third of the subjects were aware of their condition. Out of those who were aware, 70% were seeking treatment. Only a third of the treated subjects with hypertension had their blood pressure adequately controlled (Figure 1). Females were marginally more aware of their hypertensive status as compared to male counterparts (see Table 4, history of hypertension). As age, education status, and socioeconomic status were advancing, the awareness of hypertensive status

Table 2: Background characteristics of the study subjects (*N* 640).

Variables	*N* (640)	Proportion%
Age group		
25–34	204	31.9
35–44	179	28.0
45–54	133	20.8
55–64	124	19.4
Sex		
Male	301	47.0
Female	339	53.0
Caste		
Gen	313	48.9
OBC	305	47.7
SC/ST	22	3.4
Religion		
Hindu	619	96.7
Non-Hindu	21	3.3
Education		
Illiterate	64	10.0
Primary	85	13.3
Secondary	182	28.4
Graduate & above	309	48.3
Marital status		
Unmarried	60	9.4
Married	545	85.2
Others	35	5.5
Occupation		
Government	86	13.4
Private	155	24.2
Self-employed	109	17.0
Retired	27	4.2
Homemaker	229	35.8
Others	34	5.3
Family type		
Nuclear	311	48.6
Joint	329	51.4
Number of family members		
1–5	401	62.7
≥6	239	37.3
Socioeconomic status		
Lower class	41	6.4
Lower middle class	105	16.4
Middle class	120	18.8
Upper middle class	140	21.9
Upper class	234	36.6
BMI (kg/m^2)		
Overweight	186	29.1
Obese	59	9.2
Waist circumference (cm)		
Abdominal obesity	258	40.3

TABLE 3: Mean systolic and diastolic blood pressure (mm hg) and prevalence (%) of isolated systolic hypertensive and isolated diastolic hypertensive by age and gender.

Age groups (years)	*N* 640	Systolic BP (mean ± SD)			Diastolic BP (mean ± SD)		
		Male	Female	Total	Male	Female	Total
25–34	*204*	122.17 ± 9.54	114.81 ± 9.99	117.84 ± 10.44	82.92 ± 9.0	78.97 ± 7.46	80.59 ± 8.34
35–44	*179*	124.10 ± 10.77	121.71 ± 15.13	122.90 ± 13.07	85.70 ± 7.66	81.71 ± 9.30	83.75 ± 8.68
45–54	*133*	132.36 ± 13.21	127.16 ± 18.04	129.66 ± 16.05	*89.23 ± 8.16*	*83.28 ± 10.22*	*86.14 ± 9.72*
55–64	*124*	*134.66 ± 19.53*	*127.27 ± 15.74*	*130.97 ± 18.05*	86.42 ± 12.15	83.24 ± 9.32	84.83 ± 10.90
Total	*640*	127.49 ± 14.19	121.39 ± 15.26	124.25 ± 15.05	85.82 ± 9.43	81.34 ± 9.05	83.45 ± 9.49
Test of significance		*F = 15.396* *df = 3* *p = 0.001*	*F = 15.611* *df = 3* *p = 0.001*	*F = 30.466* *df = 3* *p = 0.001*	*F = 5.801* *df = 3* *p = 0.001*	*F = 4.921* *df = 3* *p = 0.002*	*F = 11.174* *df = 3* *p = 0.001*
Age groups (years)	*N* 559	Isolated systolic HTN (*N* = 59)#			Isolated diastolic HTN (*N* = 110)#		
		Male	Female	Total	Male	Female	Total
25–34	202	3 (3.6)	1 (0.8)	4 (6.8)	14 (16.7)	10 (8.5)	24 (21.8)
35–44	166	11 (12.9)	7 (8.6)	18 (30.5)	25 (29.4)	10 (12.3)	35 (31.8)
45–54	101	9 (18.4)	6 (11.5)	15 (25.4)	22 (44.9)	8 (15.4)	30 (27.3)
55–64	90	16 (35.6)	6 (13.3)	22 (37.3)	13 (28.9)	8 (17.8)	21 (19.1)
Total		*39 (14.8)*	*20 (6.8)*	*59 (10.6)*	*74 (28.1)*	*36 (12.2)*	*110 (19.7)*
Test of significance		$\chi^2 = 24.461$ *df = 3* *p = 0.001*	$\chi^2 = 11.974$ *df = 3* *p = 0.007*	$\chi^2 = 36.114$ *df = 3* *p = 0.001*	$\chi^2 = 12.355$ *df = 3* *p = 0.006*	$\chi^2 = 3.338$ *df = 3* *p = 0.342*	$\chi^2 = 15.160$ *df = 3* *p = 0.002*

#Excluding known hypertensive.

TABLE 4: Prevalence of hypertension and prehypertension by gender and age groups among the study subjects (*N* 640).

Category	*n*	Age groups (years)				Test of significance
		25–34	35–44	45–54	55–64	
Men (n 263)		*84*	*85*	*49*	*45*	
Normal	*40*	18 (45.0)	10 (25.0)	3 (7.5)	9 (22.5)	
Prehypertension	*138*	51 (37.0)	48 (34.8)	21 (15.2)	18 (13.0)	$\chi^2 = 22.297$ *df = 9* *p = 0.008*
HTN stage 1	*69*	12 (17.4)	23 (33.3)	19 (27.5)	15 (21.7)	
HTN stage 2	*16*	3 (18.8)	4 (25.0)	6 (37.5)	3 (18.8)	
History of HTN	*38*	0 (0.0)	6 (15.8)	15 (39.5)	17 (44.7)	
Women (n 296)		*118*	*81*	*52*	*45*	
Normal	*122*	59 (48.4)	33 (27.0)	17 (13.9)	13 (10.7)	
Prehypertension	*129*	48 (37.2)	35 (27.1)	25 (19.4)	21 (16.3)	$\chi^2 = 13.983$ *df = 9* *p = 0.123*
HTN stage 1	*37*	10 (27.0)	10 (27.0)	7 (18.9)	10 (27.0)	
HTN stage 2	*8*	1 (12.5)	3 (37.5)	3 (37.5)	1 (12.5)	
History of HTN	*43*	2 (2.5)	13 (16.0)	32 (39.5)	34 (42.0)	

among study subjects was also increasing (not shown in the table).

4. Discussion

India is a developing country and like other developing countries, it is going through a rapid demographic and epidemiological transition. In all such transitions, nutrition is the key ingredient and plays prime role. This cross-sectional community based study identified a high prevalence of prehypertension and hypertension in urban areas of Varanasi, which was 41.7% and 32.96%, respectively. Only a quarter of subjects were in the normal category, which highlights the escalating burden of this silent killer.

The prevalence of hypertension in the present study (32.96%) was higher in comparison with the prevalence reported in other studies [4, 6, 10, 19–22]. Few studies reported the results in line with the present study [23, 24]. According to World Health Organization (2015), the overall prevalence of hypertension in India was 23.5% and gender specific prevalence was 24.2% and 22.7% among the men and women, respectively [25].

The prevalence of prehypertension in the present study was 41.7% (male: 45.9% and female: 38.05%). The prevalence estimated in the present study was much higher than that estimated by Nellore (22.3%) [10] and Bihar (37.95%) [20]. The difference of prevalence observed between the present study and other studies with respect to hypertension and prehypertension could be due to social and cultural differences, dietary and lifestyle factors, and also the age span as well as the research methodology used.

Men exhibit higher prevalence of hypertension and prehypertension than their female counterparts (M: 40.9% and F: 26.0%) and (M: 45.9% and F: 38.05%), respectively. Similarly, various studies came out with the higher percentage of hypertension in men than women [20, 22, 23, 26–29].

Table 5: Prevalence of prehypertension and hypertension* according to sociodemographic characteristics and behavioral risk factors.

Variables	Total *N* 559	Normal	Prehypertension	Hypertension	Test of significance
Sex					
Male	*263*	40 (15.2)	138 (52.5)	85 (32.3)	$p = 0.001$ $df = 2$ $\chi^2 = 52.352$
Female	*296*	122 (41.2)	129 (43.6)	45 (15.2)	
Age					
25–34	*202*	77 (38.1)	99 (49.0)	26 (12.9)	$p = 0.001$ $df = 6$ $\chi^2 = 28.822$
35–44	*166*	43 (25.9)	83 (50.0)	40 (24.1)	
45–54	*101*	20 (19.8)	46 (45.5)	35 (34.7)	
55–64	*90*	22 (24.4)	39 (43.3)	29 (32.2)	
Caste					
Gen	*263*	62 (23.6)	140 (53.2)	61 (23.2)	$p = 0.087$ $df = 4$ $\chi^2 = 8.12$
OBC	*275*	93 (33.8)	118 (42.9)	64 (23.3)	
SC/ST	*21*	7 (33.3)	9 (42.9)	5 (23.8)	
Marital status					
Unmarried	*58*	22 (37.9)	27 (46.6)	9 (15.5)	$p = 0.033$ $Df = 4$ $\chi^2 = 10.501$
Married	*473*	126 (26.6)	231 (48.8)	116 (24.5)	
Others	*28*	14 (50.0)	9 (32.1)	5 (17.9)	
Occupation					
Government	*75*	4 (5.3)	40 (53.3)	31 (41.3)	$p = 0.001$ $df = 10$ $\chi^2 = 51.488$
Private	*142*	36 (25.4)	75 (52.8)	31 (21.8)	
Self-employed	*100*	27 (27.0)	45 (45.0)	28 (28.0)	
Retired	*15*	4 (26.7)	7 (46.7)	4 (26.7)	
Homemaker	*194*	82 (42.3)	87 (44.8)	25 (12.9)	
Others	*33*	9 (27.3)	13 (39.4)	11 (33.3)	
Education					
Illiterate	*57*	23 (40.3)	18 (31.6)	16 (28.1)	$p = 0.009$ $df = 6$ $\chi^2 = 17.049$
Primary	*71*	25 (35.2)	34 (47.9)	12 (16.9)	
Secondary	*157*	53 (33.7)	67 (42.7)	37 (23.6)	
Graduate & above	*274*	61 (22.3)	148 (54.0)	65 (23.7)	
Socioeconomic status					
Lower	*38*	11 (28.9)	15 (39.5)	12 (31.6)	$p = 0.001$ $df = 8$ $\chi^2 = 30.454$
Lower middle	*99*	42 (42.4)	37 (37.4)	20 (20.2)	
Middle	*112*	37 (33.0)	51 (45.5)	24 (21.4)	
Upper middle	*120*	39 (32.5)	64 (53.3)	17 (14.2)	
Upper	*190*	33 (17.4)	100 (52.6)	57 (30.0)	
Tobacco use					
Nonusers	*391*	127 (32.5)	188 (48.1)	76 (19.4)	$\chi^2 = 13.685$ $df = 2$ $p = 0.001$
Users	*168*	35 (20.8)	79 (47.0)	54 (32.1)	
Alcohol use					
Nonusers	*498*	149 (29.9)	240 (48.2)	109 (21.9)	$\chi^2 = 5.239$ $df = 2$ $p = 0.073$
Users	*61*	13 (21.3)	27 (44.3)	21 (34.4)	
Physical activity					
Inactive	*55*	10 (18.2)	36 (65.5)	9 (16.4)	$\chi^2 = 7.968$ $df = 2$ $p = 0.021$
Active	*504*	152 (30.2)	231 (45.8)	121 (24.0)	

*Excluding known hypertensive.

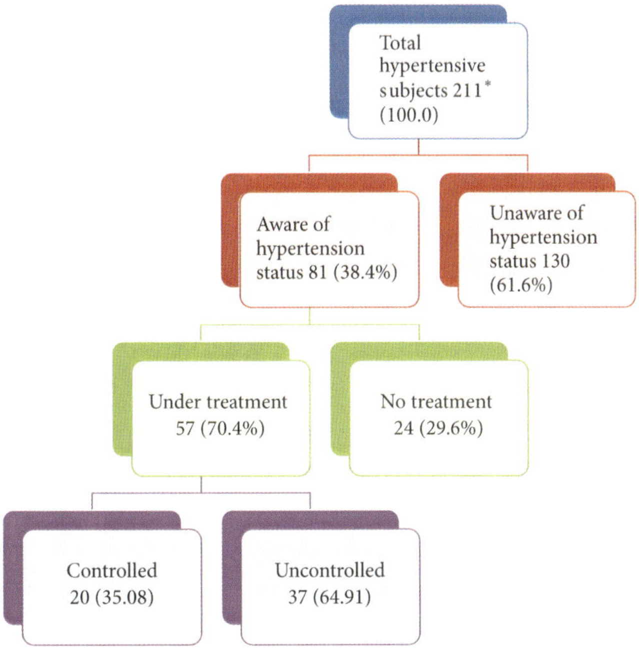

*Total hypertensive subjects = new identified hypertensive (130) + prediagnosed hypertensive (81) = 211

FIGURE 1: Flow diagram showing awareness, treatment, and adequacy of control of hypertension among study subjects.

One of the possible explanations for this gender disparity in hypertension prevalence could be partially due to biological sex difference and partially due to behavioral risk factors like smoking, alcohol consumption, or physical activity. We speculate that absentia from alcohol and smoking might be few of those protective factors against hypertension in women. Other than that, women are more interested in health care services utilization and also more frequently report their poor health and therefore they are more likely to have better health [6, 30].

Age was found to be an important risk factor for hypertension. As the age was advancing so did the prevalence of hypertension among both the sexes. Similar findings were reported by few other studies also where advancing age was positively related to hypertension [1, 6, 19, 21, 22, 26, 31, 32]. With increasing age, the aorta and arteries walls will be stiffened and this contributes to the high prevalence of hypertension in older age groups [4].

In the present study, marital status, education, occupation, socioeconomic status, BMI, abdominal obesity, tobacco use, alcohol use, and physical activity were significantly associated with the hypertension.

Low literacy level and being too rich were associated with hypertension. The higher education level was negatively correlated to hypertension in the present study. These studies also supported this finding [6, 12, 33]. We speculate that it could be due to the reason that higher education imparts better knowledge and information about hypertension and subsequently those people with higher education had a healthier lifestyle.

Table 5 revealed that education was significantly associated with hypertension ($\chi^2 = 17.049$, df = 6 and p value = 0.009); however, when adjusted effect of education on hypertension was observed by logistic regression, then no statistical association was observed. Though some studies had shown a significant association of these two variables [6, 12], in the study performed in the state of Kerala [33], insignificant association between education and hypertension was observed. We speculate that this insignificant association could be due to very few subjects in the illiterate and less educated category. There are so many studies which do not refute the finding of the present study that higher socioeconomic status is a risk for hypertension [3, 22, 24, 32, 34–36]. We assume that better socioeconomic status imparts people with more purchasing power on fast and convenience foods and less physical activity which are already proven to be contributing risk factors for overweight and obesity that subsequently linked to hypertension.

The different anthropometric measurements like BMI, waist circumference, and hip circumference were taken into account to measure overweight, obesity, and central or abdominal obesity. This study showed that overweight and obesity measured by both BMI and waist circumference were major modifiable risk factors to develop hypertension. Overweight subjects had twofold risk of being hypertensive and obese had more than threefold risk for the same in comparison to underweight subjects in this study. There was positive relation observed between increasing BMI and increasing rate of hypertension, which was consistent with other studies [1–4, 6, 12, 20, 21, 23, 32, 36–39]. South Asians have

Table 6: Univariate analysis for the association of hypertension and sociodemographic characteristics, anthropometric measurements, and behavioral risk factors (*N* 640).

Variables	Odds ratio (95% CI)	*p* value
Sex		
Male	1.97 (1.41–2.75)	0.001
Female	1.0 (reference)	
Age groups		
25–34	1.0 (reference)	
35–44	2.64 (1.58–4.41)	0.001
45–54	6.38 (3.77–10.77)	0.001
55–64	6.49 (3.814–11.05)	0.001
Marital status		
Unmarried	1.0 (reference)	
Married	2.34 (1.19–4.61)	0.014
Others	2.32 (0.89–6.04)	0.084
Education		
Graduate & above	1.0 (reference)	
Illiterate	1.17 (0.66–2.06)	0.580
Primary	0.92 (0.54–1.54)	0.756
Secondary	1.08 (0.73–1.59)	0.698
Occupation		
Private	1.0 (reference)	
Government	2.40 (1.39–4.16)	0.002
Self-employed	1.29 (0.76–2.19)	0.336
Retired	3.66 (1.57–8.52)	0.003
Homemaker	0.89 (0.56–1.41)	0.636
Others	1.37 (0.62–3.01)	0.426
Socioeconomic status		
Lower class	1.0 (reference)	
Lower middle class	0.57 (0.26–1.23)	0.156
Middle class	0.63 (0.29–1.33)	0.230
Upper middle class	0.62 (0.29–1.30)	0.208
Upper class	1.31 (0.66–2.61)	0.432
BMI		
Underweight	1.0 (reference)	
Normal	1.27 (0.65–2.47)	80.480
Overweight	1.99 (1.00–3.97)	0.049
Obese	3.57 (1.59–8.00)	0.002
Abdominal obesity		
No	1.0 (reference)	
Yes	1.73 (1.24–2.42)	0.001
Tobacco use		
Nonusers	1.0 (reference)	0.001
Users	1.86 (1.31–2.64)	
Alcohol use		
Nonusers	1.0 (reference)	0.092
Users	1.55 (0.93–2.57)	
Physical activity		
Inactive	0.63 (0.34–1.17)	0.146
Active	1.0 (reference)	
Eating habits		
Vegetarian	1.0 (reference)	
Nonvegetarian	1.10 (0.78–1.54)	0.569
Ovo-vegetarian	0.34 (0.11–1.02)	0.055

tendency of developing centralized obesity without developing generalized obesity and because of this waist circumference and waist-hip ratio are better measures of body fat [40]. Abdominal obesity (OR: 1.73) also found to be positively linked to high blood pressure in the present study. Various epidemiological and pathophysiological mechanisms explained the link between obesity and hypertension. One of the probable reasons behind this positive relation between obesity and hypertension could be that increased weight increases cardiac output and increased peripheral resistance of arterioles. Other than that, urbanization is also a cause of changes in dietary habits and reduced physical activity which leads to obesity and subsequently results in hypertension [4].

Interestingly, we have found inverse association between physical activity and hypertension. Hypertension was more among physically active subjects as compared to inactive subjects (OR: 0.63) but no statistically significant difference was found. Similar result was reported by other study conducted in Turkey [1]. The exact reason behind this is unknown and yet to be explored. We speculate that they had started physical activity probably under medical advice after being diagnosed for hypertension or other risk factors like overweight or obesity.

As per WHO report, alcohol consumption was the third largest risk factor in the developed countries and tobacco use was being the second major cause of death worldwide [17]. This study indicated the positive association between alcohol and tobacco use and hypertension. Hypertension was more prevalent in tobacco users (OR: 1.86) and alcohol users (OR: 1.55) as compared to nonusers. This finding is supported by other studies also [19, 23, 32, 36]. But there are several other studies with contradictory findings [1, 21, 41]. Although not statistically significant, odds of being hypertensive were more among nonvegetarian (OR: 1.10) subjects, while vegetarian diet was proved to be protective against hypertension in this study. Several other studies reported the same result [3, 19, 33, 34]. A study conducted in Bihar [20] refutes this finding and reported that vegetarian diet was positively associated with hypertension.

A recent review study revealed that hypertension awareness rate has been doubled from less than 30% in 1980s to around 60% in present among urban populations and less than 10% in 1980s to 35–40% presently among rural population. However, the treatment and control status is still low at around 30% in urban and 20% in rural areas [42]. Rate of awareness, treatment, and control in the present study was observed as 38.4%, 70.4%, and 35.08%, respectively. Previous study conducted in rural Varanasi reported hypertension awareness, treatment, and control (26.5%, 55.6%, and 40%), respectively [7].

5. Conclusion & Recommendation

From the results of this study, it can be concluded that the prevalence of both prehypertension and hypertension is very high in urban Varanasi. This makes the people of this area vulnerable to several chronic diseases and other unbearable health consequences. Specifically men are at more risk of being hypertensive than female. Increasing age is proved to be an independent risk factor for hypertension. Programs are needed to improve the surveillance systems and implementation of community based screening programs for early detection of hypertension is also needed. As the awareness of the hypertension status among hypertensive cases was very poor, improving health literacy to increase the awareness of hypertension is also the need of the hour. Interventions like weight management, increased physical activity, increased fruits and vegetables consumption, and reduction in tobacco and alcohol use are required and recommended.

Additional Points

Limitations of the Study. This study suffers from few of the following limitations. (i) One of the main limitations of this study was the cross-sectional design of the study which restricts examining causal associations. (ii) The study was only conducted in urban areas. (iii) Stress is a major risk factor for hypertension. It could also be considered in the present study for better results.

Acknowledgments

The authors would like to thank all the participants for participating in the study.

References

[1] C. Erem, A. Hacihasanoglu, M. Kocak, O. Deger, and M. Topbas, "Prevalence of prehypertension and hypertension and associated risk factors among Turkish adults: trabzon hypertension study," *Journal of Public Health*, vol. 31, no. 1, pp. 47–58, 2009.

[2] A. Ahmed, M. Rahman, R. Hasan et al., "Hypertension and associated risk factors in some selected rural areas of Bangladesh," *International Journal of Research in Medical Sciences*, vol. 2, no. 3, p. 925, 2014.

[3] C. P. Mishra and S. Kumar, "Risk factors of hypertension in a rural area of Varanasi," *Indian Journal of Preventive and Social Medicine*, vol. 42, no. 1, pp. 101–111, 2011.

[4] S. M. Abebe, Y. Berhane, A. Worku, and A. Getachew, "Prevalence and associated factors of hypertension: a crossectional community based study in Northwest Ethiopia," *PLoS ONE*, vol. 10, no. 4, Article ID e0125210, 2015.

[5] S. Mendis, "Global status report on non communicable diseases 2010," Tech. Rep., World Health Organisation, 2010, http://www.who.int/nmh/publications/ncd_report2010/en/.

[6] J. S. Tabrizi, H. Sadeghi-Bazargani, M. Farahbakhsh, L. Nikniaz, and Z. Nikniaz, "Prevalence and associated factors of prehypertension and hypertension in Iranian population: the lifestyle promotion project (LPP)," *PLoS ONE*, vol. 11, no. 10, Article ID e0165264, 2016.

[7] M. R. Kumar, R. Shankar, and S. Singh, "Hypertension among the adults in rural Varanasi: a cross-sectional study on prevalence and health seeking behavior," *Indian Journal of Preventive and Social Medicine*, vol. 47, no. 1-2, pp. 78–83, 2016.

[8] A. V. Chobanian, G. L. Bakris, H. R. Black et al., "Seventh report of the Joint National Committee on prevention, detection, evaluation, and treatment of high blood pressure," *Hypertension*, vol. 42, no. 6, pp. 1206–1252, 2003.

[9] Wikipedia, Hypertension, https://en.wikipedia.org/wiki/Hypertension.

[10] J. Prabakaran, N. Vijayalakshmi, and E. VenkataRao, "Prevalence of hypertension among urban adult population (25–64 years) of Nellore," *International Journal of Research & Development of Health*, vol. 1, no. 2, pp. 42–49, 2013.

[11] N. D. Fisher and G. H. Williams, "Hypertensive vascular disease," in *Harrison's Principles of Internal Medicine*, D. L. Kasper, E. Braunwald, A. S. Fauci et al., Eds., pp. 1463–1481, McGraw-Hill, New York, NY, USA, 16th edition, 2005.

[12] R. Rani, V. Mengi, R. K. Gupta, and H. K. Sharma, "Hypertension and its risk factors—a cross sectional study in an urban population of a North Indian District," *Public Health Research*, vol. 5, no. 3, pp. 67–72, 2015.

[13] World Health Organization, "Urbanization and health," *Bulletin of the World Health Organization*, vol. 88, no. 4, pp. 245-246, 2010.

[14] C. Angkurawaranon, N. Wattanatchariya, P. Doyle, and D. Nitsch, "Urbanization and Non-communicable disease mortality in Thailand: an ecological correlation study," *Tropical Medicine & International Health*, vol. 18, no. 2, pp. 130–140, 2013.

[15] International Institute for Population Sciences. Ministry of Health and Family Welfare, Government of India. National family Health Survey (NFHS-4) 2015-16 Factsheet, India, http://rchiips.org/NFHS/pdf/NFHS4/India.pdf.

[16] World Health Organization (WHO), "Obesity: preventing and managing the global epidemic," WHO Technical Report Series 894, World Health Organization, Geneva, Switzerland, 1998.

[17] World Health Organization, "WHO STEPS surveillance manual: the WHO STEP wise approach to chronic disease risk factor surveillance," Tech. Rep., World Health Organization, Geneva, Switzerland, 2005.

[18] A. Mangal, V. Kumar, S. Panesar, R. Talwar, D. Raut, and S. Singh, "Updated BG Prasad socioeconomic classification, 2014: a commentary," *Indian Journal of Public Health*, vol. 59, no. 1, pp. 42–44, 2015.

[19] S. S. Reddy and G. R. Prabhu, "Prevalence and risk factors of hypertension in adults in an Urban Slum, Tirupati, A. P," *Indian Journal of Community Medicine*, vol. 30, no. 3, pp. 84–86, 2005.

[20] R. Singh, R. K. Sinha, C. Mani, R. Singh, and R. Pal, "Burden and vulnerability of hypertension in a rural population of Patna, Bihar, India," *South East Asia Journal of Public Health*, vol. 1, no. 1, 2013.

[21] Costa et al., "Hypertension prevalence and its associated risk factors in adults: a population-based study in Pelotas," *Arq Bras Cardiol*, vol. 88, no. 1, pp. 54–59, 2007.

[22] Y. Gao, G. Chen, H. Tian et al., "Prevalence of hypertension in China: a cross-sectional study," *PLoS ONE*, vol. 8, no. 6, Article ID e65938, 2013.

[23] R. R. Dhungana, A. R. Pandey, B. Bista, S. Joshi, and S. Devkota, "Prevalence and associated factors of hypertension: a community-based cross-sectional study in municipalities of Kathmandu, Nepal," *International Journal of Hypertension*, vol. 2016, Article ID 1656938, 2016.

[24] A. Galav, R. Bhatanagar, S. Meghwal, and M. Jain, "Prevalence of hypertension among rural and urban population in Southern Rajasthan," *Indian Journal of Community Medicine*, vol. 6, no. 2, pp. 41–45, 2015.

[25] World Health Organization, "Global Health Observatory data repository 2015," Tech. Rep., 2015, http://apps.who.int/gho/data/view.main.2464EST?lang=en.

[26] K. Thankappan, G. Mini, M. Daivadanam, G. Vijayakumar, P. Sarma, and M. Nichter, "Smoking cessation among diabetes patients: results of a pilot randomized controlled trial in Kerala, India," *BMC Public Health*, vol. 13, no. 1, 2013.

[27] A. Krishnan, B. Shah, V. Lal, D. K. Shukla, E. Paul, and S. K. Kapoor, "Prevalence of risk factors for non-communicable disease in a rural area of Faridabad district of Haryana.," *Indian Journal of Public Health*, vol. 52, no. 3, pp. 117–124, 2008.

[28] A. Bhagyalaxmi, T. Atul, and J. Shikha, "Prevalence of risk factors of non-communicable diseases in a district of Gujarat, India," *Journal of Health, Population and Nutrition*, vol. 31, no. 1, pp. 78–85, 2013.

[29] J. Prabakaran, N. Vijayalakshmi, and N. Ananthaiah Chetty, "Risk Factors of Non-Communicable Diseases in an Urban Locality of Andhra Pradesh," *National Journal of Research in Community Medicine*, vol. 2, no. 1, p. 28, 2013.

[30] B. Everett and A. Zajacova, "Gender differences in hypertension and hypertension awareness among young adults," *Biodemography and Social Biology*, vol. 61, no. 1, pp. 1–17, 2015.

[31] M. Priya and C. Mishra, "Prevalence of hypertension in an area of urban Varanasi, India and its association with selected demographic factors," *International Journal of Community Medicine and Public Health*, pp. 1600–1605, 2016.

[32] J. F. Wamala, Z. Karyabakabo, D. Ndungutse, and D. Guwatudde, "Prevalence factors associated with hypertension in Rukungiri District, Uganda—a community-based study," *African Health Sciences*, vol. 9, no. 3, pp. 153–160, 2009.

[33] A. Vimala, S. A. Ranji, M. T. Jyosna, V. Chandran, S. R. Mathews, and J. M. Pappachan, "The prevalence, risk factors and awareness of hypertension in an urban population of Kerala (South India)," *Saudi Journal of Kidney Diseases and Transplantation*, vol. 20, no. 4, pp. 685–689, 2009.

[34] A. S. Ingale and J. V. Dixit, "Prevalence of hypertension, awareness & health seeking behaviour among adults residing in field practice area of urban health training centre, government medical college Aurangabad," *National Journal of Community Medicine*, vol. 8, no. 1, pp. 31–36, 2017.

[35] S. S. Todkar, V. V. Gujarathi, and V. S. Tapare, "Period prevalence and sociodemographic factors of hypertension in rural Maharashtra: a cross-sectional study," *Indian Journal of Community Medicine*, vol. 34, no. 3, pp. 183–187, 2009.

[36] J. Kishore, N. Gupta, C. Kohli, and N. Kumar, "Prevalence of hypertension and determination of its risk factors in rural Delhi," *International Journal of Hypertension*, vol. 2016, Article ID 7962595, 6 pages, 2016.

[37] M. Naresh, S. Viral, K. Sudham, C. Mahesh, G. Kalpesh, and Y. Sudha, "Assessment of risk factors of hypertension," *Journal of Evolution of Medical and Dental Sciences*, vol. 1, no. 4, pp. 519–526, 2012.

[38] M. E. Hendriks, F. W. N. M. Wit, M. T. L. Roos et al., "Hypertension in Sub-Saharan Africa: cross-sectional surveys in four rural and urban communities," *PLoS ONE*, vol. 7, no. 3, Article ID e32638, 2012.

[39] A. Dzudie, A. P. Kengne, W. F. T. Muna et al., "Prevalence, awareness, treatment and control of hypertension in a self-selected sub-Saharan African urban population: a cross-sectional study," *BMJ Open*, vol. 2, no. 4, Article ID e001217, 2012.

[40] S. Srivastava and A. Chakravarty, "Correlation between anthropometric measurements and nutrient intake of different weight status of women," *Asian Journal of Home Science*, vol. 5, no. 1, pp. 145-48, 2010.

[41] K. Peltzer and N. Phaswana-Mafuya, "Hypertension and associated factors in older adults in South Africa," *Cardiovascular Journal of Africa*, vol. 24, no. 3, pp. 66–71, 2013.

[42] R. Gupta and S. Gupta, "Hypertension in India: Trends in prevalence, awareness, treatment and control," *RUHS Journal of Health Sciences*, vol. 2, no. 1, pp. 40–46, 2017.

23

Factors Influencing Compliance and Health Seeking Behaviour for Hypertension in Mukono and Buikwe in Uganda: A Qualitative Study

Geofrey Musinguzi,[1,2] Sibyl Anthierens,[2] Fred Nuwaha,[1] Jean-Pierre Van Geertruyden,[3] Rhoda K. Wanyenze,[1] and Hilde Bastiaens[2]

[1]*Department of Disease Control and Environmental Health, School of Public Health, Makerere University, Kampala, Uganda*
[2]*Primary and Interdisciplinary Care, University of Antwerp, Antwerp, Belgium*
[3]*International Health, University of Antwerp, Antwerp, Belgium*

Correspondence should be addressed to Geofrey Musinguzi; mgeof@musph.ac.ug

Academic Editor: Omotayo O. Erejuwa

Background and Methods. Hypertension is a global public health challenge and a leading risk factor for cardiovascular morbidity and mortality. Hypertension control rates are low worldwide, and delay in seeking care is associated with increased mortality. *Methods.* In a qualitative study, known hypertensive patients were interviewed to explore factors influencing compliance and health seeking behaviour (HSB). Data was analyzed following a semantic thematic analysis approach. *Results.* Patients sought various channels of care for their hypertension. Self-medication and access to antihypertensive drugs with or without prescription were common as well as use of herbal remedies. Regular monitoring of blood pressure was not a common practice. Factors influencing HSB were related to health systems and the patient socioeconomic and structural environment. The main system issues were related to availability and attitudes of staff and shortage of supplies and medicines. The patient factors were related to awareness, perceived severity, perceived effectiveness of therapy, adverse effects, and perceived fears of lifelong dependence on medicines. The patient socioeconomic status played a role as did the marketing of traditional medicine. *Conclusion.* Patients seek varied channels of care for their hypertension. Strategies to address the multifactorial dimensions that affect HSB are needed to improve hypertension control in this population.

1. Introduction

Hypertension is a leading risk factor for cardiovascular morbidity and mortality worldwide [1]. A comparative risk analysis of the burden of disease and injury associated with 67 risk factors revealed that hypertension (also known as high blood pressure) is the leading risk factor for mortality with 7% of deaths attributable to it [1]. It is predicted that, by 2025, the number of adults with hypertension will increase by about 60% to a total of 1.56 billion and most of the cases will occur in low and middle income countries (LMIC) [2]. Urbanization and the epidemiological transition characterised by an aging population, physical inactivity, obesity, increasing alcohol consumption, and high salt intake are contributing to the increasing rates of hypertension in LMIC [3]. Hypertension is a "silent killer" [4] and data suggests that hypertensive heart disease could be the most common form of cardiovascular disease (CVD) in Africa [5]. Unfortunately, most cases of hypertension are asymptomatic and as a result, hypertensive patients often seek medical attention late or when they have developed complications such as strokes, heart attacks, heart failure, and kidney failure [3]. In their publication, Cruickshank et al. on the rule of halves reported that 50% of the hypertensives are known, of the known hypertensives, half are on treatment and of those on treatment, half are controlled [5]. The World Health Organization (WHO) projected that, over the next ten years, Africa will experience the largest increase in death rates from CVDs. Consequently, the negative economic impact of CVDs will be felt more on the African continent [6] and the cost of handling chronic illness will lead many households to poverty [7].

Health seeking behaviour (HSB) has been defined as any activity undertaken by individuals who perceive themselves to have a health problem or to be ill for the purpose of finding an appropriate remedy. The desired HSB is responding to an illness by seeking help from a trained allopathic doctor in a recognized health care center [8]. It is well established that HSB is influenced by manifestation of symptoms [9, 10]. However, many hypertensive individuals may not be aware and may not have any symptoms to compel them to seek care. Even among those presenting with symptoms and those who are aware hypertensive, their HSB is suboptimal [11, 12]. Hypertension control remains very low [13] and attributable reasons revolve around noncompliance due to side effects of the medication, lack of information and support, difficulty obtaining the medication, poverty, low education, and poor access to health care [14–16]. In addition, health system deficiencies such as lack of antihypertensive medication, the physicians' inertia in treating hypertension, and long distance to the health facilities have been implicated in affecting HSBs and control of hypertension [13, 17, 18]. Delays in seeking care for hypertension are associated with increased mortality [19] and the benefits of early treatment and control are also well established [20–22].

Like most of Sub-Saharan Africa, Uganda's health care system was established with a greater orientation towards communicable diseases. It is only in the past 15 years that the NCD agenda started featuring in the national health strategic plan of the Ministry of Health [23]. The current health service delivery system has a number of gaps ranging from lack of preventive services for NCDs to lack of essential supplies for managing NCDs [24].

Over the last 20 years, Uganda has witnessed an increasingly aging population which has ushered in increasing rates of lifestyle-related chronic noncommunicable diseases [25]. Notably, increasing cases of obesity, diabetes mellitus, and hypertension, along with such complications as stroke, and heart diseases are reported [25]. Data from the Health management information system (HMIS) suggests that hypertension is the most reported NCD and community surveys also suggest that one in five of every adult $\geq$ 18 years have uncontrolled hypertension [26]. The detailed reasons for low levels of hypertension control and inadequate HSB in this setting are not well understood.

We explored compliance and HSBs for hypertension using qualitative approach in order to understand reasons for low levels of hypertension control. Understanding the HSB for hypertension is vitally important in designing programs for hypertension control and enhancing quality standards in healthcare delivery [8].

2. Methods

2.1. Setting and Design. From August to October 2014, we conducted a community descriptive qualitative study and performed semistructured individual interviews with 48 patients with known hypertension in Mukono and Buikwe districts in Uganda. According to the Uganda population and housing census area specific profiles, 78% and 72% of the population in Buikwe and Mukono, respectively, live in rural areas [27]. The Uganda National Health System is made up of the Public and the Private sectors. Uganda implements a level based healthcare delivery system with a referral framework from a lower facility (Health Center (HC) II, III, IV) through hospitals at the district, regional, or national level. Mukono and Buikwe districts combined have six (6) hospitals, 4 HCIV, 27 HCIIIs, and 57 HCIIs. Moreover, most of these facilities are ill-equipped to provide services for hypertension. For example, essential ingredients including diagnostic equipment, antihypertensive medicines, and personnel are scarce [28]. Secondly, conducting this study in this setting would provide incremental evidence to our previously conducted WHO Stepwise Approach to Chronic Disease Risk Factor Surveillance (STEPS) study [29]. In the STEPS study, we observed an unacceptably high prevalence rate of hypertension and suboptimal treatment and control [29].

2.2. Sampling. A purposive sample of patients with known hypertension was identified from the database gathered two years before [29]. The STEPS, conducted in 2012, enrolled 4653 study participants of whom 258 were hypertensive patients and aware of their hypertension. The data set for the 258 patients was organised by gender, residential status, and district to select patients for enrolment into the current study. To generate a wide range of experiences, a fairly big sample size (48) comprising of a varied group of patients (males' and females, urban and rural, Buikwe and Mukono districts) were interviewed. The final sample is comprised of equal number of patients drawn from both districts of Mukono and Buikwe, 17 males, and 24 rural residents. All participants consented except two males.

2.3. Data Collection. Data were collected by one of the lead investigators (GM) and three graduate research assistants who underwent a rigorous and extensive 5-day training to standardise data collection procedures. The training entailed a review of the study objectives, conduct of qualitative inquiries, blood pressure measurement using a validated automated digital sphygmomanometer (Omron model M3W) with an appropriate cuff size, interpersonal communication skills, ethics, confidentiality, and informed consent, seminars on one-on-one interviewing techniques, and detailed instructions on using the semistructured interview protocol. The use of semistructured interview guides (Appendix) enabled data gathering on background characteristics of the study patients, compliance, and HSBs for hypertension. Interviews were conducted at the participants' homes. Each interview lasted one hour on average after which the patients' blood pressure was measured thrice one minute apart. Measuring blood pressure after the interview allowed the patient to relax and also prevented any biased responses that would arise if measurements were done before the interviews. All interviews were audio-recorded with consent from each patient and the average of the three readings was used to estimate the patient blood pressure.

2.4. Ethics Statement. Ethical approval was granted by Makerere University School of Public Health Higher Degrees-Research and Ethics Committee and the Uganda National Council of Science and technology. Each participant provided written informed consent.

2.5. Data Management. All qualitative data were transcribed verbatim and then translated into English from the local language. Each transcript was reviewed by at least two research assistants and one of the investigators (GM) for content and completeness. Final transcripts were stored securely on pass-worded external drives and later exported to ATLAS.ti version 7, qualitative data management software for further management.

2.6. Data Analysis. To identify the factors influencing compliance and health seeking behaviours for hypertension, we analysed the data following a semantic approach in thematic analysis [30]. Using free coding options in ATLAS.ti, GM read each transcript and extracted relevant data to generate codes related to compliance and health seeking behaviours. The codes were reviewed to identify patterns within the data [31] and iteratively compared with the original transcripts. Following the review and with use of code families' options in ATLAS.ti, the codes were sorted into groups (to generate subthemes) and where appropriate were split or dropped or renamed if better subthemes were obtained. The subthemes were further reanalysed to generate themes and overarching themes. For quality control, and to ensure that the interpretation was close to the content and to support reflexivity, the process of analysis and output at every stage of the analysis was regularly reviewed and discussed with SA and HB.

3. Results

3.1. Participants and Context. Table 1 shows study participants' characteristics and their current blood pressure profiles as measured at the time of the interviews.

As shown in Table 1, 48 patients were interviewed between August and October 2014. Of these, 17 were males, 24 were rural residents, 35 were married, and 23 had attained post-primary education. The median age was 54 (males 54, females 51.5). Very few patients, 8, had their hypertension under control (SBP < 140 mmHg and DBP < 90 mmHg). Majority ($n = 20$) were stage one hypertensive and sizable proportions were stage 2 ($n = 11$) and stage 3 ($n = 9$) hypertensive. Self-medication and access to antihypertensive drugs with or without prescription from drug outlets were common as well as use of herbal remedies. Some patients also reported engaging in life style interventions such as cessation of alcohol consumption, increased physical activity, and dietary modifications. Regular monitoring of blood pressure was not a common practice. Modern healthcare for hypertension was sought widely from all levels of health facilities including drug shops, pharmacies, private health clinics, health centers (II, III, and IV) and hospitals. Herbal remedies in use included garlic, ginger, pumpkin leaves *(essunsa)*, herbal mixtures (names unknown), African eggplant *(Katunkuma)*, Moringa, *Mumbwa*, spider plant *(ejjobyo)*, aloe vera *(kigaji)*, dried banana leaves, neem tree, chlorophyll extracts, human urine, Tianshi (Chinese herbal), and African night shade (Nakati).

Table 1

Characteristics	Number
Sex	
Male	17
Female	31
Residential status	
Rural	24
Urban	24
Education status	
Primary or less	25
Post primary	23
Marital status	
Single	13
Married	35
Age	
Overall median age	54
Median age (female)	51.5
Median age (male)	54
Measured BP on the interview date	
(SBP < 140 mmHg and DBP < 90 mmHg)	8
Stage 1 (SBP = 140–159/ DBP = 90–99)	20
Stage 2 (SBP = 160–179/ DBP = 100–109)	11
Stage 3 (SBP ≥ 180/DBP ≥ 110)	9

3.2. Factors Influencing Compliance and Health Seeking Behaviour for Hypertension. The 3 thematic key issues influencing HSB for hypertension were related to the health system, the patient, and the broader socioeconomic and structural environment. Consequently, we organise the key findings (themes and subthemes) under each of these three overarching thematic areas. Figure 1 illustrates the schema of the identified themes and subthemes.

3.2.1. Health System Factors. Under the overarching theme of health system factors, five themes influencing compliance and HSBs were identified: (1) availability of medicines, personnel, and diagnostic supplies; (2) high burden of acute care at health facilities; (3) traditional medicines; (4) perceived provider abilities/behaviours and overall quality of care, and (5) patient waiting times at the facilities.

(1) Availability of Medicine, Personnel, and Diagnostic Supplies

Medicines. Patients noted that availability of or the assumption of [modern] medicines was readily available at health facilities and related costs played a key role in their seeking behaviours for hypertension. In private health facilities and private pharmacies, patients reported that antihypertensive drugs were readily available. However, high costs of these medicines were a deterrent to access. As such, they echoed that only those who had the money accessed the medicines as illustrated by the following patient in a local proverb.

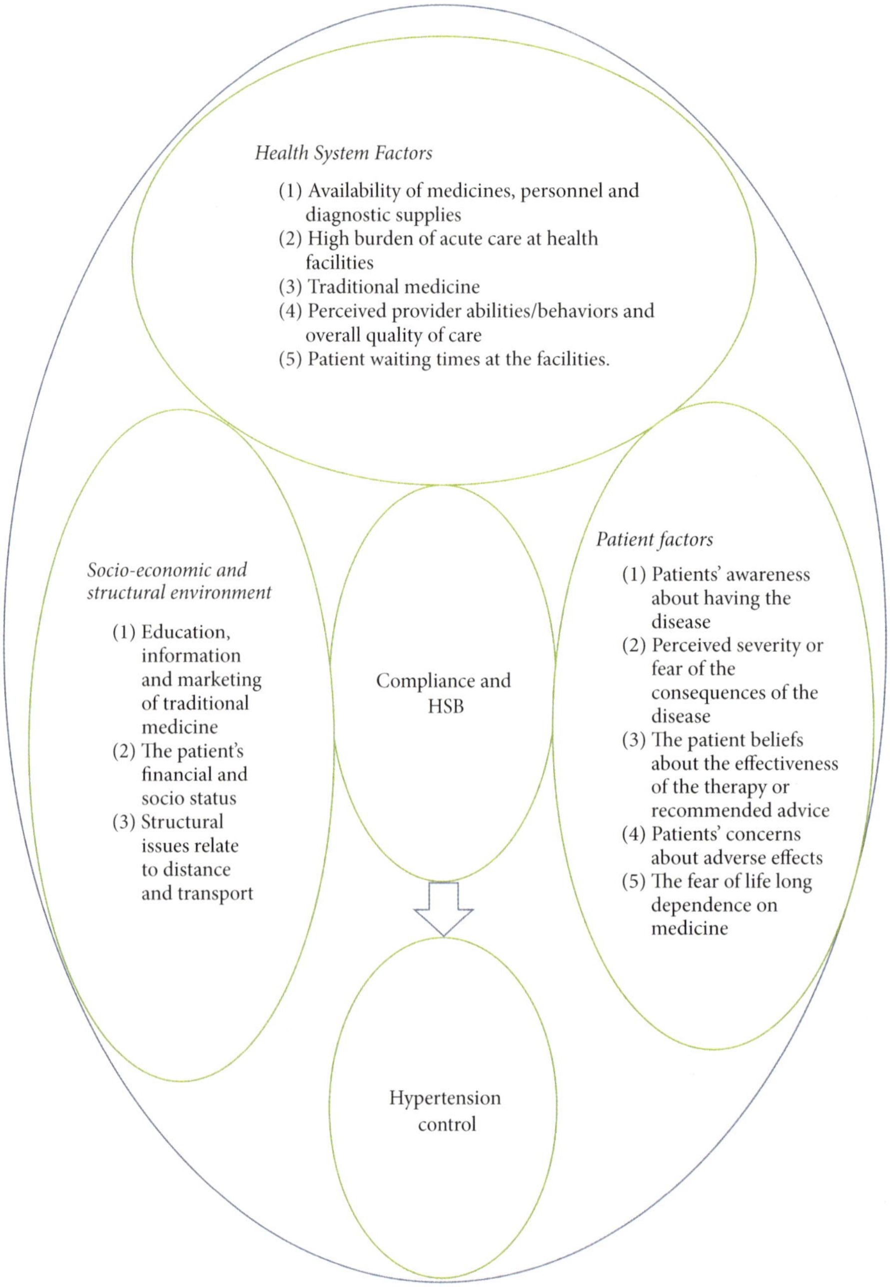

Figure 1: Factors influencing compliance and health seeking behaviours for hypertension among patients in Mukono and Buikwe Districts in Uganda.

> *When you are a poor man, you don't prick a Swahili ban [local bread] or else you get beaten if you prick and don't buy.* (8 Bulamba-Bugungu_Male 1-*Buikwe, Rural*)

As a caveat to turn away from high costs, self-medication was commonly reported from drug outlets, which dispensed medicines with or without prescription and in any quantities depending on the patients' affordability. But even with this option, cost still deterred patients from access as illuminated by the following patient.

> *Apart from the medicine he gave me. I failed to buy the medicine he had prescribed; even the last time I went to him; I failed to buy the medicine because it's expensive. One tablet costs 2,000 shs; and yet I had to swallow one per day for one month. I calculated and it was 60,000 shs; so I only swallowed the medicine he gave me; and then stopped.* (19 Kanyogoga_Male 2-*Buikwe, Urban*)

The costs of antihypertensive medicine were offset when the health facilities provided the medicine free of charge to patients. Indeed, patients attested that finding medicines at the health facilities was a motivation for their health seeking behaviours. However, lack of medicines had a negative implication on their compliance and health seeking behaviours. Patients expressed a sense of disappointment when they visited a health facility in anticipation of getting free medicines only to be given prescriptions to go and buy medicine elsewhere.

> *I went there four times; the first two times I got the medicine; while the other two times I was told that there was no medicine. So I realized that I was wasting time and stopped going there.* (20 Kateete_Femalel)

> Another also echoed, "they gave me that medicine that I have told you [valium] and they told me to buy the other drugs since it was out of stock in the hospital. I didn't buy it; the truth is that the medicine was expensive" (12 Geregere Majjani_Female 1-*Buikwe, Urban*).

Personnel. Finding a service provider at a health facility was also critical in influencing health seeking behaviour of hypertensive patients. Patients were motivated to go to a health facility where they were sure of finding health workers. Most acknowledged that the situation was improving with establishment of specialised clinics especially at the national referral hospital, which run most days of the week.

> *Previously I only saw a doctor once a month but now, I can see the doctor any day between Monday to Friday.* (1 Anthony_Male 1)

> Some, however, were still hindered by lack of providers at health facilities.

> *Doctors would come once in a month so I didn't have the vigor to go to hospital for care.* (16 Kabumba_female 1-*Mukono, Rural*)

Lack of personnel as a barrier to health seeking behaviour was mainly reported by patients from the rural areas. However, some also stressed that their district hospital operated a one-day clinic in a week for diabetes and hypertension which limited access to specialised health workers for hypertension.

Diagnostic Supplies. Supply issues entailed the availability or lack of/or inadequacies in diagnostic equipment. It was common for patients in rural areas to report that they lacked a place where they could have their hypertension routinely monitored.

> *... the clinics here in the village do not have the BP machines ... all they do is to ask you; 'what are you suffering from'? Then they base on what you have told them to give you a few tablets to relieve you from the pain.* (6 Bukamunye B_Female 2-*Buikwe, Urban*)

> Another patient reported, "the biggest challenge we are facing as people with hypertension in this village is lack of somewhere we can go for emergency blood pressure monitoring" (41 Ssaza_female 3- *Mukono, Urban*).

(2) High Burden of Acute Care at Health Facilities. It was quite interesting to note that some patients did not seek care because they thought health workers would not attend to them since they [patients] did not have severe symptoms to warrant attention. This was especially in relation to those who desired regular BP monitoring. They said that hospitals were full of the severely ill meaning that a visit to health facilities for routine hypertension monitoring would be an additional burden to an already overwhelmed system. This subtheme was best illuminated by a patient (33 Malongwe Ajjija_male 2-*Buikwe, Urban*) who reported that it was difficult to just walk into a health facility and request a BP measurement. He said that such a daring would be considered luxurious because most of the facilities focus their efforts and resources on the very ill not the healthy looking individuals who walk in for BP measurements. The participant exemplified as follows:

> *One challenge has been the monitoring of blood pressure ... It's hard to just walk up to a health worker and tell them you would like to check your blood pressure ... It's hard for the health worker to really give you attention ... because you would have gone there for luxury and not as a patient. So when I would request for a blood pressure check-up; they would ask what the problem was. They cannot work on a person like me yet there are many patients who need help.* (33 Malongwe Ajjija_male 2-*Buikwe, Urban*)

(3) Traditional Medicine. With respect to the challenges surrounding access to modern health services, some patients resorted to using alternative medicines and seeking care from traditional practitioners. Most patients seeking complimentary medicines used herbs and some reported that they consulted traditional healers for their hypertension. Patients considered herbs easily accessible and to a certain extent comparably affordable. Planting them in the back yards enhanced access to herbs. In addition, most of the herbal remedies reported were readily available on the local market. However, it was also noted that some special herbs including those exported from abroad were sometimes difficult to access and expensive and that some traditional healers asked for certain items such as chicken and goats, which deterred patients from consulting them.

> *At first I tried local medicine like mumbwa but when the traditional healers started asking goats from me I couldn't manage that because I didn't have the money to buy these goats so I stopped visiting traditional healers* (47 Vvuluga_female 1-*Buikwe, Urban*). *It was Chinese medicine; ... my brother brought it for me. I drank it ... in fact I improved slightly; the fast heart beats stopped and my head also stopped hurting; only that I failed to use it because of my finances.* (14 Jagary Cable_female 1-*Buikwe, Urban*)

It was also observed that traditional healers do not necessary stay in the same communities where they provide their services. In some cases, patients reported that they abandoned their local treatment remedies because their providers [traditional healers] were out of reach. This patient alluded as follows:

> *From the time I would buy their medicine it would take like two to three months before they [traditional healers] returned to our village, this stopped me from using their medicine.* (16 Kabumba_female 1-*Buikwe, Urban*)

(4) Perceived Provider Abilities and Behaviours and Overall Quality of Care. This theme comprises the four subthemes: (1) patients' perceptions about their providers' abilities in terms of skills and knowledge competences; (2) perceived providers' attitudes towards work and the feeling of being treated with or without respect; (3) providers' advising role towards their patients' health seeking behaviours; and (4) perceived quality of care.

Patients' Perceptions about Their Providers' Abilities in Terms of Skills and Knowledge Competences. Whereas most patients perceived their providers to have sufficient knowledge and the required skills to manage hypertension, some had reservations. Those who had reservations depicted their providers as not having sufficient competencies. They felt the providers focused on treating symptoms rather than conducting a proper disease diagnosis prior to treatment.

> *... it is better for the health worker to know the disease they are treating by examining the patient, but for them [referring to health workers] they just dish [give] medicine to patients based on whatever disease the patients mentions ... If you tell them [health workers]; 'I have headache due to over sleeping or that I have headache because I have fever', that is it – then he/she [health worker] will give you tablets to treat that.* (6 Bukamunye B_Female 2-*Buikwe, Rural*)

Providers implicated with such incompetence were mainly those operating at the lower level health facilities especially drug outlets, pharmacies, and rural health facilities. On the other hand, most patients had confidence in medical doctors. They also felt that hospitals were better prepared in managing hypertension compared to private and lower health facilities.

Perceived Provider Attitudes towards Work and the Feeling of Being Treated with or without Respect. Patients noted that providers exhibited different attitudes towards their work and their patients. They felt very comfortable seeking care from providers who were friendly. Some providers were implicated in having unwelcoming behaviours and negative attitudes towards patients. Examples of negative behaviours reported in this study included barking at patients, treating patients disrespectfully, and being unconcerned. Patients noted that it was common to find such behaviours in the public facilities. Most patients complemented private health facilities for their welcoming and caring attitudes. In fact, one patient stated that, in the private clinics, they are treated as customers which motivates them to seek care from the private clinics although he was also quick to speculate that the warm care was possibly because of the financial incentives [since patients pay for the service] and the strict leadership. Some patients also noted that they did not appreciate the decision making process that their providers followed while helping them to get appropriate remedy for their ailments. They felt that providers exhibited unnecessary delays, which resulted in negative health outcomes. One patient expressed dissatisfaction and wondered why the healthcare workers could not agree on the next course of action and refer her in a timely manner given that they were failing to diagnose and manage her condition.

> *Nurse ... 'her case cannot be handled here' ... 'we have to refer her to Mulago hospital; she will die here.' She would continue to tell the others to allow me go to Mulago stressing that they cannot handle me ... But there was a nurse who would prescribe medicine and tell me, 'These will work for you' so that's how I was. I would always go back to them complaining of not sleeping well; it was like that every time; until I got the doctor from Mulago.* (37 Namengo Female 1- *Buikwe, Urban*)

Providers' Advising Role towards Their Patients. In spite of the reported challenges with some modern health care providers, patients were to a greatest extent likely to follow the advice they received from their providers. Certain patients said that they were using herbal remedies because they had been advised to do so by their healthcare providers. However, others said that they were not using herbal remedies because their healthcare providers advised them against arguing that concurrent use of herbal and modern medicine could result in contraindications and that the efficacy and effectiveness of such medicines were not established. On the other hand, some traditional practitioners were also discouraging their patients from using modern medicines arguing that they were not effective.

> *I left Nagalaama [hospital] with some medicine and when I reached the herbalists' place they stopped me from taking modern medicine.* (17 Kabumba_female 2-*Mukono, Rural*)

Health care providers also advised patients on lifestyle modification. Some patients were advised on salt intake, dietary modification, physical activity, alcohol consumption, and smoking. But the patients were also keen on reporting that although they put effort in following their providers' advice, some of the advices were not contextually feasible.

> *... he told me not to eat many things; and yet I cannot stop eating some of those that he mentioned; he told me not to eat 'posho'; sweet potatoes ... and told me not to eat one meal; which is difficult in a village.* (20 Kateete Female 1-*Mukono Rural*)

Perceived Quality of Care. This theme generated conflicting reports. Some respondents felt that government hospitals provided high quality services compared to private health facilities in spite of the high patient loads and the long waiting time. On the other hand, patients commended private health providers for being swift in service provision, although they had concerns with regard to provider competencies in private facilities. Meanwhile, the majority felt that modern medicine had an edge over traditional medicine, although some respondents noted that the quality of traditional medicine is improving especially in terms of practice, dosing, and packaging.

Patient Waiting Time at the Facility. Patients noted that it was very stressful to spend the whole day at a health facility waiting to be treated. The long waiting time was attributed to (1) high patient volume vis-a-vis the limited number of health workers; (2) sluggishness and being unconcerned on the side of the healthcare workers, and (3) a lack of clear patient flow protocol that was characterised with favouritism and lack of respect.

> *it is because by the time you go to the hospital very early in the morning, you were feeling unwell but in the process of queuing in the hospital, there can come someone who knows the doctor and the person overtakes you – one thing that is annoying because you come to the hospital after you have slept unwell and only to be disappointed – do you see such a thing?* (Njeru_Female 1 *Buikwe, Rural*)

As a consequence, some patients stopped going to certain hospitals because of the long time they spend trying to get a service. Moreover, they reported that they had to cue at every service point (consultation room, laboratory room, and dispensing room). They felt very high workload and long waiting times were most prominent at public health facilities.

3.2.2. Patient Related Factors. Another overarching theme influencing compliance and health seeking behaviour for hypertension was "patient related factors." The subthemes building up this theme: (1) awareness about having the disease; (2) perceived severity or fear of the consequences of the disease; (3) beliefs about the effectiveness of the therapy; (4) concerns about adverse effects; and (5) the fear of dependency on long-term medication.

Patients' Awareness about Having the Disease. Awareness "the state of being aware or having knowledge that one is hypertensive" played critical role in HSB. Some patients reported presenting with no symptoms at the time of diagnosis, whereas others reported mild or severe symptoms as depicted by the following patients.

> *When I went to the first clinic, they checked me and they said that I was hypertensive – I couldn't believe it. I went to another clinic and they still measured my BP and they told me that I was hypertensive, I still didn't believe it. I went to the third clinic where they measured my BP again and they found me hypertensive and they even started me on the drugs to treat it.* (10 DFI_female 2-*Mukono, Urban*)
>
> Another patient reported, "I did not have any symptom; I was like any other normal person. I did not have rapid heartbeats" (14 Jagary Cable Female 1), and another one also narrated, "I really think that I had been hypertensive for quite a long time though I was unaware" (41 Ssaza_female 3-*Mukono, Urban*).

Respondents felt that creating awareness was dependent on having the patients' blood pressure measurements taken at a health facility or during a community outreach. However, they noted that opportunities to have their blood pressure measurements at the facilities or outreach sites were scarce. Because of the limited opportunities, and the asymptomatic nature of hypertension, most patients got to learn about their hypertension after experiencing severe symptoms or presenting with signs of end organ damage such as stroke.

> *I took long to know that I was hypertensive ... One time in 2000, I was taking my agricultural produce to Kampala for sale, while travelling I got a 'stroke' in the car. I was then taken to a KCC health facility in Kampala. They (health workers) checked and found that I had hypertension, so that's when it started. From that day I knew that I had hypertension. I went on receiving treatment up to this day.* (26 Kyamabale_male 1-*Buikwe, Rural*)

Perceived Severity or Fear of the Consequences of the Disease. Patients who had mild symptoms perceived themselves to be at low risk and were likely not to seek care for their hypertension.

> *... here in the village as long as you are still able to walk, there is no need of you monitoring your BP because you have hope that it will subside and you will get back to normal* (6 Bukumunye B_female 2). *I had the disease, but because it was not very serious I kept postponing going to the health facility. (31 Lusozi_male 3-Buikwe, Urban)*

Because of the low risk perceptions, such patients mainly depended on self-medication to treat symptoms or embraced a do nothing scenario. On the other hand, patients who perceived their disease to be severe especially after experiencing life-threatening symptoms were more likely to seek care promptly from bigger hospitals and avoid self-medication

> *... after surviving death, I no longer self-treat or cover up an illness [delay diagnosis]. (41 Ssaza_female 3-Mukono, Urban)*

The Patient Beliefs about the Effectiveness of the Therapy or Recommended Advice. Some patients' HSB and compliance were dependent on their perceptions about the effectiveness of the treatment or recommended provider advice. Effective remedies encouraged patients to return to their providers for refills, whereas patients who reported otherwise commonly reported trying out alternatives in search for better therapies.

> *I have managed to treat this disease (Hypertension) for the many years I have lived with*

> *it. I have used various treatment methods. I first started with the modern method then later traditional medicine until now. However the traditional (medicine) has helped me more than the modern medicine.* (8 Bulamba_Bugungu_male 1-*Buikwe, Rural*)

Compliance based on perceived effectiveness of therapy applied both to modern as well as herbal medicine. Those who perceived herbal medicines to be effective in relieving their symptoms were likely to report usage of such remedies.

> *I use the onions and the small egg plants – they help me a lot because whenever they bring them for me, I tend to feel better after using them* (34 Mayugwe Ssi_female 1-*Buikwe, Rural*). *It's very bitter and I know that hypertension can be controlled with bitter substances. When you take aloe vera, you feel well.* (6 Bulamba_Bugungu_male 1-*Buikwe, Rural*)

Similarly, those who perceived modern medicines to be effective were likely to report modern medicine usage.

> *Well I went to the hospital and they diagnosed me with hypertension and they started me on the drugs and later in the process of seeking care from the modern health facility, there was someone who advised me to also use the traditional herbal medicine which I used for a short time and later realized that it was useless. So I returned to the modern health facility and they gave me the drugs to take.* (P 16: Ngogwe_Kikoota_ female 1-*Buikwe, Rural*)

A third category reported using both. This category perceived that using both modern and herbal remedies had complimentary effectiveness and resulted in better health outcomes.

> *For the modern medicine, they can tell you to take one tablet a day (1 × 1) of which I have already taken it in the morning at around 8.00 AM. So by evening when I feel my BP raised due to the constant movements, that is when I take that Aloe Vera - it normalizes it and I finally sleep. (2 Bugga female 1-Buikwe, Rural)*

Patients' Concerns about Adverse Effects. Patients reported that some therapies were not tolerable. They were associated with unpleasant outcomes. Some noted that adverse effects of some medicines were worse off than their hypertension. On the other hand, if the remedy was tolerable, usage was more likely. These concerns were reported for modern medicines as well as herbal medicines.

> *In the beginning they introduced me to start using herbal medicine; but when I started using it I realized that it had bad side effects; my hands and legs were swelling. So I stopped and remained on the modern medicine (14 Jagary_cable_female 1-Buikwe, Urban). I do not like the [modern] medicine they provide; the medicine is bitter; others are tiny others are big. It makes 'you' weak, and dizzy; even if 'you' have a baby crying next to 'you'; it's hard to carry the baby because 'you' get weak.* (29 Lusozi_female 2-*Buikwe, Urban*)

The Fear of Life Long Dependence on Medicine. Lifelong dependence on antihypertensive was perceived as a burden and some patients could not believe that they were ready for such a course of action. As a result, some patients reported that they swallowed drugs occasionally to try and avoid over dependency on medicine in controlling their hypertension.

3.2.3. The Socioeconomic and Structural and Cultural Environment. Besides, the healthcare and the patient related factors and several other issues were reported that influenced HSBs. We have summarized these factors under the socioeconomic and structural/cultural environment issues. More specifically, three topics were discussed: (1) education, information, and marketing of traditional medicine, (2) the patients' financial and social status, and (3) distance and transport.

(1) Education, Information, and Marketing of Traditional Medicine. Education, information, and marketing greatly influenced the use of alternative medicine for hypertension in this population. Patients reported that traditional practitioners, distributors, and proponents of herbal medicines embraced the power of sociomarketing, education, and active information sharing about their products. The most popular avenues of communication and promotion of herbal remedies included media houses such as radios and television, door-to-door information and drug distribution, and use of public address system in populated areas such as markets and assembly places.

> *They give us the herbal medicine that is packed in the bottles and sold on the cars that pass by advertising the herbal medicine for the people to buy. They say that their medicines heal every sickness. So I buy those Rwenzori bottles with herbal medicine and take.* (23 Kikoota_female 1 – *Buikwe Rural*)
>
> Another patient stated, "I would listen to him (traditional health practitioner) over the radio – that was before he went to the television; because up to date he is still on the radio and on the television. I listened to him and then I got his telephone contact and first I rang him and then I went there to see him" (11 DFI_male 1-*Mukono, Urban*).

On the other hand, no data was generated about efforts to use education, information, and marketing strategies to promote modern health care for hypertension.

(2) The Patient's Financial and Social Status. Financial and socioeconomic status of the patients was critical in influencing compliance and HSBs of patients with hypertension. Specifically, financial and social aspects included the ability of the patients to meet their healthcare needs, family support,

and advice from significant others. Most patients reported that hypertension was a lifetime disease that in the long run was too expensive. In fact some of them said they were already struggling with more pressing basic needs of life such as food and children school fees, which took precedence over their hypertension problems. For example, this patient narrated her story:

> *... its money; because you may have the money and think you will go [to the hospital] at the end of the week and then there comes a person who needs the money more than you do, for example your child calls saying mammy send me money; there is this problem; so you decide to send the money to them; so you postpone and say I will go next week. So it gets to that; you later realize you spent two months without treatment.* (20 Kateete_female 1-*Mukono, Rural*)

On the other hand, those who had better financial standing were more likely to seek care for their hypertension.

> *I don't have money problem to buy medicine. I have my work which earns me money that I use to buy medicine.* (1 Anthony male 1-*Mukono, Urban*)

In addition, patients with family members [children or other relatives] with better financial standing were reportedly supported to enhance their HSBs for hypertension.

> *In fact my children and my brothers' money have been spent big time – most especially my son's money has been spent so much because he wishes me to get better but all in vain.* (Mayugwe_Female 2-*Buikwe, Rural*)

Family members also provided patients with psychosocial and moral support as well as reminding them about their scheduled appointments, drug refills, and taking the medicines. Moreover, acquaintances such as friends, community members with similar challenges, or community resource persons such as religious leaders were also reported. These particularly played a key role in providing guidance to patient on whether to use modern or traditional medicine.

(3) Distance and Transport. The study shows that transport, distance, and related costs influenced health seeking behaviour of patients for hypertension. Patients from far-off areas (mainly rural) incurred higher costs of transport compared to their counterparts from urban neighbourhoods and those near the health facilities. Moreover, means of transport were not always reliably available in some settings. Consequently, rural residents commonly reported transport as a key barrier to seeking care, including adhering to scheduled hospital appointments.

> *The only challenge I faced was lack of transport; the place was really far so it was hard to go there on foot.* (P 8: 16 Kabumba_female 1-*Mukono Rural*)

On the other hand, urban resident either did not mention transport as a barrier or they reported ease of access to health facilities as a motivator to seek care for their hypertension.

> *It's because I am near the hospital so I don't spend on transport to go to Kawolo hospital. I just walk to the hospital.* (P 6: 14 Jagary_cable_ female 1-*Mukono, Rural*)

4. Discussion

The study shows that most patients in this setting utilise varied channels of care for their hypertension. In spite of the varied health seeking behaviours (HSBs), 8 in 10 patients interviewed in this qualitative study had uncontrolled hypertension. Insufficient hypertension control is prevalent in most of Sub-Saharan Africa [13] and data suggest that these high levels of uncontrolled hypertension are attributed to noncompliance, difficulty in obtaining medication, poverty, and poor access to health care [14–16]. In addition, health system deficiencies such as lack of antihypertensive medication and long distance to facilities have been implicated in affecting HSBs and control of hypertension [13, 17, 18]. Similarly, our study found that a range of health system challenges such as inadequate services, high cost of services and medicines, frequent drug stock outs, and quality concerns were strongly attributed to noncompliance and poor HSB patterns for hypertension.

In addition, HSBs were influenced by awareness, perceived severity, perceived effectiveness of recommended intervention/therapy, concerns about adverse effects, and fear of long-term dependence on medication. The influence of awareness on HSBs for hypertension is well established [11, 32]. Being aware of one's hypertension status is critical in initiation of care and impacts on self-care management practices [32] and is associated with reduced hypertension related complications and mortalities. However, availability and access to BP monitors were reported as a challenge in this study. However, perceived disease severity was critical in determining treatment compliance and HSB. In fact some of the patients reported that it was not necessary for them to continue with treatment or go to hospital if they felt well. On the other hand, manifestation of symptoms enhanced their compliance and HSBs. With mild symptoms, they mostly self-treated with herbal or modern medicines or consulted with providers at lower level health facilities including drug shops and pharmacies, whereas patients with severe symptoms reportedly sought care from hospitals or higher level health centers. The behaviours of these patients are consistent with those of the Koreans in the stroke study whose choice of care depended on their perceived severity of symptoms. For those who perceived themselves to have mild symptoms, they used over-the-counter drugs and folk remedies or visited health care facilities such as drugstores, public health agency, herbal clinic, or hospital [33]. These findings confirm the assertion that signs and symptoms influence people to seek diagnosis and treatment. The patients contemplate about the symptoms and then decide to take appropriate actions according to their perceived degree of disease severity [33]. When they perceive that the disease is very severe, they seek more specialised care but if they feel that the disease is less severe, they embark on self-care to try and resolve the discomfort.

HSBs were also influenced by the perceived effectiveness of the recommended treatment advice and this factor applied to modern as well as herbal alternative usage. Similar findings have been reported before [34–36]. In our previous study, use of traditional medicine was associated with the perception that herbal medicines were effective [34] and in Nigeria, patients strongly considered herbal medicines as viable alternative for a cure for their hypertension [37].

Another key factor was experiencing adverse reactions. Some patients reported that they experienced terrible side effects which were regarded worse off than their hypertension. Likewise, patients in Nigeria stopped medication as a result of experienced side effects [36]. Additional studies in Nigeria [11, 36], Democratic Republic of Congo [14], and Vietnam [3] have reported similar findings.

Health seeking behaviour was to a greater extent also influenced by the socioeconomic status of patients and structural and cultural factors. Patients with better socioeconomic standing had better compliance and better health seeking behaviour. The former were more likely to afford both the direct and indirect costs of health care, whereas the later, even basic amenities of life such as food, was sometimes a problem. Osamor argued that when people are hungry, nothing else matters to them except food [36]. Similar findings related to socioeconomic status and its influence on compliance and health seeking behaviour have been reported in other settings [38, 39]. In South Africa, authors reported that patients with greater economic resources were more likely to seek treatment from private doctors and spend considerably more for all types of health services compared to their counterparts in the low socioeconomic index [39]. Likewise in Nigeria, poor socioeconomic status, low level of education, unemployment, lack of effective social support networks, unstable living conditions, long distance from treatment center, and high cost of transport negatively influenced treatment compliance and health seeking behaviours for hypertension [38].

5. Implications for Policy and Practice

These findings have significant policy and practical implications on the delivery of services for hypertension. These revolve around the need for educating both the patients and the general population on hypertension, conducting routine screening, ensuring continuity of care, adherence to treatment, patient provider relations, organisation of services to minimize multiple movements across service points, availing services, and enhancing competences of staff.

Although the multiple channels of care for hypertension increase the reach of the services, the channels make it difficult for providers to monitor treatment success rates. Nonetheless, it is unlikely that the patients' behaviour of seeking care from various channels will stop in the near future as long as the comparative advantages of the different care pathways remain. For example, self-medication is comparatively cheaper and saves a lot of patients' time. Yet, it denies the patient the opportunity to receive professional management of the disease which may result in disease complication due to poor management. Therefore, empowering lower level facilities including private drug outlets through training, support supervision, and regulations may be harnessed to reduce risks of self-medication and enhance screening and monitoring, drug refills, and referral compliance. This empowerment would also reduce the challenges related to distance and access especially among the rural folks. On the other hand, higher level facilities should progressively be exempted from routine screening and monitoring which contributes to high patient volumes but instead be equipped and motivated to deal with referral cases in a timely manner. Meanwhile, it is also desirable to enhance the integration of traditional health practice with modern practice to bridge the gaps. Such integration would reduce bickering and situations where traditional health practitioners advice patients not to use prescribed modern medicines. Moreover, increased integration would increase interest in understanding traditional medicine and exploring its efficacy and effectiveness. With the increasing burden of chronic disease, a more sustainable financing mechanism is also warranted. A life time disease like hypertension in the long run becomes unaffordable even to the middle income category in this population. Hence, noncompliance and poor seeking behaviour and related negative health outcomes are inevitable. Exploring feasibility of instituting insurance schemes for chronic disease is recommended.

The patient related barriers have also significant implications. Jin and colleagues recommend that therapy related concerns should be addressed to contribute positively in improving patient's compliance. Prescribing medication with noninvasive route of administration and simple dosing regimens might motivate patients to be compliant [40]. Long duration of treatment period and medication side effects might compromise patient's beliefs about medication effectiveness. Therefore, healthcare providers should consider therapy related problems when designing the therapy plan and involve the patients in the process to minimize the possible therapeutic barriers [40].

6. Strengths and Limitations

This qualitative study highlights the factors influencing compliance and health seeking behaviour for hypertension among aware hypertensive patients in Mukono and Buikwe Districts in Uganda. The strength of the study lies in accruing the patients in their natural environment and learning from their experiences by using interviews in the community at the patients' homes. The patients were purposively selected to obtain a varied sample comprising of different gender, residential status, and district of residence. Limited transferability can be claimed given the small scale sized nature of the study which was conducted in only two districts in Uganda. Despite these limitations, the findings are insightful and of practical importance for programs and intervention trials aimed at feasible strategies to lower hypertension in this population.

7. Conclusions

Hypertension control among aware hypertensive patients in this setting is very low with eight in ten of patients aware of their hypertension not controlled. These control levels are attributable to poor compliance and health seeking behaviours which in turn are influenced by a number of factors which are closely related to the health system, the patient, and the socioeconomic circumstances and the culture of using traditional medicines. Strategies are needed to improve hypertension control in this population. Such strategies should leverage the opportunities at the various levels and traditions of care and address the barriers to health seeking behaviours.

Appendix

Factors Influencing Health Seeking Behaviours of Hypertensive Patients in Mukono and Buikwe in Uganda

Qualitative Interview Guide

(1) For how long have you had (known that you have) hypertension?

(2) What are you're own thoughts about the cause of your hypertension?

(3) How did you get to know that you had hypertension?

- (a) Probe for symptoms and diagnosis.
- (b) How did you deal with those symptoms before you got diagnosed?
  - (i) Probe for things the patient did before he/she got actually diagnosed with hypertension (selftreatment, traditional healers, ...)
- (c) How and when did you decide to seek treatment, what changed?
  - (i) Probe for change in symptoms, or things that might have encouraged them to actually go and seek help
  - (ii) How did they actually seek help, who helped them in making that decision where to go
  - (iii) how was the process of seeking help (meaning did you see many different people before actually seeing a doctor, how did you become diagnosed with hypertension)

(4) Can you explain the care and treatment process from the time you discovered that you are hypertensive?

- (a) Probe for access to treatment and care (traditional healers, drug shops, self medication with herbs or modern medicine, health care facilities)
  - (i) Probe for barriers and facilitators
- (b) frequency of blood pressure monitoring and who monitors this?
- (c) Who helps you deal with your hypertension (family, neighbours, Village health team member (VHT))
- (d) What do they help you with?
- (e) Adherance to treatment and defaults.

(5) Since you became hypertensive, have you used any other methods to treat your hypertension?

- (a) Probe for herbs or other things that they might have tried
  - (i) If yes, where do you get them from?
  - (ii) Does that interfere with your other medication (if used)
  - (iii) Why do you use herbs for your hypertension?
  - (iv) Can you explain how you came to use these products (who introduced you to these methods)

(6) Since you became hypertensive, have you visited or consulted a traditional healer for your hypertension?

- (a) Probe for advice and treatment received, experience with the treatment or advice
- (b) What influenced your decision to go to the traditional healer for your hypertension?
- (c) How were you treated?

(7) Since you became hypertensive, have you been to a modern healthcare facility (health center, hospital or private clinic) for your hypertension? If yes:

- (a) Probe for treatment and advice recieved, level of satisfaction
- (b) What influcend your decision to go to a modern healthcare facility for your hypertension?
- (c) How where you treated?

(8) What is your preferred healthcare service provider (modern or traditional)? Explain your preference, why do you choose one over the other or both and why?

(9) What recommendations would you make that can help hypetensive patients to seek care from modern healthcarefacility?

We are now at the end of the interview and the questions I wanted to ask you. Are there any other issues you find important regarding this topic that we did not talk about? What?

Thank you for your valuable time and accepting to participate in this study.

Disclosure

The funders had no role in study design, data collection and analysis, decision to publish, or preparation of the manuscript.

Authors' Contributions

Geofrey Musinguzi contributed to the study design and conception, study implementation, data analysis, and interpretation of results, wrote the initial draft of the manuscript, and edited the final submitted version. Sibyl Anthierens contributed to conceptualisation, development of study tools, and interpretation of results, conducted data analysis, and participated in peer writing. Fred Nuwaha contributed to study design, conceptualisation, and training research assistants, reviewed the draft manuscript, and provided useful comments. Jean-Pierre Van Geertruyden contributed to data analysis, interpretation, and manuscript writing. Rhoda K. Wanyenze contributed to interpretation of results, manuscript writing, and critical review of the manuscript. Hilde Bastiaens contributed to conceptualisation, development of study tools, data analysis, and interpretation of results and participated in peer writing. All authors have read and approved the final manuscript.

Acknowledgments

The authors would like to acknowledge the research assistants, the mobilisers, the study participants, and district health officers of Mukono and Buikwe. This study has received funding from the European Union's Horizon 2020 Research and Innovation Programme under Grant agreement no. 733356 (SPICES project) and the Flemish Interuniversity Council (VlIR-UOS) through the HEFS Platform Harvest Call (ZIUS2013VOA0902).

References

[1] S. S. Lim, T. Vos, A. D. Flaxman, G. Danaei, K. Shibuya et al., "comparative risk assessment of burden of disease and injury attributable to 67 risk factors and risk factor clusters in 21 regions, 1990–2010: a systematic analysis for the Global Burden of Disease Study 2010," *The Lancet*, vol. 380, no. 9859, pp. 2224–2260, 2012.

[2] P. M. Kearney, M. Whelton, K. Reynolds, P. Muntner, P. K. Whelton, and J. He, "Global burden of hypertension: analysis of worldwide data," *The Lancet*, vol. 365, no. 9455, pp. 217–223, 2005.

[3] PT. Son, *Hypertension in Vietnam from Community-Based Studies to A National Targeted Programme*, 2012.

[4] D. Hoel, "Hypertension Stacking the silent killer," *Postgraduate Medical Journal*, vol. 101, no. 2, pp. 116–121, 1997.

[5] J. K. Cruickshank, J. C. Mbanya, R. Wilks et al., "Hypertension in four African-origin populations: Current 'Rule of Halves', quality of blood pressure control and attributable risk of cardiovascular disease," *Journal of Hypertension*, vol. 19, no. 1, pp. 41–46, 2001.

[6] WHO, *Global Status Report on Noncommunicable Diseases 2010*, World Health Organization, Geneva, 2011.

[7] WHO, *Impact of out-of-pocket payments for treatment of non-communicable diseases in developing countries: A review of literature WHO Discussion Paper*, World Health Organization, Geneva, 2011.

[8] Conner M. N. P., "The theory of planned behaviour and health behaviours," in *Predicting Health Behaviours: Research and Practice with Social Cognition Models*, M. Conner and P. Norman, Eds., pp. 121–162, Open University Press, Buckingham, 1996.

[9] K. Hjelm and F. Atwine, "Health-care seeking behaviour among persons with diabetes in Uganda: an interview study," *BMC International Health and Human Rights*, vol. 11, no. 1, article 11, 2011.

[10] M. Ali and A. de Muynck, "Illness incidence and health seeking behaviour among street children in Rawalpindi and Islamabad, Pakistan - A qualitative study," *Child: Care, Health and Development*, vol. 31, no. 5, pp. 525–532, 2005.

[11] B. S. Godfrey and S. I. I. Iyalomhe, "Hypertension-related knowledge, attitudes and life-style practices among hypertensive patients in a sub-urban Nigerian community," *Journal of Public Health and Epidemiology*, vol. 2, no. 4, pp. 71–77, 2010.

[12] J. Benson and N. Britten, "What effects do patients feel from their antihypertensive tablets and how do they react to them? Qualitative analysis of interviews with patients," *Journal of Family Practice*, vol. 23, no. 6, pp. 80–87, 2006.

[13] J. Kayima, R. K. Wanyenze, A. Katamba, E. Leontsini, and F. Nuwaha, "Hypertension awareness, treatment and control in Africa: a systematic review," *BMC Cardiovascular Disorders*, vol. 13, article 54, 2013.

[14] J.-P. F. Lubaki, L. Mabuza, N. Malete, P. Maduna, and J. V. Ndimande, "Reasons for non-compliance among patients with hypertension at Vanga hospital, Bandundu Province, Democratic Republic of Congo: A qualitative study," *African Journal of Primary Health Care and Family Medicine*, vol. 1, no. 1, pp. 107–111, 2009.

[15] P. A. Bourne, "Impact of poverty, not seeking medical care, unemployment, inflation, self-reported illness, and health insurance on mortality in Jamaica," *North American Journal of Medical Science*, pp. 99–109, 2009.

[16] P. Bourne, "Health literacy and health seeking behavior among older men in a middle-income nation," *Patient Related Outcome Measures*, p. 39.

[17] J. E. Pires, Y. V. Sebastião, A. J. Langa, and S. V. Nery, "Hypertension in Northern Angola: Prevalence, associated factors, awareness, treatment and control," *BMC Public Health*, vol. 13, no. 1, article no. 90, 2013.

[18] I. I. Ulasi, C. K. Ijoma, B. J. C. Onwubere, E. Arodiwe, O. Onodugo, and C. Okafor, "High prevalence and low awareness of hypertension in a market population in Enugu, Nigeria," *International Journal of Hypertension*, vol. 2011, Article ID 869675, 5 pages, 2011.

[19] J. Moodley, "Maternal deaths associated with hypertension in South Africa : lessons to learn from the Saving Mothers report, 2005-2007," *Cardiovascular Journal of Africa*, pp. 31–35, 2011.

[20] C. Lenfant, A. V. Chobanian, D. W. Jones, and E. J. Roccella, "Seventh report of the Joint National Committee on the prevention, detection, evaluation, and treatment of high blood pressure (JNC 7): resetting the hypertension sails," *Hypertension*, vol. 41, no. 6, pp. 1178-1179, 2003.

[21] P. Isaakidis, M.-E. Raguenaud, C. Say et al., "Treatment of hypertension in rural Cambodia: Results from a 6-year programme," *Journal of Human Hypertension*, vol. 25, no. 4, pp. 241–249, 2011.

[22] R. Beaglehole, J. Epping-Jordan, V. Patel et al., "Improving the prevention and management of chronic disease in low-income and middle-income countries: a priority for primary health care," *The Lancet*, vol. 372, no. 9642, pp. 940–949, 2008.

[23] MoH, *Health Sector Strategic and Investment Plan 2010/11–2014/15*, Ministry of Health, Kampala, Uganda, 2010.

[24] R. W. Mayega, S. Etajak, E. Rutebemberwa, G. Tomson, and J. Kiguli, "'Change means sacrificing a good life': Perceptions about severity of type 2 diabetes and preventive lifestyles among people afflicted or at high risk of type 2 diabetes in Iganga Uganda," *BMC Public Health*, vol. 14, no. 1, article no. 864, 2014.

[25] D. Maher, L. Smeeth, and J. Sekajugo, "Health transition in Africa: Practical policy proposals for primary care," *Bulletin of the World Health Organization*, vol. 88, no. 12, pp. 943–948, 2010.

[26] G. Musinguzi, J.-P. Van Geertruyden, H. Bastiaens, and F. Nuwaha, "Uncontrolled hypertension in Uganda: A comparative cross-sectional study," *The Journal of Clinical Hypertension*, vol. 17, no. 1, pp. 63–69, 2015.

[27] UBOS, *National Population and Housing Census 2014 Area Specific Profiles Uganda Bureau of Statistics*, 2014.

[28] G. Musinguzi, H. Bastiaens, R. K. Wanyenze, A. Mukose, J.-P. Van Geertruyden, and F. Nuwaha, "Capacity of health facilities to manage hypertension in Mukono and Buikwe districts in Uganda: Challenges and recommendations," *PLoS ONE*, vol. 10, no. 11, Article ID e0142312, 2015.

[29] G. Musinguzi, F. Nuwaha, and N. Ashton, "Prevalence, awareness and control of hypertension in Uganda," *PLoS ONE*, vol. 8, no. 4, Article ID e62236, 2013.

[30] V. Braun and V. Clarke, "Using thematic analysis in psychology," *Qualitative Research in Psychology*, vol. 3, no. 2, pp. 77–101, 2006.

[31] H. F. Hsieh and S. E. Shannon, "Three approaches to qualitative content analysis," *Qualitative Health Research*, vol. 15, no. 9, pp. 1277–1288, 2005.

[32] T. S. Ferguson, M. K. Tulloch-Reid, N. O. Younger, S. R. McFarlane, D. K. Francis, and R. J. Wilks, "Prehypertension in Jamaica: A review of data from recent studies," *West Indian Medical Journal*, vol. 60, no. 4, pp. 429–433, 2011.

[33] H.-S. Oh and H.-A. Park, "Decision-tree model of treatment-seeking behaviors after detecting symptoms by Korean stroke patients.," *Taehan Kanho Hakhoe chi*, vol. 36, no. 4, pp. 662–670, 2006.

[34] F. Nuwaha and G. Musinguzi, "Use of alternative medicine for hypertension in Buikwe and Mukono districts of Uganda: A cross sectional study," *BMC Complementary and Alternative Medicine*, vol. 13, article no. 301, 2013.

[35] D. A. Oke and E. O. Bandele, "Misconceptions of hypertension," *Journal of the National Medical Association*, vol. 96, no. 9, pp. 1221–1224, 2004.

[36] P. E. Osamor, *Health Care Seeking For Hypertension In South West Nigeria*, Medical Sociology Online, 2011.

[37] D. A. Oke and E. O. Bandele, "Misconceptions of hypertension," *J Natl Med Assoc*, vol. 96, pp. 1221–1224, 2004.

[38] M. R. Akpa, D. I. Agomuoh, and O. J. Odia, "Drug compliance among hypertensive patients in Port Harcourt, Nigeria," *Nigerian Journal of Medicine*, vol. 14, no. 1, pp. 55–57, 2005.

[39] R. J. Petrella, E. P. Merikle, and J. Jones, "Prevalence, treatment, and control of hypertension in primary care: gaps, trends, and opportunities.," *Journal of clinical hypertension (Greenwich, Conn.)*, vol. 9, no. 1, pp. 28–35, 2007.

[40] J. Jin, G. E. Sklar, O. V. Min Sen, and L. S. Chuen, "Factors affecting therapeutic compliance: a review from the patient's perspective," *Therapeutics and Clinical Risk Management*, vol. 4, no. 1, pp. 269–286, 2008.

24

The Effects of Socioeconomic Determinants on Hypertension in a Cardiometabolic At-Risk European Country

Sarah Cuschieri,[1] Josanne Vassallo,[2] Neville Calleja,[3,4] Nikolai Pace,[1] and Julian Mamo[3]

[1] *Department of Anatomy, Faculty of Medicine and Surgery, University of Malta, Msida, Malta*
[2] *Faculty of Medicine and Surgery, University of Malta, Msida, Malta*
[3] *Department of Public Health, Faculty of Medicine and Surgery, University of Malta, Msida, Malta*
[4] *Department of Health Information and Research, Ministry of Health, Guardamangia, Malta*

Correspondence should be addressed to Sarah Cuschieri; sarah.cuschieri@um.edu.mt

Academic Editor: Franco Veglio

Background. A relationship has been established between socioeconomic status and hypertension. The aim of this study was to determine the prevalence of hypertension and to explore the links between hypertension and socioeconomic factors in the adult population of Malta. *Methods.* A national representative cross-sectional health examination study was performed between 2014 and 2016. Sociodemographic and medical history data was gathered by validated questionnaires while blood pressure was measured. Prevalence rates of known hypertension, newly hypertension, and global hypertension were calculated. Associations between sociodemographic characteristics and hypertension were identified through logistic regression models. *Results.* Hypertension contributed to 30.12% (CI 95%: 28.71–31.57) of the study population, with a male preponderance. The majority was known hypertensive (73.59% CI 95%: 71.01–76.02), with only three-quarters on medication. Multivariant analyses showed that increasing age and body mass index, male gender, and living in Gozo, Western district, and Northern Harbour district were associated with having hypertension. *Conclusion.* Hypertension is a problem in Malta especially in the male population and with increasing age and body mass index. Education did not exhibit any associated risk for having hypertension, which is inconsistent with the literature, while habitat localities played a role in hypertension development.

1. Introduction

High blood pressure is a serious public health concern, with the World Health Organization (WHO) reporting a hypertension global mortality rate of 13% [1]. Hypertension is estimated to contribute to 25% of all European myocardial infarctions [2]. In fact, the WHO European Region document *Health 2020 Policy* gave hypertension high priority in order to tackle the epidemic and to reduce its prevalence [3]. High blood pressure is a preventable disease and has been associated directly with lifestyle habits, including tobacco smoking, a lack of physical activity, and alcohol consumption [2]. In fact, the relationship between hypertension and socioeconomic status has been well established [4].

Socioeconomic status (SES) is a complex term combining a number of variables, including employment status, educational level, income, and wealth as well as place of residence. SES is a well-established cardiovascular risk factor and means for predicting behaviour [5, 6]. The educational level has been established as the best marker of SES since it offers the most stable measure at an individual level and does not have the problem of reverse causation such as income and wealth status [6].

Malta is a Mediterranean island at crossroads between Europe and Africa, with 40.1% of the mortality rate attributed to cardiovascular disease [7]. Considering the small size of this island and its crucial location, a representative adult health examination cross-sectional study was considered feasible to provide much needed information on health effects. The aim of this study was to determine the prevalence of hypertension and to explore the links between hypertension and socioeconomic factors in the adult population of Malta.

2. Method

A cross-sectional study was conducted by the University of Malta between November 2014 and January 2016, with the survey name of "SAHHTEK" *(your health)*. The detailed survey methodology was described elsewhere [8]. In summary, a randomized stratified sample, by age (18 to 70 years) and gender, representing approximately 1% of the total population from each Maltese town, was invited to participate in the health examination survey. A validated sociodemographic and medical history questionnaire was filled in during the survey [8]. The health examination consisted of three consecutive blood pressure readings after a 20-minute rest (sitting down), besides anthropometric measurements. The average of the three blood pressure readings was recoded and used for this study. Informed consent was obtained from every participant. Ethical and data protection approvals were granted from the University of Malta Research Ethical Committee (UREC) and the Information and Data Protection Commissioner, respectively.

The population reporting a history of hypertension or who was on antihypertensive medication was labeled as *"known hypertensive."* Participants with a systolic blood pressure over 140 mmHg or a diastolic blood pressure above 90 mmHg and who were not *known hypertensives* were labeled as *"newly hypertensive."* Those reporting to suffer from *known hypertension* but did not report to be on treatment and were found to have a normal blood pressure during health examination were labeled as *normotensive*. All population with no history of hypertension and a normal blood pressure during health examination was also labeled as *normotensive*.

The *known hypertensive* and the *newly hypertensive* subpopulations were considered collectively as the global *hypertension population* for this study. The prevalence rates of *known hypertension, newly hypertension,* and the global *hypertension population* were calculated. The study population was age-stratified by 10-year age groups (20 to 69 years), and considering the representative prevalence rates in these age groups, an estimate of the total Maltese adult population suffering from hypertension was calculated.

The links between self-reported sociodemographic, lifestyle variables (residing district, highest educational level, employment status, smoking habits, alcohol consumption habits, and physical activity levels), body mass index (BMI), and hypertension were explored. Univariate and multiple variant logistic regression models were performed to assess any associations between these sociodemographic characteristics and hypertension.

3. Results

The survey response rate was of 49% ($n = 3947$), out of which 30.12% (CI 95%: 28.71–31.57) contributed to the hypertension population ($n = 1189$). Hypertensive males accounted for 35.04% (CI 95%: 32.97–37.15) of the total study male population, while hypertensive females accounted for 25.09% (CI 95%: 23.21–27.06) of the total female study population.

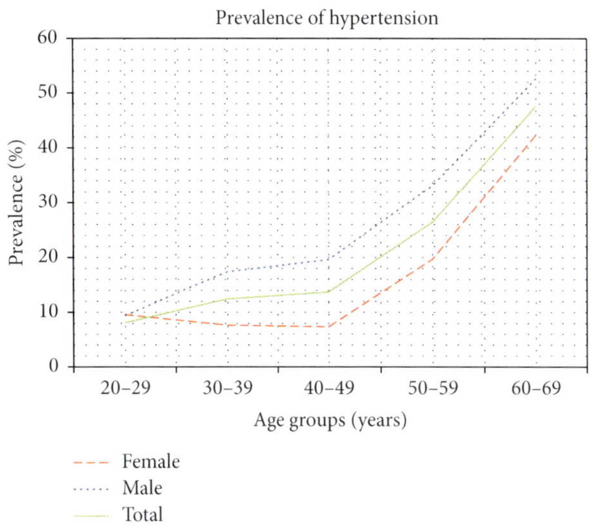

FIGURE 1: Distribution of hypertension prevalence by age groups and gender.

On age and gender stratification, a male predominance was present throughout all age groups, as seen in Figure 1. With increasing age in the 20- to 39-year bracket, males had higher blood pressure levels, while the female population actually had slightly lowered prevalence with increasing age in this bracket. However, from the age of 40 years, a higher prevalence rate of hypertension was exhibited for both genders with every age increase. On applying the prevalence rates for each age group and gender to the total Maltese population by age and gender [9], an estimated distribution of hypertension within the Maltese population was established, as seen in Table 1.

The majority of the hypertension population consisted of *known hypertensives* (73.59% CI 95%: 71.01–76.02), with the male prevalence of 71.29% (CI 95%: 67.82–74.52) and a female prevalence of 76.89% (CI 95%: 72.95–80.42). Among the *known hypertensives*, 85.60% (CI 95%: 83.11–87.78) were on medication. However, 5.34% (CI 95%: 3.93–7.21) were found to have uncontrolled systolic blood pressure (>140 mmHg) while 1.20% (CI 95%: 0.60–2.30) had uncontrolled diastolic blood pressure (>90 mmHg) during the health examination survey. Out of those reporting to suffer from hypertension, 5.52% (CI 95%: 4.19–7.23) did not report to be on treatment and were found to have a normal blood pressure during the health examination. This subgroup may have exhibited an error in their medical history recall and were therefore considered to be normotensive.

The *newly hypertensive* population contributed to 26.41% (CI 95%: 23.98–28.99) of the hypertension population. The majority (64.01% CI 95%: 58.56–69.13) of the newly diagnosed hypertensives were male. Table 2 demonstrates different hypertension characteristics by gender. The Maltese males tend to be more likely to have an elevated blood pressure, be unaware of their hypertension, be untreated, or have uncontrolled blood pressure.

Table 1: Distribution of the estimated Maltese hypertension population, by age groups and gender.

(a)

Total Maltese population by age*		Total population with hypertension	Percentage with hypertension, by age
20–29	55,218	5,345	9.68%
30–39	56,184	7,193	12.80%
40–49	48,406	6,466	13.36%
50–59	57,291	15,223	26.57%
60–69	55,986	26,395	47.15%
Total	273,085	60,622	

(b)

Total male Maltese population by age*		Male with hypertension	Percentage with hypertension, by age
20–29	28,228	2,646	9.38%
30–39	28,837	5,005	17.36%
40–49	24,546	4,796	19.54%
50–59	28,822	9,529	33.06%
60–69	27,388	14,384	52.52%
Total	137,821	36,360	

(c)

Total female Maltese population by age*		Female with hypertension	Percentage with hypertension, by age
20–29	26,990	2,699	10.00%
30–39	27,347	2,188	8.00%
40–49	23,860	1,670	7.00%
50–59	28,469	5,694	20.00%
60–69	28,598	12,011	42.00%
Total	135,264	24,262	

*Demographic data 2013.

Table 2: Demonstrating hypertension characteristics, by gender.

Hypertension characteristics	Male (%) [n = 1998]	Female (%) [n = 1949]	Total (%) [n = 3947]
Normotensive	1298 (64.96)	1460 (74.91)	2758 (69.88)
Hypertensive *(global hypertension)*	700 (35.04)	489 (25.09)	1189 (30.12)
Unaware *(newly hypertensive)*	201 (10.06)	113 (5.80)	314 (7.96)
Aware *(known hypertensive)*	499 (24.97)	376 (19.29)	875 (22.17)
Untreated	81 (4.05)	45 (2.31)	126 (3.19)
Treated	418 (20.92)	331 (16.98)	749 (18.98)
Uncontrolled	32 (1.60)	15 (0.77)	47 (1.19)
Controlled	386 (19.32)	316 (16.21)	702 (17.79)
Total with elevated blood pressure	668 (33.43)	474 (24.32)	1142 (28.93)

4. Hypertension Population and Sociodemographic Characteristics

On comparing the sociodemographic characteristics and lifestyle factors to the hypertensive and normotensive populations, significant differences were observed. These differences are outlined in Table 3.

Multivariant analyses showed that increasing age and increasing BMI, the male gender, physical activity, and living in Gozo, Western district, and Northern Harbour were associated with the development of hypertension (Table 4).

Alcohol consumption, smoking habit, education level, and employment status were not found to have a significant associated risk on hypertension after adjustment for all sociodemographic and lifestyle habits.

5. Discussion

Hypertension is one of the leading causes of cardiovascular disease and mortality worldwide [10]. The prevalence of hypertension varies from one global region to another, with the highest prevalence being in the African region (46%) and

Table 3: Distribution of the sociodemographic characteristics in the normotensive and the hypertensive populations by gender.

		Hypertensive (total)	Normotensive	p value*	Hypertensive		p value*
					Male ($n = 729$)	Female ($n = 529$)	
Locality	Southern Harbour	585	215	**0.0001**	124	91	**0.0001**
	Northern Harbour	731	340		195	145	
	Southeastern	382	220		122	97	
	Western	360	186		109	77	
	Northern	423	163		91	72	
	Gozo	208	134		87	46	
Education	Low educational level	361	273	**0.0001**	160	201	**0.0001**
	Medium educational level	497	1034		284	213	
	High educational level	399	1382		285	114	
Employment status	Employed	625	1898	**0.0001**	473	153	**0.0001**
	Not in employment	632	791		256	376	
Smoking habit	Smoking	268	691	**0.003**	192	76	**0.001**
	Nonsmoking	990	1999		537	453	
Alcohol consumption	Alcohol consumption	1487	625	**0.001**	458	167	**0.0001**
	No-alcohol consumption	1203	633		271	361	
Physical activity	No activity	290	98	**0.015**	45	53	0.084
	Walk	522	230		138	91	
	Moderate activity	1585	783		458	325	
	Vigorous activity	292	147		88	59	

*Chi-square.

TABLE 4: Demonstrates the crude and adjusted sociodemographic independent variables for the development of hypertension.

Sociodemographic factors	Crude analysis			Adjusted analysis		
	OR	CI	*p* value	OR	CI	*p* value
Male	1.521	1.332–1.737	**0.0001**	1.83	1.544–2.168	**0.0001**
Female*	Reference			Reference		
High educational level	0.218	0.181–0.264	**0.0001**	0.935	0.731–1.195	0.592
Medium educational level	0.369	0.307–0.445	**0.0001**	0.923	0.741–1.149	0.471
Low educational level*	Reference			Reference		
No-alcohol use	1.247	1.093–1.423	**0.001**	1.018	0.866–1.197	0.827
Alcohol use*	Reference			Reference		
Nonsmoking	1.285	1.097–1.505	**0.002**	0.981	0.815–1.181	0.839
Smoking*	Reference			Reference		
Vigorous activity	1.433	1.065–1.929	**0.018**	1.492	1.057–2.104	**0.023**
Moderate activity	1.41	1.111–1.789	**0.005**	1.341	1.023–1.758	**0.034**
Walk	1.264	0.965–1.655	0.09	1.143	0.842–1.553	0.391
No activity*	Reference			Reference		
Gozo	1.727	1.329–2.245	**0.0001**	1.771	1.303–2.408	**0.0001**
Northern	1.032	0.817–1.304	0.794	1.124	0.857–1.474	0.399
Western	1.424	1.125–1.802	**0.003**	1.473	1.121–1.937	**0.005**
Southeastern	1.541	1.229–1.9332	**0.0001**	1.674	1.287–2.178	**0.0001**
Northern Harbour	1.241	1.02–1.51	**0.031**	1.204	0.961–1.509	0.107
Southern Harbour*	Reference			Reference		
Not in employment	2.421	2.114–2.772	**0.0001**	1.181	0.974–1.432	0.091
Employed*	Reference			Reference		
BMI	1.127	1.113–1.141	**0.0001**	1.104	1.088–1.210	**0.0001**
Age	1.07	1.07–1.08	**0.0001**	1.066	1.058–1.073	**0.0001**

*Reference category.

the lowest in America (35%), with the European region prevalence rate reported to be somewhere in between these two continents [11, 12]. The male gender, in our study, exhibited the highest hypertension prevalence, which is consistent with what is normally found within high-income countries [13].

On comparing the hypertension prevalence found in our study to a Pan-European study conducted in 5 European countries, Malta exhibited the highest hypertension prevalence [14]. This Pan-European study had reported that Germany had the highest hypertension prevalence among UK, Italy, France, and Spain. Malta showed higher prevalence rates for each gender (Germany male: 25.1%, female: 22.9%; Malta male: 36.49%, female: 27.14%), although one needs to keep in mind that different age bands (Malta study: 18 to 70 years, Pan-European study: 20–79 years) were examined in both studies [14]. Conversely, our study population reported Maltese hypertensives having a higher antihypertensive pharmacological prescription frequency when compared to the average European prescription frequency [15, 16]. Nonadherence to antihypertensive medication is a global issue and leads to loss of clinical efficacy as well as to loss of economic efficiency resulting in an increase in hospitalization costs [16].

Hypertension determinants are well established and include age, gender, sociodemographic factors, obesity, smoking, excess alcohol, and sedentary lifestyle [17, 18]. On univariant analysis, education level, which is considered as the most stable determinant of socioeconomic status, was found to exhibit an associated protective effect against having hypertension in our study. This effect was lost on adjusting for age and gender, which could be the result of a change in education opportunities over time and more females are continuing their education. This finding is inconsistent with other association reports where the level of education was found to have an inverse association with blood pressure [19, 20].

The female gender in our study was found to exhibit an associated protective effect on hypertension. This is partially consistent with findings from other studies within other high-income countries [21]. However, this protective effect exhibited by our female population was previously reported in middle-income countries and not high-income countries like Malta [22–24].

Intense physical activity was found to increase the risk of having hypertension in our study, which is not consistent with the literature [25]. A possible reason to this finding follows the fact that the Maltese population is well known to be at high risk of metabolic diseases. A proportion of the population follows lifestyle interventions to try to halt the development of these noncommunicable diseases, which may have led to this finding.

A link was established between three different districts (Gozo, Western, and Northern Harbour) and having hypertension. Further research is required to assess whether an environmental or a genetic cause may be contributing to this relationship. However, a possible explanation for the link between the Northern Harbour and hypertension could result from the fact that the majority of the Maltese population lives in this district.

A link has been reported between alcohol consumption and blood pressure, with chronic drinkers having a longer impact on blood pressure outcomes [26]. A linear relationship had been reported between alcohol intake and blood pressure [27]. This was not the case in our study, where non-alcohol drinkers were found to be at risk of having hypertension. However, this associated effect of alcohol consumption on hypertension development was lost once various confounder factors were adjusted for, suggesting that no direct link between alcohol and hypertension was evident in our population.

6. Study Limitations and Strengths

The response rate for the health examination was rather low due to the invasive blood measurement required, which may have affected the results. The demographic data and lifestyle habits were self-reported by participants. This predisposes the risk of human bias or inaccurate recollection of information. Blood pressure measurement is very sensitive; accuracy may have been affected by the behaviour of the participant, the environment of the setup, and the aneroid sphygmomanometer device used even though sphygmomanometers were calibrated regularly. Auscultation fieldworker observer errors may have occurred including systematic error in auscultation method if the observer did not hear well enough or had slow reactions to auditory and visual cues, even though fieldworkers were trained and their readings double checked with other experienced blood pressure measurers prior to initiation of the fieldwork. Measurement of blood pressure was taken after 20 minutes of sitting down; this avoided any blood pressure fluctuations. All participants were asked to sit up straight with both feet touching the floor and their arms resting at the heart level, where these techniques were found to enable more accurate readings. The study was a cross-sectional study, which does not adjust for changes in behaviour after the diagnoses of hypertension or other diseases. There is thus great difficulty in linking exposures with outcomes from this study in any causative way.

7. Conclusion

Approximately a third of the adult population in Malta (mostly males) suffered from hypertension. Aging males, increase in BMI, and living in Gozo, Western district, and Northern Harbour exhibited a higher associated risk to develop hypertension. Education levels were not found to be associated with the hypertension development.

Disclosure

The funding body had no influence on the protocol of the survey or on the data analysis. No author received any personal funding.

Acknowledgments

The authors are extremely grateful for the strong support forthcoming from the University of Malta (through the Medical School and Research Innovative Development Trust Department) and from the Alfred Mizzi Foundation as major sponsors, as well as that of a host of others, including Atlas Health Insurance (Malta). The in-kind support and encouragement of the Parliamentary Secretariat for Health of the Government of Malta are also gratefully acknowledged.

References

[1] WHO, *Global Health Risks: Mortality And Burden of Disease Attributable to Selected Major Risks*, WHO, Geneva, Switzerland, 2009.

[2] WHO, *High Blood Pressure - Country Experience And Effective Interventions Utilized across The European Region*, WHO, Copenhagen, Denmark, 2013.

[3] WHO, *Health 2020: A European Policy Framework Supporting Action across Government And Society for Health And Well-Being*, WHO, Copenhagen, Denmark, 2012.

[4] B. Leng, Y. Jin, G. Li, L. Chen, and N. Jin, "Socioeconomic status and hypertension: a meta-analysis," *Journal of Hypertension*, vol. 33, no. 2, pp. 221–229, 2015.

[5] C. S. P. Lam, "The socioeconomics of hypertension: How $50 000 may buy a drop in blood pressure," *Hypertension*, vol. 58, no. 2, pp. 140-141, 2011.

[6] D. Minor, M. Wofford, and S. B. Wyatt, "Does socioeconomic status affect blood pressure goal achievement?" *Current hypertension reports*, vol. 10, no. 5, pp. 390–397, 2008.

[7] Department of Health Information and Research, *Annual Mortality Report National Mortality Registry. Gwardamangia*, Department of Health Information and Research, Gwardamangia, Malta, 2013.

[8] S. Cuschieri, J. Vassallo, N. Calleja, N. Pace, and J. Mamo, "Diabetes, pre-diabetes and their risk factors in malta: a study profile of national cross-sectional prevalence study," *Global Health, Epidemiology and Genomics*, vol. 1, 2016.

[9] NSO, *Demographic Review 2013*, NSO: National Statistics Office, Valletta, Malta, 2015.

[10] L. Tao, C. Pu, S. Shen, H. Fang, X. Wanf, and Q. Xuan, "Tendency for age-specific mortality with hypertension in the European Union from 1980 to 2011," *International Journal of Clinical and Experimental Medicine*, vol. 8, no. 2, pp. 1611–1623, 2015.

[11] G. Stevens, M. Mascarenhas, and C. Mathers, "Global health risks: progress and challenges," *Bulletin of the World Health Organization*, vol. 87, no. 9, p. 646, 2009.

[12] K. Wolf-Maier, R. S. Cooper, J. R. Banegas et al., "Hypertension prevalence and blood pressure levels in 6 European countries, Canada, and the United States," *The Journal of the American Medical Association*, vol. 289, no. 18, pp. 2363–2369, 2003.

[13] K. T. Mills, J. D. Bundy, T. N. Kelly et al., "Global disparities of hypertension prevalence and control," *Circulation*, vol. 134, no. 6, pp. 441–450, 2016.

[14] F. Eichmann, P. Potthoff, and M. Schmidt, "PCV115 burden of hypertension in selected EU countries: 2010-2025," *Value in Health*, vol. 15, no. 7, p. A383, 2012.

[15] L. Breitscheidel, B. Ehlken, K. Kostev, M. S. A. Oberdiek, A. Sandberg, and R. E. Schmieder, "Real-life treatment patterns, compliance, persistence, and medication costs in patients with hypertension in Germany," *Journal of Medical Economics*, vol. 15, no. 1, pp. 155–165, 2012.

[16] F. S. Mennini, A. Marcellusi, J. M. von der Schulenburg et al., "Cost of poor adherence to anti-hypertensive therapy in five European countries," *The European Journal of Health Economics*, vol. 16, no. 1, pp. 65–72, 2015.

[17] M. Joffres, E. Falaschetti, C. Gillespie et al., "Hypertension prevalence, awareness, treatment and control in national surveys from England, the USA and Canada, and correlation with stroke and ischaemic heart disease mortality: a cross-sectional study," *BMJ Open*, vol. 3, no. 8, Article ID e003423, 2013.

[18] R. S. Vasan, M. G. Larson, E. P. Leip, W. B. Kannel, and D. Levy, "Assessment of frequency of progression to hypertension in non-hypertensive participants in the Framingham Heart Study: a cohort study," *The Lancet*, vol. 358, no. 9294, pp. 1682–1686, 2001.

[19] Y. Wang, J. Chen, K. Wang, and C. L. Edwards, "Education as an important risk factor for the prevalence of hypertension and elevated blood pressure in Chinese men and women," *Journal of Human Hypertension*, vol. 20, no. 11, pp. 898–900, 2006.

[20] B. H. Brummett, M. A. Babyak, I. C. Siegler et al., "Systolic blood pressure, socioeconomic status, and biobehavioral risk factors in a nationally representative us young adult sample," *Hypertension*, vol. 58, no. 2, pp. 161–166, 2011.

[21] H. M. Colhoun, H. Hemingway, and N. R. Poulter, "Socio-economic status and blood pressure: an overview analysis," *Journal of Human Hypertension*, vol. 12, no. 2, pp. 91–110, 1998.

[22] N. L. Fleischer, A. V. Diez Roux, M. Alazraqui, H. Spinelli, and F. De Maio, "Socioeconomic gradients in chronic disease risk factors in middle-income countries: Evidence of effect modification by urbanicity in Argentina," *American Journal of Public Health*, vol. 101, no. 2, pp. 294–301, 2011.

[23] A. Cois and R. Ehrlich, "Analysing the socioeconomic determinants of hypertension in South Africa: a structural equation modelling approach," *BMC Public Health*, vol. 14, article 414, 2014.

[24] World Bank, Malta, 2016, Available at: http://data.worldbank.org/country/malta.

[25] K. M. Diaz and D. Shimbo, "Physical activity and the prevention of hypertension," *Current Hypertension Reports*, vol. 15, no. 6, pp. 659–668, 2013.

[26] M. G. Marmot, P. Elliott, M. J. Shipley et al., "Alcohol and blood pressure: the INTERSALT study," *British Medical Journal*, vol. 308, no. 6939, pp. 1263–1267, 1994.

[27] J. B. Saunders, D. G. Beevers, and A. Paton, "Alcohol-induced hypertension," *The Lancet*, vol. 318, no. 8248, pp. 653–656, 1981.

25

Tracking of Blood Pressure in Children and Adolescents in Germany in the Context of Risk Factors for Hypertension

Giselle Sarganas,[1,2] **Angelika Schaffrath Rosario**,[1] **Claudia Niessner**,[3] **Alexander Woll**,[3] and **Hannelore K. Neuhauser**[1,2]

[1] *Robert Koch Institute, Department of Epidemiology and Health Monitoring, Berlin, Germany*
[2] *DZHK (German Center for Cardiovascular Research), Partner Site Berlin, Germany*
[3] *Institute for Sports and Sport Science, Karlsruhe Institute of Technology, Karlsruhe, Germany*

Correspondence should be addressed to Giselle Sarganas; sarganas-margolisg@rki.de

Academic Editor: Tomohiro Katsuya

Blood pressure (BP) tracking from childhood to adulthood has two aspects: the ranking stability relative to others over time and the prediction of future values. This study investigates BP tracking in children and adolescents in Germany in the context of hypertension risk factors. BP was measured and analyzed in 2542 participants of the German Health Examination Survey for Children and Adolescents (t_0 2003-2006; 3 to 17-year olds) and of a six year follow-up "Motorik Modul" (t_1 2009-2012; 9 to 24-year olds). BP tracking coefficients were calculated from Spearman's rank-order correlations. Predictive values and logistic regression models were used to forecast t_1-BP above the hypertension threshold from t_0-BP as well as from baseline and follow-up hypertension risk factors. BP tracking was moderate (0.33-0.50 for SBP and 0.19-0.39 for DBP) with no statistically significant differences between sex and age groups. Baseline hypertensive BP was the strongest independent predictor of hypertensive BP at follow-up (OR 4.3 and 3.4 for age groups 3-10 and 11-17 years) after adjusting for sex, BMI trajectories, birthweight, parental hypertension, and age-group dependent-sports/physical activity. However, the positive predictive value of baseline hypertensive BP for hypertensive BP at follow-up in 3- to 10-year olds was only 39% (34% in 11- to 17-year olds) and increased only moderately in the presence of additional risk factors. Our analysis with population-based data from Germany shows that BP in children and adolescents tracks only moderately over six years. BP in childhood is the strongest independent predictor of future BP but its predictive value is limited.

1. Introduction

Blood pressure (BP) elevation is much more common among children and adolescents than previously thought. Moreover, BP in childhood correlates with BP in adulthood [1]; hence children with elevated BP have a higher probability of developing hypertension in adulthood than children with lower BP. However, the usefulness of universal pediatric BP screening is strongly debated due to the only moderate BP tracking correlation from childhood to adulthood [1–4].

BP tracking correlation has two aspects: the stability of BP ranking relative to others over a specified period of time (calculated as tracking coefficients) and the predictability of future values from baseline values. Meta-analyses have reported moderate tracking coefficients of 0.42-0.38 for SBP and 0.41-0.28 for DBP from childhood to adulthood [1, 3]. While several studies have investigated BP tracking in children and adolescents and have compared different age groups as well as BP tracking over different time periods, little is known on whether having risk factors for hypertension, such as overweight and obesity, low birthweight, or parental hypertension, is associated with higher BP tracking correlation from childhood to adolescence/young adulthood. Moreover, the predictability of BP measurements from hypertension risk factors in clinically meaningful terms such as positive and negative predictive values has been reported only in the context of screening, not of tracking [5].

Therefore, the aim of this study is twofold: (1) to investigate six year BP tracking correlation coefficients from childhood to adolescence/young adulthood in a large population-based sample with a broad baseline age range of 3 to 17 years and to illustrate whether this aspect of tracking is stronger in subgroups with additional hypertension risk factors; and (2) to analyse the predictability of future BP values above the hypertension threshold from previous BP and hypertension risk factors and to quantify this predictability using different measures of association including odds ratios (OR) and predictive values.

2. Methods

2.1. Study Population. The German Health Interview and Examination Survey for Children and Adolescents (KiGGS) is a nationwide study based on a stratified population-registry sample of 17,641 participants aged 0–17 years living in Germany (response rate 67%), including 14,835 participants aged 3-17 years [6]. Details on the baseline and follow-up surveys including its several parallel study modules were published previously [6–8]. At baseline, about half of the participants were invited to take part in the "Motorik Modul Study" (MoMo; response rate 58%) [7]. The six-year MoMo follow-up had a response rate of 48% [7]. The present analysis includes data from 2686 children and adolescents who participated in the KiGGS baseline study KiGGS0 (t_0 2003-2006; participants aged 3 to 17 years) and the MoMo follow-up (t_1 2009-2012; participants aged 9 to 24 years) with complete BP data sets and who have not taken antihypertensive medication at t_0 (unfortunately we do not have information on medication use at t_1). The proportion of complete data sets was higher for those 3-10 years old at t_0 than for those 11-17 years old. Analyses were stratified by age group: 3-10 years at t_0 and 9-17 years at t_1 vs. 11-17 years at t_0 and 18-24 years at t_1. We therefore excluded 144 participants who did not fall into these two groups in order to have a clear cutoff in the age group analysis and not mix both hypertension definitions (percentile and mmHg based; see below), leaving 2542 participants (1269 males and 1273 females) for analysis. Additional follow-up data were available from the telephone interview KiGGS1 2009-2012 [8].

BP measurement methods were standardized and followed the same protocol in KiGGS0 2003-2006 (t_0) and in the MoMo study 2009-2012 (t_1). At both time-points, BP measurements were taken in the sitting position on a height-adjustable chair with a backrest, the right forearm resting on a table at the level of the heart, the elbow slightly bent, the legs uncrossed, and the feet placed firmly on the floor. Four cuff sizes (cuff bladder in cm 6 × 12, 9 × 18, 12 × 23, or 17 × 38.6) were available, which had to cover at least two-thirds of the upper arm length (from the axilla to the antecubital fossa). Two readings of systolic (SBP), diastolic blood pressure (DBP), mean arterial BP, and heart rate were obtained at a two-minute interval with an automated upper arm oscillometric device (Datascope Accutorr Plus, Mahwah, NJ) after a nonstrenuous part of the examination and an additional 5-minute rest in both surveys [9, 10]. The mean of the 2 systolic and diastolic measurements was used for this analysis.

BP in children is age, gender, and height dependent; therefore, it is not possible, as for adults, to designate a single BP threshold to define hypertension. BP reference percentiles [11] based on KiGGS data from nonoverweight children were used according to German guidelines [12]: hypertensive BP measurement was SBP or DBP at or above the 95th age-, sex-, and height-specific percentile for children and adolescents under 18 years, or BP ≥ 140/90 mmHg irrespective of the percentile. For young adults aged 18 years or older, the absolute cutoff for hypertension (≥140/90 mmHg) was applied. Since percentile-based cutoffs in children and the 140/90 mmHg cutoff in adults are not equivalent, analyses were stratified accordingly: baseline ages 3 to 10 years with t_1-ages 9 to 17 years vs. baseline ages 11 to 17 years with t_1-ages 18 to 24 years.

In addition, weight and height were measured at t_0 and t_1 according to a common protocol. Weight was measured in underwear to the nearest 0.1 kg with a calibrated scale (Seca, Birmingham, United Kingdom) according to a standardized protocol [6]. BMI was calculated as the ratio of weight (in kg) by height^2 (in m^2) and rounded to 3 digits. BMI was categorized as underweight, normal weight, overweight, and obese according to the International Obesity Task Force (IOTF) cutoffs defined by the age-specific percentiles in <18-year olds, which at the age 18 and older correspond to the adult cutoff points for overweight 25 kg/m^2 and obesity 30 kg/m^2 [13]. BMI trajectory was defined as the BMI course between t_0 and t_1 in 4 categories: "persistently low or normal" defined as under- or normal weight at t_0 and at t_1; "resolution" as overweight or obese at t_0 and normal or underweight at t_1; "persistently overweight/obesity" (at t_0 and at t_1); and "incident overweight/obesity" as under- or normal weight at t_0 and overweight or obese at t_1.

Information on physical activity was collected only in t_0: in children aged 3 to 10 years it was assessed through parent-reported frequency of sports activities per week (categories: 3 or more, 1-2, and less than once) [14] and in children aged 11 to 17 years through self-reported leisure time physical activities that makes them sweat or get out of breath (categories: ≤2.0, 2.1-4.9, and 5.0-31.0 hours per week) [15].

Birth weight (in g) was reported by the mother at t_0; we have classified the variable into less than 2500 g, as low birth weight, or greater than 2500 g.

Parental hypertension was collected at t_1 with the question: has the mother or father of the study participant ever been diagnosed by a doctor as having hypertension or high blood pressure?

2.2. Statistical Analysis. The analysis was performed in two parts. First, BP tracking was estimated by calculating Spearman's rank-order correlation coefficients stratified by sex and age and potential hypertension risk factors (overweight/obesity, birthweight and parental hypertension). For this purpose, four age groups were chosen: 3 to 6, 7 to 10, 11 to 14, and 15 to 17 years. In the first two age groups, the rank order of t_0-percentiles was correlated with the rank order of t_1-percentiles. For the last two groups, the rank order of t_0-percentiles were correlated with the rank order of t_1 mmHg values.

For testing statistical differences between correlation coefficients, we have used the software cocor (http://comparingcorrelations.org/) [16].

In the second part of the analysis, we determined the proportion of participants with hypertensive BP measurement

Table 1: Characteristics of the 2542 study participants (1269 males and 1273 females) at baseline (2003-2006) and at follow-up (2009-2012).

Characteristics Age range (years)	Males Baseline (t_0) (3-17)	Males Follow-up (t_1) (9-24)	p-value	Females Baseline (t_0) (3-17)	Females Follow-up (t_1) (9-24)	p-value
Mean age*	8.5 (8.3-8.7)	14.7 (14.5-14.9)	0.000	8.5 (8.3-8.7)	14.8 (14.6-15.0)	0.000
SBP (mmHg)*	102.8 (102.2-103.4)	117.6 (116.8-118.5)	0.000	102.8 (102.3-103.4)	114.7 (114.0-115.4)	0.000
DBP (mmHg)*	62.1 (61.7-62.5)	66.2 (65.7-66.7)	0.001	62.7 (62.3-63.1)	66.0 (65.5-66.5)	0.001
Hypertensive BP&	8.5% (7.1-10.2)	15.7% (13.8-17.8)	0.001	8.6% (7.2-10.3)	14.0% (12.2-16.0)	0.000
BMI (kg/m^2)*	17.1 (16.9-17.2)	20.7 (20.4-20.9)	0.000	17.1 (17.0-17.3)	20.5 (20.3-20.8)	0.000
Underweight	9.8% (8.3-11.6)	6.1% (4.9-7.5)	0.001	11.3% (9.7-13.2)	9.4% (7.9-11.1)	0.104
Normal-weight	78.9% (76.6-81.1)	72.5% (70.0-74.9)	0.000	74.0% (71.6-76.4)	72.6% (70.0-75.0)	0.372
Overweight	9.1% (7.6-10.8)	16.3% (14.4-18.5)	0.000	12.2% (10.5-14.1)	13.8% (12.0-15.8)	0.238
Obese	2.2% (1.5-3.2)	5.1% (4.0-6.5)	0.000	2.4% (1.7-3.4)	4.3% (3.3-5.5)	0.011
Sports activities (3 or more times/week) (3-10 years)	43.2% (40.1-46.4)	-	-	35.5% (32.4-38.6)	-	-
Sports activities (h/week)* (11-17 years)	7.6 (6.5-8.8)	-	-	5.2 (4.7-5.7)	-	-
Parental hypertension	-	28.1% (25.7-30.8)	-	-	30.3% (27.7-32.9)	-
Low birthweight (<2500 g)	5.0% (3.9-6.4)	-	-	6.3% (5.1-7.8)	-	-

*mean (95% CI).
&SBP or DBP at or above the 95th age-, sex-, and height-specific percentile for children and adolescents under 18 years, or BP ≥140/90 mmHg irrespective of the percentile. For young adults aged 18 years or older, the absolute cutoffs for hypertension (≥140/90 mmHg) were applied.

at t_0 and t_1. For calculating the positive predictive value (PPV) of hypertensive BP at t_0 for future hypertensive BP (six years later at t_1), as well as the negative predictive value (NPV) of normotensive BP at t_0 for future normotensive BP, we used the software MedCalc (https://www.medcalc.org/calc/diagnostic_test.php). We calculated the PPV and NPV also for risk factor combinations, e.g., for having hypertensive BP and being obese at t_0. In sensitivity analyses, we checked whether the results were altered when using weighting factors in the analysis. These weights take selective participation in the MoMo study and the drop-out between t_0 and t_1 into account. They are the inverse of the probability to participate in the MoMo study/the follow-up, estimated in a logistic regression model including several relevant KiGGS variables as predictors. Since no weights are available for the exact population under study here, we used three existing sets of weights: longitudinal weights adjusting the KiGGS follow-up to the KiGGS baseline, longitudinal weights adjusting the MoMo follow-up to the MoMo baseline, and cross-sectional MoMo weights adjusting the MoMo follow-up to the KiGGS1 follow-up.

Furthermore, we investigated the prediction of hypertensive t_1-BP from t_0-BP and other baseline and follow-up risk factors for hypertension, using logistic regression models. Models were run separately for the t_0-age-group 3 to 10 years (percentile-defined t_1-hypertension) and the t_0-age-group 11 to 17 years (140/90 mmHg threshold t_1-hypertension). STATA SE14.1 was used for the analyses.

3. Results

The characteristics of the 2542 study participants (1269 males and 1273 females) at baseline (2003-2006) and six year follow-up (2009-2012) are presented in Table 1. At six-year follow-up, mean SBP had significantly increased by 14.8 mmHg in males and by 11.9 mmHg in females. In addition, the proportion of overweight in males and obesity in both sexes was at follow-up statistically significantly greater compared to baseline (Table 1).

Spearman rank-order correlations for BP tracking from childhood to adolescence/young adulthood are shown in Table 2. Tracking coefficients were higher for SBP (ranging for sex-age groups from 0.33 to 0.50) than for DBP (ranging for sex-age groups from 0.19 to 0.39). Although tracking coefficients increased with age in males, this increase was not statistically significant. Other differences between sex and age groups were as well not statistically significant.

Table 2: Spearman rank-order correlation coefficients for six year-tracking of BP in children and adolescents in Germany.

Baseline age	n	Tracking coefficients SBP	DBP
3-6 years[1]			
All	1063	0.38	0.24
Male	530	0.33	0.19
Female	533	0.44	0.30
7-10 years[1]			
All	953	0.42	0.36
Male	481	0.41	0.30
Female	472	0.42	0.42
11-14 years[2]			
All	320	0.34	0.34
Male	155	0.43	0.32
Female	165	0.36	0.38
15-17 years[2]			
All	206	0.47	0.36
Male	103	0.50	0.34
Female	103	0.46	0.39

[1] t_0-BP and t_1-BP in age-, sex-, and height-specific percentiles; [2] t_0-BP in percentiles and t_1-BP in mmHg.
All Spearman rank-order¡sup/¿correlation coefficients were statistically significant at a p-value <0.001.

The BP tracking coefficients stratified by birthweight, parental hypertension and BMI trajectories remained in the order of magnitude of the tracking coefficients for the overall sex-age groups; i.e., children with these hypertension risk factors did not have substantially higher SBP or DBP tracking correlation coefficients compared to children without these risk factors (data not shown).

We investigated the prevalence of hypertensive BP measurement at baseline and at follow-up in a younger age group (baseline age 3 to 10 years, pediatric percentile-based definition of hypertensive BP at t_1) and an older age group (baseline age 11 to 17 years, adult definition of hypertensive BP at t_1) (Figure 1). Among children aged 3 to 10 years, 7.9% (95% CI 6.7-9.1) had hypertensive BP at baseline. Of these, 39% (n = 62 out of 159) also had hypertensive BP at follow-up. The proportion of children with persistent hypertensive BP (at t_0 and t_1) accounted for 3.1% of this age group; incident hypertensive BP (children with normal BP at t_0 and hypertensive BP measurement at t_1) was observed in 11.6%; resolution of hypertensive BP (children with hypertensive BP at t_0 and a normal BP at t_1) was observed in 4.8% and the proportion of persistently normal BP in the 3- to 10-year-old group accounted for 80.5%. Among children and adolescents aged 11 to 17 years, 11.2% (95% CI 8.6-14) had hypertensive BP at baseline. Of these, 34% (n = 20 out of 59) also had hypertensive BP at follow-up. In this age group, persistent hypertensive BP accounted for 3.8%; incident hypertensive BP was observed in 12%; resolution of hypertensive BP in 7.4% and persistently normal BP in 77% of the study population (Figure 1).

The univariate and multivariable logistic regression (Table 3) showed the factors associated with having hypertensive BP at t_1. In the models for both the younger and the older age group hypertensive BP at t_0 was one of the major determinants (OR 4.25 (95% CI 2.90-6.23) and OR 3.35 (95% CI 1.60-7.01)). Further, increasing age was also identified as a risk factor for hypertensive BP at follow-up in both age groups. In the 3- to 10-year-old group, children with a persistently overweight/obesity as well as those with an incident overweight/obesity were more likely to have hypertensive BP at t_1 (OR 2.70 (95% CI 1.78-4.12) and OR 4.44 (95% CI 3.08-6.42), respectively) compared to children who had a persistently low or normal BMI. A gender difference was found only in the 11- to 17-year-old group, in which females were less likely to have hypertensive BP at t_1 compared with their male peers. Moreover, only in the 11- to 17-year-old group, parental hypertension was found to be a determinant for hypertensive BP at follow-up.

The probability of having hypertensive BP at six year follow-up increased with baseline BP percentile (Figure 2) but did not exceed 50% with the exception of a small subgroup (n = 8) of 11- to 17-year-old males having a SBP between 90th and 94.9th percentile (prehypertensive at t_0) with a probability of 88% (95% CI 47-99.7) of having hypertensive BP at t_1.

The positive (PPV) and negative predictive values (NPV) according to age at baseline and risk factors are presented in Table 4. The PPV of baseline hypertensive BP for hypertensive BP six years later was 39% (95% CI 32-46) for 3- to 10-year-old children and 34% (95% CI 24-45) for 11- to 17-year olds. The NPV of non-hypertensive baseline BP was 87% (95% CI 87-88) and 87% (95% CI 85-88) respectively. In the 3- to 10-year-old group, the PPV increased as risk factors were combined: for instance, 53% (95% CI 30-76) of 3- to 10-year-old children with a hypertensive BP and obesity at baseline also had hypertensive BP six years later. In the 11- to 17-year-old group, similar probabilities of having hypertensive BP at

TABLE 3: Predictors of hypertensive BP* at six-year follow-up in children and adolescents in Germany.

	univariable analysis		multivariable analysis	
3- to 10-year-olds (at baseline)	**OR (95% CI)**	**p-value**	**OR (95% CI)**	**p-value**
Sex				
Male	Ref	0.50	Ref	0.19
Female	1.09 (0.85-1.39)		1.21 (0.91-1.59)	
Age	1.14 (1.08-1.21)	<0.001	1.15 (1.08-1.23)	<0.001
BP t_0				
normal (<P95)	Ref	<0.001	Ref	<0.001
hypertensive (≥P95)	4.44 (3.14-6.28)		4.25 (2.90-6.23)	
BMI trajectory (t_0 to t_1)				
persistently low or normal	Ref	<0.001	Ref	<0.001
resolution	1.74 (0.96-3.16)		1.64 (0.86-3.11)	
persistently overweight/obesity	3.87 (2.67-5.61)		2.70 (1.78-4.12)	
incident overweight/obesity	3.95 (2.83-5.51)		4.44 (3.08-6.42)	
Sport activities (times/week)				
<1	Ref	0.14	Ref	0.07
1-2	1.21 (0.85-1.73)		1.30 (0.87-1.92)	
≥3	1.42 (0.99-2.02)		1.58 (1.06-2.35)	
Parental hypertension				
No	Ref	0.02	Ref	0.48
Yes	1.38 (1.06-1.80)		1.11 (0.83-1.49)	
Low birthweight (<2500g)				
No	Ref	0.59	Ref	0.69
Yes	1.14 (0.70-1.88)		1.12 (0.64-1.96)	
11- to 17-year-olds (at baseline)				
Sex				
Male	Ref	<0.001	Ref	<0.001
Female	0.37 (0.22-0.61)		0.33 (0.18-0.61)	
Age	1.22 (1.07-1.40)	<0.01	1.21 (1.03-1.42)	0.02
BP t_0				
normal (<P95)	Ref	<0.001	Ref	0.001
hypertensive (≥P95)	3.41 (1.87-6.23)		3.35 (1.60-7.01)	
BMI trajectory (t_0 to t_1)				
persistently low or normal	Ref	0.07	Ref	0.32
resolution	1.82 (0.58-5.70)		0.85 (0.17-4.19)	
persistently overweight/obesity	2.23 (1.19-4.16)		1.96 (0.89-4.29)	
incident overweight/obesity	1.50 (0.73-3.08)		1.59 (0.65-3.88)	
Physical activities (hours/week)				
≤2.0	Ref	0.24	Ref	0.42
2.1-4.9	1.76 (0.76-4.07)		1.75 (0.69-4.40)	
5.0-31.0	1.93 (0.90-4.13)		1.70 (0.74-3.91)	
Parental hypertension				
No	Ref	0.03	Ref	0.04
Yes	1.78 (1.07-2.95)		1.85 (1.02-3.33)	
Low birthweight (<2500g)				
No	Ref	0.46	Ref	0.56
Yes	0.57 (0.13-2.50)		0.62 (0.12-3.16)	

*Hypertensive BP: SBP or DBP at or above the 95th age-, sex-, and height-specific percentile for children and adolescents under 18 years or BP ≥140/90 mmHg irrespective of the percentile; for adults aged 18 or older: ≥140/90 mmHg.
OR = odds ratio BP = blood pressure.

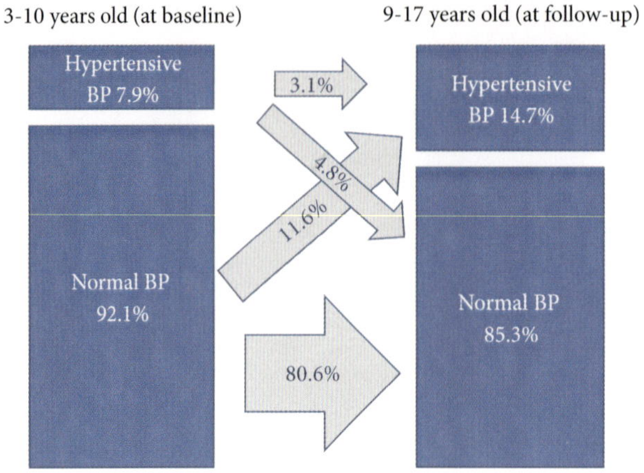

Hypertensive BP: SBP or DBP ≥95th percentile or ≥140/90 mmHg

(a) Distribution of 2016 study participants at baseline (2003-2006) and at follow-up (2009-2012) according to the BP measures

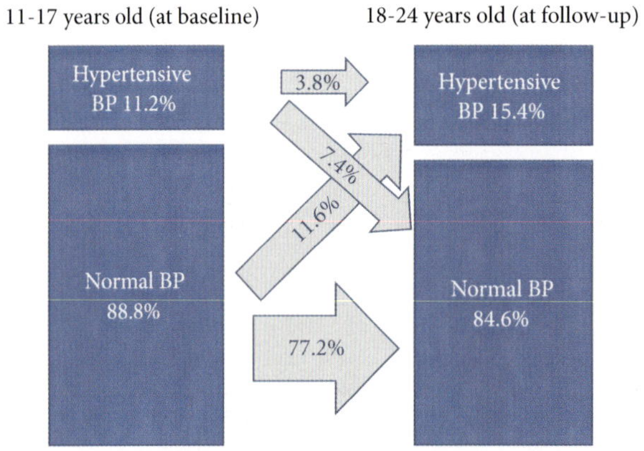

Hypertensive BP at t_0: SBP or DBP ≥95th percentile or ≥140/90 mmHg
Hypertensive BP at t_1 (≥18 year olds): ≥140/90 mmHg

(b) Distribution of 526 study participants at baseline (2003-2006) and at follow-up (2009-2012) according to the BP measures

FIGURE 1: Blood pressure in 2542 study participants at baseline (2003-2006) and at follow-up (2009-2012).

follow-up were observed in obese children at baseline (50%; 95% CI 27-74) and children with a hypertensive BP at baseline and parental hypertension (48%; 95% CI 30-67) (Table 4).

4. Discussion

This study investigates different aspects of BP tracking from childhood to adolescence/young adulthood with recent population-based data from Germany. Applying various metrics for assessing tracking including correlation coefficients, positive predictive values, and ORs from multivariable predictive modelling, BP tracking from childhood to adolescence and young adulthood was generally moderate. Our results confirm previous findings that BP in childhood and adolescence is one of the strongest predictors of future BP; however, it is one of the strongest predictors among several moderate or weak predictors. Among children and adolescents aged 3 to 17 years with hypertensive BP at baseline (mean of two measurements taken on one occasion), about one in three had hypertensive BP six years later. In population subgroups of children with additional hypertension risk factors such as overweight or parental hypertension, the PPV of baseline hypertensive BP increased but was not much higher than 50%.

In line with previous findings, we found moderate BP tracking coefficients, higher for SBP than for DBP [1–3]. Stratified by age and sex, we found a SBP tracking correlation in the range of 0.33 to 0.50 and for DBP in the range of 0.19 to 0.39, which was similar to the meta-analysis of Chen et al. [1] who found a mean correlation coefficient of 0.38 for SBP and of 0.28 for DBP.

One could ask whether BP tracking coefficients become larger among children with additional risk factors for hypertension, but in fact mathematically they are expected to remain similar or even become smaller, as verified with data from this study (results not shown). This happens since in subgroups with additional hypertension risk factors, BP values are more similar than in an unselected group and

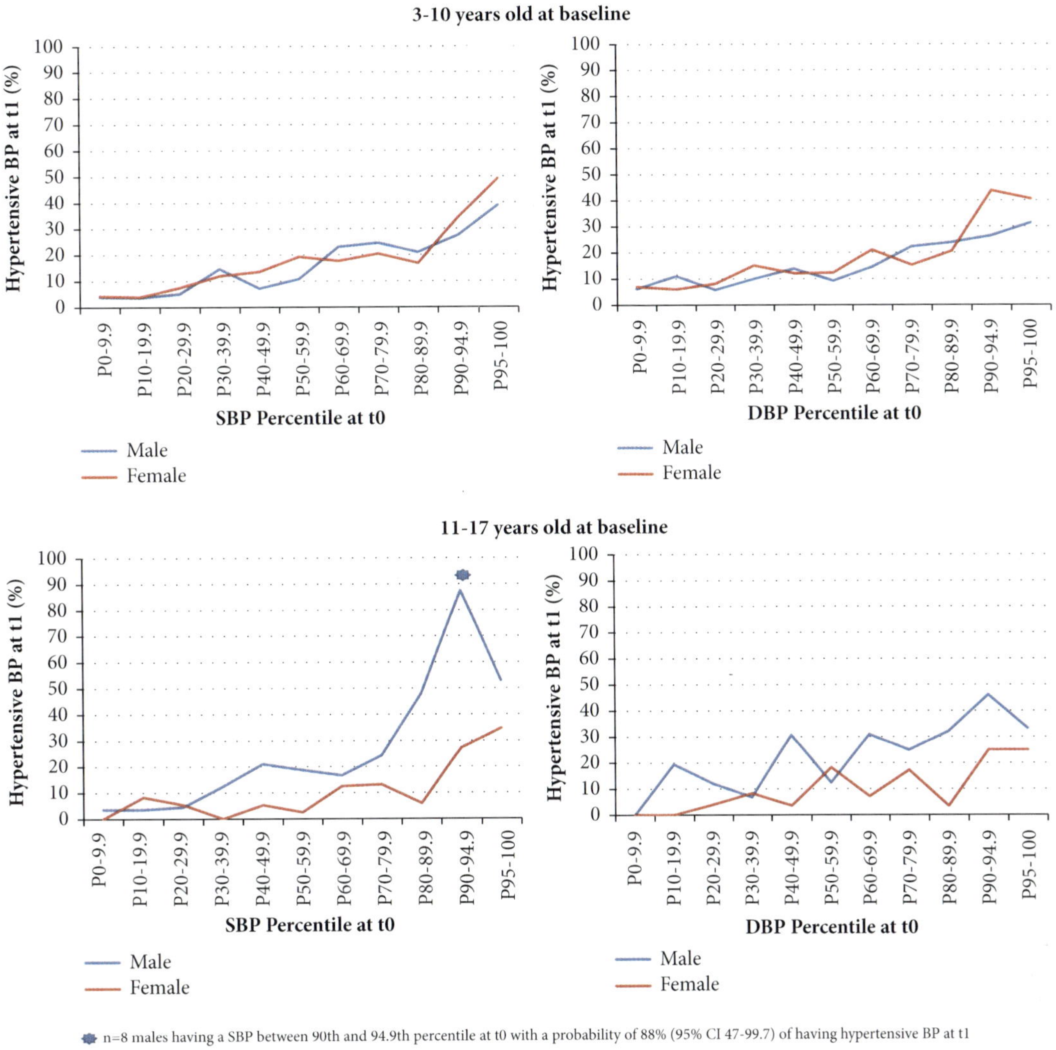

FIGURE 2: Probability of having hypertensive BP at six year follow-up (t1) according to baseline BP percentiles.

ranking to a greater extent due to chance. In other words, for combinations of risk factors, tracking coefficients are not an appropriate measure for assessing the predictability of future BP values.

Our results confirm previous findings that risk factors for hypertensive BP in young adulthood can be identified in childhood and adolescence [2, 17]. However, the associations were moderate. After adjusting for various hypertension risk factors including overweight/obesity and parental hypertension, a child aged 3 to 10 years with hypertensive BP was more likely to have hypertensive BP six years later than a child in the same age group with a normal BP (OR 4.25, 95% CI 2.90-6.23). For the age group 11 to 17 years the respective adjusted OR was 3.35 (95% CI 1.60-7.01).

The association between overweight/obesity and hypertension in children was observed in several studies [18–20]. Our study showed that 36% of 3- to 10-year-old and 50% of 11- to 17 year-old obese children at baseline had a hypertensive BP at follow-up. The multivariable logistic regression analyses revealed that 3- to 10-year-old participants with a persistently or incidentally overweight/obesity were more likely to have a hypertensive BP at follow-up compared to participants with a persistently low or normal BMI trajectory, suggesting a potential action for prevention of future hypertension. In this regard, other studies have shown that children with higher BMI at follow-up changed BP standard deviation scores from initially normal to higher BP values [21]. Moreover, it has been observed that changes in BMI during growth predicted BP levels during adolescence [22]; for instance, the study of Kelly et al. [2] showed that the resolution of elevated BP in the transition from childhood to adulthood could be partially explained by improvements in associated factors such as by decreasing the BMI z-score between childhood and adulthood.

Our univariable logistic regression analysis showed that children with hypertensive parents were at higher risk of hypertension at follow-up compared to children without hypertensive parents. However, this was only confirmed in the multivariable analysis of 11-17-year olds. Children and adolescents with parental hypertension had an 18% and

Table 4: Positive (PPV) and negative predictive value (NPV) of various hypertension risk factors or risk factor combinations for hypertensive BP* at six-year follow-up.

	n	Proportion at t_0 % (95% CI)	PPV % (95% CI)	NPV % (95% CI)
Baseline age 3 to 10 years				
Hypertensive BP at t_0	2016	7.9 (6.8-9.1)	39 (32-46)	87 (87-88)
Overweight or obesity at t_0	2011	12 (11-14)	27 (22-32)	87 (86-88)
Obesity at t_0	2011	2.2 (1.7-3.0)	36 (23-50)	86 (85-86)
Parental hypertension	1942	29 (27-31)	18 (15-20)	87 (86-88)
Hypertensive BP and overweight or obesity at t_0	2011	2.0 (1.5-2.7)	48 (33-62)	86 (86-86)
Hypertensive BP and obesity at t_0	2011	0.7 (0.4-1.2)	53 (30-76)	86 (85-86)
Hypertensive BP at t_0 and parental hypertension	1942	2.6 (2.0-3.4)	51 (38-64)	86 (86-87)
Baseline age 11 to 17 years				
Hypertensive BP at t_0	526	11 (8.8-14)	34 (24-45)	87 (85-88)
Overweight or obesity at t_0	525	17 (14-20)	24 (17-33)	87 (85-88)
Obesity at t_0	525	2.7 (1.6-4.5)	50 (27-74)	86 (85-87)
Parental hypertension	481	32 (28-36)	21 (16-26)	87 (85-89)
Hypertensive BP and overweight or obesity at t_0	525	3.2 (2.0-5.1)	35 (17-59)	85 (85-86)
Hypertensive BP and obesity at t_0	525	0.6 (0.2-1.8)	§	85 (85-85)
Hypertensive BP at t_0 and parental hypertension	481	4.8 (3.2-7.1)	48 (30-67)	86 (85-87)

§ n<=10 subjects

* Hypertensive BP: SBP or DBP at or above the 95th age-, sex-, and height-specific percentile for children and adolescents under 18 years or BP ≥140/90 mmHg irrespective of the percentile; for adults aged 18 or older: ≥140/90 mmHg.

21% probability of having a hypertensive BP at follow-up (Table 4). A familial predisposition for hypertension was reported in previous studies [23, 24]; furthermore, it has been evaluated whether BP screening should target only children with a parental hypertension instead of all children (universal screening), with the conclusion that this may not be a substantially better strategy [5].

In our data, obesity of the child/adolescent at t_0 was a significantly stronger predictor for hypertension at t_1 than parental hypertension in both age groups (Table 4).

Consistent with the literature [25–27] we observed male sex as a risk factor for hypertension in young adults: Figure 2 showed that 11- to 17-year-old males at baseline had a higher probability for having a hypertensive BP at follow-up (18 to 24 years) compared to females and Table 3 presented an OR = 0.33 (95% CI 0.18-0.61) for 11- to 17-year-old females at baseline, where they were less likely to have a hypertensive BP at follow-up compared to their male peers.

Contrary to other reports [28, 29], our study did not find a significant association between low birthweight and hypertension.

Even though we did not find significant associations between physical activity at t_0 and hypertensive BP at follow-up, our estimates showed the tendency of a negative correlation between these two variables, which is in line with other studies [30, 31].

Our study does not intend to estimate the prevalence of hypertension in children, as the diagnosis of hypertension requires, among other things, BP measurements on several occasions; however, the proportion of children and adolescents with persistently elevated BP in our study was 3.1% for 3- to 10-year olds at baseline and 3.8% for 11- to 17-year olds, which is in line with studies reporting prevalences of sustained hypertension in children and adolescents of 1% to 5% [32–34].

Major strengths of this study are the large national population database, coverage of a wide age range (3 to 17 years), the six-year follow-up, and standardized BP measurements according to the same protocol at baseline and follow-up examinations. However, despite using the same BP measurement devices, identical resting times, and the same measurement protocol, including performing BP measurements before motor performance testing, we cannot exclude the possibility that the environment and expectation of an extensive motor testing like in the MoMo study could have influenced BP at follow-up, leading to somewhat higher BP values and somewhat lower tracking indices. Another limitation is the possible selection bias arising from selective participation in the MoMo study and from longitudinal dropout. Sensitivity analyses with weights that partially account for this selection showed somewhat lower predictive values and thus did not alter the main conclusions. A further limitation is that the rule for KiGGS0 (2003-2006) was that the cuff should cover at least two-thirds of the upper arm length while current recommendations (2016 ESH guidelines [4]) suggest that the cuff size should cover 80-100% of the individual's arm circumference. Another limitation is that we had only two time points for assessment of the tracking; however, the KiGGS study just completed its second wave, allowing a future analysis of BP trajectories over a 10-year follow-up [35].

In conclusion, our analysis with recent population-based data from Germany shows that BP in children and adolescents tracks only moderately over six years; however, BP in childhood is the strongest independent predictor for future hypertensive BP measurements.

Acknowledgments

The authors thank the participants of the KiGGS and MoMo studies and all their colleagues who conducted and contributed with these studies: partial presentation of the manuscript (abstract) for DGEpi Congress 2017 in Gesundheitswesen 2017; 79(08/09): 656-804 DOI: 10.1055/s-0037-1605847. The study has been financed by the Robert Koch Institute, DZHK and the Institute for Sports and Sport Science.

References

[1] X. Chen and Y. Wang, "Tracking of blood pressure from childhood to adulthood: A systematic review and meta-regression analysis," *Circulation*, vol. 117, no. 25, pp. 3171–3180, 2008.

[2] R. K. Kelly, R. Thomson, K. J. Smith, T. Dwyer, A. Venn, and C. G. Magnussen, "Factors Affecting Tracking of Blood Pressure from Childhood to Adulthood: The Childhood Determinants of Adult Health Study," *Journal of Pediatrics*, vol. 167, no. 6, pp. 1422–1428, 2015.

[3] A. M. Toschke, L. Kohl, U. Mansmann, and R. Von Kries, "Meta-analysis of blood pressure tracking from childhood to adulthood and implications for the design of intervention trials," *Acta Paediatrica*, vol. 99, no. 1, pp. 24–29, 2010.

[4] E. Lurbe, E. Agabiti-Rosei, J. K. Cruickshank et al., "2016 European Society ofHypertension guidelines for themanagement of high blood pressure in children and adolescents," *Journal of Hypertension*, vol. 34, no. 10, pp. 1887–1920, 2016.

[5] C. Bloetzer, F. Paccaud, M. Burnier, P. Bovet, and A. Chiolero, "Performance of parental history for the targeted screening of hypertension in children," *Journal of Hypertension*, vol. 33, no. 6, pp. 1167–1173, 2015.

[6] B.-M. Kurth, P. Kamtsiuris, H. Hölling et al., "The challenge of comprehensively mapping children's health in a nation-wide health survey: Design of the German KiGGS-Study," *BMC Public Health*, vol. 8, 2008.

[7] M. O. Wagner, K. Bös, D. Jekauc et al., "Cohort Profile: The Motorik-Modul Longitudinal Study: Physical fitness and physical activity as determinants of health development in German children and adolescents," *International Journal of Epidemiology*, vol. 43, no. 5, pp. 1410–1416, 2014.

[8] M. Lange, H. G. Butschalowsky, F. Jentsch et al., "The first KiGGS follow-up (KiGGS Wave 1): Study conduct, sample design, and response," *Bundesgesundheitsblatt - Gesundheitsforschung - Gesundheitsschutz*, vol. 57, no. 7, pp. 747–761, 2014.

[9] H. Neuhauser and M. Thamm, "Blood pressure measurement in the German Health Interview and Examination Survey for Children and Adolescents (KiGGS): Methodology and initial results," *Bundesgesundheitsblatt - Gesundheitsforschung - Gesundheitsschutz*, vol. 50, no. 5-6, pp. 728–735, 2007.

[10] A. Worth, A. Woll, C. Albrecht et al., *MoMo-Längsschnittstudie ,,Physical Fitness and Physical Activity as Determinants of Health Development in Children and Adolescents*, Karlsruhe Germany: Karlsruher Institut für Technologie (KIT), 2015.

[11] H. K. Neuhauser, M. Thamm, U. Ellert, H. W. Hense, and A. S. Rosario, "Blood pressure percentiles by age and height from nonoverweight children and adolescents in Germany," *Pediatrics*, vol. 127, no. 4, pp. e978–e988, 2011.

[12] A. Hager, E. Wühl, G. Bönner, M. Hulpke-Wette, S. Läer, and J. Weil, *S2k Leitlinie Pädiatrische Kardiologie, Pädiatrische Nephrologie und Pädiatrie: Arterielle Hypertonie: Deutsche Gesellschaft für Pädiatrische Kardiologie*, 2015.

[13] T. J. Cole and T. Lobstein, "Extended international (IOTF) body mass index cut-offs for thinness, overweight and obesity," *Pediatric Obesity*, vol. 7, no. 4, pp. 284–294, 2012.

[14] K. Manz, S. Krug, A. Schienkiewitz, and J. D. Finger, "Determinants of organised sports participation patterns during the transition from childhood to adolescence in Germany: Results of a nationwide cohort study," *BMC Public Health*, vol. 16, no. 1, 2016.

[15] J. D. Finger, G. B. M. Mensink, W. Banzer, T. Lampert, and T. Tylleskär, "Physical activity, aerobic fitness and parental socioeconomic position among adolescents: The German Health Interview and Examination Survey for Children and Adolescents 2003-2006 (KiGGS)," *International Journal of Behavioral Nutrition and Physical Activity*, vol. 11, no. 1, article no. 43, 2014.

[16] B. Diedenhofen and J. Musch, "Cocor: A comprehensive solution for the statistical comparison of correlations," *PLoS ONE*, vol. 10, no. 4, 2015.

[17] R. M. Lauer and W. R. Clarke, "Childhood risk factors for high adult blood pressure: The Muscatine study," *Pediatrics*, vol. 84, no. 4, pp. 633–641, 1989.

[18] R. Din-Dzietham, Y. Liu, M.-V. Bielo, and F. Shamsa, "High blood pressure trends in children and adolescents in national surveys, 1963 to 2002," *Circulation*, vol. 116, no. 13, pp. 1488–1496, 2007.

[19] B. Falkner, S. S. Gidding, G. Ramirez-Garnica, S. A. Wiltrout, D. West, and E. B. Rappaport, "The relationship of body mass index and blood pressure in primary care pediatric patients," *Journal of Pediatrics*, vol. 148, no. 2, pp. 195–200, 2006.

[20] R.-C. Huang, S. Burrows, T. A. Mori, W. H. Oddy, and L. J. Beilin, "Lifecourse adiposity and blood pressure between birth and 17 years old," *American Journal of Hypertension*, vol. 28, no. 8, pp. 1056–1063, 2015.

[21] A. Miersch, M. Vogel, R. Gausche et al., "Blood pressure tracking in children and adolescents," *Pediatric Nephrology*, vol. 28, no. 12, pp. 2351–2359, 2013.

[22] A. Kollias, K. Pantsiotou, N. Karpettas, L. Roussias, and G. S. Stergiou, "Tracking of blood pressure from childhood to adolescence in a Greek cohort," *European Journal of Public Health*, vol. 22, no. 3, pp. 389–393, 2012.

[23] T. J. Niiranen, E. L. McCabe, M. G. Larson et al., "Risk for hypertension crosses generations in the community: Amulti-generational cohort study," *European Heart Journal*, vol. 38, no. 29, pp. 2300–2308, 2017.

[24] R. F. Theodore, J. Broadbent, D. Nagin et al., "Childhood to Early-Midlife Systolic Blood Pressure Trajectories: Early-Life Predictors, Effect Modifiers, and Adult Cardiovascular Outcomes," *Hypertension*, vol. 66, no. 6, pp. 1108–1115, 2015.

[25] H. K. Neuhauser, C. Adler, A. S. Rosario, C. Diederichs, and U. Ellert, "Hypertension prevalence, awareness, treatment and control in Germany 1998 and 2008-11," *Journal of Human Hypertension*, vol. 29, no. 4, pp. 247–253, 2015.

[26] G. Sarganas and H. K. Neuhauser, "The persisting gender gap in hypertension management and control in Germany: 1998 and 2008-2011," *Hypertension Research*, vol. 39, no. 6, pp. 457–466, 2016.

[27] K. Wolf-Maier, R. S. Cooper, J. R. Banegas et al., "Hypertension prevalence and blood pressure levels in 6 European countries, Canada, and the United States," *The Journal of the American Medical Association*, vol. 289, no. 18, pp. 2363–2369, 2003.

[28] M. Gamborg, L. Byberg, F. Rasmussen et al., "Birth weight and systolic blood pressure in adolescence and adulthood: Meta-regression analysis of sex- and age-specific results from 20 nordic studies," *American Journal of Epidemiology*, vol. 166, no. 6, pp. 634–645, 2007.

[29] M. Mu, S.-F. Wang, J. Sheng et al., "Birth weight and subsequent blood pressure: A meta-analysis," *Archives of Cardiovascular Diseases*, vol. 105, no. 2, pp. 99–113, 2012.

[30] L. B. Andersen, "Tracking of risk factors for coronary heart disease from adolescence to young adulthood with special emphasis on physical activity and fitness. A longitudinal study," *Danish Medical Journal*, vol. 43, no. 5, pp. 407–418, 1996.

[31] D. A. Jenner, R. Vandongen, and L. J. Beilin, "Relationships between blood pressure and measures of dietary energy intake, physical fitness, and physical activity in Australian children aged 11-12 years," *Journal of Epidemiology and Community Health*, vol. 46, no. 2, pp. 108–113, 1992.

[32] B. Falkner, "Hypertension in children and adolescents: epidemiology and natural history," *Pediatric Nephrology*, vol. 25, no. 7, pp. 1219–1224, 2010.

[33] A. R. Marras, P. P. Bassareo, and M. Ruscazio, "The prevalence of paediatric hypertension, emphasising the need to use specific population references: The Sardinian Hypertensive Adolescents Research Programme Study," *Cardiology in the Young*, vol. 19, no. 3, pp. 233–238, 2009.

[34] P. P. Bassareo and G. Mercuro, "Pediatric hypertension: An update on a burning problem," *World Journal of Cardiology*, vol. 6, no. 5, p. 253, 2014.

[35] E. Mauz, A. Gößwald, P. Kamtsiuris et al. et al., "New data for action. Data collection for KiGGS Wave 2 has been completed," *Journal of Health Monitoring*, vol. 2, pp. 2–27, 2017.

26

Blood Pressure and Haematological Indices in Twelve Communities in Ashanti, Ghana

Jacob Plange-Rhule,[1,2] Sally M. Kerry,[3] John B. Eastwood,[1] Frank B. Micah,[4] Sampson Antwi,[5] and Francesco P. Cappuccio[6]

[1]*Division of Clinical Sciences, Renal Medicine, St George's, University of London, Cranmer Terrace, London SW17 0RE, UK*
[2]*School of Medical Sciences, Kwame Nkrumah University of Science and Technology, Kumasi, Ghana*
[3]*Blizard Institute, Barts and The London School of Medicine and Dentistry, Queen Mary University of London, 58 Turner Street, London E1 2AB, UK*
[4]*Department of Medicine, Komfo Anokye Teaching Hospital, P.O. Box 1934, Kumasi, Ghana*
[5]*Department of Paediatrics, Komfo Anokye Teaching Hospital, P.O. Box 1934, Kumasi, Ghana*
[6]*Division of Health Sciences, Warwick Medical School, University of Warwick, Gibbet Hill Road, Coventry CV4 &AL, UK*

Correspondence should be addressed to Jacob Plange-Rhule; jprhule@gmail.com

Academic Editor: Franco Veglio

Hypertension is the most important risk factor for cardiovascular mortality and morbidity in Sub-Saharan Africa. In western populations, high haemoglobin levels are associated with raised BP unlike in Sub-Saharan Africa where there is a paucity of data. Our study examines the association between haematological indices with BP variables. Weight, height, BP, and whole blood indices of viscosity (Hb, haematocrit, RBC count, and MCV) were measured in 921 adults (340 men, 581 women; aged 40–75) in 12 communities in Ghana. Mean values for Hb (12.3 g/dl ± 1.7 SD), haematocrit (36.7% ± 5.2), RBC (4.10 million/μL ± 0.64), and MCV were lower than reference values used in Sub-Saharan Africa. Mean BMI was 21.1 ± 4.1 indicating a lean population. Systolic BP increased by 1.0 mmHg (95% CI 0.5–1.5), $p < 0.001$, for women and 0.5 (0.1–1.0), $p = 0.027$, for men per unit increase in haematocrit. Similar relationships were found for Hb and RBC but not for MCV or platelets. The relationships were weaker when adjusted for BMI, 0.7 mmHg (0.2–1.2) in women and 0.5 (0.0–1.0) in men. Findings for diastolic BP were similar. Overall haematological indices were low. We have found a significant, positive relationship between BP, Hb, Haematocrit, and RBC count in our population.

1. Introduction

Cardiovascular disease has become an important cause of premature death and disability in Sub-Saharan Africa [1, 2]. Hypertension is known to be the major contributor [3] and is itself a consequence of increasing urbanisation and an increasingly western lifestyle, exemplified by increasing obesity, higher salt intake, and a sedentary lifestyle.

Another contributory factor to hypertension may be blood viscosity. Plasma and whole blood viscosity have been suggested as important determinants of arterial blood pressure [4–9] both in normotensive individuals and in those with untreated hypertension. Others, meanwhile, have suggested that both blood pressure and viscosity are themselves secondary to factors such as obesity, mental stress, smoking, and physical inactivity [10]. Nonetheless, it is possible that whole blood viscosity plays a part in the genesis of stroke and coronary artery disease [11–15] and cardiac hypertrophy [16]. Of the factors contributing to whole blood viscosity, haematocrit, red cell aggregability, red cell rigidity, and plasma viscosity, haematocrit is thought to be the most important, being responsible for at least 70% of the contribution [17]. However, others have not found a correlation between blood pressure and blood viscosity in normotensives [18, 19].

Most of the evidence relating blood pressure to blood viscosity is derived from studies from the developed world. There is very little data on the relationship between blood pressure and blood viscosity from Sub-Saharan Africa [20].

In Sub-Saharan Africa, individuals have lower haemoglobin, RBC count and haematocrit [21, 22] as a result of chronic infection, malaria, and malnutrition so blood viscosity is likely to be reduced. The question is whether blood viscosity, even within the lower ranges of haemoglobin found in Sub-Saharan Africa, exhibits any relationship to blood pressure.

The study described here examines the association of haematological indices (haemoglobin, haematocrit, mean cell volume, and red cell count) with BP variables in a population-based sample of Ghanaians, with a view to determine any relation between blood viscosity and systolic and diastolic blood pressure and to explore whether any such relationships are explained by differences in body mass index (BMI).

2. Methods

2.1. Population. Adults aged 40–75 years from 12 communities (6 semiurban, 6 rural) in the Ejisu-Juaben and Kumasi Districts of the Ashanti region of Ghana took part in the study.

In brief, there were 16,965 individuals [6,597 rural, 10,368 semiurban] living in 1,460 households [750 in rural and 710 in semiurban communities]. The 12 communities had an average population [all ages] of 1,414 per community [range 562–1,966]. The adult population [≥16 years of age] was 38% in rural and 33% in semiurban communities. The population structure of these communities was comparable to that reported for Ghana as a whole. There were 2,743 adults aged 40–75 years [23]. A stratified random sample of 1,896 inhabitants aged 40–75 years was invited to take part in the study. Stratification was by age and sex within community so that the total sample selected matched the overall population structure, and there were no differences between the communities in the age and sex distribution. The proportion of the invited community population varied according to community size, with a higher proportion in smaller communities [24].

The original study referred to above [24] was intended to determine prevalence, participant awareness, treatment, and control of blood pressure and to study the effect of dietary salt reduction advice on urinary sodium and blood pressure (Control and Intervention Communities) [25].

Since this was an intervention study we chose the lower end of the age-range to be 40 years of age. This was to minimise any risk of pregnancy and its complications in participants in the "reduced salt intake" (Intervention) communities. The upper end of the age-range of 75 years was chosen as there was a steep fall in numbers of potential participants in the older age groups.

2.2. Questionnaire. The participants attended a registration centre set up in their community. After obtaining written informed consent, each participant was helped to complete a questionnaire to obtain information on demographic background and medical history. The Committee on Human Research Publication and Ethics of the School of Medical Sciences, Kwame Nkrumah University of Science and Technology, Kumasi, Ghana, and the Ethics Committee of St George's Healthcare NHS Trust, London, UK approved the study protocol.

2.3. Measurements. Height was measured without shoes using a wooden platform and a height rule to the nearest 0.5 cm. Weight was measured to the nearest 0.5 kg with manual Seca 761 scales (Vogel & Halke, Germany) after the participants had removed their outer garments and footwear. BMI was calculated as weight (kg) divided by the square of height (m^2).

After participants had been in a relaxed sitting position for 5 minutes, blood pressure was measured using an automatic device (OMRON HEM705CP sphygmomanometer; Omron Matsusaka Co. Ltd, Japan). The appropriate cuff size (13×23 cm or 16×30 cm) was used. Three readings were taken one minute apart; the first was discarded, and the mean of the second and third readings was used in the analysis [25].

2.3.1. Fasting Blood Samples. A fasting venous blood sample was taken from each participant. The samples were put into EDTA-containing vacutainer tubes and transported without delay to Komfo Anokye Teaching Hospital and refrigerated at 4°C until analysed for full blood count, haemoglobin (Hb), packed cell volume (PCV)/haematocrit, mean corpuscular volume (MCV), red cell count (RBC), and platelets using the Cell-Dyn 3700 Haematology Analyzer (Abbott Diagnostics) and also for fasting blood glucose. A diagnosis of diabetes was made if a single fasting blood glucose sample was >7.0 mmol/L or the participant was on treatment for diabetes.

2.4. Statistics. Men and women were compared using a random effects model. First the relationship between each viscosity variable and blood pressure was estimated using random effects regression in both men and women separately, and allowing for clustering by community. Age, BMI, and smoking were then added to the model. BMI was fitted as a linear and quadratic term as previous research has shown this relationship may not be linear and a quadratic term gives a better fit [26, 27]. Interactions terms were added to see if the relationship between blood pressure and viscosity was significantly different in men and women. The relationships between blood pressure and age and body mass index tend to be different in men and women in this population [26]. Interactions terms with sex were fitted for all main effect. Regression coefficients for the relationship between blood pressure and each viscosity are presented with 95% confidence intervals. Mean values of systolic and diastolic blood pressure were calculated for each quintile of haematocrit for men and women separately and displayed graphically.

Blood pressure readings were adjusted for time of day [25]. Summary statistics are given as mean (SD). p values less than 0.05 were considered significant.

All analyses were conducted using Stata Statistical Software (StataCorp. Stata statistical software: release 4.0. College Station, TX: StatCorp; 1995).

3. Results

Of the 1,896 subjects invited to participate, 1,013 took part in the study. Full haematological measurements were available

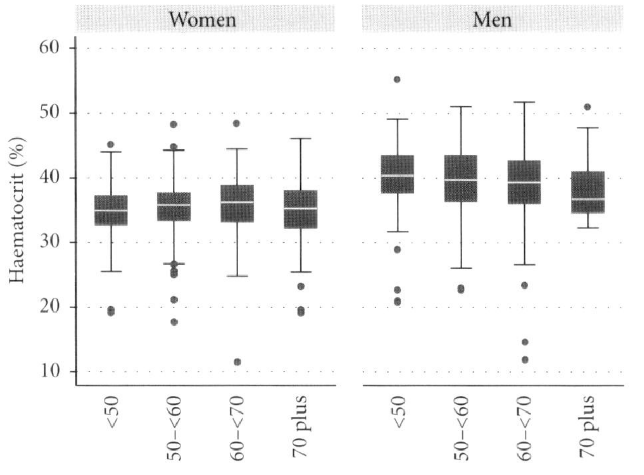

FIGURE 1: Haematocrit by age and sex; box and whisker plot showing median and interquartile range of haematocrit by age for 340 men and 581 women.

in 921 (340 men, 581 women). The majority of the participants (94%) were from the Ashanti tribe. Farming and trading were the main occupations [23].

Mean values for all haematological indices except MCV were at or below the bottom of the corresponding reference range (Table 1) and some individuals had values well below the normal ranges (Figure 1). Whilst haematocrit falls with age in men, it first rises and then falls in women (Figure 1).

Overall haematocrit, haemoglobin, red blood count, and mean corpuscular volume were significantly higher in men than in women.

Mean BMI was 21.1 (4.1) kg/m^2. BMI, though relatively low in both, was higher in the women than the men (21.6 v 20.3 kg/m^2 $p < 0.05$); mean blood pressure was 128 (26) mmHg (systolic) and 76 (13) mmHg (diastolic); both systolic and diastolic blood pressures were similar in men and women.

Table 2 shows all the models used in our study to investigate the relationship between measures of blood viscosity and blood pressure. For women, systolic blood pressure increased by 1.0 mm Hg for each unit increase in haematocrit. (95% confidence interval 0.5 to 1.5); $p < 0.001$. After adjusting for age and body mass index, the figure fell to 0.7 mmHg per unit increase in haematocrit (95% CI 0.2 to 1.2); $p = 0.004$. Similar relationships were found for haemoglobin and red blood count with both systolic and diastolic blood pressure.

Slopes in the women were consistently steeper than in the men but none of the interactions achieved statistical significance.

There was no evidence of a relationship with blood pressure for either mean corpuscular volume or platelets (Table 2). Adjusting for age, body mass index and smoking in men did not alter these findings (data not shown).

Figure 2 shows the mean blood pressure for quintiles of haematocrit. The data indicate that where men and women have the same values for haematocrit, the slopes of blood pressure are similar. However, for higher values of haematocrit, the rise in BP with a unit increase in haematocrit is less than at lower values.

The relationship between blood pressure and mean corpuscular volume or platelet count was not statistically significant for either men or women. Smoking rates among the participants were low and those that smoked only smoked an average of 4 cigarettes a day. Adjusting for smoking made a negligible difference to the relationships between blood pressure and viscosity.

4. Discussion

In our study, in 12 communities in the Ashanti Region of Ghana, we have described the haematological indices for healthy Ghanaians. We have shown that the subjects had low levels of haematocrit and haemoglobin, with values similar to what has been in found in populations in other countries in Sub-Saharan Africa [28, 29]. The haematological indices reported in this study are low in comparison to the frequently quoted reference ranges determined from studies in the developed world [30, 31].

In this population, in both men and women, we have shown a significant increase in both systolic and diastolic blood pressure with higher values of haematocrit, haemoglobin, and red blood count even after allowing for age and body mass index. Systolic blood pressure increased by 1.0 (0.5 to 1.5) mm Hg for each unit increase in haematocrit for women and 0.5 (0.1 to 1.0). After adjusting for age and body mass index, the figure fell to 0.7 (0.2 to 1.2) mmHg per one percent increase in haematocrit in women but remained unchanged at 0.5 (0.0 to 1.0) in men.

A number of studies have demonstrated that both measured blood viscosity and haematocrit increased with increasing blood pressure [4, 13]; and haematocrit correlated significantly with both systolic and diastolic blood pressure [13, 32]. The relationship was true both in normotensives and in untreated hypertensives. In a population study, a similar relationship was found between haematocrit and blood pressure with mean haematocrit being significantly higher in hypertensives than in normotensives for both sexes, after adjusting for age [33]. In this study untreated hypertensives and drug-treated hypertensives were found to have similar haematocrit but a significantly lower blood pressure in the treated group. This finding persisted on exclusion of hypertensives treated with diuretics from the analysis. Thus, the possible diuretic treatment-induced reductions in plasma volume did not seem to have any effect on mean haematocrit in this group.

Devereux et al. [10] found that whole blood viscosity was higher in untreated hypertensives than in normotensives. However, the authors failed to find a relationship between haematocrit and whole blood viscosity in their hypertensive subjects. One possible explanation for this in our study could be that mechanisms other than through a raised whole blood viscosity may be responsible for the positive association between blood pressure and blood haematocrit described in our study. Indeed, important factors contributing to whole blood viscosity other than haematocrit are circulating fibrinogen, red cell aggregation, and red cell deformability. Support for the effect of fibrinogen in raising blood pressure was suggested by Fowkes et al. [7], an association that was found to be independent of smoking, alcohol intake, and BMI.

TABLE 1: Height, weight, BMI, and systolic and diastolic BP versus gender. Results are means (SD).

		Men (n = 340)	Women (n = 581)	All (n = 921)
Age	Years	54.6 (10.8)	54.9 (11.6)	54.8 (11.3)
Height	Cm	167 (7)***	157 (7)	160 (8)
Weight	Kg	56 (10)***	53 (12)	54 (11)
BMI	kg/m^2	20.2 (3.0)***	21.6 (4.6)	21.1 (4.1)
Systolic BP	mm Hg	128 (25)	128 (27)	128 (26)
Diastolic BP	mm Hg	77 (14)	76 (13)	76 (13)
Current smoker	n (%)	64 (19)	1 (0)	65 (7)
Haematocrit/packed cell volume	%	39.3 (5.5)***	35.2 (4.4)	36.7 (5.2)
Haemoglobin	g/dL	13.2 (1.9)***	11.8 (1.4)	12.3 (1.7)
Red blood count	$\times 10^{12}/L$	4.33 (0.69)***	3.96 (0.58)	4.10 (0.64)
Mean corpuscular volume	Fl	91.0 (8.5)**	89.5 (7.7)	90.0 (8.0)
Platelets	$\times 10^{12}/L$	160 (90)*	175 (89)	169 (89)

Significance tests for *Men* versus *Women* given under *Men*. $^{*}p < 0.05$; $^{**}p < 0.01$; $^{***}p < 0.001$.

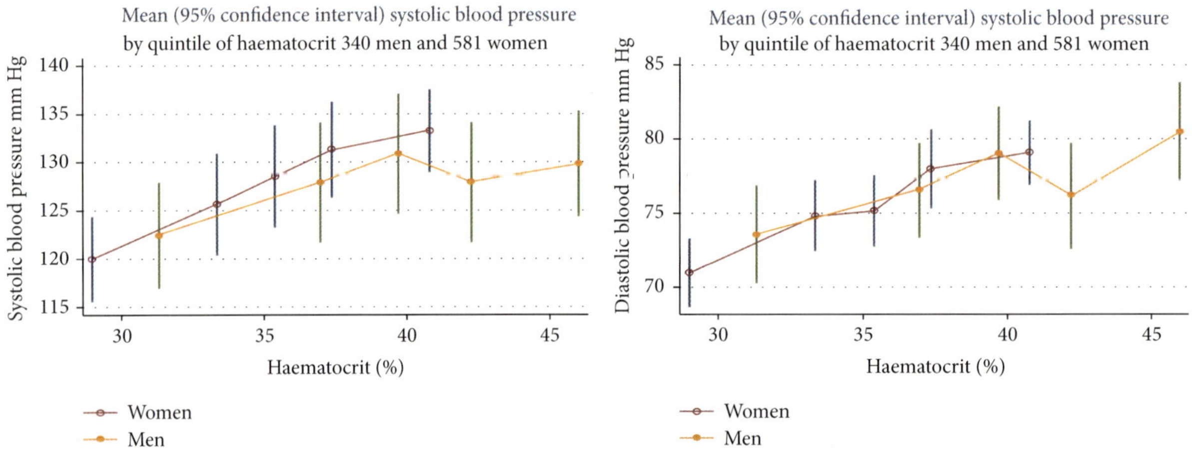

FIGURE 2: Mean blood pressure by quintile of haematocrit for men and women.

Salazar-Vazquez et al. [34], in a study of diabetics, found a statistically significant U-shaped/bimodal relationship between haematocrit and mean arterial blood pressure; the control subjects showed a nonsignificant increase in blood pressure with an increase in haematocrit. In contrast, De Simone et al. [6] have shown an inverse relationship between systolic blood pressure and whole blood viscosity and haematocrit in a homogeneous population of American Indians greater than 80% of who were either overweight or frankly obese and many of whom were Type II diabetics (43%) or smokers (30%). They demonstrated no relationship between diastolic blood pressure and haematocrit. The high percentage of Type II diabetes mellitus and smoking in the population used in the study by De Simone et al. [6] may have influenced the measures of blood viscosity and hence the relationship between blood viscosity and hypertension.

In summary, our data support those of Gori et al. [5] but do not support either a U-shaped curve [31] or an inverse relationship between blood pressure and haematocrit [6].

Our study was carried out in a group of unselected individuals from African communities. The population was unusually homogeneous (94% Ashanti tribe) and lean and only 30 of the 921 participants were taking antihypertensive drugs. We have therefore been able to observe the relationship between blood pressure and indirect measures of viscosity virtually uninfluenced by ethnic differences and drug treatment. Few participants in the study suffered from diabetes (4.0%) and smoking rates were relatively low (7%) so the possible influence of smoking and diabetes mellitus on haematocrit and the results of this study were minimised.

In our study, we used haemoglobin, haematocrit, and red blood cell count as indirect measures of blood viscosity to assess the relationship between viscosity and blood pressure and did not determine whole blood viscosity. We also did not measure plasma proteins.

The importance of our study is that it details the haematological indices of healthy Africans. As many of the values fall outside the standard reference values in common use in

Table 2: Systolic BP and diastolic BP (adjusted and unadjusted for BMI) by gender versus measures of viscosity: regression coefficients.

	Men ($n = 340$)	Women ($n = 581$)	Interaction[5] ($n = 921$)
Systolic blood pressure			
Haematocrit (%)			
Haematocrit only[1]	0.54 (0.06 to 1.01)*	1.00 (0.51 to 1.49)***	0.47 (−0.22 to 1.16)
Adjusted for age[2]	0.67 (0.20 to 1.14)**	0.91 (0.44 to 1.37)***	0.24 (−0.42 to 0.90)
Adjusted for age, BMI[3]	0.50 (0.03 to 0.97)*	0.69 (0.22 to 1.15)***	0.17 (−0.50 to 0.83)
Adjusted for age, BMI, smoking[4]	0.49 (0.02 to 0.96)*	#	#
Haemoglobin (g/dL)			
Haemoglobin only[1]	1.58 (0.16 to 3.00)*	3.43 (1.90 to 4.95)***	1.85 (−0.23 to 3.94)
Adjusted for age[2]	2.03 (0.63 to 3.44)**	3.33 (1.90 to 4.76)***	1.33 (−0.67 to 3.33)
Adjusted for age, BMI[3]	1.46 (0.05 to 2.87)*	2.73 (1.27 to 4.19)***	1.25 (−0.78 to 3.29)
Adjusted for age, BMI, smoking	1.47 (0.06 to 2.87)*	#	#
Red blood count ($\times 10^{12}$/L)			
Red blood count only[1]	4.6 (0.8 to 8.4)*	7.3 (3.6 to 11.0)***	2.70 (−2.67 to 8.07)
Adjusted for age[2]	5.7 (2.0 to 9.5)**	7.0 (3.5 to 10.4)***	1.27 (−3.89 to 6.43)
Adjusted for age, BMI[3]	4.3 (0.6 to 8.1)*	5.5 (2.0 to 9.0)***	1.20 (−4.01 to 6.37)
Adjusted for age, BMI, smoking	4.3 (0.6 to 8.1)*	#	#
Mean corpuscular volume (fL)			
Mean corpuscular volume only	−0.04 (−0.36 to 0.27)	−0.09 (−0.38 to 0.20)	0.03 (−0.40 to 0.45)
Platelets ($\times 10^{12}$/L)			
Platelets only	0.01 (−0.02 to 0.04)	−0.01 (−0.03 to 0.02)	0.02 (−0.02 to 0.06)
Diastolic blood pressure			
Haematocrit (%)			
Haematocrit only[1]	0.44 (0.18 to 0.71)***	0.66 (0.42 to 0.90)***	0.19 (−0.16 to 0.54)
Adjusted for age[2]	0.45 (0.19 to 0.72)***	0.64 (0.40 to 0.88)***	0.15 (−0.20 to 0.50)
Adjusted for age, BMI[3]	0.36 (0.09 to 0.62)**	0.51 (0.27 to 0.75)***	0.11 (−0.24 to 0.46)
Adjusted for age, BMI, smoking	0.35 (0.08 to 0.61)**	#	#
Haemoglobin (g/dL)			
Haemoglobin only[1]	1.36 (0.58 to 2.14)***	2.25 (1.51 to 2.99)***	0.90 (−0.16 to 1.96)
Adjusted for age[2]	1.40 (0.61 to 2.19)***	2.23 (1.50 to 2.96)***	0.83 (−0.22 to 1.89)
Adjusted for age, BMI[3]	1.07 (0.27 to 1.86)**	1.82 (1.07 to 2.56)***	0.77 (−0.31 to 1.84)
Adjusted for age, BMI, smoking	1.09 (0.30 to 1.88)**	#	#
Red blood count ($\times 10^{12}$/L)			
Red blood count only[1]	3.50 (1.40 to 5.60)***	4.38 (2.57 to 6.20)***	0.85 (−1.90 to 3.60)
Adjusted for age[2]	3.61 (1.48 to 5.74)***	4.31 (2.52 to 6.11)***	0.65 (−2.10 to 3.39)
Adjusted for age, BMI[3]	2.83 (0.71 to 4.96)**	3.33 (1.53 to 5.12)***	0.44 (−2.31 to 3.19)
Adjusted for age, BMI, smoking	2.83 (0.71 to 4.95)**	#	#
Mean corpuscular volume (fL)			
Mean corpuscular volume only	−0.03 (−0.20 to 0.14)	−0.02 (−0.16 to 0.13)	−0.00 (−0.22 to 0.22)
Platelets ($\times 10^{12}$/L)			
Platelets only	0.00 (−0.01 to 0.02)	0.00 (−0.01 to 0.02)	−0.00 (−0.02 to 0.02)

[1]Model: $BP = \beta_0 + \beta_1 \times V$ where V is viscosity variable; [2]Model: $BP = \beta_0 + \beta_1 \times V + \beta_2 \times \text{age}$; [3]Model: $BP = \beta_0 + \beta_1 \times V + \beta_2 \times \text{age} + \beta_3 \times BMI + \beta_4 \times BMI^2$; [4]Model: $BP = \beta_0 + \beta_1 \times V + \beta_2 \times \text{age} + \beta_3 \times BMI + \beta_4 \times BMI^2 + \beta_3 \times \text{smoking}$; [5]Model includes all interactions with sex for main effects in model. #There was only one female smoker hence there is no regression coefficient given for adjusting for smoking in women; $^{*}p < 0.05$; $^{**}p < 0.01$; $^{***}p < 0.001$.

Ghana, there will be implications for clinical decision-making and patient care.

Currently, anaemia is common in many populations in Sub-Saharan Africa but as Africa-wide public health initiatives directed at improving health begin to take effect it is likely that the prevalence of anaemia will fall, particularly in women. If the relationship between blood pressure and haematocrit is causal then the correction of anaemia will tend to be accompanied by a population rise in blood pressure. Such an increase in blood pressure is likely to be exacerbated by the continuing migration of rural Africans to cities, with the consequent accompanying increase in body mass index. The importance of our results is that higher levels of haematological indices are associated with higher blood pressure independent of BMI.

We hope that the findings of this study will inform the WHO, Governments, and other policy-makers in formulating their plans for reducing the burden of noncommunicable diseases, especially hypertension, in Africa.

5. Conclusions

We have measured haematological indices in healthy Ghanaians living in rural and semiurban communities and found that the values are significantly lower than reference values originating in the developed world but in current use in most of Sub-Saharan Africa.

We have found that blood pressure rises as blood viscosity measured by indirect measures (haemoglobin, haematocrit, and red cell count) rises for both men and women.

Authors' Contributions

Francesco P. Cappuccio, Sally M. Kerry, Jacob Plange-Rhule, and John B. Eastwood contributed to fund raising, idea for and design of the study, collection of data, and interpretation of results. Jacob Plange-Rhule and John B. Eastwood drafted the paper. Frank B. Micah and Sampson Antwi contributed to collection of data and interpretation of results. All authors contributed to the critical revision of the paper. Francesco P. Cappuccio had full access to all the data in the study and takes responsibility for the integrity of the data and the accuracy of the data analysis.

Acknowledgments

The authors thank the many workers in Ghana who have contributed to the study whose names are listed elsewhere [19]. They would also like to thank the Chiefs and Elders of the 12 communities for their help. The study was supported by The Wellcome Trust (060415/Z/00/Z). Frank B. Micah was supported by a Wellcome Trust Master's Research Training Fellowship (069500/Z/02/Z).

References

[1] M. A. B. van der Sande, H. M. Inskip, K. O. Jaiteh et al., "Changing causes of death in the West African town of Banjul, 1942–19497," *Bulletin of the World Health Organization*, vol. 79, pp. 133–141, 2001.

[2] S. Kadiri, "Tackling cardiovascular disease in Africa," *British Medical Journal*, vol. 331, no. 7519, pp. 711-712, 2005.

[3] R. S. Cooper and A. G. Amoah, "High blood pressure: the foundation for epidemic cardiovascular disease in African populations," *Ethnicity & Disease*, vol. 13, no. 2, supplement 2, pp. S48–S52, 2003.

[4] J. O. Mugisha, K. Baisley, G. Asiki, J. Seeley, and H. Kuper, "Prevalence, Types, Risk Factors and Clinical Correlates of Anaemia in Older People in a Rural Ugandan Population," *PLoS ONE*, vol. 8, no. 10, Article ID e78394, 2013.

[5] T. Gori, P. S. Wild, R. Schnabel et al., "The distribution of whole blood viscosity, its determinants and relationship with arterial blood pressure in the community: Cross-sectional analysis from the Gutenberg Health Study," *Therapeutic Advances in Cardiovascular Disease*, vol. 9, no. 6, pp. 354–365, 2015.

[6] G. De Simone, R. B. Devereux, M. Chinali, L. G. Best, E. T. Lee, and T. K. Welty, "Association of blood pressure with blood viscosity in American Indians: The Strong Heart Study," *Hypertension*, vol. 45, no. 4, pp. 625–630, 2005.

[7] F. G. R. Fowkes, G. D. O. Lowe, A. Rumley, S. E. Lennie, F. B. Smith, and P. T. Donnan, "The relationship between blood viscosity and blood pressure in a random sample of the population aged 55 to 74 years," *European Heart Journal*, vol. 14, no. 5, pp. 597–601, 1993.

[8] F. Atsma, I. Veldhuizen, W. De Kort, M. Van Kraaij, P. Pasker-De Jong, and J. Deinum, "Hemoglobin level is positively associated with blood pressure in a large cohort of healthy individuals," *Hypertension*, vol. 60, no. 4, pp. 936–941, 2012.

[9] S.-G. Lee, J. H. Rim, and J.-H. Kim, "Association of hemoglobin levels with blood pressure and hypertension in a large population-based study: The Korea National Health and Nutrition Examination Surveys 2008-2011," *Clinica Chimica Acta*, vol. 438, pp. 12–18, 2015.

[10] R. B. Devereux, D. B. Case, M. H. Alderman, T. G. Pickerung, S. Chien, and J. H. Laragh, "Possible role of increased blood viscosity in the hemodynamics of systemic hypertension," *American Journal of Cardiology*, vol. 85, pp. 1265–1267, 2000.

[11] L. Bogar, "Hemorheology and hypertension: Not "chicken or egg" but two chickens from similar eggs," *Clinical Hemorheology and Microcirculation*, vol. 26, no. 2, pp. 81–83, 2002.

[12] G. D. O. Lowe, A. J. Lee, A. Rumley, J. F. Price, and F. G. R. Fowkes, "Blood viscosity and risk of cardiovascular events: the Edinburgh Artery Study," *British Journal of Haematology*, vol. 96, no. 1, pp. 168–173, 1997.

[13] W. Koenig, M. Sund, B. Filipiak, A. Döring, H. Löwel, and E. Ernst, "Plasma viscosity and the risk of coronary heart disease: Results from the MONICA-Augsburg cohort study, 1984 to 1992," *Arteriosclerosis, Thrombosis, and Vascular Biology*, vol. 18, no. 5, pp. 768–772, 1998.

[14] W. Koenig, M. Sund, H. Löwel, A. Döring, and E. Ernst, "Association between plasma viscosity and all-cause mortality: Results from the MONICA-Augsburg Cohort study 1984-92," *British Journal of Haematology*, vol. 109, no. 2, pp. 453–458, 2000.

[15] J. Danesh, R. Collins, R. Peto, and G. D. O. Lowe, "Haematocrit, viscosity, erythrocyte sedimentation rate: meta-analyses of prospective studies of coronary heart disease," *European Heart Journal*, vol. 21, no. 7, pp. 515–520, 2000.

[16] R. B. Devereux, J. I. M. Drayer, S. Chien et al., "Whole blood viscosity as a determinant of cardiac hypertrophy in systemic hypertension," *American Journal of Cardiology*, vol. 54, no. 6, pp. 592–595, 1984.

[17] G. De Simone, R. B. Devereux, S. Chien, M. H. Alderman, S. A. Atlas, and J. H. Laragh, "Relation of blood viscosity to demographic and physiologic variables and to cardiovascular risk factors in apparently normal adults," *Circulation*, vol. 81, no. 1, pp. 107–117, 1990.

[18] B. Y. S. Vázquez, "Blood pressure and blood viscosity are not correlated in normal healthy subjects," *Vascular Health and Risk Management*, vol. 8, no. 1, pp. 1–6, 2012.

[19] C. Irace, F. Scavelli, A. Loprete, and V. Merante, "Lack of association between systolic blood pressure and blood viscosity in normotensive healthy subjects," *Clinical Hemorheology and Microcirculation*, vol. 51, no. 1, pp. 35–41, 2012.

[20] J. B. Rasmussen, D. L. Mwaniki, L. U. Kaduka et al., "Hemoglobin levels and blood pressure are associated in rural black africans," *American Journal of Human Biology*, vol. 28, no. 1, pp. 145–148, 2016.

[21] S. Tatala, U. Svanberg, and B. Mduma, "Low dietary iron availability is a major cause of anemia: A nutrition survey in the Lindi District of Tanzania," *American Journal of Clinical Nutrition*, vol. 68, no. 1, pp. 171–178, 1998.

[22] O. A. Awodu and A. A. Famodu, "Haemostatic variables and their relationship to body mass index and blood pressure in adult Nigerians with the sickle cell trait," *Clinical Hemorheology and Microcirculation*, vol. 36, no. 1, pp. 89–94, 2007.

[23] J. Plange-Rhule, F. P. Cappuccio, L. Emmett et al., "A community study of health promotion in rural West Africa: Details of a household survey and population census," *QJM: Monthly Journal of the Association of Physicians*, vol. 95, no. 7, pp. 445–450, 2002.

[24] F. P. Cappuccio, F. B. Micah, L. Emmett et al., "Prevalence, detection, management, and control of hypertension in Ashanti, West Africa," *Hypertension*, vol. 43, no. 5, pp. 1017–1022, 2004.

[25] F. P. Cappuccio, S. M. Kerry, F. B. Micah, J. Plange-Rhule, and J. B. Eastwood, "A community programme to reduce salt intake and blood pressure in Ghana," *BMC Public Health*, vol. 6, article 13, pp. 1–11, 2006.

[26] S. M. Kerry, F. B. Micah, J. Plange-Rhule, J. B. Eastwood, and F. P. Cappuccio, "Blood pressure and body mass index in lean rural and semi-urban subjects in West Africa," *Journal of Hypertension*, vol. 23, no. 9, pp. 1645–1651, 2005.

[27] J. S. Kaufman, M. C. Asuzu, J. Mufunda et al., "Relationship between blood pressure and body mass index in lean populations," *Hypertension*, vol. 30, no. 6, pp. 1511–1516, 1997.

[28] E. S. Lugada, J. Mermin, and F. Kaharuza, "Population-based hematologic and immunologic reference values for a healthy Ugandan population," *Clinical and Diagnostic Laboratory Immunology*, vol. 11, no. 1, pp. 29–34, 2004.

[29] E. Saathoff, P. Schneider, V. Kleinfeldt et al., "Laboratory reference values for healthy adults from southern Tanzania," *Tropical Medicine & International Health*, vol. 13, no. 5, pp. 612–625, 2008.

[30] C. W. Tsang, R. Lazarus, W. Smith, P. Mitchell, J. Koutts, and L. Burnett, "Hematological indices in an older population sample: Derivation of healthy reference values," *Clinical Chemistry*, vol. 44, no. 1, pp. 96–101, 1998.

[31] K. Usman, Z. Ali Syed, and AA. Rao, "Reference range values of haematological parameters in healthy Pakistani adults," *Pakistan Journal of Physiology*, vol. 3, no. 1, pp. 19–22, 2007.

[32] B. O. Gobe, A. S. Gobel, B. Weisser, K. Gldnzer, H. Vetter, and R. Düsing, "Arterial blood pressure correlation with erythrocyte count, hematocrit, and hemoglobin concentration," *American Journal of Hypertension*, vol. 4, no. 1, pp. 14–19, 1991.

[33] M. Cirillo, M. Laurenzi, M. Trevisan, and J. Stamler, "Hematocrit, blood pressure, and hypertension: The Gubbio Population Study," *Hypertension*, vol. 20, no. 3, pp. 319–326, 1992.

[34] B. Y. Salazar-Vazquez, M. Intaglietta, M. Rodŕiguez-Moŕan, and F. Guerrero-Romero, "Blood pressure and hematocrit in diabetes and the role of endothelial responses in the variability of blood viscosity," *Diabetes Care*, vol. 29, no. 7, pp. 1523–1528, 2006.

Epidemiology of Hypertensive State among Chinese Migrants: Effects of Unaffordable Medical Care

Ming Guan [1,2]

[1] *Family Issues Center, Xuchang University, Road Bayi 88, Xuchang, Henan, China*
[2] *School of Business, Xuchang University, Road Bayi 88, Xuchang, Henan, China*

Correspondence should be addressed to Ming Guan; gming0604@163.com

Academic Editor: Tomohiro Katsuya

Hypertension is a major risk factor for heart disease and stroke. Affordability of medical care affects hypertension prevention, treatment, and control, but limited information is available for Chinese migrants with hypertensive state. Using Longitudinal Survey on Rural Urban Migration in China 2009 data, 2468 Chinese migrants reported hypertensive status. On the basis of comparison between medical payment and job income, participants were categorized as unaffordable and affordable. Thus, unaffordable expenses and unaffordable services were defined based on a public available survey. The descriptive statistics showed that 24.96% were at risk of prehypertension and mild-moderate-severe hypertension among 2468 Chinese migrants from 15 cities. Small part of the sample was not affordable to pay medical expenses and services. There were significant differences of hypertensive states between gender, marital status, regular smoker, and economic unaffordability. Multiple logistic regressions indicated that economic unaffordability had associations with abnormal weight, poor health assessment, and unhealthy hypertensive status. The alarming results may necessitate targeted interventions, even among people with good health status.

1. Introduction

Hypertension was an important public health burden in China, and control of hypertension was still suboptimal [1]. The trend of an increase in prevalence of hypertension in China was striking in young people and rural populations [2]. Hypertension prevalence in north China was 9.1% (95% CI: 4.1–14.1), which was higher than south China [3]. The treatment and control status of incident hypertension, while improved, remained very poor [4]. Rates of awareness and treatment of hypertension remained low and blood pressure was poorly controlled [5]. There was an urgent need for public health strategies with more emphasis on improvement of primary healthcare in China [6]. Inadequate counseling, lack of understanding on the disease, difficulties in accessing specialist care, and poor medication adherence were the barriers to optimal blood pressure control [7]. In addition, many cases of hypertension were going undetected and untreated under the effective health system in China [8]. Inadequate health insurance coverage for the high hypertension-risk migrants remained a challenge for the Chinese health reform [9].

Clinically, hypertension transits from normal blood pressure (normal pressure) to prehypertension, moderate hypertension, and severe hypertension. Normal pressure was defined as 90 mm Hg < systolic blood pressure < 120 mm Hg and 60 mm Hg < diastolic blood pressure < 80 mm Hg [10]. Prehypertension referred to a systemic BP of 120–139 mm Hg systolic and/or 80–89 mm Hg diastolic [11]. Prehypertension was often associated with other cardiovascular risk factors and independently increases the risk of hypertension and subsequent cardiovascular events [12]. Mild-and-moderate hypertension also was defined (mean sitting systolic BP/mean sitting diastolic BP, mild: 140–179/90–109 mmHg) [13]. Thus, severe hypertension was defined as (mean sitting systolic BP/mean sitting diastolic BP, severe: 180–/110– mmHg).

The primary care was effective in managing hypertension irrespective of management and operation models in urban China [14]. The migrants, the poor, and the vulnerable remained in the edge of the health insurance system [15]. Thus, subjects from rural migrants in urban China can be considered as a specifically medical and clinical targeted group.

The objective of this study was to assess the relationship between healthcare affordability and its association with change of hypertensive state among the Chinese migrants. Hypertensive state was defined under the combination of systolic pressure and diastolic pressure. Multiple logistic regressions were conducted to compute association of economic unaffordability with BMI, health assessment, and hypertensive states.

2. Methods

2.1. Data Source. This study used data from the Longitudinal Survey on Rural Urban Migration in China (RUMiC) organized by Professor Xin Meng at Australian National University. Detailed information is available at https://datasets.iza.org/. The core component was conducted in 15 Chinese cities (Guangzhou, Dongguan, Shenzhen, Zhengzhou, Luoyang, Hefei, Bengbu, Chongqing, Shanghai, Nanjing, Wuxi, Hangzhou, Ningbo, Wuhan, and Chengdu).

2.2. Main Variables. Unaffordability was defined based on the following questions: (a) Expenses: "how much were your total medical expenses on the disease in the last three months?" (b) Services: "what was the total amount of your cash expenditure on medical services in 2007?" (c) Income: "what is your average monthly income from current primary job?" Thus, two variables, "unaffordable expenses" and "unaffordable services," were constructed after income minus the two types of expenditure, respectively. Subsequently, "unaffordable expenses" and "unaffordable services" were also dichotomized into 1 and 0, when they were above 0 and equal to or below 0. Negative values were defined as unaffordability, while zero and positive values were defined as affordability.

Sociodemographic characteristics collected were age (9–25, 26–40, and ≥41 years), sex, marital status (married and other), current work status (employed and other), and BMI. Obesity was defined using BMI according to the Chinese criteria: underweight (less than 18.5 kg/m^2), normal (18.5–23.9 kg/m^2), overweight (24.0–27.9 kg/m^2), and obese (equal to or more than 28.0 kg/m^2) [16].

2.3. Statistical Analysis. The distributions of normal pressure, prehypertension, and mild-moderate-severe (MMS) hypertension were assessed by sociodemographic characteristics. Using unaffordable expenses and services as covariates, logistic regression models were mainly used to assess the associations of hypertensive state, while adjusting for age, sex, marital status, current work status, and education. All analyses accounted for the RUMiC complex sample design by using STATA 14.0 for Windows (STATA Corp, College Station, TX, USA).

3. Results

Overall, 63.25% of the sample was males among 2468 individuals aged ≥18 years included in the study. The participants had the mean age of 32.37 years (95% CI 31.26–33.46, range 18–72 years), with mean systolic blood pressure of 119.22 mm Hg (95% CI 118.78–119.66, range 90.01–191.67 mm Hg), and mean diastolic blood pressure of 75.90 mm Hg (95% CI 75.58–76.22, range 60.02–124.67 mm Hg).

In Table 1, there were significant differences of hypertensive state among age, gender, marital status, regular smoker, unaffordable expenses, and unaffordable services. Among the 2468 participants, 19.85% was risk of prehypertension, and 5.11% was risk of MMS hypertension. 1.30% was unaffordable to pay medical expenses. 8.47% was unaffordable to pay medical services. The migrants who could not afford medical services were more than migrants who could not afford medical expenses.

In Table 2, unaffordable services were significantly associated with being underweight, overweight, and obese. But, the odds ratios were below 1. In Table 3, unaffordable expenses were significantly associated with average and poor health assessment. Unaffordable services were associated with excellent, good, average, poor, and very poor health assessment. But, the odds ratios were below 1. This suggested that increase in unaffordable services would produce decrease in dimensions in health assessment.

In Table 4, age range 26–40 was associated with normal pressure (AOR: 1.380; 95 CI: 1.150–1.657), prehypertension (AOR: 0.598; 95 CI: 0.494–0.723), and MMS hypertension (AOR: 0.097; 95 CI: 0.069–0.137). Age ≥41 was associated with prehypertension (AOR: 0.560; 95 CI: 0.428–0.732) and MMS hypertension (AOR: 0.418; 95 CI: 0.310–0.565). This suggested that young migrants would be more likely to be in risk of hypertension than old migrants did. Female was associated with normal pressure (AOR: 3.823; 95 CI: 3.059–4.777), prehypertension (AOR: 0.263; 95 CI: 0.207–0.335), and MMS hypertension (AOR: 0.206; 95 CI: 0.140–0.301). Never married status was associated with normal pressure (AOR: 3.519; 95 CI: 2.865–4.323), prehypertension (AOR: 0.266; 95 CI: 0.214–0.330), and MMS hypertension (AOR: 0.034; 95 CI: 0.019–0.060). Regular smoker was associated with normal pressure (AOR: 1.258; 95 CI: 1.012–1.564), prehypertension (AOR: 0.780; 95 CI: 0.621–0.978), and MMS hypertension (AOR: 0.474; 95 CI: 0.331–0.678). Unaffordable services were associated with normal pressure (AOR: 0.659; 95 CI: 0.462–0.940) and prehypertension (AOR: 1.672; 95 CI: 1.153–2.425). This suggested that female, never married, regular smokers with higher age were not likely to be at risk of prehypertension and MMS hypertension. Persons with unaffordable services were likely to be at risk of prehypertension. Due to the smallest odds ratio in the table, never married subjects face the highest risk of hypertension.

4. Discussion

The findings of this study indicate that hypertensive state has been very prevalent in Chinese migrants. Part of Chinese migrants suffering from hypertension was accompanied by unaffordable expenses and services. With respect to high medical fees, affordable coverage could not be available to each migrant. Even worse, this affliction falls particularly hard on low-wage workers due to high cost of medical services. Thus, Chinese migrants with hypertension were less likely to report affordable medical expenses and services

TABLE 1: Demographic characteristics among adults with hypertensive state, N (%).

	Normal pressure	Prehypertension	MMS hypertension	chi2	p value
Age				207.6162***	0.000
9–25	756 (30.63)	111 (4.50)	12 (0.49)		
26–40	829 (33.59)	258 (10.45)	40 (1.62)		
≥41	267 (10.82)	121 (4.90)	74 (3.00)		
Gender				98.7121***	0.000
Male	973 (39.42)	370 (14.99)	94 (3.81)		
Female	879 (35.62)	120 (4.86)	32 (1.30)		
Marital status				126.4450***	0.000
Married	967 (39.18)	346 (14.02)	104 (4.21)		
Remarried	14 (0.57)	4 (0.16)	2 (0.08)		
Cohabited	21 (0.85)	0 (0.00)	0 (0.00)		
Divorced	32 (1.30)	11 (0.45)	2 (0.08)		
Widowed	9 (0.36)	5 (0.20)	5 (0.20)		
Never married	809 (32.78)	124 (5.02)	13 (0.53)		
Physical disabilities				0.9726	0.615
No	1,781 (72.16)	467 (18.92)	122 (4.94)		
Yes	71 (2.88)	23 (0.93)	4 (0.16)		
Sick injured				2.5501	0.279
No	1,514 (61.35)	395 (16.00)	96 (3.89)		
Yes	338 (13.70)	95 (3.85)	30 (1.22)		
Regular smoker				33.5242***	0.000
No	1,369 (55.47)	303 (12.28)	77 (3.12)		
Yes	483 (19.57)	187 (7.58)	49 (1.99)		
Unaffordable expenses				8.3172**	0.016
No	1,835 (74.35)	478 (19.37)	123 (4.98)		
Yes	17 (0.69)	12 (0.49)	3 (0.12)		
Unaffordable services				12.7682***	0.002
No	1,715 (69.49)	429 (17.38)	115 (4.66)		
Yes	137 (5.55)	61 (2.47)	11 (0.45)		

$^{**}p < 0.05$; $^{***}p < 0.01$.

which produced inadequate healthcare access. This study suggested that, even among those who afforded medical expenses and services, barriers to receiving affordable healthcare were still a challenge.

A possible explanation for the unaffordable expenses was due to lack of basic health insurance which dramatically increased the risk of depression based on northwestern Chinese community samples [17]. It is a common sense that mental disorders are risk factors for hypertension. China has achieved high population coverage rate over a short time period, starting with a limited benefit package. However, poor people have less benefit from New Cooperative Medical Scheme (NCMS) in terms of health service utilization [18]. The prices, availability, and affordability of medicines in China were not equitable access to basic medical treatments, especially for the poor [19]. Thus, psychiatric disorders produced by socioeconomic factors increased the risk of hypertension, when the migrants were out of the protection of social, health, and medical insurance.

Unaffordable medical care can be explained by marketization of health and social service organizations. The finding that a significantly higher proportion of married, employed, and women migrants aged 36 to 44 years had unaffordable medical care suggested that factors other than individual (such as employer) were also related to insurance status. Moreover, the insured still paid high amount of out-of-pocket medical expenditure [20]. NCMS improved the situation of receiving healthcare services but did not reduce the high healthcare fees [21]. The rapid increase of public funding to subsidize health insurance in China did not mitigate the out-of-pocket payment for healthcare over the past decade [22]. Thus, organizational, institutional, and employers' power dominate affordability, accessibility, and availability of Chinese migrants' healthcare.

This finding was consistent with those of earlier studies. For example, a study concluded that rural-urban migrant workers might well be left out of sharing the social and economic development [23]. Another study indicated that young migrant male workers appeared to be most vulnerable in their psychological well-being [24]. A published literature also argued that health systems governance was criticized as ineffective and inefficient in the development and operation

Table 2: Association between BMI and economic unaffordability.

	Underweight		Normal weight		Overweight		Obese	
	AOR	95 CI	AOR	95 CI	AOR	95 CI	AOR	95 CI
Unaffordable expenses	0.358	0.074–1.734	1.361	0.631–2.935	0.891	0.366–2.166	0.577	0.102–3.260
Unaffordable services	0.144***	0.093–0.222	1.242	0.927–1.664	0.345***	0.248–0.481	0.077***	0.044–0.132

*** $p < 0.01$.

TABLE 3: Association between health assessment and economic unaffordability.

	Excellent		Good		Average		Poor		Very poor	
	AOR	95 CI	AOR	95 CI	AOR	95 CI	AOR	95 CI	AOR	95 CI
Unaffordable expenses	0.391	0.128–1.193	1.190	0.557–2.544	0.344*	0.126–0.939	3.470*	1.207–9.974	1.503	0.120–18.892
Unaffordable services	0.331***	0.237–0.463	0.480***	0.352–0.656	0.511***	0.376–0.694	0.095***	0.057–0.158	0.018***	0.007–0.045

*$0.05 < p < 0.10$; ***$p < 0.01$.

TABLE 4: Association between hypertensive states with economic unaffordability.

	Normal pressure AOR (95% CI)	Prehypertension AOR (95% CI)	MMS hypertension AOR (95% CI)
Age			
9–25	1.00 (reference)	1.00 (reference)	1.00 (reference)
26–40	1.380*** (1.150–1.657)	0.598*** (0.494–0.723)	0.097*** (0.069–0.137)
≥41	0.847 (0.660–1.086)	0.560*** (0.428–0.732)	0.418*** (0.310–0.565)
Gender			
Male	1.00 (reference)	1.00 (reference)	1.00 (reference)
Female	3.823*** (3.059–4.777)	0.263*** (0.207–0.335)	0.206*** (0.140–0.301)
Marital status			
Married	1.00 (reference)	1.00 (reference)	1.00 (reference)
Remarried	0.874 (0.301–2.542)	0.918 (0.286–2.945)	1.586 (0.325–7.747)
Divorced	1.103 (0.574–2.121)	1.028 (0.535–1.974)	0.430 (0.085–2.169)
Widowed	0.473 (0.162–1.378)	1.226 (0.379–3.968)	2.589 (0.740–9.052)
Never married	3.519*** (2.865–4.323)	0.266*** (0.214–0.330)	0.034*** (0.019–0.060)
Physical disabilities			
No	1.00 (reference)	1.00 (reference)	1.00 (reference)
Yes	1.098 (0.677–1.781)	1.007 (0.605–1.676)	0.472 (0.173–1.290)
Sick injured			
No	1.00 (reference)	1.00 (reference)	1.00 (reference)
Yes	1.049 (0.810–1.358)	0.861 (0.651–1.138)	0.997 (0.620–1.602)
Regular Smokers			
No	1.00 (reference)	1.00 (reference)	1.00 (reference)
Yes	1.258* (1.012–1.564)	0.780* (0.621–0.978)	0.474*** (0.331–0.678)
Unaffordable expenses			
No	1.00 (reference)	1.00 (reference)	1.00 (reference)
Yes	0.595 (0.246–1.436)	1.710 (0.703–4.156)	1.800 (0.402–8.064)
Unaffordable services			
No	1.00 (reference)	1.00 (reference)	1.00 (reference)
Yes	0.659* (0.462–0.940)	1.672** (1.153–2.425)	0.588 (0.274–1.263)

*$p < 0.10$; **$p < 0.05$; ***$p < 0.01$.

of Cooperative Medical Scheme and New Rural Cooperative Medical Scheme [25]. Thereby, poor connection between urban and rural insurance system was partially responsible for the omission of the migrants' health support plans.

Together, these findings show that the healthcare system should seek to reduce the barriers for these patients to achieve BP control. Enrolled in the Urban Employee Basic Health Insurance scheme, people with hypertension in Shanghai, China, had no access to publicity of hypertension prevention knowledge [26]. For the floating population, health insurance coverage needs to be improved [27]. The fragmented health insurance schemes generated inequitable healthcare utilization and health outcomes for the elderly [28]. In order to effectively control hypertension, a study highlighted better health insurance packages [29]. These findings may encourage employment service agencies to expand the coverage of health service from a specific targeted population to general population included migrants.

This finding was in line with the previous research that unaffordable expenses, unaffordable insurance, and unaffordable services were related to income inequality. Based on the China Health and Nutrition Survey (1991–2006), health disparities in China were related to rising income inequality and in particular to the adverse health and income experience of older (wo)men [30]. Based on US data from four waves of the Panel Study of Income Dynamics, low wages were risk factors for hypertension among working people for women and persons aged 25–44 years [31]. Comparing 2009 with 2006, the income inequality in health insurance coverage was largely corrected in China through rapid expansion in rural areas and initiation of urban resident basic medical insurance in urban areas [32]. This combination of findings provided some support for the intuition that income inequality caused by poor distribution of wealth resources led to health vulnerabilities of the marginalized persons.

This study had several limitations. First, all hypertension information collected from the RUMiC was from measurement of systolic pressure and diastolic pressure. In fact, most of the Chinese migrants with hypertension were unaware of the condition, leading to under-reporting of barriers to care in this population. In addition, Chinese migrants with hypertension were unaware of blood control. Second, the

RUMiC did not provide information on antihypertensive care and cure. Thus, the expenditure of antihypertensive cure and hypertension affordability could not be assessed and estimated scientifically. Third, the survey provided no information about the affordable medical expenditure as a proportion of household income. Thus, a method of more accurate unaffordable measure could not be conducted. Finally, given that only 15 cities were surveyed, the data may not be nationally representative.

5. Conclusion

In conclusion, the hypertensive states were serious in the Chinese migrants. There were significant differences between hypertensive states among the migrants with respect to affordable and unaffordable medical expenses and services. Also, part of Chinese migrants with hypertension was likely to report unaffordable care under the condition that there were significant differences between hypertensive states among the migrants with respect to specific sociodemographic factors. Among the Chinese migrants, economic unaffordability was associated with abnormal weight, poor health status, and hypertensive states. Subsequently, some policies and interventions suggested were highlighted.

References

[1] J. Wang, L. Zhang, F. Wang, L. Liu, and H. Wang, "Prevalence, awareness, treatment, and control of hypertension in China: results from a national survey," *American Journal of Hypertension*, vol. 27, no. 11, pp. 1355–1361, 2014.

[2] Y. Gao, G. Chen, H. Tian et al., "Prevalence of hypertension in China: a cross-sectional study," *PLoS ONE*, vol. 8, no. 6, Article ID e65938, 2013.

[3] X. Wang, M. L. Bots, F. Yang, A. W. Hoes, and I. Vaartjes, "Prevalence of hypertension in China: A systematic review andmeta-regression analysis of trends and regional differences," *Journal of Hypertension*, vol. 32, no. 10, pp. 1919–1927, 2014.

[4] Y. Liang, R. Liu, S. Du, and C. Qiu, "Trends in incidence of hypertension in Chinese adults, 1991–2009: the China Health and Nutrition Survey," *International Journal of Cardiology*, vol. 175, no. 1, pp. 96–101, 2014.

[5] C. Dong, P. Ge, X. Ren, H. Fan, and X. Yan, "Prevalence, awareness, treatment and control of hypertension among adults in rural north-western China: A cross-sectional population survey," *Journal of International Medical Research*, vol. 41, no. 4, pp. 1291–1300, 2013.

[6] X. Chen, W. Wei, S. Zou et al., "Trends in the prevalence of hypertension in island and coastal areas of China: a systematic review with meta-analysis," *American Journal of Hypertension*, vol. 27, no. 12, pp. 1503–1510, 2014.

[7] Y.-B. Wang, D.-G. Kong, L.-L. Ma, and L.-X. Wang, "Patient related factors for optimal blood pressure control in patients with hypertension," *African Health Sciences*, vol. 13, no. 3, pp. 579–583, 2013.

[8] X. L. Feng, M. Pang, and J. Beard, "Health system strengthening and hypertension awareness, treatment and control: data from the China Health and Retirement Longitudinal Study," *Bulletin of the World Health Organization*, vol. 92, no. 1, pp. 29–41, 2014.

[9] K. K. F. Lam and J. M. Johnston, "Health insurance and healthcare utilisation for Shenzhen residents: A tale of registrants and migrants?" *BMC Public Health*, vol. 12, no. 1, article no. 868, 2012.

[10] A. V. Chobanian, G. L. Bakris, H. R. Black et al., "The seventh report of the joint national committee on prevention, detection, evaluation, and treatment of high blood pressure: the JNC 7 report," *The Journal of the American Medical Association*, vol. 289, no. 19, pp. 2560–2572, 2003.

[11] C. Tripolino, A. Gnasso, C. Carallo, F. B. Scavelli, and C. Irace, "Hemorheological profiles of subjects with prehypertension," *Hypertension Research*, vol. 39, no. 7, pp. 519–523, 2016.

[12] W. J. Elliott and H. R. Black, "Prehypertension," *Nature Clinical Practice Cardiovascular Medicine*, vol. 4, no. 10, pp. 538–548, 2007.

[13] G. Mancia, G. de Backer, and A. Dominiczak, "2007 Guidelines for the Management of Arterial Hypertension: The Task Force for the Management of Arterial Hypertension of the European Society of Hypertension (ESH) and of the European Society of Cardiology (ESC)," *Journal of Hypertension*, vol. 25, no. 6, pp. 1105–1187, 2007.

[14] H. Li, X. Wei, M. C. Wong et al., "A comparison of the quality of hypertension management in primary care between Shanghai and Shenzhen: A cohort study of 3196 patients," *Medicine (United States)*, vol. 94, no. 5, p. e455, 2015.

[15] Y. Jin, Z. Hou, and D. Zhang, "Determinants of health insurance coverage among people aged 45 and over in China: Who buys public, private and multiple insurance," *PLoS ONE*, vol. 11, no. 8, Article ID e0161774, 2016.

[16] Ministry of Health of the People's Republic of China, *The guidelines for prevention and control of overweight and obesity in Chinese adults*, People's Medical Publishing House, 2006.

[17] D. Tian, Z. Qu, X. Wang et al., "The role of basic health insurance on depression: An epidemiological cohort study of a randomized community sample in Northwest China," *BMC Psychiatry*, vol. 12, article no. 151, 2012.

[18] X. Liu, S. Tang, B. Yu et al., "Can rural health insurance improve equity in health care utilization? a comparison between China and Vietnam," *International Journal for Equity in Health*, vol. 11, no. 1, article no. 10, 2012.

[19] M. Jiang, S. Yang, K. Yan, J. Liu, J. Zhao, and Y. Fang, "Measuring Access to Medicines: A Survey of Prices, Availability and Affordability in Shaanxi Province of China," *PLoS ONE*, vol. 8, no. 8, Article ID e70836, 2013.

[20] Y. Wang, Y. Jiang, Y. Li, X. Wang, C. Ma, and S. Ma, "Health insurance utilization and its impact: Observations from the middle-aged and elderly in China," *PLoS ONE*, vol. 8, no. 12, Article ID e80978, 2013.

[21] X. Wang, X. He, A. Zheng, and X. Ji, "The effects of China's New Cooperative Medical Scheme on accessibility and affordability of healthcare services: an empirical research in Liaoning Province," *BMC Health Services Research*, vol. 14, no. 1, 2014.

[22] Q. Long, L. Xu, H. Bekedam, and S. Tang, "Changes in health expenditures in China in 2000s: Has the health system reform

improved affordability," *International Journal for Equity in Health*, vol. 12, no. 1, article no. 40, 2013.

[23] L. Xu, Y. Wang, C. D. Collins, and S. Tang, "Urban health insurance reform and coverage in China using data from National Health Services Surveys in 1998 and 2003," *BMC Health Services Research*, vol. 7, article no. 37, 2007.

[24] Z. Zeng, Y. Guo, L. Lu, L. Han, W. Chen, and L. Ling, "Mental health status and work environment among workers in small- and medium-sized enterprises in Guangdong, China - A cross-sectional survey," *BMC Public Health*, vol. 14, article no. 1162, 2014.

[25] B. Yuan, W. Jian, L. He, B. Wang, and D. Balabanova, "The role of health system governance in strengthening the rural health insurance system in China," *International Journal for Equity in Health*, vol. 16, no. 1, article no. 44, 2017.

[26] X. Zhang, Y. Zhang, X. Xiao, X. Ma, and J. He, "The relation between health insurance and management of hypertension in Shanghai, China: A cross-sectional study," *BMC Public Health*, vol. 16, no. 1, article no. 959, 2016.

[27] Y. Zhao, B. Kang, Y. Liu et al., "Health insurance coverage and its impact on medical cost: Observations from the floating population in China e111555," *PLoS ONE*, vol. 9, no. 11, Article ID e111555, 2014.

[28] X. Liu, H. Wong, and K. Liu, "Outcome-based health equity across different social health insurance schemes for the elderly in China," *BMC Health Services Research*, vol. 16, no. 1, article no. 1261, 2016.

[29] Y. Liao, S. Gilmour, and K. Shibuya, "Health insurance coverage and hypertension control in China: Results from the China health and nutrition survey," *PLoS ONE*, vol. 11, no. 3, Article ID e0152091, 2016.

[30] S. Baeten, T. Van Ourti, and E. van Doorslaer, "Rising inequalities in income and health in China: Who is left behind?" *Journal of Health Economics*, vol. 32, no. 6, pp. 1214–1229, 2013.

[31] J. P. Leigh and J. Du, "Are low wages risk factors for hypertension?" *European Journal of Public Health*, vol. 22, no. 6, pp. 854–859, 2012.

[32] J. Liu, L. Shi, Q. Meng, and M. M. Khan, "Income-related inequality in health insurance coverage: Analysis of China Health and Nutrition Survey of 2006 and 2009," *International Journal for Equity in Health*, vol. 11, no. 1, article no. 42, 2012.

28

High Prevalence of Hypertension in Ethiopian and Non-Ethiopian HIV-Infected Adults

Maya Korem,[1] Tali Wallach,[2] Michael Bursztyn,[3] Shlomo Maayan,[4] and Karen Olshtain-Pops [1]

[1] *AIDS Unit, Department of Clinical Microbiology and Infectious Diseases, Hadassah-Hebrew University Medical Center, Jerusalem, Israel*
[2] *Department of Pediatrics, Kaplan Medical Center, Rehovot, Israel*
[3] *Hypertension Unit, Department of Medicine, Hadassah-Hebrew University Medical Center, Mount Scopus, Jerusalem, Israel*
[4] *Infectious Diseases and Infection Control Unit, Barzilai Medical Center, Ashkelon, Israel*

Correspondence should be addressed to Karen Olshtain-Pops; kerenop@hadassah.org.il

Academic Editor: Roberto Pontremoli

Objectives. Prevalence of hypertension has not been studied in the Ethiopian HIV-infected population, which represents 60% of the patients in our AIDS unit. Our aim was to identify risk factors and characterize the prevalence of hypertension in the population monitored at our unit. *Methods.* A retrospective chart review categorized subjects according to their blood pressure levels. Hypertension prevalence was determined and stratified according to variables perceived to contribute to elevated blood pressure. *Results.* The prevalence of hypertension in our study population was significantly higher compared to the general population (53% versus 20%, $P < 0.0001$) and was associated with known risk factors and not with patients' viral load and CD4 levels. Ethiopian HIV-infected adults had a prominently higher rate of blood pressure rise over time as compared to non-Ethiopians ($P = 0.016$). *Conclusions.* The high prevalence of hypertension in this cohort and the rapid increase in blood pressure in Ethiopians are alarming. We could not attribute high prevalence to HIV-related factors and we presume it is part of the metabolic syndrome. The lifelong cardiovascular risk associated with HIV infection mandates hypertension screening and close monitoring in this population.

1. Introduction

The increased use of highly active antiretroviral therapy (HAART) in recent decades has led to a reduction in morbidity and mortality among people living with Human Immunodeficiency Virus (HIV) and has modified the course of HIV to a chronic infection with long-term complications, one of which is cardiovascular disease (CVD) [1, 2]. Among HIV-infected individuals, CVD is a main cause of morbidity and mortality, comprising 10% of non-AIDS-related mortalities [3].

The increased risk of CVD is attributed to a combination of factors. Prolonged viremia is associated with elevated systemic inflammatory markers [4–6], hypercoagulation, damage to the endothelium [7], and premature atherosclerosis [8]. Prolonged HAART administration is associated with a linear increase in cardiovascular-related mortality for up to 5 years of HAART exposure [9, 10]. This increase is related to the occurrence of lipodystrophy and metabolic derangements such as elevated cholesterol and triglyceride levels [11], insulin resistance, and impaired glucose tolerance [9, 10, 12].

Fifty percent of coronary heart disease in developed countries is attributed to hypertension (HTN) [13]. HTN is increased in subjects with diabetes and dyslipidemia, which are more prevalent among HIV-infected individuals than in the general population [3, 14, 15], and has become a potentially significant cause of morbidity in this population [16]. HTN in HIV-infected adults is associated with a higher frequency of persistent proteinuria, coronary heart disease, and myocardial infarction compared to nonhypertensive HIV-infected subjects [17].

The reported prevalence of HTN in HIV-infected adults shows great variance. It has been described as ranging from 8% to 34% [18, 19] and was not found to be consistently higher than the levels found in matched HIV-negative adults [20]. An increased incidence of HTN was observed in HIV-infected adults treated with HAART for 48 weeks, as compared with HIV-infected HAART-naïve adults (26% versus 7%, resp.) [19]. In a recent meta-analysis of seven hypertension studies, the prevalence of abnormal diurnal blood pressure (BP) pattern that may contribute to the high CVD risk ranged from 29 to 82% among HIV-infected individuals, compared to 15–53% in their HIV-negative counterparts [21].

Ethnic origin is a known factor affecting BP. Numerous studies conducted in the US found increased incidence and severity of HTN in African Americans compared with Caucasians [22, 23]. The Ethiopian population is Semitic in origin and not frequently studied in HTN trials. A large meta-analysis of HTN in Equatorial African countries, which included studies from 1998 to 2008, estimated the incidence of HTN in Ethiopia as 10.6% [24]. In a study conducted in young Ethiopian immigrants in Israel, BP was significantly higher among young male Ethiopian immigrants compared with a group of Israeli students, despite a dramatically lower body mass index (BMI). In addition, the prevalence of HTN was higher in Ethiopian immigrants after 2 years of residence in Israel, compared to <3 months' residency in the same boarding schools [25].

The HIV unit at the Hadassah Medical Center is unique in that Ethiopian immigrants constitute 60% of the patients monitored in the clinic. This high rate allows for a HTN evaluation study in this population.

The goal of this retrospective study was to estimate the prevalence of elevated blood pressure (BP) among our cohort of HIV-infected adults and to compare its prevalence in Ethiopians and non-Ethiopians. In addition, we aimed to identify risk factors for the occurrence of elevated BP. To our knowledge, no previous studies have yet focused on BP in Ethiopian HIV-infected adults.

2. Methods

2.1. Study Population. The observational analytical cross-sectional study was based on data retrieved from medical records of HIV-infected adults aged ≥18 years, who had been followed up at the AIDS unit in the outpatient clinic of the Hadassah (Ein Karem) Medical Center during the years 2000–2012. This adult HIV center, the only one in Jerusalem, monitors approximately 400 HIV-infected adults every 3 months. Each visit includes BP measurement, routine blood tests (including viral load and CD4 levels), an interview, and a physical examination.

As a control to our study population, we used BP data from a survey conducted by the Ministry of Health and the Central Bureau of Statistics in Israel during 2003-2004, which included approximately 10,000 participants (Supplement 1).

The research protocol for this study was approved by the Research Ethics Committee of the Hadassah-Hebrew University Medical Center.

2.2. Blood Pressure Measurement, Definition, and Collection. Blood pressure (BP) was measured at each visit in the clinic using a digital blood pressure machine (General Electric, DINAMAP ProCare 120). Measurements were taken by the staff nurse, after at least 5 minutes of rest, on the right upper arm, in the sitting position. BP levels were categorized into four levels, based on the seventh report of the Joint National Committee (JNC7) [26]: normal (systolic BP < 120 mm Hg, diastolic < 80 mm Hg); prehypertension (systolic BP 120–139 mm Hg, diastolic BP 80–89 mm Hg); stage 1 HTN (systolic BP 140–159 mm Hg, diastolic BP 90–99 mm Hg), and stage 2 HTN (systolic BP ≥ 160 mm Hg, diastolic BP ≥ 100 mm Hg). The term HTN was generally used in this work for patients classified as HTN stage 1 or 2 as measured during two separate visits in the clinic over the follow-up period, or when antihypertensive medication was used for treating hypertension regardless of BP level in the clinic.

BP data from four time points during follow-up were collected from patient files: close to HIV diagnosis, at the time of the lowest recorded CD4 count, at the time the highest BP was recorded, and at the last visit.

2.3. Clinical Data Collection and Risk Factor Definitions. Clinical and laboratory data were obtained from the medical records. Basic clinical data included age, gender, ethnic origin, height, antiretroviral treatment, duration of HIV infection from the date of diagnosis, CVD risk factors, and family history of CVD. Laboratory data included CD4 cell counts, categorized as <200, 200–349, 350–500, and >500 cells/μl, and HIV-1 RNA or viral load, categorized as undetectable, ≤1000, >1000–10,000, >10,000–100,000, ≥100,000 copies/ml, HDL cholesterol, triglycerides, and fasting plasma glucose. Weight and all laboratory data were recorded at the same 4 time points as BP data. BMI ≥ 25 kg/m^2 was defined as overweight. Metabolic syndrome was defined according to the criteria of the National Cholesterol Education Program (NCEP) Adult Treatment Panel III (ATP III) 2005 [27]. In cases where diabetes mellitus had not been diagnosed, we used ADA criteria for the diagnosis [28]. Tobacco use was defined as any current or previous use. Family history of CVD was defined as development of atherosclerotic CVD in a first-degree relative younger than 55 (males) or 65 (females).

2.4. Statistical Methods. All statistical analyses were conducted using SPSS software version 21.0. Statistical significance was assessed at the 0.05 level, and 2-sided P values are reported.

One-sample chi-square test was used to compare the prevalence of hypertension in the study group and in the general population. The t-test was used to compare quantitative variables between two independent groups. The association between two categorical variables was tested by a chi-square test and Fisher's exact test as appropriate.

The correlation between two quantitative variables was estimated by calculating the Pearson correlation coefficient.

Variables found to have a statistically significant association with the dependent variable (HTN) in a univariate analysis were examined in a multivariate model of logistic regression. To test which factors had impact on blood pressure over a period of time, a variability analysis model with repeated measurements was used.

3. Results

The study cohort consisted of 297 patients living with HIV, monitored at the Hadassah AIDS Center between January 2000 and December 2012. Within this group, 257 (86%) patients were on HAART according to accepted guidelines [29].

3.1. Study Population Characteristics. Two hundred and seventy-eight subjects were included in the final analysis, representing 94% of the patients followed up at the clinic during the study period. The remaining 19 patients did not have sufficient follow-up information in their files. Mean age of study participants was 42 (range: 22–80 years). Most subjects were of Ethiopian origin (172/278, 61.8%). Overall, 157 (56%) were men, but the proportion of men was significantly lower in Ethiopian (73/172, 42%) than in non-Ethiopian (84/106, 79%) patients ($P < 0.001$). Mean CD4 count at baseline for all participants was 350 ± 255 cells/ml; 30% had a CD4 count below 200 cells/ml. Mean follow-up time was 7 years.

3.2. Prevalence of HTN. Fifty-three percent (147/278) of the subjects were categorized as having HTN according to the highest recorded BP, which is significantly higher than the 20% prevalence in the general Israeli population, according to the national health survey conducted by the Central Bureau of Statistics (CBS) in 2003-2004 ($P < 0.0001$). This discrepancy remained significant when gender and age (21–44 and ≥45 years) were stratified. BP data from the last visit in the clinic showed a lower prevalence of HTN, 63/278 (22.6%), which is similar to the prevalence in the general population.

HTN rate was similar in Ethiopian and non-Ethiopian HIV-infected subjects (93/172, 54% versus 54/106, 51%, resp.).

3.3. Prevalence of HTN by Stratified Characteristics and Risk Factors. Table 1 describes the stratification of participants' characteristics according to three levels of blood pressure (normal, pre-HTN, and HTN) that were measured at two follow-up time points: (1) when the highest BP was measured and (2) at the last visit in the clinic.

The prevalence of HTN was significantly higher in males than in females. Subjects with metabolic syndrome or diabetes showed a greater propensity for HTN (94.5% and 87.5%, resp.; $P < 0.001$), as did obese (68.8%, $P < 0.01$) or older (73.6%, $P < 0.001$) participants.

However, when multivariate analysis was used, the only factor that associated significantly with HTN was the presence of metabolic syndrome ($P < 0.001$).

3.4. Prevalence of HTN by Disease Parameters. No significant association was found between viral load or CD4 levels measured at nadir and HTN ($P > 0.05$) (Table 2).

The duration of HIV before HTN diagnosis was estimated using 2 parameters: (1) the duration of time measured between HIV diagnosis and maximal BP measurement and (2) the CD4 level at nadir, which is considered an indirect measure of disease duration. Both parameters had no significant effect on the prevalence of HTN.

3.5. Impact of Ethnic Origin and the Time Elapsed from HIV Diagnosis to the Highest Recorded BP on the Prevalence of HTN. The highest BP was recorded on average 7 years (range: 1–20 years) after HIV diagnosis. The mean maximal BP was 141/83, significantly higher than that measured at baseline (122/77, $P < 0.001$).

No significant correlation was found between duration of the period since HIV diagnosis to the highest recorded BP, or to HTN diagnosis, and there was no significant difference in HTN prevalence between Ethiopian and non-Ethiopian HIV-infected subjects between these two time points. However, we found a significant interaction between time and ethnic origin: the rate of diastolic and systolic BP rise over time was significantly higher in Ethiopian than in non-Ethiopian HIV-infected subjects ($P = 0.016$).

4. Discussion

This study describes the prevalence of HTN in HIV-infected adults in an urban setting in Israel, with a focus on patients of Ethiopian origin, a population that has not been thoroughly studied.

Prevalence of HTN in all study subjects was significantly higher among HIV-infected adults (53%) compared to the general population (20%, $P < 0.0001$). Male gender and age were significantly associated with HTN, as reported for non-HIV populations [30]. This high prevalence was found at the point of the highest recorded BP, as well as at CD4 nadir. This finding is in concordance with results from a study conducted in Italy [31], which showed that the incidence of HTN is significantly higher among HIV-infected adults, compared to a control cohort of healthy blood donors (34.2% and 11.2%, resp.). The authors suggest that the higher resistance to insulin found among HIV-infected adults as compared with the controls (HOMA index 1.2 ± 3.3 versus 0.9 ± 2, resp.; $P < 0.001$) could explain this finding. In addition, higher HOMA indices were found among HIV-infected adults with HTN as opposed to those without HTN (3.7 ± 1 versus 1.2 ± 3.1, $P < 0.001$).

Other studies have also reported high rates of insulin resistance among HIV-infected adults treated with HAART [32, 33]. Hyperinsulinemia contributes to HTN by several mechanisms, including increased effect of angiotensin II on aldosterone and vascular contraction [34]. It is also linked to the metabolic syndrome, a strong independent cardiovascular risk factor [35] with increased prevalence among HIV-infected adults [36]. Insulin resistance was also predictive of the development of hypertension in lean, young Ethiopian immigrants in Israel [37].

A correlation between HAART and increased prevalence of HTN in HIV-infected adults has been reported [31, 34]. In a study conducted in Spain [19], which included patients who began HAART, a statistically significant rise in systolic and diastolic BP was found after 48 weeks of treatment. However, we did not find a significant association between HAART and

TABLE 1: Participants' characteristics by three levels of BP at two time points of follow-up.

Characteristics	Number of patients (% of total cohort) Highest BP Normal	Pre-HTN	HTN	Last visit BP Normal	Pre-HTN	HTN
Ethnicity						
Ethiopian	12 (7)	67 (39)	93 (54)	59 (34.3)	73 (42.4)	40 (23.2)
Non-Ethiopian	2 (1.9)	50 (47.2)	54 (51)	33 (31.1)	50 (47.2)	23 (21.7)
			$P = 0.2$			$P = 0.87$
Gender						
Female	9 (7.4)	61 (50.4)	51 (42.2)	51 (42.1)	50 (41.3)	20 (16.5)
Male	5 (3.2)	56 (35.7)	96 (61.2)	41 (26.1)	73 (46.4)	43 (27.3)
			$P < 0.01$			$P < 0.05$
Age (years)						
21–44	10 (5.4)	94 (51)	80 (44.1)	74 (39.5)	77 (41.1)	36 (19.2)
≥45	4 (4.2)	23 (24.4)	67 (71.2)	18 (19.7)	46 (50.5)	27 (29.6)
			$P < 0.001$			$P < 0.01$
Overweight						
No	5 (7.1)	33 (47.1)	32 (45.7)	29 (42)	26 (37.7)	14 (20.2)
Yes	0 (0)	15 (31.3)	63 (68.8)	8 (16.7)	24 (50)	16 (33.3)
			$P^1 = 0.01$			$P^1 = 0.01$
Metabolic syndrome						
No	5 (5.4)	46 (50)	41 (44.5)	33 (36.3)	44 (48.4)	14 (15.4)
Yes	0 (0)	1 (5.6)	17 (94.5)	0 (0)	6 (33.3)	12 (66.7)
Diabetes mellitus	0 (0)	1 (12.5)	7 (87.5)	2 (25)	2 (25)	4 (50)
			$P < 0.001$			$P^1 < 0.001$
Family history of CVD						
No	5 (4.9)	45 (43.7)	53 (51.4)	34 (33.3)	46 (45.1)	22 (21.5)
Yes	0 (0)	4 (23.5)	13 (76.5)	2 (11.8)	6 (35.3)	9 (53)
			$P^1 = 0.26$			$P^1 = 0.02$
Tobacco use						
No	1 (3.1)	16 (50)	15 (46.8)	14 (43.8)	13 (40.6)	5 (15.6)
Yes	5 (5.6)	35 (38.9)	50 (55.5)	25 (28.1)	39 (43.8)	25 (28.1)
			$P^1 = 0.3$			$P^1 = 0.41$
CD4 count (cells/μl)						
≤200 ($n = 131$)	8 (6.1)	51 (38.9)	72 (54.9)	46 (34.3)	56 (42.7)	30 (23)
>200 ($n = 147$)	6 (4)	66 (44.8)	75 (51)	46 (29.9)	67 (47.6)	33 (22.4)
			$P = 0.64$			$P = 0.64$
Use of HAART						
No ($n = 38$)	4 (10.8)	16 (43.2)	17 (45.9)	15 (33.3)	22 (48.8)	8 (17.7)
Yes ($n = 240$)	10 (4.1)	101 (41.9)	130 (53.9)	77 (33)	101 (43.3)	55 (23.6)
			$P = 0.38$			$P = 0.69$

[1]Fisher's exact test was performed for low prevalence; BP: blood pressure; HTN: hypertension; CVD: cardiovascular disease; HAART: highly active antiretroviral treatment.

the presence of HTN. The lack of agreement among the studies may be related to the inclusion of HIV-infected adults with initially lower CD4 values in other studies [19]. Commencing HAART in these subjects may have led to weight gain and consequently to HTN. Another explanation is the low rate of HIV-infected adults that were not treated with HAART in our study.

We found obesity, family history, advanced age, diabetes, and metabolic syndrome to be associated with HTN. These are the known risk factors for HTN, closely related to insulin resistance in the general population [38], and therefore support the reliability of our findings. Yet, we could not point to a clear reason for the higher prevalence of HTN in this population. Possibly, the HIV associated chronic inflammatory process is responsible for an increased prevalence of the metabolic syndrome in HIV patients and for the higher prevalence of HTN found in this cohort, which we assume is part of the metabolic syndrome.

Table 2: Prevalence of HTN measured at the time of the lowest recorded CD4 count according to categorized CD4 and viral load levels ($P > 0.05$).

	Number of patients (% of total cohort) BP status		Total
	No HTN	HTN	
CD4 count (cells/μl)			
<200	70 (47.9)	76 (52)	146 (100)
200–349	37 (43.5)	48 (56.5)	85 (100)
350–499	15 (50)	15 (50)	30 (100)
≥500	9 (53)	8 (47)	17 (100)
Total	131 (47.1)	147 (52.8)	278 (100)
VL[1] (copies/ml)			
<50	23 (40.4)	34 (59.6)	57
50–1000	9 (39.1)	14 (60.9)	23
>1000–10,000	16 (42.1)	22 (57.9)	38
>10,000–100,000	34 (54.8)	28 (45.2)	62
>100,000	31 (48.4)	33 (51.6)	64
Total	113	131	244 (100)

[1]Data was missing for $n = 34$; BP: blood pressure; HTN: hypertension; VL: viral load.

A recent study [39] found nadir CD4 values below 50 cells/μl to be an independent risk factor for the development of HTN in HIV-infected adults. Possible explanations for these results are inflammation of the small intestine found at low CD4 levels (HIV enteropathy) with activation of the immune system and release of inflammatory mediators, contributing to elevation of angiotensin II and salt accumulation [40, 41]. We did not find nadir CD4 values to be associated with a high prevalence of HTN, possibly because we categorized CD4 counts to higher values, which were chosen according to the guidelines for starting HAART therapy [29].

In our cohort, no association was found between viral load or CD4 levels at nadir and the presence of HTN. Both parameters are indirect measures of disease duration and do not accurately reflect the duration of viremia.

Unlike results from other studies [22, 23], no significant correlation was found between ethnic origin and the presence of HTN. However, the rate of BP increase over time was significantly higher in Ethiopian than in non-Ethiopian HIV-infected subjects. This finding may be related to lifestyle and dietary modifications as a result of immigration and is supported by a research conducted in Israel among Ethiopian adolescents, which pointed to the impact of an adopted new lifestyle on BP [25]. It is important to note that in this study the proportion of male patients of Ethiopian origin was significantly lower than in the non-Ethiopian group (42% versus 79%, $P < 0.001$). Since male patients had a significantly higher prevalence of HTN, this may have resulted in an underestimation of HTN prevalence among patients of Ethiopian origin.

A limitation of this study resides in its retrospective nature, which prevents determining the cause of HTN. Current guidelines define HTN as the average of two or more properly measured readings at each of two or more office visits after an initial screen [26]. With multiple measurements, high BP tends to decrease during subsequent visits [26, 42]. However, elevated BP may be predictive of future BP elevations [43], and the high prevalence of HTN was recorded at two different time points under identical conditions during the whole follow-up period. This somewhat reduces the probability of inconsistency between measurements. Although HTN data obtained at the last visit was similar to the values in the general population (63/278, 22.6%), this may have been the result of antihypertensive medication provided to patients with high BP during follow-up.

5. Conclusions

HIV-infected adults have an increased risk of cardiovascular morbidity and related risk factors, such as the metabolic syndrome.

Our study reports increased prevalence of HTN in this population in comparison with the general population and points to an increased rate of BP rise in Ethiopian HIV-infected adults. Despite the lack of a clear explanation for this finding, we postulate that prolonged replication of the virus and the resulting inflammatory process may lead to metabolic syndrome and related hypertension. Raising awareness of the treating physicians to the significance of this risk factor will allow better monitoring and earlier treatment, reducing the impact of this risk factor on cardiovascular mortality.

Acknowledgments

Michele Hauzi-Bashan, Head Nurse at the Hadassah AIDS Center, performed all blood pressure measurements, as part of her routine clinical responsibilities.

References

[1] J. S. Currier, A. Taylor, F. Boyd et al., "Coronary heart disease in HIV-infected individuals," *Journal of Acquired Immune Deficiency Syndromes*, vol. 33, no. 4, pp. 506–512, 2003.

[2] P. Y. Hsue, K. Squires, A. F. Bolger et al., "Screening and assessment of coronary heart disease in HIV-infected patients," *Circulation*, vol. 118, no. 2, pp. e41–e47, 2008.

[3] V. A. Triant, H. Lee, C. Hadigan, and S. K. Grinspoon, "Increased acute myocardial infarction rates and cardiovascular risk factors among patients with human immunodeficiency virus disease," *The Journal of Clinical Endocrinology & Metabolism*, vol. 92, no. 7, pp. 2506–2512, 2007.

[4] G. K. Hansson, "Inflammation, atherosclerosis, and coronary artery disease," *The New England Journal of Medicine*, vol. 352, no. 16, pp. 1685–1695, 2005.

[5] J. S. Reingold, C. Wanke, D. P. Kotler et al., "Association of HIV infection and HIV/HCV coinfection with C-reactive protein levels: The fat redistribution and metabolic change in HIV infection (FRAM) study," *Journal of Acquired Immune Deficiency Syndromes*, vol. 48, no. 2, pp. 142–148, 2008.

[6] P. C. Tien, A. I. Choi, A. R. Zolopa et al., "Inflammation and mortality in HIV-infected adults: Analysis of the FRAM study cohort," *Journal of Acquired Immune Deficiency Syndromes* 55, no. 3, pp. 316–322, 2010.

[7] J. Baker, H. Quick, K. H. Hullsiek et al., "Interleukin-6 and d-dimer levels are associated with vascular dysfunction in patients with untreated HIV infection," *HIV Medicine*, vol. 11, no. 9, pp. 608-609, 2010.

[8] S. Subramanian, A. Tawakol, T. H. Burdo et al., "Arterial inflammation in patients with HIV," *Journal of the American Medical Association*, vol. 308, no. 4, pp. 379–386, 2012.

[9] N. Friis-Møller, C. A. Sabin, R. Weber et al., "Combination antiretroviral therapy and the risk of myocardial infarction," *New England Journal of Medicine*, vol. 349, pp. 1993–2003, 2003.

[10] A. Carr, K. Samaras, A. Thorisdottir, G. R. Kaufmann, D. J. Chisholm, and D. A. Cooper, "Diagnosis, prediction, and natural course of HIV-1 protease-inhibitor-associated lipodystrophy, hyperlipidaemia, and diabetes mellitus: a cohort study," *The Lancet*, vol. 353, no. 9170, pp. 2093–2099, 1999.

[11] E. Fontas, F. Van Leth, C. A. Sabin et al., "Lipid profiles in HIV-infected patients receiving combination antiretroviral therapy: are different antiretroviral drugs associated with different lipid profiles?" *The Journal of Infectious Diseases*, vol. 189, no. 6, pp. 1056–1074, 2004.

[12] G. Behrens, A. Dejam, H. Schmidt et al., "Impaired glucose tolerance, beta cell function and lipid metabolism in HIV patients under treatment with protease inhibitors," *AIDS* 13, no. 10, pp. F63–F70, 1999.

[13] M. Rayner, S. Allender, and P. Scarborough, "Cardiovascular disease in Europe," *European Journal of Cardiovascular Prevention & Rehabilitation*, vol. 16, supplement 2, pp. S43–S47, 2009.

[14] C. Grunfeld, M. Pang, W. Doerrler, J. K. Shigenaga, P. Jensen, and K. R. Feingold, "Lipids, lipoproteins, triglyceride clearance, and cytokines in human immunodeficiency virus infection and the acquired immunodeficiency syndrome," *The Journal of Clinical Endocrinology & Metabolism*, vol. 74, no. 5, pp. 1045–1052, 1992.

[15] T. T. Brown, S. R. Cole, X. Li et al., "Antiretroviral therapy and the prevalence and incidence of diabetes mellitus in the multicenter AIDS cohort study," *JAMA Internal Medicine*, vol. 165, no. 10, pp. 1179–1184, 2005.

[16] F. J. Palella Jr., K. M. Delaney, A. C. Moorman et al., "Declining morbidity and mortality among patients with advanced human immunodeficiency virus infection," *The New England Journal of Medicine*, vol. 338, no. 13, pp. 853–860, 1998.

[17] O. Jung, M. Bickel, T. Ditting et al., "Hypertension in HIV-1-infected patients and its impact on renal and cardiovascular integrity," *Nephrology Dialysis Transplantation* , vol. 19, no. 9, pp. 2250–2258, 2004.

[18] M. Baekken, I. Os, L. Sandvik, and O. Oektedalen, "Hypertension in an urban HIV-positive population compared with the general population: Influence of combination antiretroviral therapy," *Journal of Hypertension*, vol. 26, no. 11, pp. 2126–2133, 2008.

[19] R. Palacios, J. Santos, A. García et al., "Impact of highly active antiretroviral therapy on blood pressure in HIV-infected patients. A prospective study in a cohort of naive patients," *HIV Medicine*, vol. 7, no. 1, pp. 10–15, 2006.

[20] B. M. Bergersen, L. Sandvik, O. Dunlop, K. Birkeland, and J. N. Bruun, "Prevalence of Hypertension in HIV-Positive Patients on Highly Active Retroviral Therapy (HAART) compared with HAART-Naïve and HIV-Negative Controls: results from a Norwegian Study of 721 patients," *European Journal of Clinical Microbiology & Infectious Diseases*, vol. 22, no. 12, pp. 731–736, 2003.

[21] S. T. Kent, S. G. Bromfield, G. A. Burkholder et al., "Ambulatory blood pressure monitoring in individuals with HIV: A systematic review and meta-analysis," *PLoS ONE*, vol. 11, no. 2, Article ID e0148920, 2016.

[22] A. P. Carson, G. Howard, G. L. Burke, S. Shea, E. B. Levitan, and P. Muntner, "Ethnic differences in hypertension incidence among middle-aged and older adults: The multi-ethnic study of atherosclerosis," *Hypertension*, vol. 57, no. 6, pp. 1101–1107, 2011.

[23] H. Kramer, C. Han, W. Post et al., "Racial/ethnic differences in hypertension and hypertension treatment and control in the Multi-Ethnic Study of Atherosclerosis (MESA)," *American Journal of Hypertension*, vol. 17, no. 10, pp. 963–970, 2004.

[24] M. Twagirumukiza, D. De Bacquer, J. G. Kips, G. de Backer, R. V. Stichele, and L. M. van Bortel, "Current and projected prevalence of arterial hypertension in sub-Saharan Africa by sex, age and habitat: an estimate from population studies," *Journal of Hypertension*, vol. 29, no. 7, pp. 1243–1252, 2011.

[25] M. Bursztyn and I. Raz, "Blood pressure, glucose, insulin and lipids of young ethiopian recent immigrants to israel and in those resident for 2 years," *Journal of Hypertension*, vol. 11, no. 4, pp. 455–459, 1993.

[26] A. V. Chobanian, G. L. Bakris, H. R. Black et al., "The seventh report of the joint national committee on prevention, detection, evaluation, and treatment of high blood pressure: the JNC 7 report," *The Journal of the American Medical Association*, vol. 289, no. 19, pp. 2560–2572, 2003.

[27] S. M. Grundy, J. I. Cleeman, S. R. Daniels et al., "Diagnosis and management of the metabolic syndrome: an American Heart Association/National Heart, Lung, and Blood Institute scientific statement," *Circulation*, vol. 112, no. 17, pp. 2735–2752, 2005.

[28] American Diabetes Association, "Diagnosis and classification of diabetes mellitus," *Diabetes Care*, vol. 33, supplement 1, pp. S62–S69, 2010.

[29] M. A. Thompson, J. A. Aberg, J. F. Hoy et al., "Antiretroviral treatment of adult HIV infection: 2012 recommendations of the International Antiviral Society-USA panel," *The Journal of the American Medical Association*, vol. 308, no. 4, pp. 387–402, 2012.

[30] D. E. Vance, M. Mugavero, J. Willig, J. L. Raper, and M. S. Saag, "Aging with HIV: a cross-sectional study of comorbidity prevalence and clinical characteristics across decades of life," *Journal of the Association of Nurses in AIDS Care*, vol. 22, no. 1, pp. 17–25, 2011.

[31] C. Gazzaruso, R. Bruno, A. Garzaniti et al., "Hypertension among HIV patients: prevalence and relationships to insulin resistance and metabolic syndrome," *Journal of Hypertension*, vol. 21, no. 7, pp. 1377–1382, 2003.

[32] M. Fantoni, C. Del Borgo, C. Autore, and G. Barbaro, "Metabolic disorders and cardiovascular risk in HIV-infected patients treated with antiretroviral agents," *Italian Heart Journal*, vol. 3, no. 5, pp. 294–299, 2002.

[33] S. Grinspoon, "Insulin resistance in the HIV-lipodystrophy syndrome," *Trends in Endocrinology & Metabolism*, vol. 12, no. 9, pp. 413–419, 2001.

[34] N. Hejazi, M. S. Huang, K. G. Lin, and L. C. K. Choong, "Hypertension among HIV-infected adults receiving highly active antiretroviral therapy (HAART) in Malaysia," *Global Journal of Health Science*, vol. 6, no. 2, pp. 58–71, 2014.

[35] B. Isomaa, P. Almgren, T. Tuomi et al., "Cardiovascular morbidity and mortality associated with the metabolic syndrome," *Diabetes Care*, vol. 24, no. 4, pp. 683–689, 2001.

[36] C. Gazzaruso, P. Sacchi, A. Garzaniti, P. Fratino, R. Bruno, and G. Filice, "Prevalence of metabolic syndrome among HIV patients," *Diabetes Care*, vol. 25, no. 7, pp. 1253-1254, 2002.

[37] M. Bursztyn and I. Raz, "Prediction of hypertension by the insulinogenic index in young Ethiopian immigrants," *Journal of Hypertension*, vol. 13, no. 1, pp. 57–61, 1995.

[38] A. R. Dyer, K. Liu, M. Walsh, C. Kiefe, D. R. Jacobs Jr., and D. E. Bild, "Ten-year incidence of elevated blood pressure and its predictors: The CARDIA Study," *Journal of Human Hypertension*, vol. 13, no. 1, pp. 13–21, 1999.

[39] I. W. Manner, M. Trøseid, O. Oektedalen, M. Baekken, and I. Os, "Low nadir CD4 cell count predicts sustained hypertension in HIV-infected individuals," *The Journal of Clinical Hypertension*, vol. 15, no. 2, pp. 101–106, 2013.

[40] D. G. Harrison, T. J. Guzik, H. E. Lob et al., "Inflammation, immunity, and hypertension," *Hypertension*, vol. 57, no. 2, pp. 132–140, 2011.

[41] W. Jiang, M. M. Lederman, P. Hunt et al., "Plasma levels of bacterial DNA correlate with immune activation and the magnitude of immune restoration in persons with antiretroviral-treated HIV infection," *The Journal of Infectious Diseases*, vol. 199, no. 8, pp. 1177–1185, 2009.

[42] R. D. S. Watson, R. Lumb, M. A. Young, T. J. Stallard, P. Davies, and W. A. Littler, "Variation in cuff blood pressure in untreated outpatients with mild hypertension—implications for initiating antihypertensive treatment," *Journal of Hypertension*, vol. 5, no. 2, pp. 207–211, 1987.

[43] I. Bidlingmeyer, M. Burnier, M. Bidlingmeyer, B. Waeber, and H. R. Brunner, "Isolated office hypertension: A prehypertensive state?" *Journal of Hypertension*, vol. 14, no. 3, pp. 327–332, 1996.

The MentalPlus® Digital Game Might Be an Accessible Open Source Tool to Evaluate Cognitive Dysfunction in Heart Failure with Preserved Ejection Fraction in Hypertensive Patients: A Pilot Exploratory Study

Valeria Fontenelle Angelim Pereira and Livia Stocco Sanches Valentin

Department of Cardiopneumology, Heart Institute, School of medicine, University of São Paulo, São Paulo, Brazil

Correspondence should be addressed to Valeria Fontenelle Angelim Pereira; valeria@angelim.com.br

Academic Editor: Francesco Cappuccio

Introduction. Cognitive dysfunction with heart failure with reduced ejection fraction (HFrEF) is well studied. However, there are few comparative studies with heart failure and preserved ejection fraction (HFpEF). Cognitive dysfunction diagnosis usually demands a long neuropsychological battery. We developed MentalPlus® digital game to overwhelm that issue. *Methods.* As a pilot study, we evaluated 60 patients with systemic hypertension and HFpEF. They were submitted to TICS (Telephone Interview Cognitive Status) to evaluate the general cognitive function and 25 minutes of MentalPlus® digital game evaluation. *Results.* The results disclosed 60 hypertensive patients. All of them presented with HFpEF. Patients presented a mean age of 56±10 years; 46% male; LVMi (g/m^2) mean of 110±20; educational attainment of 9 years or more; mean income of 8 Brazilian minimum wages. The TICS results disclosed 28 ±3.7. MentalPlus® digital game evaluation disclosed preserved values for the phases I, III, IV, V, VI, and VII. Phase II, short-term memory related, was below the normals values that were assigned. This group of patients presented a normal general cognition by both evaluations, except for specific functions displayed above, disclosed by MentalPlus®. The MentalPlus® was designed to possibly evaluate specific cognitive functions separately, like attention, memory, executive function, and language, because each phase evaluates specific functions shortly. *Conclusion.* Hypertensive HFpEF patients presented in general a normal cognition, except for some aspects related to short-term memory. The MentalPlus® digital game, compared with TICS, presented similar general results. It is an advantage that MentalPlus® software could be used to assess cognitive function, in general and individually, and be an open tool shortly.

1. Introduction

Heart failure (HF) is a major health problem in developed countries that affects 1%–2% of the adult population with rising prevalence in people over 65 years or older [1].

There is a strong association with increased mortality and morbidity, frequent hospital admissions, and reduced quality of life and functional status [2]. It is important to bear in mind that most randomized controlled trials in HF specifically exclude patients with significant comorbidities or HFpEF, yet this group constitutes a significant proportion of older people with HF [3–5].

Up to 75 % of >65-year-old patients will have multiple chronic conditions that will impact HF management; [4, 6] comorbidity is one of the strongest independent predictors of rehospitalization and mortality[7]. One of the key factors less frequently considered as comorbidities in patients with HF is cognitive impairment.

The impaired cognitive function is associated with poor levels of self-care and functional decline [8] and predicts nonengagement in HF management programmers. Patients may not recognize or understand a change in symptoms or function, with negative consequences for overall care.

Identifying cognitive impairment allows patient, caregivers, and clinicians to plan management strategies and clinicians should be vigilant for its presence. Observational data suggest that informal assessment of cognition by cardiologists is insensitive, with approximately three in four HF patients with important cognitive problems not recognized during their routine consultations. [9] Nearly half of all patients with HF symptoms, like breathlessness on exertion, have a preserved EF, exceeding 50%. Its prevalence is rising, with morbidity, mortality, and healthcare costs following the same trends of HF with reduced EF (HFrEF). HFpEF patients also present multiple common comorbidities, such as hypertension, diabetes mellitus, renal disease, atrial fibrillation, and metabolic syndrome, which have a major impact on the syndrome and mortality. [6, 10–13]

Cognitive function is a superior cortical function involving multiple brain activities that permit that human being perceives information, learn it, and remember specific knowledge. It can enable us to solve problems and plan actions during daily life. There are some cognitive functions, including memory, attention, executive function, language, and visuospatial ability. [14]The most frequently measured cognitive domains in HF studies are attention, working memory, long-term memory, learning, executive function, and psychomotor speed, with approximately 28%–58% of individuals with HF demonstrating impairment of one or more of those cognitive domains. [15] There are many neuropsychologic tests, used to measure different cognitive domains. The main impairment is that it is a time-consuming process. It usually deserves around 2 hours to have a complete evaluation, and only specialists can make it. Moreover, at least in our country, Brazil, the majority of these tests can be known and applied only by psychologists and neuropsychologists. Other health professionals interested in evaluating the cognitive function of patients are not allowed to use them. The restriction to use and time-consuming applicability of the neuropsychological tests has led the scientific community to a constant search for alternative diagnostic methods to evaluate cognition. As an alternative to overcome those issues, we developed a digital game named MentalPlus® as a possible open tool to assess cognition. Previous studies have shown that digital games might stimulate cognitive functions and enhance skills such as creativity, the search for strategies, decision-making, and skills aimed at visuoperception. In clinical trials, the games have been applied for neuropsychological function skill improvement. They have been able to modify the structure and functioning of the brain architecture. [16, 17]

However, the use of virtual games for assessing the integrity of neuropsychological functions is insufficient or nonexistent. The development and validation of an easy neuropsychological open test application as a digital game can contribute to a better cognition knowledge in different clinical situations, as in HFpEF.

The primary objective of this study aimed to evaluate general cognitive status comparing the MentalPlus® digital game to Telephone Interview Cognition Status (TICS). Afterward, the secondary objective of the study would be to describe specific cognitive function status in this pilot study group and stimulate the continuous study to validate that simple, open source tool to be used by colleagues in various health fields to access cognitive dysfunction in earlier states. One of the most important social conditions would be its application mainly where the sociodemographic conditions are low and give a chance to those patients to have rehabilitation and possible inclusion in society.

2. Materials and Methods

2.1. Study Design and Subject Enrollment. The study conceived as a pilot exploratory study, received the approval of the Ethics Committee for Research Project Analysis (CAPPesq) of the Clinical Board, Hospital das Clínicas da Faculdade de Medicina da Universidade de São Paulo (HC-FMUSP) (S1 File).

There were 60 hypertensive treated patients, presenting exertion dyspnea, enrolled to be submitted to TICS, and play a free digital game, MentalPlus®, after invitation acceptance and a signed written informed consent. The volunteer recruitment to the study was from May 2016 to August 2016. The neuropsychological assessment phase study finished in September 2016.

Inclusion criteria were hypertensive treated patients who accepted the invitation to play a free digital game, MentalPlus®, and receive TICS test. They should present dyspnea on exertion and a normal left ventricular systolic function (Figure 1).

60 transthoracic echocardiography examinations performed with a 2D, M-Mode, pulse wave Doppler, and tissue Doppler echocardiography by using an ACUSON X300™ ultrasound system, Mountain View (California, USA) with a 1.4–5.6 MHz frequency bandwidth transducer. The echocardiographic measurements were according to American Society of Echocardiography: guidelines: http://asecho.org/guidelines/guidelines-standards/. Myocardial velocity profiles of the lateral mitral annulus are obtained by placing a 6 mm sample volume at the junction of the mitral annulus and lateral myocardial wall. Left ventricular mass (LVM) was calculated using the Devereux Formula [18], where $LVM = 0.8(1.04(IVST + LVID + LPWT)^3 - (LVID)^3 + 0.6)$, LVST is interventricular septal thickness, LVID is left ventricular internal dimension, and LPWT is left posterior wall thickness. The left ventricular mass index (LVMI) calculus used the formula, LVM/(height). [18, 19] The systolic ventricular function was assessed by 2D biplane Simpson's rule. Left ventricular ejection fraction (LVEF) ≥ 50 % has been defined as preserved or normal left ventricular (LV) systolic function.

The exclusion criteria were the presence of a history of brain disease or dementia, psychiatric disorders that affect cognition, and the presence of some grade of visuomotor ability impairment to play video games and a not preserved left ventricular systolic function.

The Telephone Interview Cognition Status (TICS) was applied to all patients before MentalPlus®. The test consists of an interview script with 11 items that assess spatial and temporal orientation skills, mind control, memory, general information, language, and calculations (S2 File). The TICS total score is a sum of the individual item scores. It provides a measure of global cognitive functioning and can be used to monitor changes in cognitive functioning over time. TICS results are reported using a qualitative

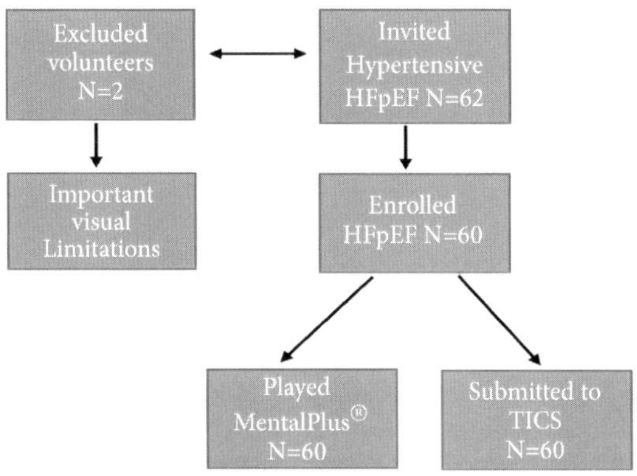

FIGURE 1: **Study fluxogram.** HFpEF: heart failure with preserved ejection fraction; MentalPlus®: Open Tool Virtual Game; TICS: Telephone Interview Cognition Status.

impairment range and *T* scores (TICS normal range for Brazilian population 27.7±3.3). The appropriate normative reference group for interpretation will depend on the reason for the evaluation and the examinee's age and level of education [20–22]. The study followed the CONSORT criteria (http://www.consort-statement.org/) (S3 File).

2.2. The Video Game MentalPlus® Characteristics. MentalPlus® is a digital game developed to evaluate and stimulate neuropsychological functions, patented and registered with the National Library Foundation by Law no. 9,610/98, under copyright no. 663,707. This digital game identifies the neuropsychological deficits in functions, Attention/Memory/Executive. Attention, resistance to distractor stimulus, sustaining attention, and memory evaluation consist of a series of tasks in 8 digital game phases. We show the game phases in detail in the video (S4 File).

2.3. Sociodemographic Evaluation. Demographic data were analyzed, including age, education, and family income. The education evaluation was an index derived from the schooling years and the family income based on Brazilian minimum wages.

3. Statistical Analyses

The qualitative characteristics were described using absolute and relative frequencies and the quantitative characteristics were described using summary measures (mean, standard deviation, median, minimum, and maximum) (Kirkwood and Sterne, 2006).

The domains of cognition assessed by MentalPlus were described according to each assessed personal and clinical qualitative trait and compared among the categories using Mann-Whitney tests (Kirkwood and Sterne, 2006) to verify construct validation of MentalPlus.

The Spearman (Kirkwood and Sterne, 2006) correlations of the MentalPlus domains with quantitative characteristics, age, and MAP (presence of HFpEF and presence of diastolic dysfunction) were also calculated for construct validation as well as for TICs for the concurrent validation of the MentalPlus domains with another cognition scale. But as that study was a descriptive and exploratory one, the group had still not the pretension to evaluate the power of the test at that study stage. We have the intention of developing larger studies in a newer future. At that time, surely, a precise sample size as confidence intervals and power calculations will be executed for more precise results. With that pilot study, the main objective was to show some data with hypertensive patients with HFpEF that could stimulate the scientific community to study cognitive function deeply in many heart groups, possibly with the open tool MentalPlus® digital game.

The analyses were performed using IBM-SPSS for Windows software version 20.0 and tabulated using Microsoft-Excel 2003 software and tests were performed with a significance level of 5% [23].

4. Results

According to Figure 1, we recruited 60 hypertensive patients under treatment with HFpEF and excluded two patients due to limiting visual problems. Patients presented treated hypertension and dyspnea on exertion. There was no history of anemia or COPD. Table 1 discloses sociodemographic and clinical data, with the mean and standard deviation (SD). The 60 study participants presented a mean age of 56±10 years (mean; SD). 46% were male. They had a school level mean of 13±3 years (mean; SD) and 72 % received a mean income ≥ ten while 28% received an amount corresponding to ≥ 5 and < 10 Brazilian minimum wages per month. The drugs used were thiazide diuretics, calcium channel blockers, beta-blockers, angiotensin-converting enzyme (ACE) inhibitors, and angiotensin II receptor blockers (ARB). Table 2 presented some clinical and echocardiographic parameters. Mean medium arterial pressure (MAP) was 94±9mmHg (mean; SD), with antihypertensive medication. They all presented EF ≥ 50% by 2D biplane Simpson's rule and 100% disclosed an abnormal diastolic function by tissue Doppler velocity measurements. Left ventricular hypertrophy was present in 53%, with a left ventricular mass index (LVMi) >90 and 110 g/m^2 for women and men, respectively. Left atrium volume per square meter was larger than 30 ml in 53% of them. Different professionals supervised both tests for each patient. We have not evaluated NT-proBNP.

In the neuropsychological evaluation, the HFpEF group exhibited TICS score of 28±3 (mean; SD), for an expectation of more than 25±3 (mean; SD) for the normal population [23].

Table 3 displayed that there was no statistically significant correlation between the MentalPlus domains and the age of the hypertensive patients (p> 0.05) and only the inverse correlation between short-term memory, MentalPlus® Phase II with mean arterial pressure (MAP) (r = -0.290 and p = 0.025). That implies that the higher the MAP, the lower the values for short-term memory. Although the correlation was low, it was statistically significant. TICs showed no statistically significant correlation with any of the MentalPlus

Table 1: Sociodemographic and clinical data.

Age(years) (Mean; SD)	56±10
Male Gender (%)	46
School level in years (13±3) (Mean; SD) (%)	100%
Mean Income ≥10 minimum wage (%)	75%
Dyspnea on exertion (%)	100%
Presence of anemia (%)	0%
Presence of POCD (%)	0%
Past history of heart failure (%)	0%
Presence of Type II Diabetes (%)	25%
Presence of 26≤ BMI ≤ 33	00%
Presence of Hypertension (%)	00%
Use of thiazide diuretics, calcium channel blockers, ARB, ACE inhibitors, beta-blockers (alone or in combination)	100%
Number of evaluated patients	60

SD: standard deviation; BMI: Body Mass Index; ARB: angiotensin receptor blocker; ACE: angiotensin converting enzyme inhibitors.

Table 2: Parameters of echocardiography evaluation.

MAP (mmHg) (Mean; SD)	VMI>90g/m^2 for female or >115g/m^2 for male (percentage)	LVEF (Simpson)≥50% (percentage)	LA volume (ml/m^2)≥30 (percentage)	E/A filling pressure>1 (percentage)	E/e′ ≥13 or E/e′ ≤8 (percentage)
(94;9)	53%	100%	53%	47%	100%

MAP: mean arterial pressure; SD: standard deviation; VMI: ventricular mass index; LVEF: left ventricular ejection fraction; Simpson: Simpson's method; LA: left atrium.

domains (p> 0.05). We tried to show that patients with hypertension and HFpEF with normal general cognitive function, evaluated by TICS, could have specific deficiencies as showed by MentalPlus® phase, like short memory function.

5. Discussion

This study found evidence that we might use MentalPlus® digital game in an HFpEF group of patients, for neuropsychological evaluation. It can be an open diagnostic tool of cognitive dysfunction for mnemonic, attentional, and executive functions. Data analysis yielded interesting findings. There was a good agreement for selective and alternate attention, long-term memory, inhibitory control, executive function, and visuoperception and visuoconstruction. Only short-term memory displayed an inverse correlation with MAP. Although the correlation was low, it was statistically significant (Table 3).

The use of the game in patients with HFpEF disclosed a normal general cognition, except for some aspects of the memory. That might be a sign that even in patients with normal ventricular systolic function, some factors that might be more intensively evaluated by MentalPlus® digital game can disclose characteristics that TICS by itself is not able to identify. The main interest in developing that possible open tool for cognitive function evaluation is its convenience when compared with extensive and time-consuming psychological battery usually undertaken to that end.

The digital game presents many advantages through the extensive psychological battery usually performed to evaluate those patients. It only requires about 25 minutes to be played through all its phases (S4). It would be enough to have an oriented health professional to apply the video game. The MentalPlus® has the proposal to evaluate attention, short- and long-term memory, executive function, language, and visuoconstruction. We can have both general and individualized evaluation of cognitive function. It can be used many times during cognitive evaluation follow-up and follow small changes in cognitive functions separately. Other usual cognitive tests, like Mini-Mental State Examination (MMSE), could be speculated to be applied. Otherwise, the content of the MMSE is highly verbal, lacking sufficient items to measure both visuospatial and constructional praxis adequately. It brings some limitations as evaluation of low cognitive impairment as small changes. Hence, its utility to detect impairment caused by focal lesions is uncertain. We are aware that to evaluate all those cognitive functions, it would be necessary a long time to perform a neuropsychological battery.

Therefore, that justification would favor MentalPlus® digital game usefulness in a broad of clinical settings as we can observe in this pilot study with an emphasis in HFpEF, enabling a prompt cognitive dysfunction diagnosis. Future research might focus on direct neuropsychological assessment using the MentalPlus® digital game in patients for diverse underline pathologies. We already presented the game reliability in near past [23]. Now, our next step is the validation of the digital game cited in a normal population, compared with a normal neuropsychologic test battery. Although preliminary studies have shown that we can apply that digital game for that goal, there is a necessity for accurate measurements and calibrations to get reliable results of these cognitive functions.

Table 3: Spearman correlation with MentalPlus® phases, with patients age, mean arterial pressure, and TICS.

Spearman Correlation		Age (years)	Mean arterial pressure	TICS
Short Term Memory, MentalPlus Phase II	r	−0,048	−0,290	0,119
	p	0,715	**0,025**	0,363
Inhibitory Control, MentalPlus Phase II	r	0,092	0,033	0,097
	p	0,485	0,801	0,463
Visuoperception and Visuoconstruction, MP phases VI and VII	r	0,057	0,016	−0,151
	p	0,663	0,904	0,248
Selective Attention, MP phases III and IV	r	0,093	−0,044	0,097
	p	0,480	0,741	0,460
Alternate Attention, MP phases V and VI	r	−0,009	0,054	0,192
	p	0,944	0,680	0,141
Long Phase Memory, MP phase I	r	−0,182	0,033	0,122
	p	0,163	0,804	0,352
Spearman correlation				

MP: Mentalplus.

6. Conclusion

The MentalPlus® digital game already presented reliable evidence for cognition evaluation like attention, memory, and executive functions. Here we showed that in HFpEF the general and specific cognitive functions are preserved, except for a lower range of short-term memory function-MentalPlus phase II. It might have many implications but bring to the scientific community that at that level of the pathology we should make every effort to stimulate the cognitive functions, besides the maintenance of the treatment and all the risk factors. As a feasible open tool, it is possible to claim for new colleagues to use the digital game and evaluate it with us. Additional study will contribute for an effective calibration of the game as for its validation and usual open utilization.

Conflicts of Interest

The authors have declared that no conflicts of interest exist.

Authors' Contributions

Livia Stocco Sanches Valentin and Valeria Fontenelle Angelim Pereira conceived and designed the experiments; Valeria Fontenelle Angelim Pereira and Livia Stocco Sanches Valentin performed the experiments; Livia Stocco Sanches Valentin and Valeria Fontenelle Angelim Pereira analyzed the data; Valeria Fontenelle Angelim Pereira wrote the manuscript.

Acknowledgments

The authors wish to acknowledge the timely help given by Professor Simone Kühn, Max Planck Institute, and Professor Lars Simon Rasmussen, the University of Copenhagen, in the support that we received for our study with MentalPlus®. Our Research was supported by Comissão de Análise de Projetos de Pesquisa da Universidade de São Paulo, CAPpesq-FMUSP (**CAAE: 49463315.5.1001.0068**), Coordenação de Aperfeiçoamento de Pessoal de Nível Superior, CAPES, Faculdade de Medicina, FMUSP, Pró-Reitoria de Pós-Graduação da Universidade de São Paulo, PRRG/USP, and Project MentalPlus Association, A.P.M.P., a NGO, from Brazil.

Supplementary Materials

Supporting File 1 (S1): the approval of the Ethics Committee for Research Project Analysis (CAPPesq) of the Clinical Board, Hospital das Clínicas da Faculdade de Medicina da Universidade de São Paulo (HC-FMUSP). Supporting File 2 (S2): the Telephone Interview Cognition Status (TICS). Supporting File 3 (S3): the CONSORT criteria (http://www.consort-statement.org). Supporting File 4 (S4): video-demo MentalPlus®. *(Supplementary Materials)*

References

[1] P. Ponikowski, A. A. Voors, S. D. Anker et al., "2016 ESC guidelines for the diagnosis and treatment of acute and chronic heart failure: The task force for the diagnosis and treatment of acute and chronic heart failure of the European Society of Cardiology (ESC) developed with the special contribution of the Heart Failure Association (HFA) of the ESC," *European Heart Journal*, vol. 37, no. 27, pp. 2129–2200, 2016.

[2] A. P. Maggioni, U. Dahlström, G. Filippatos et al., "EURObservational Research Programme: regional differences and 1-year follow-up results of the Heart Failure Pilot Survey (ESC-HF Pilot)," *European Journal of Heart Failure*, vol. 15, no. 7, pp. 808–817, 2014.

[3] A. Donkor, J. Cleland, T. McDonagh et al., "National Heart Failure Audit, April 2014–March 2015," http://www.ucl.ac.uk/nicor/audits/heartfailure/documents/annualreports/heartfailurepublication14_15.

[4] K. Sharma and D. A. Kass, "Heart failure with preserved ejection fraction: mechanisms, clinical features, and therapies," *Circulation Research*, vol. 115, no. 1, pp. 79–96, 2014.

[5] C. W. Yancy, M. Jessup, B. Bozkurt et al., "2013 ACCF/AHA guideline for the management of heart failure: A report of the American college of cardiology foundation/American heart

association task force on practice guidelines," *Circulation*, vol. 128, no. 16, pp. e240–e327, 2013.

[6] A. S. Go, D. Mozaffarian, V. L. Roger et al., "American Heart Association Statistics Committee and Stroke Statistics Subcommittee. Heart disease and stroke statistics–2013 update: a report from the American Heart Association," *Circulation*, vol. 127, pp. e6–e245, 2013.

[7] I. Oudejans, A. Mosterd, N. P. Zuithoff, and A. W. Hoes, "Comorbidity drives mortality in newly diagnosed HF: a study among geriatric outpatients," *Journal of Cardiac Failure*, vol. 18, no. 1, pp. 47–52, 2012.

[8] K. Harkness, G. A. Heckman, N. Akhtar-Danesh, C. Demers, E. Gunn, and R. S. McKelvie, "Cognitive function and self-care management in older patients with heart failure," *European Journal of Cardiovascular Nursing*, vol. 13, no. 3, pp. 277–284, 2014.

[9] O. Hanon, J.-S. Vidal, P. de Groote et al., "Prevalence of memory disorders in ambulatory patients aged ≥70 years with chronic heart failure (from the EFICARE Study)," *The American Journal of Cardiology*, vol. 113, no. 7, pp. 1205–1210, 2014.

[10] B. A. Steinberg, X. Zhao, P. A. Heidenreich et al., "Trends in patients hospitalized with heart failure and preserved left ventricular ejection fraction: Prevalence, therapies, and outcomes," *Circulation*, vol. 126, no. 1, pp. 65–75, 2012.

[11] T. E. Owan, D. O. Hodge, R. M. Herges, S. J. Jacobsen, V. L. Roger, and M. M. Redfield, "Trends in prevalence and outcome of heart failure with preserved ejection fraction," *The New England Journal of Medicine*, vol. 355, no. 3, pp. 251–259, 2006.

[12] R. S. Bhatia, J. V. Tu, D. S. Lee et al., "Outcome of heart failure with preserved ejection fraction in a population-based study," *The New England Journal of Medicine*, vol. 355, no. 3, pp. 260–269, 2006.

[13] L. Liao, J. G. Jollis, K. J. Anstrom et al., "Costs for heart failure with normal vs reduced ejection fraction," *Arch Intern Med*, vol. 166, no. 1, pp. 112–118, 2006.

[14] M. D. Lezak, *Neuropsychological assessment*, vol. 3, Oxford University Press, NY, USA, 2004.

[15] L. Bauer, B. Pozehl, M. Hertzog, J. Johnson, L. Zimmerman, and M. Filipi, "A brief neuropsychological battery for use in the chronic heart failure population," *European Journal of Cardiovascular Nursing*, vol. 11, no. 2, pp. 223–230, 2017.

[16] C. Green and D. Bavelier, "Learning, Attentional Control, and Action Video Games," *Current Biology*, vol. 22, no. 6, pp. R197–R206, 2012.

[17] F. Fernández-Aranda, S. Jiménez-Murcia, J. J. Santamaría et al., "Video games as a complementary therapy tool in mental disorders: playMancer, a European multicentre study," *Journal of Mental Health*, vol. 21, no. 4, pp. 364–374, 2012.

[18] R. B. Devereux, D. R. Alonso, and E. M. Lutas, "Echocardiographic assessment of left ventricular hypertrophy: comparison to necropsy findings," *American Journal of Cardiology*, vol. 57, no. 6, pp. 450–458, 1986.

[19] C. A. Feldstein, M. Akopian, A. O. Olivieri, A. P. Kramer, M. Nasi, and D. Garrido, "A comparison of body mass index and waist-to-hip ratio as indicators of hypertension risk in an urban Argentine population: A hospital-based study," *Nutrition, Metabolism & Cardiovascular Diseases*, vol. 15, no. 4, pp. 310–315, 2005.

[20] T. G. Fong, M. A. Fearing, R. N. Jones et al., "Telephone Interview for Cognitive Status: Creating a crosswalk with the Mini-Mental State Examination," *Alzheimer's & Dementia*, vol. 5, no. 6, pp. 492–497, 2009.

[21] O. L. Lopez and L. H. Kuller, "Telephone interview for cognitive status," *Neuroepidemiology*, vol. 34, no. 1, pp. 63-64, 2010.

[22] J. Brandt, M. Spencer, and M. Folstein, "The Telephone Interview for Cognitive Status," *Neuropsychiatry Neuropsychol Behav Neurol*, vol. 1, pp. 111–117, 1988.

[23] B. R. kirkwood and J. A. C. sterne, *Essential medical statistics*, Blackwell Science, Massachusetts, USA, 2nd edition, 2006.

Permissions

 Every chapter published in this book has been scrutinized by our experts. Their significance has been extensively debated. The topics covered herein carry significant findings which will fuel the growth of the discipline. They may even be implemented as practical applications or may be referred to as a beginning point for another development.

The contributors of this book come from diverse backgrounds, making this book a truly international effort. This book will bring forth new frontiers with its revolutionizing research information and detailed analysis of the nascent developments around the world.

We would like to thank all the contributing authors for lending their expertise to make the book truly unique. They have played a crucial role in the development of this book. Without their invaluable contributions this book wouldn't have been possible. They have made vital efforts to compile up to date information on the varied aspects of this subject to make this book a valuable addition to the collection of many professionals and students.

This book was conceptualized with the vision of imparting up-to-date information and advanced data in this field. To ensure the same, a matchless editorial board was set up. Every individual on the board went through rigorous rounds of assessment to prove their worth. After which they invested a large part of their time researching and compiling the most relevant data for our readers.

The editorial board has been involved in producing this book since its inception. They have spent rigorous hours researching and exploring the diverse topics which have resulted in the successful publishing of this book. They have passed on their knowledge of decades through this book. To expedite this challenging task, the publisher supported the team at every step. A small team of assistant editors was also appointed to further simplify the editing procedure and attain best results for the readers.

Apart from the editorial board, the designing team has also invested a significant amount of their time in understanding the subject and creating the most relevant covers. They scrutinized every image to scout for the most suitable representation of the subject and create an appropriate cover for the book.

The publishing team has been an ardent support to the editorial, designing and production team. Their endless efforts to recruit the best for this project, has resulted in the accomplishment of this book. They are a veteran in the field of academics and their pool of knowledge is as vast as their experience in printing. Their expertise and guidance has proved useful at every step. Their uncompromising quality standards have made this book an exceptional effort. Their encouragement from time to time has been an inspiration for everyone.

The publisher and the editorial board hope that this book will prove to be a valuable piece of knowledge for researchers, students, practitioners and scholars across the globe.

List of Contributors

Vincent Boima
School of Medicine and Dentistry, University of Ghana, Accra, Ghana
Department of Medicine, Korle Bu Teaching Hospital, Accra, Ghana

Francis Agyekum
Department of Medicine, Korle Bu Teaching Hospital, Accra, Ghana

Adebowale Dele Ademola
Department of Paediatrics, Faculty of Clinical Sciences, College of Medicine, University of Ibadan, Ibadan PMB 5017, Oyo State, Nigeria
Department of Paediatrics, University College Hospital, Ibadan PMB 5116, Oyo State, Nigeria

Aina Olufemi Odusola
Department of Medicine, General Hospital, Randle Avenue, Apapa PMB 1014, Lagos, Nigeria

Chibuike Eze Nwafor
Cardiology Division, Department of Medicine, University of Port Harcourt Teaching Hospital, Port Harcourt PMB 6173, Rivers State, Nigeria

Helen Cole
Department of Population Health, NYU School of Medicine, 227 E. 30th Street, 6th Floor, New York, NY 10016, USA

Babatunde L. Salako
Department of Medicine, Faculty of Clinical Sciences, College of Medicine, University of Ibadan, Ibadan PMB 5017, Oyo State, Nigeria
Department of Medicine, University College Hospital, Ibadan PMB 5116, Oyo State, Nigeria

Gbenga Ogedegbe
Department of Population Health, NYU School of Medicine, 227 E. 30th Street, 6th Floor, New York, NY 10016, USA
Global Institute of Public Health, New York University, New York, NY 10003, USA

Bamidele O. Tayo
Department of Public Health Sciences, Stritch School of Medicine, Loyola University Chicago, 2160 South First Avenue, Maywood, IL 60153, USA

Khwaja Mir Islam Saeed
Grant and Service Contract Management Unit (GCMU), Ministry of Public Health, Kabul, Afghanistan

Sayed Fazel Zinat Motlagh, Sayed Rashid Ghafari, Zafar Parisay, Mohamad Reza Golabi and Amin Babouei
Social Determinants of Health Research Center, Yasuj University of Medical Sciences, Yasuj, Iran

Reza Chaman
Department of Community Medicine, School of Medicine, Yasuj University of Medical Sciences, Yasuj, Iran

Ahmad Ali Eslami
Department of Health Education and Promotion, School of Health, Isfahan University of Medical Sciences, Isfahan, Iran

Richard F. W. Barnes and Thomas J. Cramer
Department of Medicine, Division of Hematology/ Oncology, University of California San Diego, San Diego, CA, USA

Afrah S. Sait
Department of Medicine, Division of Hematology/ Oncology, University of California San Diego, San Diego, CA, USA
Department of Medicine, University of British Columbia, Vancouver, BC, Canada

Rebecca Kruse-Jarres
School of Medicine, Section of Hematology/Oncology, Tulane University, New Orleans, LA, USA
Washington Center for Bleeding Disorders at Bloodworks NW, Seattle, WA, USA

Doris V. K. Quon
Orthopaedic Hemophilia Treatment Center, Orthopaedic Institute for Children, Los Angeles, CA, USA

Annette von Drygalski
Department of Medicine, Division of Hematology/ Oncology, University of California San Diego, San Diego, CA, USA
Department of Molecular and Experimental Medicine, The Scripps Research Institute, La Jolla, CA, USA

Eva Drevenhorn
Department of Health Sciences, Faculty of Medicine, Lund University, Lund, Sweden

Mirnova E. Ceïde
Montefiore Medical Center, Department of Psychiatry and Behavioral Science, 111 East 210 Street, Bronx, NY 10467, USA

Abhishek Pandey and Margaret Donat
Brooklyn Health Disparities Center, Department of Medicine, SUNY Downstate Medical Center, Brooklyn, NY 11203, USA

Gbenga Ogedegbe, Girardin Jean-Louis and Joe Ravenell
Center for Healthful Behavior Change, Department of Population Health, NYU Langone Medical Center, New York, NY 10016, USA

Rajendra Bhimma and Elaene Naicker
Department of Paediatrics and Child Health, Nelson R Mandela School of Medicine, School of Health Science, University of KwaZulu-Natal, Congella, Durban 4013, South Africa

Verena Gounden
Department of Chemical Pathology, University of KwaZulu-Natal and National Health Laboratory Services, Inkosi Albert Luthuli Central Hospital, Durban, South Africa

Louansha Nandlal
Department of Optics and Imaging, Nelson R Mandela School of Medicine, School of Health Science, University of KwaZulu-Natal, South Africa

Cathy Connolly
Department of Biostatistics, School of Public Health, University of KwaZulu-Natal, South Africa

Sudesh Hariparshad
Department of Nephrology, Nelson R Mandela School of Medicine, School of Health Science, University of KwaZulu-Natal, Congella, Durban 4013, South Africa

Esi K. Colecraft and Seth Adu-Afarwuah
Department of Nutrition and Food Science, University of Ghana, Legon, Accra, Ghana

Matilda Asante
Department of Dietetics, School of Biomedical and Allied Health Sciences, College of Health Sciences, University of Ghana, Accra, Ghana

Aaron K. Christian
Regional Institute for Population Studies, University of Ghana, Legon, Ghana

R. Bou Serhal, N. Wakim, B. Kassem, L. Abou Jaoude and N. Saleh
Department of Epidemiology and biostatistics, Faculty of Public Health, Lebanese University, Fanar, Lebanon

P. Salameh
Faculty of Pharmacy, Lebanese University, Al Hadath, Lebanon

C. Issa
Department of Nutrition and Dietetics, Faculty of Public Health, Lebanese University, Fanar, Lebanon

Kirubel Zemedkun Gebreselassie
Epidemiology and Global Health, Department of Public Health and Clinical Medicine, Umeå University, 901 85 Umeå, Sweden

Mojgan Padyab
Centre for Population Studies, Ageing and Living Conditions Programme, Umeå University,Umeå, Sweden

Stefano Omboni
Clinical Research Unit, Italian Institute of Telemedicine, 21048 Solbiate Arno, Italy

Igor N. Posokhov
Hemodynamic Laboratory, Nizhny Novgorod 603009, Russia

Anatoly N. Rogoza
Department of New Methods of Diagnostics, Russian Cardiology Research and Production Complex, Moscow 121552, Russia

Takuto Nakamura, Masanobu Yamazato, Akio Ishida and Yusuke Ohya
Department of Cardiovascular Medicine, Nephrology and Neurology, Graduate School of Medicine, University of the Ryukyus, Okinawa Prefecture, Japan

Masood Ahmad and Devan Makati
Department of Medicine, West Virginia University School of Medicine, Morgantown, WV, USA

Sana Akbar
Department of Medicine, Division of Nephrology, West Virginia University School of Medicine, Morgantown, WV, USA

Mariel VanWoudenberg, Jean Shin, Manon Bernard, Catriona Syme and Zdenka Pausova
The Hospital for Sick Children, University of Toronto, Toronto, ON, Canada M5G 1X8

Michal Abrahamowicz
Department of Epidemiology, Biostatistics and Occupational Health, McGill University, Montreal, QC, Canada H3A 0G4

Gabriel Leonard
Montreal Neurological Institute and Hospital, McGill University, Montreal, QC, Canada H3A 2B4

Michel Perron, Louis Richer and Suzanna Veillette
Université du Québec à Chicoutimi, Chicoutimi, QC, Canada G7H 2B1

Daniel Gaudet
Community Genomic Centre, Chicoutimi Hospital, Université de Montréal, Montreal, QC, Canada G7H 5H6

Tomas Paus
Rotman Research Institute, University of Toronto, Toronto, ON, Canada M6A 2E1

William K. Bosu
Department of Epidemics and Disease Control, West African Health Organisation, 01 BP 153, Bobo-Dioulasso 01, Burkina Faso

Lai-Jiang Chen and Jiu-Chang Zhong
State Key Laboratory of Medical Genomics, Ruijin Hospital, School of Medicine, Shanghai Jiao Tong University, Shanghai 200025, China
Shanghai Key Laboratory of Hypertension, Shanghai Institute of Hypertension, Shanghai 200025, China
Institute of Health Sciences, Shanghai Institute for Biological Sciences, Chinese Academy of Sciences, Shanghai 200025, China

Ran Xu and Qing Chang
State Key Laboratory of Medical Genomics, Ruijin Hospital, School of Medicine, Shanghai Jiao Tong University, Shanghai 200025, China
Shanghai Key Laboratory of Hypertension, Shanghai Institute of Hypertension, Shanghai 200025, China

Hui-Min Yu
Department of Cardiology, Guangdong General Hospital, Guangdong Academy of Medical Sciences, Guangzhou 510080, China

S. Curcio, V. García-Espinosa, I. Farro, Y. Zócalo and D. Bia
Physiology Department, Faculty of Medicine, CUiiDARTE, University of the Republic, General Flores 2125, 11800 Montevideo, Uruguay

M. Arana and G. Giachetto
Clínica Pediátrica "C", Pereira-Rossel Hospital Centre, Faculty of Medicine, University of the Republic, Bulevar Artigas 1550, 11600 Montevideo, Uruguay

P. Chiesa
Pediatric Cardiology Service, Pereira-Rossell Hospital Centre, ASSE, Bulevar Artigas 1550, 11600 Montevideo, Uruguay

Alejandro Diaz
Instituto de Investigación en Ciencias de la Salud, UNICEN, CONICET, Tandil, Argentina

Daniel Bia and Yanina Zócalo
Physiology Department, School of Medicine, Centro Universitario de Investigación, Innovación y Diagnóstico Arterial (CUiiDARTE), Republic University, General Flores 2125, 11800 Montevideo, Uruguay

Hugo Manterola, Ignacio Larrabide, Lucas Lo Vercio and Mariana Del Fresno
PLADEMA, Facultad de Ciencias Exactas, Universidad Nacional del Centro de la Provincia de Buenos Aires, Tandil, Argentina

Edmundo Cabrera Fischer
Instituto de Medicina Traslacional, Trasplante y Bioingeniería (IMETTyB),Universidad Favaloro-CONICET, Buenos Aires, Argentina

Walters Tabi Arrey
Ako District Hospital, North West Region, Cameroon

Christian Akem Dimala
Faculty of Epidemiology and Population Health, London School of Hygiene and Tropical Medicine, London, UK
Orthopaedics Department, Southend University Hospital, Essex, UK
Health and Human Development (2HD) Research Group, Douala, Cameroon

Julius Atashili and Gottlieb Lobe Monekosso
Faculty of Health Sciences, University of Buea, Buea, Cameroon

Josephine Mbuagbaw
Faculty of Health Sciences, University of Buea, Buea, Cameroon
College of Medicine, Madonna University Nigeria, Rivers State, Nigeria

Ho Anh Hien
Department of Family Medicine, Hue University of Medicine and Pharmacy, Hue University, Hue, Vietnam
Department of Family Medicine and Chronic Care, Faculty of Medicine and Pharmacy, Vrije Universiteit Brussel, Brussels, Belgium

Dirk Devroey
Department of Family Medicine and Chronic Care, Faculty of Medicine and Pharmacy, Vrije Universiteit Brussel, Brussels, Belgium

Nguyen Minh Tam
Department of Family Medicine, Hue University of Medicine and Pharmacy, Hue University, Hue, Vietnam

Vo Tam
Department of Internal Medicine, Hue University of Medicine and Pharmacy, Hue University, Hue, Vietnam

Anselme Derese
Department of Family Medicine and Primary Health Care, Faculty of Medicine and Health Sciences, Ghent University, Ghent, Belgium

Xianglong Xu, Lingli Liu, Cheng Chen and Yong Zhao
School of Public Health and Management, Chongqing Medical University, Chongqing 400016, China
Research Center for Medicine and Social Development, Chongqing Medical University, Chongqing 400016, China
The Innovation Center for Social Risk Governance in Health, Chongqing Medical University, Chongqing 400016, China

Yunshuang Rao
School of Nursing, Chongqing Medical University, Chongqing 400016, China

Zumin Shi
School of Medicine, Faculty of Health Sciences, The University of Adelaide, North Terrace, Adelaide, SA 5005, Australia

Shikha Singh and Ravi Shankar
Department of Community Medicine, Institute of Medical Sciences, Banaras Hindu University, Varanasi 221005, India

Gyan Prakash Singh
Division of Biostatistics, Department of Community Medicine, Institute of Medical Sciences, Banaras Hindu University, Varanasi 221005, India

Geofrey Musinguzi
Department of Disease Control and Environmental Health, School of Public Health, Makerere University, Kampala, Uganda
Primary and Interdisciplinary Care, University of Antwerp, Antwerp, Belgium

Sibyl Anthierens and Hilde Bastiaens
Primary and Interdisciplinary Care, University of Antwerp, Antwerp, Belgium

Rhoda K. Wanyenze and Fred Nuwaha
Department of Disease Control and Environmental Health, School of Public Health, Makerere University, Kampala, Uganda

Jean-Pierre Van Geertruyden
International Health, University of Antwerp, Antwerp, Belgium

Sarah Cuschieri and Nikolai Pace
Department of Anatomy, Faculty of Medicine and Surgery, University of Malta, Msida, Malta

Josanne Vassallo
Faculty of Medicine and Surgery, University of Malta, Msida, Malta

Neville Calleja
Department of Public Health, Faculty of Medicine and Surgery, University of Malta, Msida, Malta
Department of Health Information and Research, Ministry of Health, Guardamangia, Malta

Julian Mamo
Department of Public Health, Faculty of Medicine and Surgery, University of Malta, Msida, Malta

Giselle Sarganas and Hannelore K. Neuhauser
Robert Koch Institute, Department of Epidemiology and Health Monitoring, Berlin, Germany
DZHK (German Center for Cardiovascular Research), Partner Site Berlin, Germany

Angelika Schaffrath Rosario
Robert Koch Institute, Department of Epidemiology and Health Monitoring, Berlin, Germany

Claudia Niessner and Alexander Woll
Institute for Sports and Sport Science, Karlsruhe Institute of Technology, Karlsruhe, Germany

Jacob Plange-Rhule
Division of Clinical Sciences, Renal Medicine, St George's, University of London, Cranmer Terrace, London SW17 0RE, UK

School of Medical Sciences, Kwame Nkrumah University of Science and Technology, Kumasi, Ghana

Sally M. Kerry
Blizard Institute, Barts and The London School of Medicine and Dentistry, Queen Mary University of London, 58 Turner Street, London E1 2AB, UK

John B. Eastwood
Division of Clinical Sciences, Renal Medicine, St George's, University of London, Cranmer Terrace, London SW17 0RE, UK

Frank B. Micah
Department of Medicine, Komfo Anokye Teaching Hospital, Kumasi, Ghana

Sampson Antwi
Department of Paediatrics, Komfo Anokye Teaching Hospital, Kumasi, Ghana

Francesco P. Cappuccio
Division of Health Sciences, Warwick Medical School, University of Warwick, Gibbet Hill Road, Coventry CV4 and AL, UK

Ming Guan
Family Issues Center, Xuchang University, Road Bayi 88, Xuchang, Henan, China
School of Business, Xuchang University, Road Bayi 88, Xuchang, Henan, China

Maya Korem and Karen Olshtain-Pops
AIDS Unit, Department of Clinical Microbiology and Infectious Diseases, Hadassah-Hebrew University Medical Center, Jerusalem, Israel

Tali Wallach
Department of Pediatrics, Kaplan Medical Center, Rehovot, Israel

Michael Bursztyn
Hypertension Unit, Department of Medicine, Hadassah-Hebrew University Medical Center, Mount Scopus, Jerusalem, Israel

Shlomo Maayan
Infectious Diseases and Infection Control Unit, Barzilai Medical Center, Ashkelon, Israel

Valeria Fontenelle Angelim Pereira and Livia Stocco Sanches Valentin
Department of Cardiopneumology, Heart Institute, School of medicine, University of São Paulo, São Paulo, Brazil

Index

P

R

S

T

V